A Practical Approach to Neuroanesthesia

A Practical Approach to Neuroanesthesia

Editors

PAUL D. MONGAN, MD
Professor of Anesthesiology
University of Colorado School of Medicine
Aurora, CO

SULPICIO G. SORIANO III, MD
Boston Children's Hospital Endowed Chair in Pediatric
Neuroanesthesia
Professor of Anaesthesia
Harvard Medical School
Boston, MA

TOD B. SLOAN, MD, MBA, PhD
Professor of Anesthesiology
University of Colorado School of Medicine
Aurora, CO

. Wolters Kluwer | Lippincott Williams & Wilkins
Health

Philadelphia · Baltimore · New York · London
Buenos Aires · Hong Kong · Sydney · Tokyo

Acquisitions Editor: Brian Brown
Product Manager: Nicole Dernoski
Production Manager: David Saltzberg
Senior Manufacturing Manager: Beth Welsh
Marketing Manager: Lisa Lawrence
Design Coordinator: Doug Smock
Production Service: Aptara, Inc.

Printed in China

Library of Congress Cataloging-in-Publication Data
A practical approach to neuroanesthesia / editors, Paul D. Mongan,
Sulpicio G. Soriano, Tod B. Sloan. – 1st ed.
      p. ; cm.
   Includes bibliographical references and index.
   ISBN 978-1-4511-7315-4 (alk. paper)
   I. Mongan, Paul D. II. Soriano, Sulpicio. III. Sloan, Tod B.
   [DNLM: 1.   Anesthesia. 2.   Neurosurgical Procedures. 3.   Nervous
System Diseases–surgery.   WL 368]
   RD87.3.N47
   617.9'6748–dc23

                              2013004060

Care has been taken to confirm the accuracy of the information presented and to describe generally accepted practices. However, the authors, editors, and publisher are not responsible for errors or omissions or for any consequences from application of the information in this book and make no warranty, expressed or implied, with respect to the currency, completeness, or accuracy of the contents of the publication. Application of the information in a particular situation remains the professional responsibility of the practitioner.

The authors, editors, and publisher have exerted every effort to ensure that drug selection and dosage set forth in this text are in accordance with current recommendations and practice at the time of publication. However, in view of ongoing research, changes in government regulations, and the constant flow of information relating to drug therapy and drug reactions, the reader is urged to check the package insert for each drug for any change in indications and dosage and for added warnings and precautions. This is particularly important when the recommended agent is a new or infrequently employed drug.

Some drugs and medical devices presented in the publication have Food and Drug Administration (FDA) clearance for limited use in restricted research settings. It is the responsibility of the health care provider to ascertain the FDA status of each drug or device planned for use in their clinical practice.

To purchase additional copies of this book, call our customer service department at (800) 638-3030 or fax orders to (301) 223-2320. International customers should call (301) 223-2300.

Visit Lippincott Williams & Wilkins on the Internet: at LWW.com. Lippincott Williams & Wilkins customer service representatives are available from 8:30 am to 6 pm, EST.

10 9 8 7 6 5 4 3 2 1

CCS0413

❖

We wish to dedicate this work to those pioneers of neuroanesthesiology
who have made the subspecialty
what it is today.

Contributors

Rita Agarwal, MD, FAAP
Professor
Department of Anesthesiology
University of Colorado Denver
Denver, CO
Children's Hospital Colorado
Aurora, CO

Linda S. Aglio, MD, MS
Associate Professor
Department of Anesthesia
Harvard Medical School
Director of Neuroanesthesia
Department of Anesthesia
Brigham and Women's Hospital
Boston, MA

Verna L. Baughman, MD
Professor
Department of Anesthesiology
University of Illinois at Chicago
Director of Neuroanesthesia
Department of Anesthesiology
University of Illinois Medical Center
Chicago, IL

J. Brad Bellotte, MD, FAANS
Clinical Assistant Professor
Department of Neurosurgery
University of Pittsburgh School of Medicine
Pittsburgh, PA
Chief, Division of Neurosurgery
UPMC Hamot Medical Center
Erie, PA

Hubert A. Benzon, MD
Assistant Professor of Anesthesiology
Northwestern University Feinberg School of Medicine
Lurie Children's Hospital of Chicago
Chicago, IL

Jess W. Brallier
Assistant Professor
Department of Anesthesiology
Mount Sinai School of Medicine
New York, NY

Brenda Bucklin, MD
Professor of Anesthesiology
University of Colorado School of Medicine
Aurora, CO

James P. Chandler, MD
Professor of Neurosurgery and ENT
Department of Neurological Surgery
Northwestern Medical Faculty Foundation
Northwestern University Feinberg School of Medicine
Chicago, IL

Grace Chen, MD
Assistant Professor
Department of Anesthesiology
Oregon Health and Science University
Portland, OR

Michael Chen, MD
Clinical Associate Professor
Department of Anesthesiology
Stanford University Medical Center
Stanford University
Stanford, CA

Rosemary Ann Craen, MBBS, FANZCA, FRCPC
Associate Professor
Department of Anesthesia & Perioperative Medicine
University of Western Ontario
Director of Neuroanesthesia
Department of Anesthesia & Perioperative Medicine
University Hospital
London Health Sciences Centre
London, Ontario, Canada

Karen A. Dean, MD
Assistant Professor
Department of Anesthesiology
University of Colorado Denver
Denver, CO
Children's Hospital Colorado
Aurora, CO

Stacie Deiner, BS, MD
Assistant Professor of Anesthesia
Neurosurgery, Geriatrics and Palliative Care
Mount Sinai School of Medicine
New York, NY

John M. Dunford, MD
Walter Reed National Military Medical Center - Bethesda
Section Chief, Neuroanesthesia
Director of Neurointraoperative Monitoring
Assistant Professor of Anesthesiology
Uniformed Services University of the Health Sciences
Anesthesia Clinical Associate
Johns Hopkins Hospital
Bethesda, MD

Steven B. Edelstein, MD
Professor
Department of Anesthesiology
Stritch School of Medicine
Loyola University Chicago
Professor & Vice Chairman
Department of Anesthesiology
Loyola University Medical Center
Maywood, IL

Audrice Francois, MD
Associate Professor
Department of Anesthesiology
Loyola University Medical Center
Maywood, IL

Katherine S.L. Gil, MD
Assistant Professor of Anesthesiology and Neurological
    Surgery
Northwestern University Feinberg School of Medicine
Northwestern Memorial Hospital
Chicago, IL

Susan M. Goobie, MD, FRCPC
Assistant Professor of Anaesthesia
Harvard Medical School
Boston Children's Hospital
Boston, MA

Leslie Jameson, MD
Associate Professor
Department of Anesthesiology
School of Medicine
University of Colorado
Aurora, CO

Grace Y. Kim, MD
Clinical Instructor
Department of Anesthesia
Harvard Medical School
Staff Anesthesiologist
Department of Anesthesia
Brigham and Women's Hospital
Boston, MA

Heidi M. Koenig, MD
Professor, Academic Advisory Dean
Department of Anesthesiology and Perioperative Medicine
University of Louisville
Louisville, KY

Antoun Koht, MD
Professor of Anesthesiology, Neurological Surgery &
    Neurology
Department of Anesthesiology
Department of Neurological Surgery
The Ken & Ruth Davee Department of Neurology
Northwestern University Feinberg School of Medicine
Chicago, IL

Avinash B Kumar, MD, FCCP, FCCM
Associate Professor Anesthesia and Critical Care
Associate Fellowship Director-Critical Care
Vanderbilt University Medical Center
Nashville, TN

Penny P. Liu, MD
CEO
Vigilance Physician Services, PC
Sewickley, PA

Andreas W. Loepke, MD, PhD, FAAP
Associate Professor of Clinical Anesthesia & Pediatrics
University of Cincinnati College of Medicine
Division of Pediatric Cardiac Anesthesia
Department of Anesthesia
Cincinnati Children's Hospital Medical Center
Cincinnati, OH

Pirjo H. Manninen, MD, FRCPC
Associate Professor
Department of Anesthesia
University of Toronto
Toronto Western Hospital
University Health Network
Toronto, Ontario, Canada

Mary Ellen McCann, MD, MPH
Associate Professor of Anaesthesia
Harvard Medical School
Boston Children's Hospital
Boston, MA

Craig D. McClain, MD
Assistant Professor of Anaesthesia
Harvard Medical School
Boston Children's Hospital
Boston, MA

Petra M. Meier, MD, DEAA
Assistant Professor of Anaesthesia
Harvard Medical School
Boston Children's Hospital
Boston, MA

Mark F. Mueller, MD
Assistant Professor
Department of Anesthesiology
Division of Neuroanesthesiology
University of Illinois Medical Center
Chicago, IL

Sabin Caius Oana, MD
Assistant Professor
Department of Anesthesiology
Loyola University Medical Center
Maywood, IL

Chanannait Paisansathan, MD
Associate Professor
Department of Anesthesiology
University of Illinois at Chicago
University of Illinois at Chicago Medical Center
Chicago, IL

Jeffrey J. Pasternak, MS, MD
Assistant Professor
Chair – Division of Neuroanesthesia
Department of Anesthesiology
Mayo Clinic College of Medicine
Rochester, MN

Hélène G. Pellerin, MD, FRCPC
Assistant Clinical Professor
Department of Anesthesiology
Universite Laval
Anesthesiologist
Department of Anesthesia
CHA– Hopital de l'Enfant Jesus
Quebec, QC, Canada

Valentina Picozzi, DDS
University of Milano
Department of Biomedical, Surgical and Odontoiatric
   Sciences
Milano, Italy

Michael V. Presta, DO
Assistant Professor
Department of Anesthesiology
Stritch School of Medicine
Loyola University Chicago
Assistant Professor
Department of Anesthesiology
Loyola University Medical Center
Maywood, IL

Eiman Rahimi, MD
Department of Anesthesia
University of Toronto
Toronto Western Hospital
University Health Network
Toronto, Ontario, Canada

Chiranjeev Saha, MBBS, MS
Attending Anesthesiologist
Department of Anesthesiology
Rush University Medical Center
Chicago, IL

Francesco Sala, MD
Section of Neurosurgery
Department of Neurological and Visual Sciences
Verona, Italy

Joseph Salama-Hanna, MBBch
Pain Management Fellow
Department of Anesthesiology
Oregon Health and Science University
Portland, OR

Benjamin Scott, MD
Assistant Professor
Department of Anesthesiology
University of Colorado School of Medicine
Denver, CO

Ricky B. Shah, MD
Assistant Professor
Department of Anesthesiology
Stritch School of Medicine
Loyola University Chicago
Assistant Professor
Department of Anesthesiology
Loyola University Medical Center
Maywood, IL

Deepak Sharma, MBBS, MD, DM
Associate Professor of Anesthesiology & Pain Medicine
Chief, Division of Neuroanesthesiology & Perioperative
   Neurosciences Neuroanesthesiology
Fellowship Director Adjunct Associate Professor of
   Neurological Surgery University of Washington,
   Seattle, WA

Tod B. Sloan, MD, MBA, PhD
Professor of Anesthesiology
University of Colorado School of Medicine
Aurora, CO

Edward R. Smith, MD
Assistant Professor of Surgery (Neurosurgery)
Harvard Medical School
Boston Children's Hospital
Boston, MA

Krystal Tomei, MD, MPH
Neurosurgery Resident
Department of Neurological Surgery
UMDNJ–NJMS
Newark, NJ

Concezione Tommasino, MD
Associate Professor of Anesthesiology and Intensive Care
University of Milano
Department of Biomedical, Surgical and Odontoiatric
   Sciences
Ospedale San Paolo Medical School
Milano, Italy

Cynthia S. Tung, MD, MPH
Instructor
Department of Anaesthesia
Harvard Medical School
Boston Children's Hospital
Boston, MA

Monica S. Vavilala, MD
Professor
Departments of Anesthesiology and Pediatrics
Adjunct in Neurological Surgery
University of Washington
Seattle, WA

Cuong Vu, MD
Assistant Professor
Department of Anesthesiology
Oregon Health and Science University
Portland, OR

N. Kurt Baker-Watson, MD
Assistant Professor
Department of Anesthesiology
Loyola University Medical Center
Maywood, IL

Cristina Wood, MD, MS
Assistant Professor
University of Colorado School of Medicine
Department of Anesthesiology
Aurora, CO

Preface

THIS BOOK WAS SUGGESTED AS an addition to complement the Practical Approach series of anesthesia subspecialty texts. The goal was to create a text which provides insights into the various areas of neuroanesthesia that practitioners may encounter in a busy surgical practice. Our vision was to include aspects of the pediatric and pregnant patient to avoid the need to consult additional texts dedicated to those subspecialities. The authors have done a good job of covering the topics and providing a very current discussion of the medical and surgical issues involved. In keeping with the series, the authors have provided clinical pearls and key points (listed at the beginning of the chapter with reference numbers in the margins to identify the relevant text for each point).

The editors appreciate the wisdom of our mentors and the questions of our mentees who have challenged us to question our knowledge and expand our horizons in neuroanesthesiology. We also appreciate our families whose patience gives us the energy to do this work and our patients who give us the desire to apply the latest knowledge and techniques.

Clearly neuroanesthesia will continue to evolve from our history (as detailed by Maurice Albin) and this work presents a firm foundation for building that growth and evolution of practice. The editors are grateful for all who have made this work possible.

Paul Mongan, Sulpicio Soriano, Tod Sloan
February 2013

Foreword

Voices from the Legacies of Modern Day Neuroanesthesia

"The farther backward you can look, the farther forward you are likely to see."
(Winston Churchill)

Maurice S. Albin, MD, MSc (Anes)
Professor of Anesthesiology
University of Alabama at Birmingham
Birmingham, Alabama

THE INITIATION OF A GROUNDSWELL of interest and participation by the anesthesiology community in modern-day neurosurgical anesthesia (neuroanesthesia) can be noted in the 1960s. A review of this progress in terms of the organized effort to give structure to North American neuroanesthesia was described by Albin [1]. A look back at the still earlier origins has been described by Frost [2] and Boulton [3]. The incredible dynamic expansion of neuroanesthesia concepts in the period from 1960 to 1980 certainly needs further review. With the exception of the publication by the cerebral blood flow group at the University of Pennsylvania (Kety, Schmidt, and coworkers) in the late 1940s to early 1950s, an analysis of the *Quarterly Cumulative Index* indicated a relative poverty of information concerning anesthesia and anesthetic techniques during neurosurgical procedures when compared to a similar approach 2 decades later when the increase in the neuroanesthesia literature increased more than 1,000-fold. This foreword will attempt to show the dynamics of this lusty explosion of information in terms of its movement across geographical areas, its cross-pollination with other medical specialties especially in the neurosciences; its permeation into the core of anesthesia education, the establishment of neuroanesthesia research in academic centers; its cultural maturity as manifested by subspecialty (neuroanesthesia) organizations and development of specialty (neuroanesthesia) training; the movement from the service of neuroanesthesia in the operating room to the postoperative critical care management of neurosurgical patients, and those with neuropathology of a nonneurosurgical nature; and its extension into disciplines involving the treatment of pain and pain research, as well as the care of those without hope of survival. The foreword will not present detailed descriptions of the various areas of neuroanesthesia research and the current progress as this has been well documented by William Lanier, Andrew Kofke, and Jeffrey Pasternak with William Lanier in three extraordinarily thorough articles in the Journal of Neurosurgical Anesthesiology (JNA) of October 2012, which also celebrated the 40th anniversary of the founding of the now named Society of Neurosurgical Anesthesia and Critical Care (SNACC) [4–6].

A survey of the enormous amount of neuroanesthesia literature during the past 40 years reveals that only a small number of the authors have remained in the collective consciousness of our subspecialty in spite of the fact that we have developed extraordinary search engines with our information technology. Another impediment to an organic appreciation of our history is the lack of discipline of many of our authors today in neglecting to lay out the historical background of an event, concept, or hypothesis. Thus, important contributors of the past are in effect erased from the rolls of history. So for the readers, please do not be inhibited by the many names you will find listed, for they have all in their own way made this book possible. In fact, this foreword will be so ponderous with names that it may, for a while, resemble the first book of the Pentateuch, or Genesis, in other parlance known as the "begatting book," that is, in Genesis 11:27 "and Terah lived seventy years and begat Abram, Nahor, and Haran . . . ."

The 1960s and 1970s were extraordinary because of the huge outpouring of information in the area of neuroanesthesia. Topics such as anesthesia, anesthetics, hypothermia, air embolism, cerebral circulation and metabolism, EEG, ICP, resuscitation, spinal cord and head injury, are only a small portion of the many descriptors investigated during this period. Maurice Albin, in a talk at one of the late 1970 SNACC meetings, described this period as the equivalent of an "academic gold rush!" The geographical distribution of some of these studies can be seen in Figure 1 marked with a letter of the alphabet. I have listed below the names of the institutions and many of the contributors who made these advances possible. Because of the difficulties

A. The University of Pennsylvania, Philadelphia, PA
B. Mayo clinic, Rochester, MN
C. University of Pittsburgh, Pittsburgh, PA
D. University of California at San Diego, San Diego, CA
E. McGill University, Montreal, Quebec, Canada
F. University of Western Ontario, London, Ontario, Canada
A   G. Case Western Reserve University, Cleveland, OH

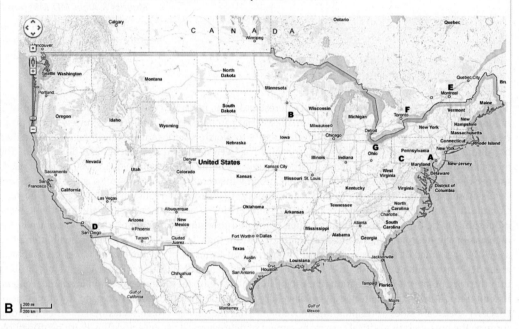

FIGURE 1 **A:** Listing of centers of neuroanesthesia studies in the United States and Canada, 1960–1980. **B:** Map showing location of centers of neuroanesthesia studies in the United States and Canada, 1960–1980.

involved in searching for this information, some of which is a half century older or more, *I ask forgiveness in the event that I have inadvertently omitted any player.*

A. *The University of Pennsylvania.* The pioneering work of Seymour Kety and Karl Schmidt in developing the nitrous oxide technique for CBF in 1945 was a cornerstone stimulus in the development of neuroanesthesia. In a similar vein, Robert D. Dripps, MD, Professor and Chairman of the Department of Anesthesiology, was the editor of a landmark 1956 report on the physiology of induced hypothermia based on the 1955 symposium sponsored by the National Academy of Sciences—National Research Council. Professor Dripps encouraged important research in the area of neuroanesthesia and believed in a multidisciplinary approach to problems. The Chairman of the Division of Neurosurgery, Tom Langfitt, was one of the early founders of NAS (The Neuroanesthesia Society), a predecessor to SNACC. He had a very vigorous program in research on head injuries, and also encouraged interdisciplinary research. Important contributions were also made by James Harp, Henry Wollman, Harvey Shapiro (a former SNACC president), Craig Alexander (a former SNACC president), Peter Cohen, Derek Bruce (a neurosurgeon and former SNACC president), A. L. Smith, L. S. Fregler, G. W. Stephen, Tom Gennarelli, Neal Cassell (a neurosurgeon and former SNACC president), Lawrence Marshall (a neurosurgeon and former SNACC president), David Smith, MD (a former SNACC president), and Brian Dunlop.

B. *The Mayo Clinic* made many early contributions to neuroanesthesia, many of them stimulated by and due to the pioneering efforts of John (Jack) Michenfelder (the first SNACC President) in the areas of air embolism, hypothermia, cerebral circulation and metabolism, EEG, the pharmacology of anesthetics, and in the development of clinical anesthetic practices, as well as in the educational area. It is to be remembered that John Silas Lundy helped to develop sodium pentothal, and was a pioneer in regional blocks. The listing of those working in the area of neuroanesthesia is considerable and includes Howard Terry, Ed Daw, Albert Faulconer, Brian Dawson, Richard Theye, Reginald Bickford, Bill Lanier (a former SNACC president), Hiroshi Takeshita, Joseph Messick, Roy Cucchiara, Alan Artru, James Milde, Susan Black, Leslie Newberg Milde, Gerald Gronert, and Kai Rehder.

C. *The University of Pittsburgh* played an important role in the development of neuroanesthesia concepts with individuals like Peter Safar, Professor and Chairman of the Department of Anesthesiology, and for many years a guiding light in resuscitation, neuroprotection, hypothermia, equipment design, and education; Maurice Albin, working in the fields of acute spinal cord injury and physiopathology, air embolism, brain retraction pressure monitoring, pharmacology of anesthetics, drug addiction, and the transcranial Doppler; Peter Jannetta, Professor and Chairman of the Department of Neurosurgery, and a former President of SNACC, pioneering in vascular compression syndromes of cranial nerves and their treatment; Joseph Maroon, neurosurgeon and pioneer in spinal cord and head injuries and primary author of the first paper (1996 with British Anesthesiologist Edmonds-Seal at Oxford University) on the use of a precordial ultrasonic Doppler detector for vascular air embolism; T. K. Hung, PhD, Professor of Civil and Biomedical Engineering, who studied the biomechanics of acute spinal cord injury; Leonid Bunegin, chemical engineer, who helped to develop the multiorifice aspiration catheter for air embolism, studies on the neurochemistry of acute spinal cord injury, and the biomechanics of acute spinal cord injury; and Ake Grenvik, who is remembered for his studies on resuscitation, brain death, and critical care medicine. Other important contributors were Howard Yonas on the use of xenon as a marker for CBF; and James Snyder for his work in critical care medicine.

D. *The University of California at San Diego.* Working in the salutary ambience created by Anesthesiology Chairmen Larry Saidman and Harvey Shapiro, a primary organizer of our very early efforts to form NAS, and who was active in neuroanesthesia at the University of Pennsylvania, a group of talented anesthesiologists gathered in San Diego and helped define many of the physiopathologic issues in neuroanesthesia including studies of the effects of volatile agents, high frequency ventilation, ICP, evoked potentials, air embolism, and effects of positional changes to name but a few of the many topics investigated. The senior members of this group were John Drummond and Michael Todd, both being preceded by the Pediatric Anesthesiologist Mark Rockoff. To this day, John Drummond is very active, now working in the area of cerebral ischemia while Michael Todd, a former editor of anesthesiology, is Professor and Chair of the Department of Anesthesiology at the University of Iowa School of Medicine. Other contributors to the important output of neuroanesthesia publications were Steven Toutant, Cliff Chadwick, Stella Tommasino, Mark Scheller, Steve Skahen, Mark Zornow, David Peterson, and Armin Schubert. When Michael Todd left for the University of Iowa, he was joined by an outstanding scientist/anesthesiologist, David Warner. Together they created yet another productive group, investigating both the basic sciences as well as the clinical applications of these findings, particularly in the areas of hypothermia, cerebral protection, and total and partial cerebral ischemia. David Warner left for Duke University in the mid-1990s to become Director of Research and Chief of the Neuroanesthesia Service where he continues his research efforts, and he was honored with the ASA Excellence in Research Award in 2005. Aside from his research and clinical accomplishments, David has trained a large number of individuals, especially Fellows from international areas.

E. *Neuroanesthesia in Canada.* Our Canadian colleagues were working in the area of neuroanesthesia in the late 1950s with R. G. B. Gilbert, Professor and Chairman of the Department of Anesthetics at *McGill University in Canada*, also Director of Anesthesia at the Montreal Neurological Institute (MNI), and Chairman of the Commission on Neuroanesthesia of the World Federation of Neurology (1961). At McGill and the MNI, the neuroanesthesiologists included William V. Cone, David Archer, Patrick Ravussin, Fred Brindle, Anibal Galindo, and Davy Trop. The writings of the eminent neurosurgeon and Nobel Laureate, Wilder Penfield, as well as the Director of the MNI, neuroanatomist, and neurophysiologist Theodore Rasmussen indicated the trusting relationship between neurosurgeons and neuroanesthetists. Professor Penfield was known for his investigative efforts on surgery for pain syndromes at the MNI. In 1965, Melzack and Wall, also from McGill, published their paper on the "gate" theory to explain the mechanism of pain propagation.

The major driving force behind the growth of neuroanesthesia at yet another academic center was the neurosurgeon Charles G. Drake, Professor of Neurosurgery at the *University of Western Ontario*. He was famous for his work in aneurysmal surgery as well as for his experience in dealing with acoustic neuromas. Dr. Drake was a most patient, honest and humble individual with a great understanding of the importance of anesthesia, and he was fortunate to have his dear friend and medical school classmate, Ronald Aitken, at his side giving anesthesia to his patients. Equally important, Ron Aitken was an innovative individual, fashioning monitoring devices way ahead of his time. Dr. Drake had an important vision of integrating all the attendant medical disciplines relating to neurologic pathology into a patient-centered framework so that all specialties in the neurosciences were available for input into the problems that the patient presented, and this concept carried over into the research area as well. I was fortunate to become a friend of Charlie Drake over the years and appreciated his sincerity, honesty, and acceptance of new ideas. His understanding of the role of the neuroanesthetist can be noted from a letter I received in 1993 (Fig. 2). It is no wonder that a neuroanesthesia culture flourished as is noted by the many outstanding neuroanesthetists that were identified with this program including Adrian Gelb and Art Lam, both still working in the neuroanesthesia vineyard and still producing interesting neuroanesthesia wine, with Adrian directing the Neuroanesthesia Program at the University of California, San Francisco, and Art working in the Seattle area. Other contributors in the London, Ontario, program were George Varkey, Pirjo Manninen, Rosemary Croen, and a host of neurosurgeons including "Skip" Peerless.

F. *Case Western Reserve University School of Medicine, Cleveland.* Working at Cleveland Metropolitan General Hospital (CMGH), Robert J. White, MD, PhD, teamed with Maurice S. Albin in 1962 to develop a clinical and basic science research program with important applications to neuroanesthesia. First working together at the Mayo Clinic, White and Albin looked at the physiologic responses to the ligation of the basilar artery in the large rhesus monkey, and started preliminary experiments on the effects of direct cooling of the spinal cord to low temperatures and the development of a cord-cooling technique with an eye of utilizing hypothermia in cases of acute spinal cord injury. At CMGH, Albin worked on standardizing a method for producing spinal cord injury and initiated a series of experiments in monkeys to test the effects of localized spinal cord cooling on an injury that would normally produce irreversible paraplegia of the lower extremities. This work indicated that significant recovery could occur if therapy was initiated within 4 hours after injury and spinal cord hypothermia carried out for 3 hours with the intrinsic spinal cord temperature lowered to 10°C. This data was presented at a meeting of the American Association of Neurological Surgeons and the paper on this subject published in the Journal of Neurosurgery in 1968.

Maurice Albin has been one of the few neuroanesthesiologists who has dedicated a major portion of his research efforts to investigating the pathophysiologic and therapeutic aspects concerning acute and chronic spinal cord injury. Robert J. White's major research was related to the total isolation, vascular transplantation, and storage of the mammalian brain at the CMGH research laboratories and reported these findings in Science and Nature in 1963, 1965, and 1966. These three papers were the basis of a nomination for the Nobel Prize in Physiology and Medicine in 2004 and 2006 by a Nobel laureate, honoring Robert White, Maurice Albin and Javier Verdura. Clinically, the neurosurgery service opened a four-bed neuro-ICU in 1964 with Albin directing this unit, and it was in all probability one of the earliest in existence. The neuro-ICU had a fully equipped blood gas laboratory with an Astrup blood gas unit, flame photometer, AO oximeter, and a lab technician. Interestingly, the neuro-ICU had well-trained nurses, most of whom with extensive ER and surgical nursing. Other projects included the cooling of the brain by oral–nasal perfusion, surface cooling for head injuries, and the use of a vascular bypass method for cooling the brain with the body at or near normothermia. Equally important, this concept of neuro-ICU care with the laboratory backup allowed for the education of both anesthesia and neurosurgical residents in these methodologies. Many of these neurosurgical residents went on to become leaders in academic neurosurgery, and Donald Becker, the developer of the "Richmond Bolt" was one of our appreciative "alumni" at CMGH. Other contributors were John Demian, Henry Brown, George Locke, Martin Weiss, Eugene Davidson, and George Dakters.

G. *The University of Glasgow* was important in the early development of neuroanesthesia, especially with the presence of Bryan Jennett, Professor and Chairman of Neurosurgery, (1968 to 1981), who later became Dean of the School of Medicine. His major interest was in the area of head injuries,

The University of Western Ontario

C.G. Drake, OC, MD, MSc, MS, FRCS(C),
FACS Richard Ivey Professor of Surgery
PastChairman, Department of Surgery

Faculty of Medicine
London, Canada
N6A SCl

20 April 1993

Dr. Maurice S. Albin,
Professor of Anesthesiology
and Neurological Surgery
University of Texas
7703 Floyd Curl Drvie
San Antonio, Texas.
78284-7838

Dear Maurice:

When I first came back to London in the November of 1951, there was little in the way of specialized anaesthesia, there being no neuro or cardiac surgery. Some anaesthetists were part time in the morning and general practice in the afternoon. Using anaesthetists of those days for craniotomy was an experience. Often I had to try to hold the brain in the skull while pleading with the anaesthetist to listen to the chest to make sure his tube had not slipped out, kinked or gone in to obstruct a main stem bronchus, or why else was the blood black and the brain swelling out of the craniotomy? As Gillingham once said - "In the early days, anaesthetists spent their time pushing the brain out of the head while now they suck it back inside". And they did not like it - it was demanding, sometimes frightening, often prolonged and boring and their income was diminished over doing frequent short easy cases. I was allowed to use the orthopaedic OR in the afternoon after Jack Kennedy finished his list. I seldom finished before late evening, even into early morning hours on elective cases! having only general surgical residents as assistants, but they were very bright and good. But it was there I recognized the gift that Ron Aitken had in anaesthesia: Jack had noticed it before. In those days one had to call one's anaesthetist and I soon tried for Ron for every case. We got along well and he seemed to enjoy the trials of neuro-anaesthesia. Gradually we became a team and he became involved in my searches for better ways to deal with aneuryms - especially hypotension in its various forms including moderate hypothermia and deeper levels under c.p. bypass with circulatory arrest, since by that time we had a good pump team.

FIGURE 2 Letter from Charles G. Drake to Maurice S. Albin on April 20, 1993, Pages 1 and 2. (*continued*)

Using moderate hypotension, I kept asking for deeper and deeper levels and he produced them-gradually, and not without concern. But soon 40 MAP was routine near and at the aneurysm and even lower in critical situations. He had an uncanny instinct for the condition of the patient and how far he could go, even better I thought, than the crude measuring instruments we had in those days for intra- arterial pressures, o_2 and co_2 electrolytes etc. He could tell me when to quit and I knew I should do so, if I was not committed. But I think even he was sometimes surprised how well the patient came out of it. Later when modern equipment arrived he became a master with it, but always with his innate sense of the patient as he saw things under the drapes.

Ron had no real "academic bones". I had to push him to write and for some reason he hated speaking from a rostrum. I think he was surprised that his one or two papers on hypotension became classics and his observation that respiratory changes in deliberate brain stem ischemia with temporary occlusion preceded B.P or cardiac irregularities, became an issue still debated.

Despite not being a "researcher" he was a superb clinical teacher, patient, practical, with tremendous experience. He seemed to have seen everything and had simple effective approaches to difficult problems.

He was one of the first two or three Canadians who became dedicated to neuroanaesthesia and it was his influence that persuaded the likes of George Varkey, Adrian Gelb, Arthur Lam and Pirjo Manninen to follow on.

With warm best wishes

Sincerely,

Charles G. Drake, OC, M.D. FRCS(C).

CGD- drn

FIGURE 2 (Continued)

and with Graham Teasdale, he developed the Glasgow Coma Scale. The Glasgow Outcome Scale resulted from the studies of Bryan Jennett and Michael Bona. Professor Jennett founded and directed the British Medical Research Council's (MRC) Cerebral Circulation Research Group and the MRC-sponsored Head Injury Research Program in Glasgow. This environment attracted many outstanding investigators from anesthesia, neurosurgery, neurology, neuropathology, physiology, and other specialties. Significant contributions were made to neuroanesthesia by Gordon McDowell, William Fitch, A. M. Harper, John Barker, Sam Galbraith, Douglas Miller, A. M. Parker, D. I. Graham, Sheila Jennett, G. M. Teasdale, A. B. M. Telfer, and J. P. Vance.

The Organization of Neuroanesthesia. The roots of the SNACC have been described by Albin and Kofke. The development of organized neuroanesthesia in Great Britain has a most interesting history, much of it involved in the establishment of the Neurosurgical Anesthetists Traveling Club (NATC) which came into existence on September 18, 1965. The first meeting was held at the Manchester Royal Infirmary with this gathering having been organized by Allan Brown of Scotland and Ian Hunter of Manchester. This was an important organization with forty anesthetists representing 20 neurosurgical units. The NATC was an informal group, though the Scottish Society of Anesthetists had been formed earlier with Allan Brown, the Senior Consultant Anesthetist to the Department of Surgical Neurology in Edinburgh as the Honorary Secretary. In reality, it was not until April 1993 that the Neuroanesthesia Society of Great Britain and Ireland was founded (NASGBI).

I urge readers to go to the literature and read the fascinating paper by Jean Horton, one of the founding members of NATC, titled "A History of the Neuroanesthesia Society of Great Britain and Ireland" [7]. Some achievements of NASGBI since 1993 have been mentioned below:

- In 2002, the Society had some 273 members including a small number of overseas, retired, associate, and trainee members
- Organization of national and international scientific meetings
- Recommendations on transfer of head injuries
- Guidelines on standards for neuroanesthesia services
- Neurointensive care database
- Recommendation for training and revalidation in neuroanesthesia and neurointensive care

In a previous communication by Albin it was stated that the first publication of a neuroanesthesiology text in English was authored by Professor Andrew R. Hunter of Manchester in 1964. However, it has come to my attention that a still earlier text written in English on neuroanesthesia was titled "A Practice of General Anesthesia For Neurosurgery" by Robert I.V. Ballentine, Consultant Anesthetist, St. Bartholomew's Hospital, and Ian Jackson, consultant Anesthetist, St. Bartholomew's Hospital, London, published by J. A. Churchill, Ltd, 1960 [8]. The foreword by J. E. A. O'Connell, MS, FRCS, neurosurgeon, defines the role of the neuro-anesthetist in terms of preoperative assessment, conduct of an anesthetic, as well as the postoperative care using a team approach. The book fills 152 pages, has 11 chapters plus an index, and includes 189 references. As an example of the progress made in neuroanesthesia, the book by Albin, "Textbook of Neuroanesthesia with Neurosurgical and Neuroscience Perspectives" published 37 years later (1997), has 38 chapters plus an index, for a total of 1,433 pages and 9,679 references!

Finalizing a Voice—The Maturation of Neuroanesthesia as a Subspecialty. Similar to a "telltale" on a sailing vessel, the initiation, struggle and success of the Journal of Neurosurgical Anesthesiology (JNA) probably parallels the development and acceptance of neuroanesthesia as a defined subspecialty throughout a large number of countries worldwide. This stand-alone journal's first issue took place in March 1989, and was preceded by the Anesthesiology Review which published many of the educational activities of SNACC and ceased publication when JNA was started. Although the JNA editorial board was international in nature and its membership list read like a who's-who of neuroanesthesia, we were fortunate to have two individuals to do the "heavy lifting" and chaperone the JNA from its initiation to the present time, James Cottrell and John Hartung (Personal communication, 2013). We do have interesting literature about the JNA, and I recommend that our readers take advantage of the paper by Albin and the one by Kofke, Lanier, and Pasternak. Having known both Cottrell and Hartung for more than 3 decades, I feel obliged to mention the importance of their *arbeit* in moving the JNA forward in spite of the many difficulties and trials. Jim Cottrell, MD, anesthesiologist, scientist, educator and former President of the American Society of Anesthesiologists conjoined with John Hartung, PhD, scientist, sociobiologist, humanist, and administrator–editor *par excellence*, never stopped in their desire to move the frontiers of neuroanesthesia forward. The accomplishments of the JNA cannot be appreciated unless one looks back and realizes that since the first issue in March 1989, the JNA has published 97 issues and is now on its 25th volume; PubMed now lists 1,283 JNA publications which includes clinical and laboratory investigations as reports, case reports, correspondence, and point-of-view contributions. Naturally, all of this material is peer-reviewed. Included in the PubMed listings are 37 editorials which are informally peer-reviewed. The JNA has also published 142 book reviews. The influence of the JNA has fortunately moved across borders and a listing of the international neuroanesthesia societies for which the JNA has become their affiliated voice as well as their date of affiliation can be seen below:

1. Neuroanesthesia Society of Great Britain and Ireland—1996
2. Association de Neuro-Anesthésiologie Réanimation de langue Française—1996
3. Wissenschaftijcher Arbeitskreis Neuroanasthesie der Deutschen Gesellschaft für Anästhesiologie und Intensivmedizin—1997
4. Arbeitsgemeinschaft Deutschsprachiger Neuroanasthesisten und Neuro-intensivmediziner—1997
5. Korean Society of Neuroanesthesia—1998

6. Japanese Society of Neuroanesthesia and Critical Care—1999
7. Cápitulo de Neuroanestesiologia del Colegio Mexicano de Anestesiologia—2000
8. Indian Society of Neuroanesthesiology and Critical Care—2002

It is my hope that this sketch acquaints one with the links to the past and makes one realize that the solid clinical and research accomplishments created in neuroanesthesia were indeed the voices of *many* reaching back in time.

Postscript

I would like to thank David Wilkinson and Bill Fitch for their help and, in particular, the sharp memory and writings of the seasoned neuroanesthesiologist, Jean Horton.

REFERENCES

1. Albin MS. Celebrating silver: The genesis of a neuroanesthesiology society. NAS→SNANSC→SNACC. *J Neurosurg Anesthesiol*. 1997;9:296–307.
2. Frost EM. History of neuroanesthesia. In: Albin MS, ed. *Textbook of Neuroanesthesia with Neurosurgical and Neuroscience Perspectives*. New York, NY: McGraw-Hill; 1997:1–20.
3. Boulton TE. *The Association of Anesthetists of Great Britain and Ireland, 1932–1992 and the Development of the Specialty of Anesthesia*. London: Association of anesthetists of Great Britain and Ireland; 1999:534.
4. Lanier WL. The history of neuroanesthesiology: The people, pursuits, and practices. *J Neurosurg Anesthesiol*. 2012;24:281–299.
5. Kofke WA. Celebrating ruby: 40 years of NAS→SNANSC→SNACC. *J Neurosurg Anesthesiol*. 2012;24:260–280.
6. Pasternak JJ, Lanier WL. Snapshot of 1973 and 1974: Critical thinkers and contemporary research ideas in neurosurgical anesthesia during the first years of SNACC. *J Neurosurg Anesthesiol*. 2012;24:300–311.
7. Horton J. A history of the neuroanesthesia society of Great Britain and Ireland. In: Lucien E. Morris, Mark E. Schroeder, and Mary E. Warner, eds. *Procedure of the Ralph M. Waters Symposium on Professionalism in Anesthesiology*. Park Ridge, IL: Wood library-museum of anesthesiology:146–151.
8. Ballentine, Robert IV. A practice of general anesthesia for neurosurgery. *Postgrad Med J*. 1960;36(419):580.

Contents

1

Brain Metabolism, Cerebral Blood Flow, and Cerebrospinal Fluid

Chanannait Paisansathan and Verna L. Baughman

KEY POINTS

1. The brain is the major energy-consuming organ in the body. Its high metabolic demand makes it very susceptible to injury from low perfusion pressure, hypoglycemia and anoxia, which may lead to cerebral ischemia, irreversible brain damage, and neurologic deficit.
2. The brain tightly regulates blood flow to meet its metabolic need. Several factors affect cerebral blood flow—activation of neuronal networks, dynamics of cerebral perfusion pressure, and the partial pressure of carbon dioxide and oxygen in arterial blood.
3. The brain is located in the rigid skull. Changes in volume of brain tissue, blood, or cerebrospinal fluid can affect the compliance within the cerebral compartment and cause a rise in intracranial pressure. Ultimately, a pathologic level of intracranial pressure could lead to fatal brain herniation.

I. Brain metabolism

A. General concepts. The brain is continuously active. Multiple systems affecting arousal operate in concert to ensure optimal brain function. Neurons from different areas of the brain, such as the ascending reticular activating system, monoaminergic neurons in the brain stem, and cholinergic neurons in the basal forebrain have been implicated in organizing brain activation. The posterior hypothalamus has only recently been recognized as a major center regulating waking. This area contains different neuronal populations with diverse neurotransmitters (histamine, dopamine, glutamate, GABA) and neuropeptides (orexins, melanin-concentrating hormone, galanin, enkephalins, substance P, and thyrotropin-releasing hormone). The different activating and inhibitory systems form an intricate neuronal network and display complex energy consumption processes [1].

The average human brain weighs about 1,500 g which represents about 2% of the body weight, yet accounts for approximately 20% of the energy consumed. The brain tightly regulates its oxygen supply and substrate availability in response to local demand arising from neuronal metabolic activity. Since brain function varies from region to region, metabolic activity is also different across brain regions. During the past 30 years a rapid growth in the use of functional imaging techniques, like positron emission tomography (PET) and functional magnetic resonance imaging (fMRI), has yielded valuable information, and controversy, regarding the relationships between cerebral blood flow (CBF) and brain metabolism in different brain regions.

1

Between 50% and 80% of the energy consumed by the brain appears to be linked to maintaining synaptic function. A large portion of that energy is devoted to supporting glutamatergic activity. There is also a low level of inhibitory GABAergic interneuron metabolic activity representing up to 10% to 15% of cerebral oxidative metabolism [2].

B. **Brain oxygen/glucose consumption and energy production**

1. **Brain oxygen tension.** Most of the energy required for ATP regeneration in the adult mammalian brain arises from the oxidation of glucose in the TCA (Krebs) cycle with oxygen as the electron acceptor in mitochondrial respiration. In normal conscious man, the cerebral metabolic rate for oxygen ($CMRO_2$) is approximately 3.5 mL/100 g tissue/min. Under resting conditions, this translates to O_2 consumption at a rate of 150 to 160 μmol/100 g/min. Average brain tissue pO_2 is in the range of 10 to 40 mm Hg. In the normal human, the critical brain tissue pO_2 is 15 to 20 mm Hg. However, an intracellular pO_2 as low as 1.5 mm Hg is sufficient to sustain the mitochondrial cytochrome c oxidase reaction [3].

2. **Substrate for cerebral energy production.** Theoretically, the brain at rest should utilize oxygen and glucose at a 6:1 ratio. Glucose is the main substrate during normal neuronal activity, and is consumed at a rate of 30 μmol/100 g/min (5 mg/100 g/min). This rate of glucose utilization (CMRglu) clearly exceeds what would be predicted by resting O_2 consumption. This "imbalance" is even greater during periods of increased brain activity. To explain why less than 6 mmol of O_2 is consumed for every mmol of glucose, Pellerin and Magistretti, in 1994, proposed the "Astrocyte Neuron Lactate Shuttle" (ANLS) model, in which glutamate that is released as a neurotransmitter during neuronal synaptic activity is taken up by astrocytes. This glutamate transport activity is associated with an increased energy demand, which is met by increased glycolysis in astrocytes with lactate as the end product. Astrocyte-derived lactate is then transferred to neurons using monocarboxylic acid transporters, where it is oxidized via the TCA, meeting the energy demands during neuronal activation [4]. However, this model does not entirely explain the decrease in the oxygen to glucose metabolic ratio, since lactate may escape oxidation by virtue of diffusion from the brain [5].

    In humans, using nuclear magnetic resonance spectroscopy (MRS), lactate contribution to brain energy metabolism was reported to be less than 10% under basal conditions. However, this increased to as much as 60% at elevated plasma lactate levels [6]. Recent meta-analysis indicated that lactate supplements glucose and supports an increase in cerebral energy metabolism during increased physical activity in humans [7].

C. **Clinical measures of cerebral oxygenation and metabolism**

1. **Jugular venous oximetry (see Chapter 28).** A catheter is inserted into an internal jugular vein and advanced to the jugular bulb. The right side is often used because it is usually dominant. Jugular venous oxygen saturation ($SjvO_2$) gives information about the balance between global brain oxygen delivery and metabolic demand. The normal $SjvO_2$ is 55% to 75%. The normal lower value of $SjvO_2$ compared to cardiac mixed venous saturation reflects high oxygen metabolism in the brain. $SjvO_2$ levels less than 55% suggest that the cerebral oxygen supply is inadequate to meet the metabolic demand, while a level higher than 80% indicates relative hyperemia. The arterial to jugular venous oxygen concentration difference ($AjvdO_2$) has been used to estimate brain metabolism. The normal $AjvdO_2$ is 4- to 8-mL O_2/100-mL blood.

2. **Brain tissue oxygen tension (see Chapter 28).** Measurement of brain tissue oxygen tension (PtO_2) using an oxygen-sensing electrode provides information regarding focal brain tissue oxygenation; although in doing so, global changes might be missed. Brain PtO_2 is related to other physiologic variables. It is increased by an increase in the inspired oxygen tension, arterial blood oxygen tension (PaO_2), red blood cell concentration, and mean arterial pressure (MAP) or cerebral perfusion pressure (CPP). There is no established critical level of brain PtO_2. Normal brain PtO_2 values are in the range of 35 to 50 mm Hg.

3. **Near infrared spectroscopy (see Chapter 28).** This noninvasive measurement is based on the transmission and absorption of near infrared light (700 to 950 nm) as it passes

through tissue. Oxygenated and deoxygenated hemoglobin have different absorption spectra and brain oxygenation can be calculated by their relative absorption of near infrared light. Near infrared spectroscopy (NIRS) interrogates all tissue within the field of view. Thus, NIRS measurements of hemoglobin saturation reflect influences from arterial, venous, and capillary blood [8]. Currently, there is no standard among commercial NIRS systems; although most provide an absolute measure of brain tissue oxygen saturation in some form and display this as a simple percentage value. The recent development of NIRS-derived measurements of cytochrome c oxidase has been validated in animal models as a measurement of cellular status. It offers a potential to assess intramitochondrial respiration in traumatic brain injury.

4. **Cerebral microdialysis.** This technique measures cellular functions through accumulation of substrates or metabolic by-products by analyzing microdialysate concentrations of glucose, lactate, pyruvate, glycerol, and/or glutamate. Cerebral ischemia or hypoxia is associated with marked increases in the lactate/pyruvate ratio and glycerol and glutamate levels [9].

CLINICAL PEARL • Critical brain tissue pO_2 is 15 to 20 mm Hg.
• Brain consumes glucose as its preferred substrate during normal resting conditions.
• Lactate supplements glucose as an energy source and is increasingly used by the brain during neuronal activation (e.g., exercise, severe hypoglycemia, and hypoxia).

II. Cerebral blood flow

A. **General concepts.** Tight regulation of CBF is important to meet the energy demands of active neurons. This process is often labeled "neurovascular coupling." Total CBF at rest in humans is about 800 mL/min (50 mL/100 g/min), which is 15% to 20% of the cardiac output. In normal physiologic states, total blood flow to the brain is remarkably constant. This is due in part to the prominent contributions of both large arteries and parenchymal arterioles to overall vascular resistance.

Neuronal function and cellular integrity can be compromised by reductions in regional cerebral blood flow (rCBF). During prolonged focal ischemia, brain tissue may develop a localized injury pattern consisting of a core of tissue destined for destruction (infarction) surrounded by a "penumbra" of metabolically semistable tissue that has the potential for full recovery, or may contribute to expansion of the zone of infarction. Initially, penumbra was proposed to be related to an area with 50% reduction in evoked potential amplitude. An increased extracellular K^+ concentration, which is linked to energy failure, contributes to cell death in the infarct core. The spread of the elevated K^+ into the penumbral zone can place further demands on energy-generating processes within penumbral cells and recruit more tissue into the infarct core. The use of PET imaging has permitted measurements of rCBF, $CMRO_2$, rCMRglu, and oxygen extraction fraction (OEF) in penumbra and infarction regions. In humans, penumbra is defined as the area where rCBF decreases to 12 to 22 mL/100 g/min, $rCMRO_2$ remains above 65 μmol/100 g/min, and OEF is increased to more than 50%. Infarction usually corresponds to rCBF below 12 mL/100 g/min and $rCMRO_2$ below 65 μm/100 g/min [10].

B. **Regulation of CBF**

1. **Myogenic response.** The myogenic response is the intrinsic property of vascular smooth muscle to react to changes in mechanical input or intravascular pressure. The smooth muscle of large cerebral arteries and small arterioles dilate in response to decreased pressure and constrict in response to increases in pressure, therefore contributing to autoregulation of blood flow. Local metabolites and release of vasoactive factors from endothelium and perivascular nerves can influence myogenic tone and vascular resistance. The myogenic response mechanism involves two processes: Myogenic tone and myogenic reactivity. An excessively high arterial pressure (above the autoregulatory range) results in

a condition known as forced dilation, which involves a marked increase in vessel diameter and loss of tone.

Initiation of the myogenic constrictor response occurs through ionic and enzymatic processes that lead to accumulation of intracellular calcium. Increased pressure causes depolarization of smooth muscle cell membrane promoting calcium influx via opening of voltage-operated calcium channels (Ca_v). Wall tension is proposed as a stimulus for an initiation of the myogenic response. Stretch-activated cation channels (i.e., transient receptor potential [TRP] channels) are thought to be the sensor. The increase in intracellular calcium leads to myosin light chain phosphorylation and promotes vasoconstriction. Other signaling mechanisms include activation of protein kinase C (PKC) and RhoA-Rho kinase pathways.

A feedback loop exists to prevent excessive myogenic constriction. This mechanism, which limits constriction-induced depolarization, is the activation of calcium-activated potassium channels (especially large-conductance BKca channels) expressed on cerebral artery smooth muscle. Activation of BKca channels causes hyperpolarization and attenuation of myogenic vasoconstrictive responses [11].

2. **Endothelial contributions.** Cerebral endothelial cells form tight junctions, establishing the blood–brain barrier. Endothelial dysfunction has been proposed to be an important factor in the pathogenesis of cardiovascular disease such as atherosclerosis, stroke, diabetes, and subarachnoid hemorrhage. The endothelium produces several vasoactive substances that can have significant influence on vascular tone: Nitric oxide (NO), endothelium-derived hyperpolarizing factor (EDHF), prostacyclin, and other eicosanoids.

   a. **Nitric oxide.** Nitric oxide synthase (NOS) is the enzyme responsible for the O_2-dependent conversion of L-arginine to NO. There are three isoforms of NOS. Neuronal (nNOS or NOS1) is constitutively expressed in neurons under normal conditions. Inducible (iNOS or NOS2) is not normally expressed in the brain but can be induced under pathologic conditions. Lastly, endothelial (eNOS, NOS3) is abundantly expressed in the endothelium. NO generated by eNOS diffuses to vascular smooth muscle where it binds to and activates soluble guanylate cyclase, resulting in increased levels of cyclic guanine monophosphate (cGMP) and activation of protein kinase G (PKG), which causes vasodilation by opening K^+ channels (BK_{ca}) and/or reducing the sensitivity of the contractile machinery to Ca^+. eNOS is regulated by calcium, heat shock protein (HSP90), serine/threonine phosphorylation, and tyrosine phosphorylation.

   The NO system is altered in many pathologic states. Under conditions of limited substrate or low levels of the cofactor tetrahydrobiopterin (BH_4), eNOS can become uncoupled from NO production leading to the production of superoxide (O_2^-) [12]. This has been implicated in brain damage arising from atherosclerosis, diabetes, and hypertension.

CLINICAL PEARL   Statins (HMG-CoA reductase blockers) improve outcome in stroke via increased eNOS expression and reduced NADPH oxidase activity. This action on eNOS involves preservation of eNOS mRNA and is unrelated to its cholesterol-lowering effect.

   b. **Endothelium-derived hyperpolarizing factor.** EDHF-mediated dilation occurs in the presence of NOS and cyclooxygenase (COX) metabolite inhibition. The EDHF response requires increased endothelial calcium and activation of small- and intermediate-conductance calcium-activated potassium channels (SK_{Ca} and IK_{Ca}). Endothelial hyperpolarization then transfers to vascular smooth muscle hyperpolarization and vasodilation; the mechanism is unclear, but may involve gap junctions [13]. Emerging evidence supports a role for EDHF as a contributing factor/mediator to resting tone in small cerebral arterioles, thus influencing resting CBF. In addition, the EDHF-mediated dilating system is upregulated after stroke and traumatic brain injury, whereas endothelium-derived NO dilating system is decreased [12]. This suggests a role for

EDHF as a compensatory vasodilating mechanism when NO contributions are diminished during pathologic conditions.

c. **Prostacyclin and other eicosanoids.** In endothelial cells and astrocytes, arachidonic acid is metabolized to vasoactive substances that are either vasoconstricting or vasodilating in nature. These products are collectively called eicosanoids. Arachidonic acid, once liberated from phospholipid membrane (via the action of phospholipase A_2) is further metabolized by COX, lipoxygenase, epoxygenase, or hydroxylase. The COX pathways have been well studied. The two principal COX isoforms are variably expressed in neurons, glial cells, and cerebral endothelial cells. The products of COX pathway can be vasodilating such as prostacyclin (PGI_2), prostaglandin E_2, and prostagladin D_2, or vasoconstricting such as prostaglandin $F_{2\alpha}$ and thromboxane A_2. PGI_2 is most studied in cerebral endothelium cell. PGI_2 diffuses to the smooth muscle where it binds to G-protein–coupled receptor and activates adenylate cyclase and protein kinase A (PKA). The increase in PKA activity can promote the opening of certain K^+ channels (BKca; inward-rectifier [Kir]) producing smooth muscle hyperpolarization and voltage-sensitive Ca^{2+} channel closure, resulting in decreased intracellular Ca^{2+} levels and vasodilation. The epoxygenase and hydroxylase pathways yield vasodilating and vasoconstricting products, respectively through actions toward BKca channels (Table 1.1).

C. **Control of CBF**

1. **Autoregulation of CBF.** Autoregulation is the ability to maintain a relatively constant blood flow over a wide range of perfusion pressures. Thus, global CBF will remain at 50 mL/100 g brain tissue/min, provided the CPP is between 60 and 70 to 160 mm Hg (with variability among individuals). CPP is equal to the difference between the MAP and intracranial pressure (ICP): CPP = MAP − ICP. Beyond this limit, cerebral autoregulation is lost and CBF becomes pressure dependent in a linear fashion. The mechanisms responsible for autoregulation in the brain are not entirely understood [13]. Regulation at the high end of the autoregulatory range is proposed to be related to the myogenic response of cerebral arterial smooth muscles, which constrict in response to elevated perfusion pressure and dilate in response to decreased perfusion pressure. Autoregulation at the lower end of the autoregulatory range is postulated to involve local release of metabolic vasodilating factors including H^+, K^+, CO_2, purines, prostanoids, NO, bradykinin, histamine; and, perhaps, mechanical factors (e.g., endothelial shear) (Fig. 1.1).

2. **Neurovascular coupling.** There is a close physical association between parenchymal arterioles and astrocytic processes, greatly exceeding the level of contacts between neurons and arterioles. Because of their close proximity to arterioles and neural synapses, astrocytes are well positioned to act as signaling conduits, linking neurons to arterioles. Increased synaptic activity may lead to the release of factors such as glutamate, K^+, and ATP. These factors, then, may interact with neighboring astrocytes [14]. The information regarding synaptic activity is then communicated to perivascular astrocytic end feet and eventually arterioles, permitting "appropriate" adjustments in arteriolar tone. The cellular components of the neuron–astrocyte–arteriole conduit are often referred to as the "neurovascular unit."

TABLE 1.1   Some factors influencing cerebrovascular tone

Vasoconstrictors	Vasodilators
Endothelin	NO, EDHF
Intracellular Ca^{++} in vascular smooth muscle cell (VSMC) $\rightarrow$ VSMC depolarization	Endothelial Ca^{++}/K^+ channel $\rightarrow$ VSMC hyperpolarization
Arachidonic acid products ($PGF_{2\alpha}$, thromboxane A_2)	Arachidonic acid products (PGI_2, PGE_2, PGD_2)
Synaptic depression	Synaptic activation
Extreme hyperoxia	Hypoxia >50 mm Hg
Hypocarbia	Hypercarbia

NO, Nitric oxide; EDHF, Endothelium-derived hyperpolarizing factor.

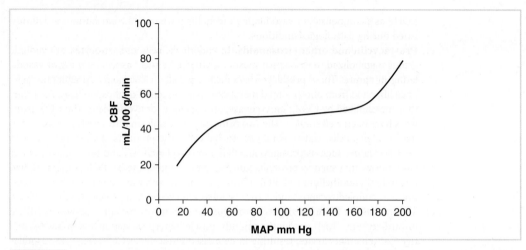

FIGURE 1.1 Over a range of cerebral perfusion pressure (CPP = MAP − ICP) cerebral blood flow remains constant at 50 mL/100 g/min.

There are multiple pathways involved in signaling via the neurovascular unit. Examples include K^+ released during synaptic activation and its subsequent spatial redistribution within astrocytes to perivascular end feet, where it is released via a Ca^{2+}-dependent process involving BKca channels. Vasodilation ensues when that released K^+ interacts with Kir channels on arteriolar smooth muscle [15]. In addition, ATP released into the extracellular milieu not only may participate in intercellular signaling, but also may be rapidly hydrolyzed to adenosine, a potent vasodilator, and mediate relaxation of cerebral arterioles.

3. **Arterial blood oxygen tension.** In the normal resting state there is a tight coupling between CBF and $CMRO_2$. Acute hypoxia is a potent dilator for cerebral circulation. However, CBF does not change until PaO_2 falls below 50 mm Hg. One possible mechanism relates to decreased ATP levels associated with acute hypoxia. This may open K_{ATP} channels on smooth muscle, causing hyperpolarization and vasodilation. Increased NO and adenosine production during hypoxia also promote smooth muscle relaxation and increase in blood flow. Cerebral vasoconstriction may occur during hyperoxic exposure. The mechanism remains unclear (Fig. 1.2).

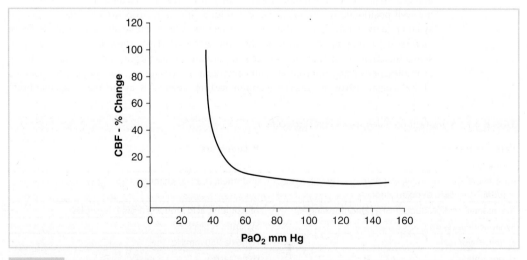

FIGURE 1.2 Cerebral blood flow remains constant until PaO_2 reaches 50 mm Hg, at which point it increases rapidly to provide adequate delivery of oxygen to the brain.

4. **Arterial blood carbon dioxide tension.** Variations in arterial blood carbon dioxide tension ($PaCO_2$) have profound effects on CBF [16]. Hypercapnia increases blood flow, while hypocapnia causes cerebral vasoconstriction and decreases blood flow. The relationship appears to be linear within $PaCO_2$ from 20 to 80 mm Hg (Fig. 1.3). Several mechanisms appear to be involved, but the exact mechanism is not completely understood [17]. A major element relates to a direct effect of extracellular H^+ on vascular smooth muscle. Other mechanisms include vasodilator prostanoids and NO, whose influence may vary according to species and developmental age.

D. **Measurement of CBF**
   1. **Nuclear medicine methods.** Nuclear medicine methods use radionucleides as tracers in combination with a tomographic approach for image reconstruction. PET is quantitative, while the single photon emission tomography (SPECT) technique is only semiquantitative. PET also allows measurement of oxygen utilization and therefore the OEF. The tracer commonly used for PET is ^{15}O-labeled water [18]. ^{99m}TcHMPAO is used for SPECT due to its long stability after being reconstituted. Xenon is also another agent commonly used in CBF measurement both with SPECT and computed tomography (CT).
   2. **Computed tomography (perfusion CT).** The appearance of iodine contrast material injection on sequential CT images permits calculation of cerebral blood volume (CBV), time to peak (TTP), mean transit time (MTT), and rCBF. This technique has gained popularity in clinical practice in stroke patients due to its rapidity for obtaining information and widespread availability.
   3. **Magnetic resonance imaging (perfusion MRI).** There are two categories of perfusion MRI: Exogenous and endogenous. The exogenous method is most commonly used. As the tracer passes through the capillary bed, the signal intensity falls and returns to baseline level as the tracer leaves the vasculature. This method provides a semiquantitative assessment of relative blood flow when TTP, MTT, and rCBV are obtained. The endogenous method uses arterial blood water as a "tracer" for perfusion imaging. This approach is termed arterial spin labeling (ASL). It is noninvasive and can be acquired as part of a multimodal MRI examination. As compared with exogenous contrast MRI, ASL has inferior signal-to-noise characteristics, but it provides more direct quantification of absolute CBF and can be used in conjunct with fMRI.
   4. **Ultrasound (see Chapter 28).** Transcranial Doppler (TCD) is noninvasive and provides real-time measurement of cerebral hemodynamics. It uses ultrasound waves to measure the velocity of blood flow through large cerebral vessels from the Doppler shift caused by

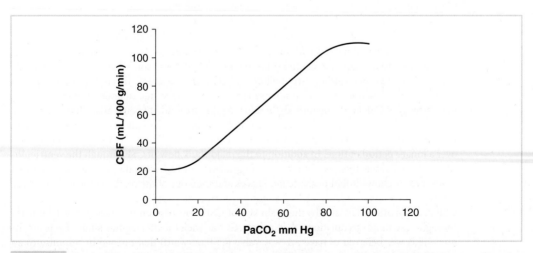

FIGURE 1.3 Cerebral blood flow varies linearly approximately 2% for each mm Hg change in $PaCO_2$ between 20 and 80 mm Hg.

red blood cells moving through the field being monitored. TCD does not provide an actual blood flow value, but is a technique for measuring relative changes in CBF.

CLINICAL PEARL • Cerebral autoregulation (maintenance of CBF between CPP of 60–70 and 160 mm Hg) becomes ineffective in hypercapnic, hypoxic, and ischemic conditions.
• Inhalation anesthetic agents suppress cerebral autoregulation in a dose-dependent manner.

III. Cerebrospinal fluid

A. General concept. The brain and the spinal cord are bathed in cerebrospinal fluid (CSF), which provides physical support and a cushion against external pressure. The CSF environment is critical for brain function. Although CSF does not provide nutrients, it facilitates movement of neuroendocrine substances and clears brain metabolic wastes such as CO_2 and lactate. The CSF acts as a fluid reservoir and is important in providing a capacitance against intracranial volume expansion.

B. CSF formation and composition. CSF is filtered and actively secreted from cerebral arterial blood. Although the main production site is the choroid plexus of the ventricular system, extrachorial sources may make up a significant amount of the total CSF formation in humans. This occurs in two steps: (i) passive filtration of fluid across choroidal capillary endothelium and (ii) regulated active secretion across a single-layered epithelium, involving pumps, cotransporters and antiporters, ion channels, and aquaporins. Net filtration is related to the hydrostatic pressure gradient between blood and choroid interstitial fluid. Transchoroidal secretion of water, ions, and macromolecules steer the CSF down the ventriculocisternal axis.

Essentially, CSF formation involves the net transport of Na^+, Cl^-, K^+, HCO_3^-, and water from plasma to choroid plexus to CSF. The biochemical composition is altered by aging and central nervous system disease. Compared to plasma, CSF has a lower concentration of K^+, Ca^{2+}, HCO_3^-, glucose and urea, and higher levels of Na^+, Cl^-, and Mg^{2+}. CSF is 99% water compared to the 92% water content of plasma. The rate of human CSF formation varies from 0.3 to 0.6 mL/min, depending upon the measurement used and the brain metabolic rate, but is independent of the ICP. Daily volume production in adult human is believed to be constant at 450 to 600 mL.

C. CSF dynamics. Pulsatile CSF flow is related to hemodynamics within the choroid plexus. CSF is secreted mainly in the lateral and third ventricles, and flows along the aqueduct of Sylvius to reach the fourth ventricle. CSF flows out of the fourth ventricle through the foramen of Magendie, and the lateral foramina of Luschka, into the subarachnoid space. This involves a network of interconnected CSF cisterns located around the basal aspect of the brain. It flows upward to the superior sagittal sinus where most of it is absorbed via the arachnoid villi. Some CSF flows downward toward the lumbar subarachnoid space. This is important for fluid exchange and pressure–volume compensation. In head injury, due to brain swelling, the normal pathway of CSF flow is disturbed; therefore a pressure gradient could arise. The critical ICP threshold is between 20 and 25 mm Hg. However, hydrocephalus patients can tolerate a rise in ICP up to 40 to 45 mm Hg without evidence of adverse effects if the increase in pressure occurs over a longer period of time. In addition to the major bulk flow of CSF through the ventriculo-subarachnoid space, there is a limited microcirculation of CSF from the cortical subarachnoid space into Virchow–Robin perivascular spaces and then out of the brain via the CSF drainage route.

D. CSF reabsorption. Classically, the main site of CSF reabsorption was thought to take place through arachnoid granulations that penetrate the walls of the sagittal sinus. Each arachnoid villus was believed to have a 1-way valve (CSF outward) that opened in response to an increased hydrostatic pressure in CSF compared to the venous blood. There are factors that could interfere with venous pressure and lead to decreased CSF reabsorption. These include coughing, straining, positive end-expiratory pressure, dural sinus thrombosis, and congestive heart failure. During the past decade, there was a paradigm shift regarding the dominant site of CSF drainage in several animal models. As such, the primary reabsorption site of CSF in rats, pigs, sheep, and even nonhuman primates is now believed to be via olfactory and optic nerves, cribriform plate, nasal mucosa, and cervical lymphatics [19]. In most mammals, the arachnoid villi are not normally the site of most CSF absorption, except perhaps under high/pathologic CSF pressure conditions [19]. Regardless of the outflow mechanism, the total CSF outflow is described by the following equation:

$$CSF_{outflow} = (ICP - P_{duralsinus})/R_{out}$$

The R_{out} is the CSF outflow resistance. R_{out} is constant in the normal ICP range. However, it can increase with age or degenerative diseases. Clinically, R_{out} has been used as a tool to select candidates for shunt surgery and is a reliable indicator of shunt malfunction.

3   **E. Intracranial pressure.** The brain is located in a different environment compared to other organs in the body. It is surrounded and protected by a rigid skull. Changes in the volume of various components (brain tissue, blood, and CSF) can raise the ICP, impede blood flow, and cause cerebral ischemia. Normal ICP in a healthy adult is within the range of 7 to 15 mm Hg. It can become negative with the mean around −10 mm Hg (but not exceeding −15 mm Hg) in the vertical position. A significant rise in ICP depends on the specific pathology.

Intracranial compliance is demonstrated by the pressure–volume curve. A compensatory reserve for brain compliance can be derived from the pressure–volume curve. The index called RAP (correlation coefficient [R] between pulse amplitude [A] and mean ICP [P]) can indicate the degree of correlation between pulse amplitude of ICP (AMP) and mean ICP over time. Theoretically, the RAP coefficient indicates the relationship between ICP and changes in cerebral volume. A RAP coefficient near 0 means no synchronization between AMP and mean ICP, where a change in volume causes no or very little change in pressure (good compensation). When the pressure–volume curve begins to increase exponentially, the RAP rises to +1, which correlates with a low compensatory reserve [20] (Fig. 1.4). Clinically, when RAP increases, signs of elevated ICP may occur (nausea, vomiting, headache, changing mental status, loss of consciousness, and in severe cases with brain herniation).

F. Measurement of ICP. Several techniques can be used to obtain ICP (intraventricular, parenchymal, subarachnoid, and subdural measurement systems). Each has different advantages and disadvantages. The fluid coupled system using an intraventricular catheter is considered to be a gold standard because it can be used both for diagnosis and therapy.

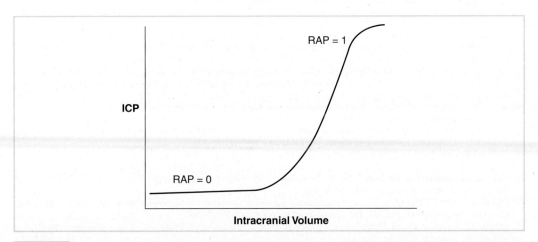

FIGURE 1.4 Relationship between intracranial pressure (ICP) and intracranial volume (ICV). ICP does not increase until a critical ICV is reached. RAP = Correlation coefficient (R) between pulse amplitude (A) and mean intracranial pressure (P).

TABLE 1.2 Normal cerebral values

Brain weight	2% body weight 1500–1600 g
Cerebral energy consumption	20% of total body energy consumption $CMRO_2$ 3.5 mL/100 g/min CMRglu 5 mg/100 g/min
Cerebral blood flow	15%–20% of cardiac output 50 cc/100 g/min
Intracranial pressure	7–15 mm Hg
Pathologic intracranial pressure	>20 mm Hg
Intracranial cerebrospinal fluid volume	150 cc
Cerebrospinal fluid production	0.3–0.6 mL/min

IV. Summary. The brain is a complex organ which requires homeostasis between cerebral metabolic demand, adequate delivery of metabolic substrates, and removal of waste products. It is the only organ in the human body that resides within a rigid bony container, and its function is sensitive to the changes in intracranial brain, blood, and CSF volumes. Normal parameters for cerebral physiology are listed in Table 1.2.

ACKNOWLEDGMENT

We wish to thank Dr. Dale Pelligrino for valuable feedback on this manuscript.

REFERENCES

1. Lin JS, Anaclet C, Sergeeva OA, et al. The waking brain: an update. *Cell Mol Life Sci.* 2011;68:2499–2512.
2. Buzsaki G, Kaila K, Raichle M. Inhibition and brain work. *Neuron.* 2007;56:771–783.
3. Masamoto K, Tanishita K. Oxygen transport in brain tissue. *J Biomech Eng.* 2009;131:074002.
4. Pellerin L, Magistretti PJ. Sweet sixteen for ANLS. *J Cereb Blood Flow Metab.* 2012;32:1152–1166. doi: 10.1038/jcbfm.2011. 149.
5. Gjedde A, Marrett S, Vafaee M. Oxidative and nonoxidative metabolism of excited neurons and astrocytes. *J Cereb Blood Flow Metab.* 2002;22:1–14.
6. Boumezbeur F, Petersen KF, Cline GW, et al. The contribution of blood lactate to brain energy metabolism in humans measured by dynamic 13C nuclear magnetic resonance spectroscopy. *J Neurosci.* 2010;30:13983–13989.
7. Rasmussen P, Wyss MT, Lundby C. Cerebral glucose and lactate consumption during cerebral activation by physical activity in human. *FASEB J.* 2011;25:2865–2873.
8. Highton D, Elwell C, Smith M. Noninvasive cerebral oximetry: is there light at the end of the tunnel? *Curr Opin Anaesthesiol.* 2010;23:576–581.
9. Smith M. Perioperative uses of transcranial perfusion monitoring. *Neurosurg Clin N Am.* 2008;19:489–502.
10. Del Zoppo GJ, Sharp FR, Heiss WD, et al. Heterogeneity in the penumbra. *J Cereb Blood Flow Metab.* 2011;31:1836–1851.
11. Cipolla MJ. *The Cerebral Circulation.* San Rafael, CA: Morgan & Claypool Life Sciences; 2009.
12. Andersen J, Shafi NI, Bryan RM Jr. Endothelial influences on cerebrovascular tone. *J Appl Physiol.* 2006;100:318–327.
13. Feletou M. *The Endothelium: Part 2: EDHF-Mediated Responses, "The Classical Pathway."* San Rafael, CA: Morgan & Claypool Life Sciences; 2011.
14. Zauner A, Daugherty WP, Bullock MR, et al. Brain oxygenation and energy metabolism: part I-biological function and pathophysiology. *Neurosurgery.* 2002;51:289–301.
15. Figley CR, Stroman PW. The role(s) of astrocytes and astrocyte activity in neurometabolism, neurovascular coupling, and the production of functional neuroimaging signals. *Eur J Neurosci.* 2011;33:577–588.
16. Paulson OB, Hasselbalch SG, Rostrup E, et al. Cerebral blood flow response to functional activation. *J Cereb Blood Flow Metab.* 2010;30:2–14.
17. Vovk A, Cunningham DA, Kowalchuk JM, et al. Cerebral blood flow responses to changes in oxygen and carbon dioxide in humans. *Can J Physiol Pharmacol.* 2002;80:819–827.
18. Okazawa H, Kudo T. Clinical impact of hemodynamic parameter measurement for cerebrovascular disease using positron emission tomography and (15)O-labeled tracers. *Ann Nucl Med.* 2009;23:217–227.
19. Johanson CE, Duncan JA 3rd, Klinge PM, et al. Multiplicity of cerebrospinal fluid functions: New challenges in health and disease. *Cerebrospinal Fluid Res.* 2008;5:10.
20. Czosnyka M, Pickard JD. Monitoring and interpretation of intracranial pressure. *J Neurol Neurosurg Psychiatry.* 2004;75:813–821.

2 Anesthetic Effects on Cerebral Blood Flow and Metabolism

Mark F. Mueller and Verna L. Baughman

KEY POINTS

1. Inhalational anesthetics cause a dose-dependent decrease in cerebral metabolism with an *increase* in cerebral blood flow (*decoupling* of flow from metabolism).
2. Nitrous oxide and ketamine are notable exceptions to these rules.
3. Intravenous anesthetics cause a dose-dependent decrease in cerebral metabolism with a *decrease* in cerebral blood flow (maintenance of flow-metabolism coupling).
4. Vasoactive medications cause a dose-dependent change in cerebral blood flow *without* a direct effect on cerebral metabolism.

INTRODUCTION

As we embark on a discussion of the interaction between physiology and pharmacology, we must bear in mind that our knowledge is imperfect, limited by the complexity of the subject and nature of the existing research. Much of the literature we have is based on animal studies alone. Where possible we attempt to emphasize human-subject research, but these also are often small studies and case-series, focused primarily on healthy subjects with otherwise intact cerebral physiology. The effects of intracranial pathology on the interaction between anesthetics and normal physiology are complex, and while some mechanisms are well preserved in all but the most severely damaged tissues, we also rely on the knowledge that most treatable cerebral insults are focal cerebral insults. This damaged tissue is surrounded by normal brain with normal responses to pharmacologic intervention, and the emphasis in neuroanesthesia lies on the protection of these as-yet uninjured neurons.

CLINICAL PEARL   The goal of the neuroanesthesiologist is to protect uninjured brain tissue in the presence of disease.

I. **Inhalational agents**
   A. **Volatile anesthetics.** As a group, the volatile anesthetics produce a dose-dependent depression in the cerebral metabolic rate for both oxygen ($CMRO_2$) and glucose (CMRglc) by virtue

TABLE 2.1 Effects of inhaled anesthetics on cerebral hemodynamics

	CBF	CMRO$_2$	Cerebral autoregulation	CO$_2$ reactivity	ICP
Sevoflurane	⇑⇑	⇓	⇓	⇔	⇑
Isoflurane	⇑	⇓⇓	⇓	⇔	⇑
Desflurane	⇑⇑⇑	⇓	⇓	⇔	⇑⇑⇑
Nitrous oxide	⇑⇑⇑	⇑⇑	⇓	⇔	⇑⇑
Xenon	⇓	⇓⇓	⇔	⇔	⇓
Carbon dioxide	⇑⇑⇑⇑⇑	⇓	⇔	—	⇑⇑⇑

CBF, cerebral blood flow; ICP, intracranial pressure.

of their anesthetic action, while simultaneously increasing cerebral blood flow (CBF) as a consequence of their direct vasodilatory properties (Table 2.1). In this way, the volatile anesthetics abolish the normal coupling of CBF to CMRO$_2$.

The decrease in metabolism seen with the volatile anesthetics is due to a reduction in organized neurotransmission, reaching a maximum reduction in CMRO$_2$ of approximately 50% when an isoelectric electroencephalogram (EEG) is achieved (Fig. 2.1). The remaining 50% of the cerebral metabolic requirement represents the energy expended in maintaining cellular integrity, and is not amenable to reduction by administration of anesthetic agents. Burst suppression, periods of isoelectric EEG interrupted by brief bursts of electrical activity, is a pattern which is seen during the transition from continuously active to continuously isoelectric EEG waveforms, and is associated with a reduction in cerebral energy requirement similar to that obtained with a completely isoelectric EEG (Fig. 2.2). This is a clinically useful target for metabolic suppression during periods of anticipated ischemia, because no additional benefit has been shown with deeper levels of anesthesia. In addition, anesthesia doses beyond those required for burst suppression increase the risk of both delayed emergence and cardiovascular collapse.

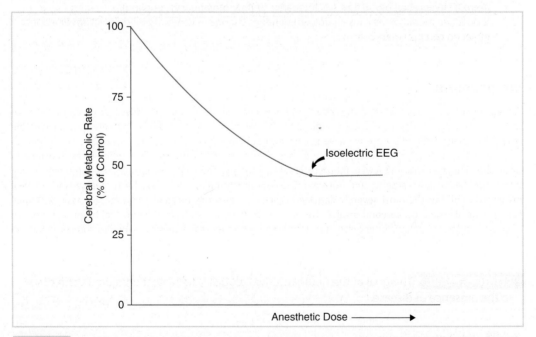

FIGURE 2.1 Cerebral metabolic rate for oxygen decreases with increasing effect-site concentration of anesthetic, to a maximum reduction of 50% of baseline. At this point an isoelectric EEG is observed. (Adapted from Newfield P, Cottrell J. *Handbook of Neuroanesthesia: Clinical and Physiologic Essentials.* 1st ed. Boston, MA: Little, Brown and Co.; 1983:21.)

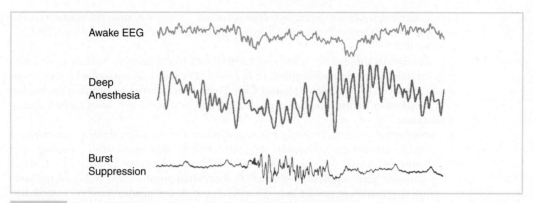

FIGURE 2.2 Representative EEG waveforms for awake, anesthetized, and burst-suppressed states. Note the periodic electrocardiographic activity visible on the burst-suppressed EEG tracing.

CLINICAL PEARL There is no evidence for improved outcomes with deeper anesthesia once burst suppression is achieved.

At high concentrations, intracranial pressure (ICP) may increase due to increases in CBF and cerebral hyperemia. However, the increase in CBF that occurs secondary to the loss of cerebral autoregulation at high anesthetic concentrations (Fig. 2.3), may be limited by a decrease in cerebral perfusion pressure (CPP) due to a reduction in the mean arterial pressure (MAP) from

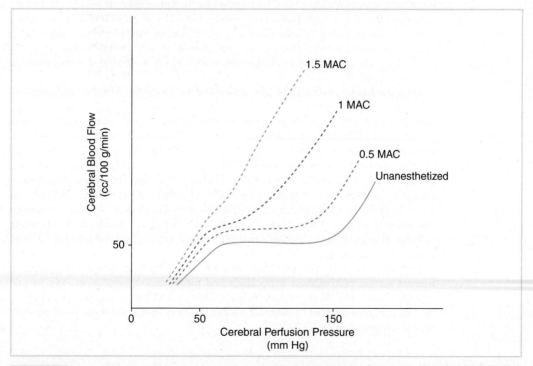

FIGURE 2.3 Attenuation of cerebral autoregulatory response by inhaled anesthetic gases. At greater than 1.5 MAC, cerebral blood flow is directly related to cerebral perfusion pressure. (Adapted from Newfield P, Cottrell J. *Handbook of Neuroanesthesia: Clinical and Physiologic Essentials.* 1st ed. Boston, MA: Little, Brown and Co.; 1983:18.)

both systemic vasodilation and myocardial depression. In addition, since the cerebrovascular response to CO_2 is generally maintained, hyperventilation may offset any increase in CBF, CBV, and thus ICP.

In addition to these direct effects on $CMRO_2$ and blood flow, the volatile agents also have variable effects on cerebrospinal fluid production and reabsorption, which independently impact ICP, CPP, and ultimately CBF. These effects, however, are slow to develop (with timeframes on the order of several hours), and in practice may be of limited clinical importance.

1. **Sevoflurane.** At concentrations less than one-half the minimum alveolar concentration (MAC), sevoflurane minimally disrupts cerebral flow-metabolism coupling and autoregulation [1]. With increasing concentration progressive decreases in $CMRO_2$ occur, with burst suppression obtained at concentrations of 1.5 to 2 MAC. At the same time, concentrations greater than 0.5 MAC cause dose-dependent cerebral vasodilation and a resulting increase in CBF, weakening the coupling of flow to metabolism [2,3]. Autoregulation and the reactivity to arterial carbon dioxide concentrations are maintained, and hyperventilation will attenuate the increases in blood flow [1,4].

    Some observers have reported epileptiform changes in the EEG during anesthesia with sevoflurane, most notably during inhalational induction and about the time burst suppression is achieved [5]. Reported activity has ranged from periodic spike and wave discharges to (rarely) frank seizure activity. While seizure activity is clearly associated with increases in $CMRO_2$ and blood flow, the clinical significance of the more often reported periodic discharges is unknown.

    Sevoflurane decreases both CSF production and reabsorption in parallel, with uncertain effects on overall CSF balance and ICP [6].

2. **Isoflurane.** The general nature of isoflurane's effect on CBF and metabolism is similar to that of sevoflurane, with maximal depression of $CMRO_2$ and increases in CBF achieved at approximately 2 MAC. For a given fraction of its respective MAC, isoflurane produces less cerebral vasodilation but greater metabolic depression than sevoflurane, making it the preferred volatile anesthetic for neuroanesthesia in some circles [2,7]. Cerebrovascular autoregulation is well maintained at concentrations less than 0.5 MAC, and may be restored at higher concentrations when combined with moderate hypocapnia [8].

    Isoflurane has no effect on CSF production and a bimodal effect on CSF reabsorption, with impaired reabsorption at low concentrations and increased reabsorption at high concentrations. The net effect promotes increased ICP at low isoflurane concentrations and decreasing ICP at high concentrations [9].

3. **Desflurane.** As compared with sevoflurane and isoflurane, desflurane produces similar cerebral vasodilation and depression of $CMRO_2$ [10], with clinically relevant effects over a range of approximately 0.5 to 2 MAC. Desflurane does, however, have slightly greater vasodilatory potency as compared with the other volatile anesthetics in common use today [7,11]. In addition, rapid increases in desflurane concentration increase sympathetic outflow, potentially compounding the anesthetic's effect in increasing CBF by elevating systemic blood pressure. Cerebral vascular response to CO_2 remains intact to at least 1 MAC of desflurane [12].

    Desflurane has little effect on CSF production or reabsorption, except in the clinically relevant setting of combined hypocapnia and intracranial hypertension [13]. In one relevant study, under those conditions desflurane increases CSF production. This has the unfortunate consequence of promoting further increases in ICP under the worst possible clinical circumstances.

CLINICAL PEARL   The cerebrovascular and cerebral metabolic effects of the potent inhalational anesthetics are similar, with minor variations on specific parameters.

B. Nitrous oxide. In contrast to the volatile inhaled anesthetics, nitrous oxide causes increases in $CMRO_2$, CBF, and ICP [14]. Increases in CBF exceed the increases in $CMRO_2$ with a nitrous oxide anesthetic, resulting in decoupling of flow from metabolism despite increases in both parameters. This effect can be attenuated by the addition of intravenous agents, including propofol, barbiturates, and opioids. Sevoflurane, on the other hand, is synergistic with nitrous oxide in increasing CBF and therefore further weakens flow-metabolism coupling. Interestingly, when cerebral electrical silence is induced with propofol, the addition of nitrous oxide may restore EEG activity [15].

Cerebrovascular reactivity to CO_2 is maintained during nitrous oxide anesthesia [16], and CSF homeostasis is unaltered.

C. Xenon. Although its use as a general anesthetic is currently limited due to scarcity and expense, xenon exhibits several favorable properties for use in neuroanesthesia. Xenon exhibits neuroprotective properties, possibly through antagonism of the N-Methyl-D-Aspartate (NMDA) receptor, which plays a role in excitotoxic cellular demise. Xenon is also noted for exceptional cardiovascular stability, and cerebrovascular autoregulation and CO_2 reactivity both appear to be maintained under xenon anesthesia at 1 MAC [17]. CBF exhibits regional variations consistent with regional variations in metabolism, with a global trend toward reductions in both, $CMRO_2$ more so than CBF [18–20]. The effects of xenon on CSF production and reabsorption are unknown.

D. Carbon dioxide. As discussed in the previous chapter and repeatedly referenced here, arterial carbon dioxide tension correlates strongly and in an inverse direction with cerebral vasomotor tone in the normal physiologic condition. This correlation is preserved under all but the most extreme physiologic derangements, both iatrogenic and pathologic.

Moderate hypercapnia is sedating, and reduces $CMRO_2$ in a dose-dependent fashion for a $PaCO_2$ of up to at least 70 mm Hg [21,22]. With higher arterial carbon dioxide tension, sympathetic activation is observed, though how this correlates with cerebral metabolic activity is unknown.

II. Intravenous anesthetics

A. Induction agents. With the exception of ketamine, intravenous induction agents uniformly generate reductions in CBF and $CMRO_2$, with maintenance of flow-metabolism coupling (Table 2.2). In addition to induction of anesthesia, these agents are often used during maintenance of anesthesia to supplement inhalational anesthetics, in order to provide burst suppression for brain protection, or as part of a total intravenous anesthetic (TIVA) to better accommodate neurophysiologic monitoring.

1. Propofol. Propofol produces dose-dependent reductions in CBF, $CMRO_2$, and thus ICP [14], to the point of abolishment of cortical electrical activity. Flow-metabolism coupling is maintained [23], with the caveat that global cardiovascular depression associated with propofol administration may reduce CPP below the lower limits of autoregulatory compensation. Vasopressor support may be required to maintain cerebral perfusion when propofol is used to induce EEG burst suppression. CO_2 reactivity is maintained, and propofol has no effect on the production or reabsorption of CSF [24].

TABLE 2.2 Effects of intravenous anesthetics on cerebral hemodynamics

	CBF	CMRO$_2$	Cerebral autoregulation	CO$_2$ reactivity	ICP
Propofol	⇓⇓⇓	⇓⇓⇓	⇔	⇔	⇓⇓
Barbiturates	⇓⇓⇓	⇓⇓⇓	⇔	⇔	⇓⇓
Etomidate	⇓⇓⇓	⇓⇓	⇔	⇔	⇓⇓
Ketamine	⇑⇑⇑	⇑⇑	⇔	⇔	⇑⇑
Benzodiazepenes	⇓⇓	⇓	⇔	⇔	⇓
Opioids	⇓	⇑	⇔	⇔	⇔
Dexmedetomidine	⇓⇓	⇓⇓	⇓	⇓	⇓

CBF, cerebral blood flow; ICP, intracranial pressure.

2. **Barbiturates.** Thiopental is the archetype for intravenous anesthetics used for metabolic suppression, and like propofol the barbiturates produce dose-dependent reductions in $CMRO_2$, CBF, and ICP, up to the point of EEG isoelectricity [25–27]. Flow-metabolism coupling and CO_2 reactivity are also maintained with these agents. High-dose barbiturates may require concomitant vasopressor support to maintain CPP, similar to propofol.

   It should be noted that while the barbiturate methohexital does induce reductions in CBF and $CMRO_2$ in a dose-dependent fashion similar to the other barbiturates, this medication has been shown to lower the seizure threshold [28,29]. As a result, seizure activity on emergence from general anesthesia with methohexital may be a concern. When it occurs, the increased metabolism associated with seizure activity far exceeds any erstwhile reductions in $CMRO_2$, and it is accompanied by large increases in CBF as a result.

3. **Etomidate.** Etomidate also produces dose-dependent reductions in $CMRO_2$, CBF, and ICP with the capacity to produce an isoelectric EEG [30,31]. Flow-metabolism coupling, autoregulation, and CO_2 reactivity are all maintained under etomidate anesthesia. Etomidate has the useful characteristic of causing less cardiovascular depression than either propofol or barbiturates; however, the fact that it causes clinically significant adrenocortical suppression has led to a decline in its use. There is also evidence that regional tissue oxygenation in the brain may decrease under burst suppression induced with etomidate [32,33], a problematic finding in the setting of neurosurgical interventions.

   Etomidate is especially useful in the setting of neurophysiologic monitoring for its ability to maintain both somatosensory evoked potential (SSEP) signal amplitude and transcranial motor evoked potential (TcMEP) thresholds [34,35].

   At low doses etomidate has no effect on CSF homeostasis, while at high doses it causes a decrease in production [36], promoting a reduction in ICP.

4. **Ketamine.** Ketamine produces increases in both CBF and $CMRO_2$ in spontaneously breathing patients, with a disruption in flow-metabolism coupling such that the increase in CBF exceeds that of $CMRO_2$ [37]. These effects are analogous to those seen with nitrous oxide. Autoregulation and CO_2 reactivity are preserved.

   The increase in CBF seen with ketamine may be due to a combination of hypoventilation and hypercarbia in spontaneously ventilated patients, direct cerebral vasodilation, and increased CPP due to sympathomimetic activity [37]. Ketamine is also an NMDA receptor antagonist that has been shown to be neuroprotective in the face of cerebral ischemia.

   Historically, induction doses of ketamine have been thought to significantly increase ICP, presumably due to the aforementioned effects, and the drug has been considered to be contraindicated in patients with increased ICP. Other studies suggest that ketamine may be safe for the patient with increased intracranial elastance so long as moderate hypocarbia is maintained [38–40], but the debate is still open and prudence would suggest the avoidance of induction doses of ketamine for patients with increased intracranial elastance (increased changes in pressure in response to changes in volume) under most circumstances.

   In patients who are sedated or anesthetized and mildly hyperventilated, however, the preponderance of evidence suggests that ketamine does not increase and in fact may lead to a reduction in ICP.

   Like etomidate, ketamine has also been found to be clinically useful during neurophysiologic monitoring to preserve SSEP signal amplitude and TcMEP thresholds under anesthesia [35,41,42].

   Ketamine also decreases reabsorption of CSF [43], and this is an additional mechanism by which it may increase ICP in some cases.

CLINICAL PEARL There is greater heterogeneity in cerebral vascular and metabolic effects amongst intravenous anesthetics than there is between inhalational anesthetics.

B. Benzodiazepines. Benzodiazepines produce reductions in both CBF and $CMRO_2$ with a modest effect on ICP reduction [44]. Midazolam serves as the most common pharmacologic model for the class due to its short half-life. Slowing but not elimination of EEG activity can be achieved, with concomitant and proportional reductions in $CMRO_2$ and CBF [45]. Cerebral autoregulation and CO_2 responsiveness are maintained [46].

While at low doses CSF production and reabsorption are unaffected, at high doses benzodiazepines do reduce CSF production [34]. The overall trend is toward reduced ICP, with the caveat that in the spontaneously breathing patient with increased intracranial elastance, oversedation and respiratory depression will result in intracranial hypertension due to CO_2-mediated cerebral vasodilation.

C. Opioids. Just as midazolam does for the benzodiazepines, remifentanil serves as the test mule for opioid pharmacology in the recent literature, and for the same reason. Reports differ as to the effect of opioids on $CMRO_2$ and CBF at clinically relevant doses, perhaps due to the variety of models and methodologies used [47]. In general it is likely that the overall effect size is small. EEG slowing but not isoelectricity can be obtained with opioids as a sole anesthetic agent. At very high doses, however, it appears that a reduction in CBF and an increase in at least regional $CMRO_2$ due to neuroexcitation may occur, and the risk of inducing seizure activity does exist. Cerebral autoregulation and CO_2 reactivity are otherwise well preserved. Respiratory depression from opioid administration in the awake patient with increased intracranial elastance may lead to marked increases in ICP secondary to hypercapnia.

D. Muscle relaxants
  1. Nondepolarizing muscle relaxants
    a. In general, nondepolarizing muscle relaxants have minimal to no impact on CBF, CBV, or ICP. There are, however, few considerations. Rapid administration of large dose pancuronium can cause tachycardia and an abrupt increase in blood pressure. If autoregulation is compromised this could adversely impact ICP. Another consideration is nondepolarizing relaxants that cause the release of histamine (metocurine, atracurium, mivacurium, curare). Histamine release can cause a decrease in the systemic blood pressure with a concomitant decrease in CVR, increase in CBF and ICP. However, judicious dosing of these medications does not result in significant histamine release.
  2. Depolarizing muscle relaxants
    a. Succinylcholine can produce an increase in ICP. However, its use is not contraindicated when there is a clinical need for rapid airway control. In addition, when carbon dioxide, hemodynamic responses, and depth of anesthesia are controlled, the ICP effect of succinylcholine is not clinically significant.

E. Dexmedetomidine. Though data regarding dexmedetomidine is more limited than for the other intravenous agents, it is clear that the drug reduces both $CMRO_2$ and CBF [48,49]. Despite initial concern over the direct vasoconstrictive effects of dexmedetomidine acting on α_2 receptors in cerebral vessels, it does not appear that the medication significantly disrupts flow-metabolism coupling. Specifically, cerebral oxygen extraction has not been found to increase during the administration of dexmedetomidine in healthy volunteers [50]. Autoregulation is impaired with dexmedetomidine, and CO_2 reactivity is reduced but not abolished [51].

III. Vasoactive medications. Though generally without effect on $CMRO_2$, vasoactive medications have the potential to significantly affect CBF through both direct effects on cerebral vasomotor tone and through their effects on CPP (Table 2.3). In addition, some medications may alter not only CBF but also cerebral blood *volume,* with significant implications for ICP, CPP, and feedback into cerebral hemodynamics.

A. Sodium nitroprusside. Sodium nitroprusside is a cerebral as well as systemic (primarily arterial) vasodilator, and CBF is often maintained despite a decrease in MAP during its administration [52,53]. Even with well-maintained global CBF, however, brain tissue oxygenation may suffer due to increased arteriovenous shunting at the expense of capillary perfusion [54].

The intracranial vasodilation from sodium nitroprusside is associated with increased intracranial blood volume, which can significantly increase ICP and so has the potential to *reduce* CBF when intracranial elastance is increased.

TABLE 2.3 Effects of vasoactive medications on systemic and cerebral hemodynamics

	Vasomotor tone	Cardiac output	Cerebral oxygen delivery
Sodium Nitroprusside	⇓⇓⇓	⇔ or ⇑	⇔ or ⇓
Nitroglycerine	⇓⇓⇓	⇔ or ⇑	⇔ or ⇓
Nicardipene	⇓⇓	⇔	⇔
Milrinone	⇓⇓	⇑⇑	⇑⇑
Dobutamine	⇓	⇑⇑	⇑⇑
Dopamine	⇑	⇑⇑⇑	⇑ or ⇓
Ephedrine	⇑	⇑	⇑
Epinephrine	⇑⇑⇑⇑	⇑⇑⇑	⇑⇑⇑
Norepinephrine	⇑⇑⇑⇑	⇑	⇑⇑
Phenylephrine	⇑⇑⇑	⇔ or ⇓	⇑ or ⇓
Vasopressin	⇑⇑⇑⇑	⇔ or ⇓	⇑ or ⇔
Esmolol	⇔	⇓⇓	⇔ or ⇓
Labetalol	⇓	⇓⇓	⇔ or ⇓

B. **Nitroglycerine.** Like nitroprusside, nitroglycerine administration produces both cerebral and systemic vasodilation, though its effect is primarily on the venous side of the circulation. In healthy subjects, nitroglycerine administration induces an increase in cerebral oxygenation as measured by near-infrared spectroscopy (NIRS) [55], though this result cannot speak to blood flow *distribution*. Of some concern, nitroglycerine causes similar increases in ICP, but greater decreases in cardiac index, than nitroprusside does during induced hypotension [53].

CLINICAL PEARL *Where* a vasoactive agent acts may be as important as *how* it acts.

C. **Nicardipine.** Nicardipine is a calcium channel antagonist which causes reductions in MAP with minimal effect on cardiac output [56]. When administered for controlled hypotension, it does not reduce cerebral oxygen saturation as measured by NIRS in otherwise healthy patients [55]. Nicardipine attenuates cerebral autoregulation to a greater degree than nitroglycerin [57], and also reduces CO_2 reactivity [58].

D. **Milrinone.** Intra-arterially, milrinone is used for relief of cerebral vasospasm by inducing local arterial vasodilatation and increasing regional blood flow [59]. Administered systemically, milrinone causes systemic arterial dilation and a reduction in MAP, with a concomitant increase in cardiac output. The specific effect of systemic milrinone on cerebral vasculature remains one of vasodilation and increased global CBF, as demonstrated by maintained or improved jugular venous saturation following milrinone infusion in patients undergoing cardiopulmonary bypass [60]. Cerebrovascular CO_2 reactivity is maintained as well.

E. **Dobutamine.** Systemic dobutamine administration causes significant increases in cardiac output along with small changes in systemic blood pressure, the direction and magnitude of which are largely dependent on the underlying vasomotor tone of the patient. The increased cardiac output seen with dobutamine administration augments global and regional CBF [61], while cerebrovascular autoregulation and CO_2 reactivity are maintained [62]. Effects on CPP are largely a result of the variable changes in MAP.

F. **Dopamine.** While dopamine administration is associated with increases in both cardiac output and MAP, it may also produce cerebral hyperemia [63,64]. Therefore, concomitant increases in ICP during its administration in patients with increased intracranial compliance may reduce or negate any potential benefits for cerebral perfusion.

G. **Ephedrine.** Ephedrine administration produces increases in MAP and cardiac output which are associated with improved cerebral perfusion [65], while cerebrovascular autoregulation and CO_2 reactivity are not affected [66]. Due to the indirect action of ephedrine, these effects may be diminished or absent in the catecholamine-depleted patient.

H. **Epinephrine.** Epinephrine produces significant increases in both cardiac output and MAP, with resultant increases in CPP and blood flow [63]. Cerebrovascular autoregulation remains intact [64].

I. **Norepinephrine.** Norepinephrine produces predominantly α-adrenergic effects in the form of systemic vasoconstriction, while cardiac output is preserved due to the drug's moderate β-adrenergic effects. This makes it an excellent choice for maintenance of hypertension during treatment for cerebral vasospasm. Norepinephrine administration generates increased CPP [63], while cerebral autoregulation remains intact [64].

CLINICAL PEARL   While CPP is classically considered to be the limiting factor with regard to CBF, adequacy of cardiac output is also significant.

J. **Phenylephrine.** Direct α-adrenergic vasoconstriction induced with phenylephrine produces an increase in MAP at the expense of decreased cardiac output. As a result, CBF and oxygenation may be impaired during phenylephrine administration despite the increase in CPP [67]. This observation implies that not only is systemic vascular resistance increased during phenylephrine administration, but that cerebrovascular resistance may also be increased due to α-adrenergic receptors in the cerebral vasculature.

K. **Vasopressin.** Vasopressin acts on V_1 receptors in vascular smooth muscle to produce peripheral vasoconstriction and augmentation of MAP, resulting in increased CPP [68]. In one study, vasopressin was found to be superior to phenylephrine for maintenance of cerebral tissue oxygenation and was associated with lower ICP [69], though concerns for increased cerebral edema due to V_1-mediated activation of cerebral ionic cotransporters remain.

L. **Esmolol.** Esmolol is an ultrashort-acting agent that selectively blocks β1-receptors but has little or no effect on β2-receptor types. While esmolol also does not affect CBF in healthy volunteers, esmolol (bolus or infusion) can blunt the postoperative increase in CBF in neurosurgical patients during emergence and extubation.

M. **Labetalol.** Labetalol is a competitive and selective α1-blocker and a nonselective β-blocker that has predominantly β effects at low doses. The onset of action is 5 minutes, and the half-life is 5.5 hours. Labetalol produces a steady, consistent drop in blood pressure without compromising CBF.

IV. **Conclusion.** The neuroanesthesiologist is routinely tasked with maintenance of adequate cerebral perfusion in the face of both cerebrovascular disease and surgical manipulation. Adequacy in this setting is defined not solely as a provision of some minimum rate of flow, but rather as a balancing of flow rate and metabolic need. The adept pharmacologic manipulation of both elements in this interaction is necessary to ensure the patient's safety and optimize his probability of achieving an excellent neurologic outcome.

REFERENCES

1. Rozet I, Vavilala MS, Lindley AM, et al. Cerebral autoregulation and CO_2 reactivity in anterior and posterior cerebral circulation during sevoflurane anesthesia. *Anesth Analg.* 2006;102(2):560–564.
2. Matta BF, Heath KJ, Tipping K, et al. Direct cerebral vasodilatory effects of sevoflurane and isoflurane. *Anesthesiology.* 1999;91(3):677–680.
3. Kuroda Y, Murakami M, Tsuruta J, et al. Preservation of the ration of CBF/metabolic rate for oxygen during prolonged anesthesia with isoflurane, sevoflurane, and halothane in humans. *Anesthesiology.* 1996;84(3):555–561.
4. Cho S, Fujigaki T, Uchiyama Y, et al. Effects of sevoflurane with and without nitrous oxide on human cerebral circulation. Transcranial Doppler study. *Anesthesiology.* 1996;85(4):755–760.
5. Constant I, Seeman R, Murat I. Sevoflurane and epileptiform EEG changes. *Paediatr Anaesth.* 2005;15(4):266–274.
6. Artru AA, Momota T. Rate of CSF formation and resistance to reabsorption of CSF during sevoflurane or remifentanil in rabbits. *J Neurosurg Anesthesiol.* 2000;12(1):37–43.
7. Holmström A, Akeson J. Desflurane increases intracranial pressure more and sevoflurane less than isoflurane in pigs subjected to intracranial hypertension. *J Neurosurg Anesthesiol.* 2004;16(2):136–143.

8. McCulloch TJ, Boesel TW, Lam AM. The effect of hypocapnia on the autoregulation of CBF during administration of isoflurane. *Anesth Analg.* 2005;100(5):1463–1467.
9. Artru AA. Concentration-related changes in the rate of CSF formation and resistance to reabsorption of CSF during enflurane and isoflurane anesthesia in dogs. *J Neurosurg Anesthesiol.* 1989;1(2):140–141.
10. Mielck F, Stephan H, Buhre W, et al. Effects of 1 MAC desflurane on cerebral metabolism, blood flow and carbon dioxide reactivity in humans. *Br J Anaesth.* 1998;81(2):155–160.
11. Holmström A, Rosén I, Akeson J. Desflurane results in higher cerebral blood flow than sevoflurane or isoflurane at hypocapnia in pigs. *Acta Anaesthesiol Scand.* 2004;48(4):400–404.
12. Luginbuehl IA, Karsli C, Bissonnette B. Cerebrovascular reactivity to carbon dioxide is preserved during hypocapnia in children anesthetized with 1.0 MAC, but not with 1.5 MAC desflurane. *Can J Anaesth.* 2003;50(2):166–171.
13. Artru AA. Rate of cerebrospinal fluid formation, resistance to reabsorption of cerebrospinal fluid, brain tissue water content, and electroencephalogram during desflurane anesthesia in dogs. *J Neurosurg Anesthesiol.* 1993;5(3):178–186.
14. Kaisti KK, Långsjö JW, Aalto S, et al. Effects of sevoflurane, propofol, and adjunct nitrous oxide on regional cerebral blood flow, oxygen consumption, and blood volume in humans. *Anesthesiology.* 2003;99(3):603–613.
15. Matta BF, Lam AM. Nitrous oxide increases cerebral blood flow velocity during pharmacologically induced EEG silence in humans. *J Neurosurg Anesthesiol.* 1995;7(2):89–93.
16. Aono M, Sato J, Nishino T. Nitrous oxide increases normocapnic CBF velocity but does not affect the dynamic cerebrovascular response to step changes in end-tidal P(CO$_2$) in humans. *Anesth Analg.* 1999;89(3):684–689.
17. Schmidt M, Marx T, Papp-Jambor C, et al. Effect of xenon on cerebral autoregulation in pigs. *Anaesthesia.* 2002;57(10):960–966.
18. Laitio RM, Kaisti KK, Låangsjö JW, et al. Effects of xenon anesthesia on CBF in humans: a positron emission tomography study. *Anesthesiology.* 2007;106(6):1128–1133.
19. Rex S, Meyer PT, Baumert JH, et al. Positron emission tomography study of regional CBF and flow-metabolism coupling during general anaesthesia with xenon in humans. *Br J Anaesth.* 2008;100(5):667–675.
20. Laitio RM, Långsjö JW, Aalto S, et al. The effects of xenon anesthesia on the relationship between cerebral glucose metabolism and blood flow in healthy subjects: a positron emission tomography study. *Anesth Analg.* 2009;108(2):593–600.
21. Prough DS, Rogers AT, Stump DA, et al. Hypercarbia depresses cerebral oxygen consumption during cardiopulmonary bypass. *Stroke.* 1990;21(8):1162–1166.
22. Xu F, Uh J, Brier MR, et al. The influence of carbon dioxide on brain activity and metabolism in conscious humans. *J Cereb Blood Flow Metab.* 2011;31(1):58–67.
23. Oshima T, Karasawa F, Satoh T. Effects of propofol on CBF and the metabolic rate of oxygen in humans. *Acta Anaesthesiol Scand.* 2002;46(7).831–835.
24. Artru AA. Propofol combined with halothane or with fentanyl/halothane does not alter the rate of CSF formation or resistance to reabsorption of CSF in rabbits. *J Neurosurg Anesthesiol.* 1993;5(4):250–257.
25. Young WL, Prohovnik I, Correll JW, et al. Thiopental effect on cerebral blood flow during carotid endarterectomy. *J Neurosurg Anesthesiol.* 1991;3(4):265–269.
26. Woodcock TE, Murkin JM, Farrar JK, et al. Pharmacologic EEG suppression during cardiopulmonary bypass: cerebral hemodynamic and metabolic effects of thiopental or isoflurane during hypothermia and normothermia. *Anesthesiology.* 1987;67(2):218–224.
27. Nordström CH, Messeter K, Sundbärg G, et al. Cerebral blood flow, vasoreactivity, and oxygen consumption during barbiturate therapy in severe traumatic brain lesions. *J Neurosurg.* 1988;68(3):424–431.
28. Gumpert J, Paul R. Activation of the electroencephalogram with intravenous Brietal (methohexitone): the findings in 100 cases. *J Neurol Neurosurg Psychiatry.* 1971;34(5):646–648.
29. Kirchberger K, Schmitt H, Hummel C, et al. Clonidine and methohexital-induced epileptic magnetoencephalographic discharges in patients with focal epilepsies. *Epilepsia.* 1998;39(8):841–849.
30. Cold GE, Eskesen V, Eriksen H, et al. Changes in CMRO2, EEG and concentration of etomidate in serum and brain tissue during craniotomy with continuous etomidate supplemented with N2O and fentanyl. *Acta Anaesthesiol Scand.* 1986;30(2):159–163.
31. Renou AM, Vernhiet J, Macrez P, et al. Cerebral blood flow and metabolism during etomidate anaesthesia in man. *Br J Anaesth.* 1978;50(10):1047–1051.
32. Edelman GJ, Hoffman WE, Charbel FT. Cerebral hypoxia after etomidate administration and temporary cerebral artery occlusion. *Anesth Analg.* 1997;85(4):821–825.
33. Hoffman WE, Charbel FT, Edelman G, et al. Comparison of the effect of etomidate and desflurane on brain tissue gases and pH during prolonged middle cerebral artery occlusion. *Anesthesiology.* 1998;88(5):1188–1194.
34. Ghaly RF, Lee JJ, Ham JH, et al. Etomidate dose-response on somatosensory and transcranial magnetic induced spinal motor evoked potentials in primates. *Neurol Res.* 1999;21(8):714–720.
35. Ubags LH, Kalkman CJ, Been HD, et al. The use of ketamine or etomidate to supplement sufentanil/N2O anesthesia does not disrupt monitoring of myogenic transcranial motor evoked responses. *J Neurosurg Anesthesiol.* 1997;9(3):228–233.
36. Artru AA. Dose-related changes in the rate of cerebrospinal fluid formation and resistance to reabsorption of cerebrospinal fluid following administration of thiopental, midazolam, and etomidate in dogs. *Anesthesiology.* 1988;69(4):541–546.
37. Långsjö JW, Maksimow A, Salmi E, et al. S-ketamine anesthesia increases cerebral blood flow in excess of the metabolic needs in humans. *Anesthesiology.* 2005;103(2):258–268.
38. Bar-Joseph G, Guilburd Y, Tamir A, et al. Effectiveness of ketamine in decreasing intracranial pressure in children with intracranial hypertension. *J Neurosurg Pediatr.* 2009;4(1):40–46.
39. Himmelseher S, Durieux ME. Revising a dogma: ketamine for patients with neurological injury? *Anesth Analg.* 2005;101(2):524–534.

40. Mayberg TS, Lam AM, Matta BF, et al. Ketamine does not increase cerebral blood flow velocity or intracranial pressure during isoflurane/nitrous oxide anesthesia in patients undergoing craniotomy. *Anesth Analg.* 1995;81(1):84–89.
41. Schubert A, Licina MG, Lineberry PJ. The effect of ketamine on human somatosensory evoked potentials and its modification by nitrous oxide. *Anesthesiology.* 1990;72(1):33–39.
42. Ghaly RF, Ham JH, Lee JJ. High-dose ketamine hydrochloride maintains somatosensory and magnetic motor evoked potentials in primates. *Neurol Res.* 2001;23(8):881–886.
43. Artru AA, Katz RA. Cerebral blood volume and CSF pressure following administration of ketamine in dogs; modification by pre- or posttreatment with hypocapnia or diazepam. *J Neurosurg Anesthesiol.* 1989;1(1):8–15.
44. Hoffman WE, Miletich DJ, Albrecht RF. The effects of midazolam on CBF and oxygen consumption and its interaction with nitrous oxide. *Anesth Analg.* 1986;65(7):729–733.
45. Baughman VL, Hoffman WE, Miletich DJ, et al. Cerebral metabolic depression and brain protection produced by midazolam and etomidate in the rat. *J Neurosurg Anesthesiol.* 1989;1(1):22–28.
46. Forster A, Juge O, Morel D. Effects of midazolam on cerebral hemodynamics and cerebral vasomotor responsiveness to carbon dioxide. *J Cereb Blood Flow Metab.* 1983;3(2):246–249.
47. Fodale V, Schifilliti D, Praticò C, et al. Remifentanil and the brain. *Acta Anaesthesiol Scand.* 2008;52(3):319–326.
48. Drummond JC, Dao AV, Roth DM, et al. Effect of dexmedetomidine on cerebral blood flow velocity, cerebral metabolic rate, and carbon dioxide response in normal humans. *Anesthesiology.* 2008;108(2):225–232.
49. Prielipp RC, Wall MH, Tobin JR, et al. Dexmedetomidine-induced sedation in volunteers decreases regional and global cerebral blood flow. *Anesth Analg.* 2002;95(4):1052–1059.
50. Drummond JC, Sturaitis MK. Brain tissue oxygenation during dexmedetomidine administration in surgical patients with neurovascular injuries. *J Neurosurg Anesthesiol.* 2010;22(4):336–341.
51. Ogawa Y, Iwasaki K, Aoki K, et al. Dexmedetomidine weakens dynamic cerebral autoregulation as assessed by transfer function analysis and the thigh cuff method. *Anesthesiology.* 2008;109(4):642–650.
52. Immink RV, van den Born BJ, van Montfrans GA, et al. Cerebral hemodynamics during treatment with sodium nitroprusside versus labetalol in malignant hypertension. *Hypertension.* 2008;52(2):236–240.
53. Maktabi M, Warner D, Sokoll M, et al. Comparison of nitroprusside, nitroglycerin, and deep isoflurane anesthesia for induced hypotension. *Neurosurgery.* 1986;19(3):350–355.
54. Hoffman WE, Edelman G, Ripper R, et al. Sodium nitroprusside compared with isoflurane-induced hypotension: the effects on brain oxygenation and arteriovenous shunting. *Anesth Analg.* 2001;93(1):166–170.
55. Choi SH, Lee SJ, Jung YS, et al. Nitroglycerin- and nicardipine-induced hypotension does not affect cerebral oxygen saturation and postoperative cognitive function in patients undergoing orthognathic surgery. *J Oral Maxillofac Surg.* 2008;66(10): 2104–2109.
56. Cheung AT, Guvakov DV, Weiss SJ, et al. Nicardipine intravenous bolus dosing for acutely decreasing arterial blood pressure during general anesthesia for cardiac operations: pharmacokinetics, pharmacodynamics, and associated effects on left ventricular function. *Anesth Analg.* 1999;89(5):1116–1123.
57. Endoh H, Honda T, Ohashi S, et al. The influence of nicardipine-, nitroglycerin-, and prostaglandin E(1)-induced hypotension on cerebral pressure autoregulation in adult patients during propofol-fentanyl anesthesia. *Anesth Analg.* 2002;94(1): 169–173.
58. Kadoi Y, Goto F. Effects of nicardipine-induced hypotension on cerebrovascular carbon dioxide reactivity in patients with diabetes mellitus under sevoflurane anesthesia. *J Anesth.* 2007;21(2):125–130.
59. Arakawa Y, Kikuta K, Hojo M, et al. Milrinone for the treatment of cerebral vasospasm after subarachnoid hemorrhage: report of seven cases. *Neurosurgery.* 2001;48(4):723–728.
60. Oh YJ, Kim SH, Shinn HK, et al. Effects of milrinone on jugular bulb oxygen saturation and cerebrovascular carbon dioxide reactivity in patients undergoing coronary artery bypass graft surgery. *Br J Anaesth.* 2004;93(5):634–638.
61. Berré J, De Backer D, Moraine JJ, et al. Dobutamine increases cerebral blood flow velocity and jugular bulb hemoglobin saturation in septic patients. *Crit Care Med.* 1997;25(3):392–398.
62. Haenggi M, Andermatt A, Anthamatten C, et al. CO(2)-dependent vasomotor reactivity of cerebral arteries in patients with severe traumatic brain injury: time course and effect of augmentation of cardiac output with dobutamine. *J Neurotrauma.* 2012;29(9):1779–1784.
63. Myburgh JA, Upton RN, Grant C, et al. The cerebrovascular effects of adrenaline, noradrenaline and dopamine infusions under propofol and isoflurane anaesthesia in sheep. *Anaesth Intensive Care.* 2002;30(6):725–733.
64. Myburgh JA, Upton RN, Grant C, et al. The effect of infusions of adrenaline, noradrenaline and dopamine on cerebral autoregulation under propofol anaesthesia in an ovine model. *Intensive Care Med.* 2003;29(5):817–824.
65. Meng L, Cannesson M, Alexander BS, et al. Effect of phenylephrine and ephedrine bolus treatment on cerebral oxygenation in anaesthetized patients. *Br J Anaesth.* 2011;107(2):209–217.
66. Moppett IK, Wild MJ, Sherman RW, et al. Effects of ephedrine, dobutamine and dopexamine on cerebral haemodynamics: transcranial Doppler studies in healthy volunteers. *Br J Anaesth.* 2004;92(1):39–44.
67. Ogoh S, Sato K, Fisher JP, et al. The effect of phenylephrine on arterial and venous CBF in healthy subjects. *Clin Physiol Funct Imaging.* 2011;31(6):445–451.
68. Muehlschlegel S, Dunser MW, Gabrielli A, et al. Arginine vasopressin as a supplementary vasopressor in refractory hypertensive, hypervolemic, hemodilutional therapy in subarachnoid hemorrhage. *Neurocrit Care.* 2007;6(1):3–10.
69. Dudkiewicz M, Proctor KG. Tissue oxygenation during management of cerebral perfusion pressure with phenylephrine or vasopressin. *Crit Care Med.* 2008;36(9):2641–2650.

3 Fluid Management During Neurosurgical Procedures

Concezione Tommasino and Valentina Picozzi

KEY POINTS

1. *Movement of water* between the normal brain and the intravascular space depends on osmotic gradients, particularly serum sodium concentration.
2. In the setting of *fluid therapy,* reducing serum osmolality induces brain edema and increases ICP. Therefore, the goal of fluid management in neurosurgery is to avoid the reduction of serum osmolality. Reduction of COP, with careful maintenance of osmolality, does not increase edema in the injured brain.
3. *Hypertonic solutions,* mannitol and hypertonic saline, decrease brain water content in the normal brain and are commonly used to reduce ICP.
4. *Glucose-containing solutions* should not be used in patients who have brain pathology, and should be avoided in patients at risk for cerebral ischemia.
5. *Fluid restriction* minimally affects cerebral edema and can lead to hemodynamic instability.

THE GOAL OF FLUID ADMINISTRATION IN NEUROANESTHESIA AND NEUROCRITICAL CARE is to avoid dehydration, to maintain an effective circulating volume, and to prevent inadequate tissue perfusion. Management of the neurosurgical patient requires careful attention to fluid and electrolyte balance over all the perioperative periods [1]. These patients can receive diuretics (e.g., mannitol, furosemide) to treat cerebral edema and to reduce intracranial pressure (ICP); at the same time, they may require large volumes of either fluid or blood as part of an initial resuscitation, treatment of cerebral vasospasm, correction of preoperative dehydration, or maintenance of hemodynamic stability.

Historical bias has favored fluid restriction in patients with brain pathology, assuming that administration of fluid might exacerbate brain edema. Brain edema, leading to an expansion of brain volume, has a crucial impact on morbidity and mortality as it increases ICP, impairs cerebral perfusion and oxygenation, and contributes to ischemic injuries (see Chapter 27). Several caveats to perioperative fluid restriction should be noted: The efficacy of fluid restriction on brain edema remains unproven, and the consequences of fluid restriction, if pursued to the point of hypovolemia, can be devastating. A negative fluid balance ($\cong$600 mL) in head trauma patients was associated with an adverse effect on outcome, independent of its relationship to ICP, mean arterial pressure, or cerebral perfusion pressure (CPP) [2].

Perioperative fluid management has undergone significant advances over the past few decades. Despite promising studies, fluid management in the neurosurgical patient remains a field where evidence-based medicine is still lacking. As long as evidence is not available, medical practice should be guided by physiologic principles.

I. Physiologic principles

A. Osmotic pressure. This is the hydrostatic force acting to equalize the concentration of water on both sides of a membrane that is impermeable to substances dissolved in that water. Water moves along its concentration gradient. This means that if a saline solution containing 10 mOsm of sodium (Na$^+$) and 10 mOsm of chloride (Cl$^-$) is placed on one side of a semipermeable membrane with water on the other, water will move "toward" the saline (NaCl) solution. The saline solution has a concentration of 20 mOsm/L, and the force driving water will be approximately 19.3 mm Hg/mOsm. Note that the driving force is proportional to the *gradient* across the membrane; if two solutions of equal concentration are placed across a membrane, there is no driving force. Similarly, if the membrane is permeable to the solutes (e.g., Na$^+$ and Cl$^-$), this reduces the gradient and hence the osmotic forces.

B. Osmolarity and osmolality. *Osmolarity* describes the molar number of osmotically active particles *per liter of solution*. In practice, this value is typically calculated by adding up the milliequivalent (mEq) concentrations of the various ions in the solution. *Osmolality* describes the molar number of osmotically active particles *per kilogram of solvent*. This value is directly measured by determining either the freezing point or the vapor pressure of the solution (each of which is reduced by a dissolved solute). Note that osmotic activity of a solution demands that particles be "independent." As NaCl dissociates into Na$^+$ and Cl$^-$, it creates two osmotically active particles. If electrostatic forces act to prevent dissociation of the two charged particles, osmolality is reduced. For most dilute salt solutions, osmolality is equal to or slightly less than osmolarity. For example, commercial lactated Ringer's solution has a calculated osmolarity of approximately 275 mOsm/L but a measured osmolality of approximately 254 mOsm/kg, indicating incomplete dissociation [1,3].

Plasma osmolality varies between 280 and 290 mOsm/L. Calculated versus measured osmolality is relevant in the clinical setting. If the technology to directly measure osmolality is not available, or it is not possible to obtain an emergency measurement 24 hours a day, osmolarity can be calculated from the osmoles that are routinely measured, such as serum sodium, blood urea nitrogen (BUN), and glucose.

Calculated plasma osmolarity:

$$2 \times [\text{Na}^+] + (\text{BUN mg/dL} \div 2.8) + (\text{glucose mg/dL} \div 18).$$

The [Na$^+$] is multiplied by 2 to account for the accompanying anions (mostly chloride and bicarbonate) that provide electroneutrality. The corrections in the glucose concentration and BUN are to convert mg/dL into mmol/L.

The plasma osmolality is primarily determined by the concentration of sodium salts with minor contributions from glucose and BUN. As BUN is lipid soluble and equilibrates across the cell membranes, it is an ineffective osmole and does not contribute to fluid distribution, and therefore it is omitted from calculation from effective plasma osmolality as follows:

Effective serum osmolality:

$$2 \times [\text{Na}^+] + (\text{glucose mg/dL} \div 18).$$

Be advised, however, that the calculation introduces a bias, overestimating osmolality in the lower ranges and underestimating it in the higher ranges [4]. Hence, the single most important factor is the serum sodium concentration.

> **CLINICAL PEARL**   Administration of large volumes of isosmolar crystalloids will dilute plasma protein concentration and result in peripheral edema, but will not generally increase brain water content (i.e., cerebral edema) or ICP.

C. **Colloid oncotic pressure (COP).** Osmolarity and osmolality are determined by the total number of dissolved "particles" in a solution, regardless of their size. COP is the osmotic pressure produced by large molecules (e.g., albumin, hetastarch, dextran). This factor becomes particularly important in biologic systems in which vascular membranes are often permeable to small ions but not to large molecules (typically plasma proteins). In such situations, proteins might be the only osmotically active particles. Normal COP is $\cong 20$ mm Hg (or equal to $\cong 1$ mOsm/kg).

D. **Starling's hypothesis.** In 1898, Starling published his equations describing the forces driving water across capillary endothelium. The major factors that control the movement of fluids between the intravascular and extravascular spaces are the transcapillary hydrostatic gradient, the osmotic and oncotic gradients, and the relative permeability of the capillary membranes that separate these spaces. The Starling equation is as follows:

$$\mathbf{FM} = k(Pc + \pi i - Pi\text{-}\pi c)$$

where FM is fluid movement, k is the filtration coefficient of the capillary wall (i.e., how leaky it is), Pc is the hydrostatic pressure in the capillaries, Pi is the hydrostatic pressure (usually negative) in the interstitial (extravascular) space, and πi and πc are interstitial and capillary osmotic pressures, respectively.

Fluid movement is, therefore, proportional to the hydrostatic pressure gradient minus the osmotic pressure gradient across a capillary wall. The magnitude of the osmotic gradient depends on the relative permeability of the vessels to solute. In the majority of the capillary beds in the human body (the periphery), the configuration of the desmosomes that connect endothelial cells creates an effective intercellular pore size of 65 Å. Small electrolyte molecules (Na^+, Cl^-) pass freely, while large molecules such as proteins (Fig. 3.1) cannot cross the membrane. As a result, π is defined only by colloids, and the Starling equation can be simplified by saying that fluid moves into a tissue whenever either the hydrostatic gradient increases (either intravascular pressure rises or interstitial pressure falls) or the osmotic gradient decreases.

In normal situations, the intravascular protein concentration is higher than the interstitial concentration, acting to draw water back into the vascular space. If COP is reduced (e.g., by dilution with large amounts of isotonic crystalloid), fluid begins to accumulate in the interstitium,

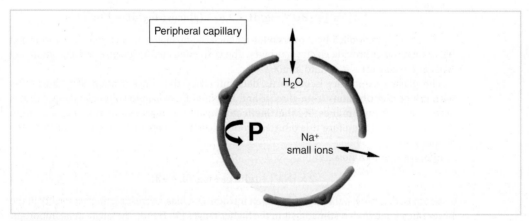

FIGURE 3.1 Schematic diagram of a peripheral capillary. The vessel wall is permeable to both water (H_2O) and small ions, but not to proteins (P).

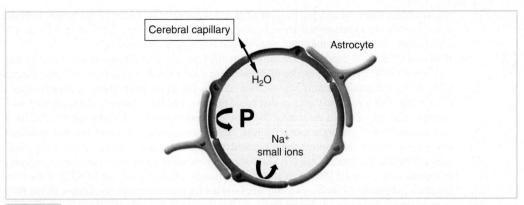

FIGURE 3.2 Schematic diagram of a cerebral capillary. The blood-brain barrier (BBB) is impermeable to small ions and proteins (P), but not to water (H_2O).

producing edema (e.g., marked peripheral edema in patients given many liters of crystalloid during surgery or resuscitation). By contrast, the blood–brain barrier (BBB) is impermeable to both ions and proteins so that osmotic pressure is determined by the total osmotic gradient, of which COP contributes only a tiny fraction ($\cong 1$ mOsm/kg) (Fig. 3.2).

E. **Interstitial clearance.** Peripheral tissues have a net outward movement of fluid (i.e., the value of FM is positive). Edema is not normally present, however, because this extravasated fluid is cleared by the lymphatics. While many researchers agree that there is some lymphatic drainage of the brain, most interstitial fluid in the brain is cleared either by bulk fluid flow into the cerebrospinal fluid (CSF) spaces or via pinocytosis back into the intravascular compartment. This is a slow process and probably does not counteract rapid fluid movement into the interstitial space.

F. **Hydrostatic forces and interstitial compliance.** In the tissues, the net hydrostatic gradient is determined by (a) intravascular pressure and (b) interstitial tissue compliance. Normally, the direction is outward (capillary to interstitium). There is no question that in the brain (or in any organ), elevated intravascular pressure, such as that produced by either high jugular venous pressure or a head-down posture, can increase edema formation. However, an often overlooked factor that influences the pressure gradient is the interstitial compliance (i.e., the tendency of tissue to resist fluid influx). The loose interstitial space in most peripheral tissues does little to impede the influx of fluid. This explains the ease with which edema develops around, for example, the face and the eyes, even with minor hydrostatic stresses (e.g., a face-down posture). By contrast, the interstitial space of the brain is extremely noncompliant, resisting fluid movement. As a result, minor changes in driving forces (either hydrostatic or osmotic/oncotic) do not produce measurable edema. However, a vicious cycle can develop so that, as edema forms in the brain, the interstitial matrix is disrupted, the compliance increases, and additional edema forms more easily. In contrast, the closed cranium and ICP can act to retard fluid influx. This may partially explain the exacerbation of edema formation that can occur after rapid decompression of the intracranial space.

1 2 G. **BBB and serum osmolality.** The endothelial cells of the cerebral microvasculature differ from other endothelial phenotypes by the absence of fenestrations and sparse pinocytic vesicular transport. They are held together by continuous tight junctions, form the BBB, and exhibit specific protective properties. The effective pore size of the BBB is only 5 to 7 Å, making this unique structure normally impermeable to all large hydrophilic molecules (e.g., plasma proteins and synthetic colloids, such as hetastarch and dextrans) and relatively impermeable to many small polar solutes (Na^+, K^+, Cl^-). The BBB functions as a semipermeable membrane that allows only water to move freely between the interstitial space and the vasculature (Fig. 3.2), according to osmotic gradients.

The reduction of serum osmolality (e.g., by infusing water or large volumes of nonisotonic crystalloid solution) increases brain water content [5]; conversely, the increase of osmolality reduces brain water content [6]. Even small changes can produce measurable changes in brain water content: In experimental animals, a reduction in plasma osmolality of as little as 5%, under otherwise normal conditions, causes brain edema and increases ICP [5].

H. BBB and COP. COP contributes to only a tiny fraction of the total osmolality (≅1 mOsm/kg) and, when the BBB is intact, can be responsible for only a small driving force. Normal plasma COP is approximately 20 mm Hg, whereas that in the brain interstitium is approximately 0.6 mm Hg. This is equal to the force that could be generated by a change in the capillary/tissue osmotic gradient of only 1 mOsm/kg. We would therefore predict that changes in COP have only minimal effect on brain water content. Several animal experiments have demonstrated that normal brain water content can be altered by small changes in osmolality but not by clinically achievable changes in COP [7]. There was no increase in brain water content (i.e., edema) in regions with an intact BBB, even after a reduction of approximately 50% in COP. If the BBB becomes permeable to both small and large molecules (i.e., complete breakdown of the BBB as is common with several clinical injuries), it is almost impossible to maintain any form of osmotic or oncotic gradient between the intravascular compartment and the brain interstitium. As a result, no changes in brain water content would be expected with a change in either gradient. Indeed, in several animal models resembling human brain injuries (e.g., implanted glioma and freezing lesion, experimental model of brain tumor and trauma, respectively), edema induced by a reduction in total serum osmolality occurred only in normal regions of the brain relatively distant from the focus of injury. In keeping with this, several studies have shown that acute hyperosmolality (as with mannitol, urea, glycerol, hypertonic saline [HS]) reduces water content only in normal brain tissue where the BBB is intact. Conversely, when the BBB is severely damaged, investigations have failed to demonstrate that reducing the COP affects brain edema [8]. In the presence of mild injury to the BBB in experimental animals, a reduction in COP may potentially aggravate brain edema. Therefore, it is possible that, with a less severe injury, the BBB *may* function similarly to the peripheral tissue [7]. In summary, injury to the brain interferes with the integrity of the BBB to varying degrees, depending on the severity of the damage. Regions where there is a complete breakdown of the BBB, there will be no osmotic/oncotic gradient. Water accumulation (i.e., brain edema) occurs because of the pathologic process itself and cannot be directly influenced by the osmotic/oncotic gradient. In other regions where there is moderate injury to the BBB (i.e., a mild opening rendering pore size similar to the periphery), it is possible that the colloid oncotic gradient is effective as in the peripheral tissue. Finally, the BBB is normal in a significant portion of the brain. The presence of a functionally intact BBB is essential if osmotherapy is to be effective.

II. Fluids for intravenous administration. The physicians can choose from among a variety of solutions suitable for intravenous use, categorized mostly on the basis of osmolality, oncotic pressure, and dextrose content (Tables 3.1 and 3.2).

A. Crystalloids are solutions of inorganic ions and small organic molecules dissolved in water, do not contain high–molecular-weight compounds and have an oncotic pressure of zero (Table 3.1). Crystalloids are inexpensive, require no special compatibility testing, and have a very low incidence of adverse reactions and no religious objections to their use. Crystalloids can be hypo-osmolar, isosmolar, or hyperosmolar with respect to plasma. Crystalloids with an ionic composition close to that of plasma may be referred to as "balanced" or "physiologic."

1. **Hypo-osmolar** crystalloids, especially in large amounts, reduce plasma osmolality, drive water across the BBB, cause brain edema even in entirely normal brain, and increase ICP. Whatever fluid regimen is chosen it should not have sufficient free water to cause reduction in osmolality. Five percent dextrose (D5W) is essentially water (as the sugar is metabolized very quickly), provides "free water" which disperses throughout the intracellular and extracellular compartments, and has little use as a resuscitative fluid. Hypo-osmolar crystalloids (0.45% NaCl or D5W) should be avoided in neurosurgical patients.

2. **Isosmolar** crystalloids such as normal saline (NS, 0.9% NaCl) and Plasmalyte have an osmolarity ≈300 mOsm/L, and do not change plasma osmolality. Potassium, calcium, and lactate may be added to more closely replicate the ionic makeup of the plasma (Table 3.1). Lactated Ringer's solution is slightly hypotonic (measured osmolarity ≈254 mOsmol/kg)

TABLE 3.1 Composition of commonly used intravenous fluids: crystalloids

Fluids	Osmolarity mOsm/L	Na$^+$ mEq/L	Cl$^+$	K$^+$	Ca^{2+}	Mg$^+$	Dextrose g/L	Lactate
5% Dextrose in H$_2$O (D5W)	278	—	—	—	—	—	50	—
5% Dextrose in 0.45% NaCl	405	77	77	—	—	—	50	—
5% Dextrose in 0.9 NaCl	561	154	154	—	—	—	50	—
5% Dextrose in Ringer's solution	525	130	109	4	3	—	50	—
Ringer's solution	309	147	156	4	4–4.5	—	—	—
Lactated Ringer's solution or Hartmann's solution	274	130	109	4	3	—	—	28
5% Dextrose in lactated Ringer's solution	525	130	109	4	3	—	50	28
Plasmalyte	298	140	98	5	—	3	—	—
0.45% NaCl	154	77	77	—	—	—	—	—
0.9% NaCl (normal saline, [NS])	308	154	154	—	—	—	—	—
3% NaCl	1,026	513	513	—	—	—	—	—
5% NaCl	1,710	855	855	—	—	—	—	—
7.5% NaCl	2,566	1,283	1,283	—	—	—	—	—
10% NaCl	3,434	1,712	1,712	—	—	—	—	—
23.4% NaCl	8,008	4,004	4,004	—	—	—	—	—
29.2% NaCl	10,000	5,000	5,000	—	—	—	—	—
20% Mannitol	1,098	—	—	—	—	—	—	—

Osmolarity = calculated value (osmol = mg ÷ molecular weight × 10 × valence).
Plasmalyte contains acetate 27 mEq/L and gluconate 23 mEq/L.
The composition of the solutions can vary slightly depending on the manufacturer.

in relation to the plasma [1,3], and can decrease serum osmolality and increase brain water content and ICP, mostly when large amounts are infused. Small volumes of lactated Ringer's (1 to 2 L) are unlikely to be detrimental and can be used safely, for example, to compensate for the changes in venous capacitance that typically accompany the induction of anesthesia. If large volumes are needed (either to replace blood loss or to compensate for some other source of volume loss), a change to a more isotonic fluid such as normal saline is probably advisable. It is also important to remember that rapid infusion of large volumes of isotonic saline can induce a dose-dependent dilutional–hyperchloremic acidosis. There is debate about the morbidity associated with this condition, and it is suggested that dilutional–hyperchloremic acidosis is a benign phenomenon, which

TABLE 3.2 Composition of commonly used intravenous fluids: colloids

	Na$^+$ mEq/L	Cl$^+$	K$^+$	Ca^{2+}	Osmolarity mOsm/L	Oncotic pressure mm Hg
Fresh frozen plasma	168	76	3.2	8.2	≈295	21
Albumin (5%)	145	130	≤2	—	≈290	20–29
Hetastarch 6% in NS	154	154	—	—	≈310	35–30
Dextran 40 (10%) in NS	145	145	—	—	≈300	168–191
Dextran 70 (6%) in NS	145	145	—	—	≈300	56–68

Osmolarity = calculated value (osmol = mg ÷ molecular weight × 10 × valence).
NS, normal saline.

usually requires no treatment, but must be differentiated from other causes of metabolic acidosis [9].

Lactated Ringer's solution and Plasmalyte contain bicarbonate precursors. These anions (e.g., lactate) are the conjugate base to the corresponding acid (e.g., lactic acid) and do not contribute to the development of acidosis, as they are administered with Na^+ rather than H^+ as the cation. The metabolism of lactate in the liver results in the production of an equivalent amount of bicarbonate.

3. **Hyperosmolar crystalloids.** Mannitol and HS. Solutions can be made hyperosmolar by the inclusion of electrolytes (e.g., Na^+ and Cl^-, as in HS) and low–molecular-weight solutes such as in mannitol (MW 182) (Table 3.1). Osmotic therapy is a cornerstone in management of ICP induced by cerebral edema. Its effectiveness depends on the integrity of the BBB, the reflection coefficient of the osmotic agent, and the osmotic gradient created.

   a. **Mannitol.** Mannitol is the primary osmotic drug for the control of increased ICP [10], and is recommended as drug of choice by both the Brain Trauma Foundation and the European Brain Injury Consortium. The recommended dose of mannitol is 0.25 to 1 g/kg, and the smallest possible dose is selected and infused over 10 to 15 minutes. The mechanism through which mannitol acts is still unknown. Very recent human PET studies do not support the hypothesis of autoregulatory cerebral vasoconstriction induced by volume expansion or by changes in blood viscosity [11]. They suggest that the ability of mannitol to lower ICP and reduce mass effect may be better explained by a reduction in brain water content, since mannitol establishes an osmotic gradient between blood and brain in the presence of a relatively intact BBB. Mannitol has several limitations. It might increase circulatory blood volume from hyperosmolality, and although this phenomenon does not occur when mannitol is given at moderate doses, care should be taken when it is given to patients with congestive heart failure. Hyperosmolality is a common problem, and a serum osmolality >320 mOsm/L is associated with adverse renal and CNS effects. The osmotic diuresis may lead to hypotension, especially in hypovolemic patients, and, although controversial, the accumulation of mannitol in cerebral tissue can reverse the brain–blood gradient with exacerbation of the edema and increased ICP. Often furosemide is used in conjunction with mannitol. In animals furosemide enhances the effect of mannitol on plasma osmolality, resulting in a greater reduction of brain water content [12]. This effect, with the decreased CSF production induced by furosemide, can explain the synergistic effect of mannitol and furosemide on intracranial compliance. In the clinical practice, the benefit of osmotic treatment with furosemide is likely to be small, if it exists at all.

   b. **Hypertonic Saline.** In humans, acute resuscitation from hemorrhagic shock with sodium-based hypertonic solution (HS) is associated with improved outcome in patients with multiple trauma and head injuries [13]. Several randomized clinical trials have suggested that HS may be superior to mannitol in reducing ICP [14]. HS is potentially more effective because the permeability of the BBB to Na^+ is low, and the reflection coefficient (selectivity of the BBB to a particular substance) of NaCl is more than that of mannitol. Moreover, HS solutions result in significant volume expansion, improved cardiac output, improved regional blood flow, and beneficial immunomodulation. A recent clinical trial has been unable to demonstrate improvement in 6-month neurologic outcome or survival in head trauma patients without evidence of shock, suggesting that HS may be better in hypotensive, brain-injured patients [15]. There is no question that HS can quickly restore intravascular volume while reducing ICP through brain water reduction in uninjured brain [6]. In animal models of head trauma, HS improves systemic hemodynamics and cerebral blood flow (CBF) and may enhance cerebral microcirculation by reducing the adhesion of polymorphonuclear cells and stimulating local release of nitric oxide. In both pediatric and adult traumatic brain injury (TBI) patients, HS has been used effectively to reduce elevated ICP unresponsive to mannitol treatment [16].

   Adverse effects after HS administration include renal failure, coagulopathy, hyperkalemia, pulmonary edema, and central pontine myelinolysis. The evidence for renal

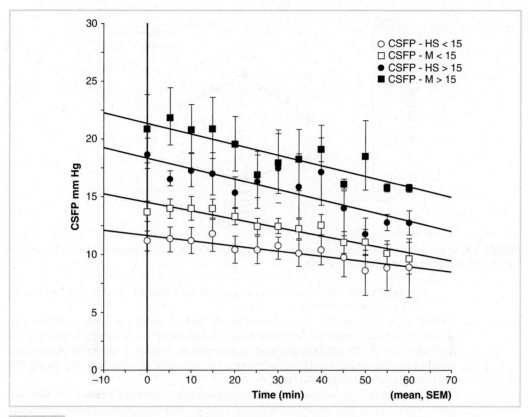

FIGURE 3.3 Cerebrospinal fluid pressure (CSFP) in patients treated with equal volume of 7.5% hypertonic saline (HS) and 20% mannitol (M), subdivided according to baseline CSFP (< or >15 mm Hg).

failure, coagulopathy, pulmonary edema, and hyperkalemia is tenuous, and it must be noted that central pontine myelinolysis has never been reported in human studies. Magnetic resonance imaging and postmortem studies failed to demonstrate central pontine myelinolysis despite maximum sodium levels of 182 mEq/L [16]. In neurosurgical patients undergoing elective supratentorial procedures, we have shown that equal volumes of 20% mannitol and 7.5% HS reduce brain bulk, as assessed by the neurosurgeon, and CSF pressure to the same extent (Fig. 3.3); serum sodium, however, increased during the HS administration and peaked at more than 150 mEq/L at the conclusion of the infusion (Fig. 3.4) [17]. The sodium load may be a concern in patients with neurologic injury and/or at risk for seizures.

c. **Glucose-containing solutions.** Salt-free solutions containing glucose (e.g., D5W) should be avoided in patients who have intracranial pathology. Free water reduces serum osmolality and increases brain water content. Furthermore, solid evidence in animals and humans indicates that excessive glucose exacerbates neurologic damage [18]. In the presence of ischemia or hypoxia, it is proposed that the impaired metabolism of excess glucose causes an accumulation of lactate, a decrease in intracellular pH, and subsequently severely compromised cellular function that may result in cell death. The reduction of adenosine levels from hyperglycemia inhibits the release of excitatory amino acids, which play a major role in ischemic cell damage. Although clinical investigations have indicated a negative relationship between patients' plasma glucose on admission and outcome after stroke, cardiac arrest, and head injury, this correlation is not necessarily one of cause and effect because the high glucose may be a concomitant of more severe CNS damage.

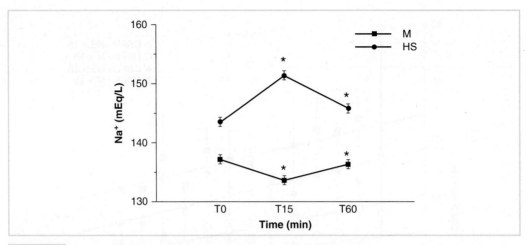

FIGURE 3.4 Serum sodium (Na^+) during administration of equal volume of 7.5% hypertonic saline (HS) and 20% mannitol (M) in patients undergoing brain surgery.

Hyperglycemia can also induce an osmotic diuresis that may lead to dehydration and electrolyte abnormalities.

B. Colloid is the term used to denote solutions that have an oncotic pressure similar to that of plasma (Tables 3.2 and 3.3). They can be divided into naturally occurring human plasma derivatives (5% or 25% albumin solutions, plasma protein fraction, fresh frozen plasma, and immunoglobulin solution) and the semisynthetic colloids (gelatins, dextrans [MW 40 and 70], and hydroxyethyl starches (HES) [19].

Safety of albumin in patients with brain pathology has been questioned. In 2004, the Saline versus Albumin Fluid Evaluation (SAFE) study concluded that critically ill patients with TBI had a higher mortality rate, if resuscitated acutely with albumin as opposed to saline [20].

HES products can induce adverse effects, such as interference with coagulation (through binding to the von Willebrand factor/factor VIII complex, causing a decreased platelet adhesion), encountered mostly with volumes exceeding 1.5 L; possible hyperoncotic renal failure (due to accumulation of large molecules in the plasma and renal tubules); and skin itching (related to accumulation of starch particles in the reticuloendothelial system) [21]. The newer colloid solutions, the tetrastarches, have a molar substitution of 0.4, compared with the older hetastarches that had a molar substitution of 0.7 (Table 3.3). This results in a lower in vivo molecular weight, leading to more rapid clearance of the starch particles, a reduced incidence of adverse effects, and a significantly improved safety profile, without any loss of volume effect compared to first- and second-generation HES preparations [22].

Third-generation HES preparation (HES 130/0.4) has been shown to reduce the inflammatory response in patients undergoing major surgery compared with a crystalloid-based volume therapy. This has been interpreted to be most likely due to an improved microcirculation with reduced endothelial activation and less endothelial damage.

Dextran (current formulations available are 10% dextran 40, and 6% dextran 70 MW) and hetastarch are dissolved in normal saline, so that the osmolality of the solution is approximately 290 to 310 mOsm/L with a sodium and chloride content of ≅154 mEq/L. Dextran 40 interferes with normal platelet function and is therefore not advisable for patients who have intracranial pathology other than to improve rheology, as in ischemic cerebrovascular diseases.

Small volumes of hypertonic/hyperoncotic solutions (typically hypertonic hetastarch or dextran solutions) can restore normovolemia rapidly, without increasing ICP. They have been successfully used to treat intracranial hypertension in TBI patients, in patients with subarachnoid hemorrhage (SAH), and in patients with stroke.

TABLE 3.3   Hydroxyethyl starch (HES) solutions

	HES 670/0.75	HES 450/0.7	HES 130/0.4
Trade name	Hextend	Hespan	Voluven
Availability	US	Europe/US	Europe/US
Concentration (%)	6	6	6
Volume effect plasma half-life (Hr)	5–6	5–6	2–3
Molecular weight (kD)	670	450	130
Molecular substitution (MS)	0.75	0.7	0.4
C2/C6 ratio	4:1	4:1	9:1
Na^+	143	140	154
Cl^-	124	118	154
Oncotic pressure (mm Hg)	25–30	25–30	36

The administration of colloids restores the intravascular volume with minimal risk of peripheral tissue edema in comparison with crystalloid solutions alone. The type of the colloid, volumes applied, aggressiveness of fluid resuscitation, and the volume status at the initial phase of administration determine their clinical responses [22].

III. **Clinical fluid management of neurosurgical patients**

A. **Fluid restriction.** Despite the lack of convincing experimental evidence that isosmolar crystalloids are detrimental, fluid restriction has been widely practiced in patients with mass lesions or cerebral edema or at risk for intracranial hypertension. Restriction has some logic, only when *hypotonic* fluids are used. The first human studies on fluid therapy in neurosurgical patients by Shenkin et al. [23] in 1976, who has generated the "restricted fluid intake" attitude in neurosurgery ("*Run them dry*"), has demonstrated that patients when given standard maintenance intravenous fluid (2 L/day of 0.45 NaCl in 5% dextrose) develop a progressive reduction in serum osmolality in the postoperative period ($\approx$275 mOsm/L). On the other hand, patients given half of this volume over about a week show a progressive increase in serum osmolality ($\approx$285 mOsm/L). While no CNS parameters were measured, the results suggest that hyposmotic solutions (0.45% NaCl) contain excess free water for the typical postoperative craniotomy patient. In this regard, fluid restriction can be viewed only as "preventing" hyposmotically driven edema. However, this does not imply that even greater degrees of fluid restriction are beneficial or that the administration of a fluid mixture that does not reduce osmolality is detrimental.

B. **Intraoperative volume replacement.** Considerable debate has occurred regarding the amount of deficit generated by the *nil per os* status (patients are presumed to develop preoperative fluid deficits secondary to continuing insensible losses and urine output) and the existence of "third space losses" (sequestration of fluid to a nonfunctional extracellular space that is beyond osmotic equilibrium with the vascular space). Strong evidence suggests that healthy adult patients will maintain normal intravascular volumes despite a prolonged fast, and that a classic "third space" does not exist [24,25]. Considering this new evidence, in the neurosurgical patient intraoperative fluids should be given at a rate sufficient to replace the urinary output and insensible losses (e.g., skin and lungs), and to maintain normovolemia. The available data indicate that intravascular volume replacement and expansion will have no effect on cerebral edema as long as normal serum osmolality is maintained and cerebral hydrostatic pressure is not markedly increased (e.g., owing to true volume overload and elevated right heart pressures). Whether this is achieved with crystalloids or colloids seems irrelevant, although the osmolality of the selected fluid is crucial. Fluid administration that results in a reduction in osmolality should be avoided. With respect to this issue, it should also be noted that lactated Ringer's solution is not strictly isosmotic (measured osmolality 252 to 255 mOsm/kg), particularly when administered to patients whose baseline osmolality has been increased by either fluid restriction or hyperosmolar fluids (mannitol, HS, etc.). Small volumes of lactated Ringer's (1 to 3 L) are unlikely to be detrimental and can be used safely, for example, to compensate

TABLE 3.4 Intravascular volume increase after fluid administration

Fluid infused	Intravascular volume increase
1 L isotonic crystalloid	~250 mL
1 L 5% albumin	~500 mL
1 L Hetastarch—Dextran	~750–800 mL

for the changes in venous capacitance that typically accompany the induction of anesthesia. If large volumes are needed (either to replace blood loss or to compensate for some other source of volume loss), a change to a more isotonic fluid such as normal saline is probably advisable, and combination of isotonic crystalloids and colloids may be the best choice.

To rationally prescribe fluid replacement, it is important to identify which compartment is depleted; specific losses should be replaced with the appropriate fluid. As a general role, isosmolar crystalloids should be administered to replace operative and ongoing fluid requirements, and colloids should be used to replace blood loss and maintain normovolemia. Table 3.4 illustrates the intravascular volume expansion obtained with different types of fluids. Volume replacement with crystalloid solutions, geared to maintain the hematocrit at approximately 33%, is calculated on a 3:1 ratio (crystalloid to intraoperative blood loss) because of the larger distribution space of the crystalloids. Transfusion may be indicated at a hemoglobin concentration of 8 g/dL, with a higher threshold being appropriate if there is evidence of tissue hypoxia or ongoing uncontrolled hemorrhage.

These recommendations should not be interpreted, however, as a license to "give all the isotonic fluid you like." Volume *overload* can have detrimental effects on ICP by increasing either cerebral blood volume (CBV) or hydrostatically driven cerebral edema formation. Moreover, a more judicious fluid management has the potential to reduce the occurrence of pulmonary complications [2,26].

C. **Postoperative period.** In the postoperative period, the patients no longer need large volumes of intravenous fluid, mostly when they can ingest sufficient water to balance urinary output. We would recommend periodic measurement of serum osmolality, particularly if the patient's neurologic status deteriorates. If cerebral edema and/or intracranial hypertension develop, further fluid restriction is unlikely to be of value and can cause hypovolemia. Instead, treatment consists of mannitol or HS and maintenance of normovolemia with fluids to sustain the increased osmolality. Inducing hypovolemia so that vasopressors are required to maintain acceptable hemodynamic parameters has little advantage (and some disadvantage).

D. **Glucose administration and glycemic control.** There is solid evidence that hyperglycemia exacerbates neurologic damage and can worsen outcome from both focal and global ischemia [18], and, on the other hand, withholding glucose from adult neurosurgical patients is not associated with hypoglycemia. Therefore, it may be prudent to withhold glucose-containing fluids from acutely injured and elective surgical patients. There is a growing consensus to selectively administer intraoperative dextrose only in those patients at greatest risk for hypoglycemia (e.g., neonates and endocrinopathies). This *caveat* does not apply to the use of alimentation in such patients, perhaps because the administration of these hyperglycemic solutions typically begins several days after the primary insult.

The control of hyperglycemia with intensive insulin therapy has been reported to improve outcome. However, a recent multicenter, prospective trial, the NICE-SUGAR study, suggests that the aggressive control of hyperglycemia by insulin therapy may increase mortality in critically ill patients [27]. Institution of strict glycemic-control protocols has been associated with an increased risk of hypoglycemia, a condition that, like hyperglycemia, can be detrimental to the brain [28]. In patients with SAH, intensive glycemic control had no effect on overall in-hospital mortality, and it was reported to increase the incidence of hypoglycemia, which was powerfully associated with mortality [29].

Blood sugar in neurosurgical patients should be controlled carefully to avoid both hypo- and hyperglycemia and to maintain glucose between 100 and 150 mg/dL. Glucose-containing solutions should be withheld, except in the case of neonates and patients who have diabetes in whom hypoglycemia can occur very rapidly and be detrimental.

IV. Hemodilution. One common accompaniment of fluid administration is a reduction in the hemoglobin and hematocrit. Several animal studies have shown that regional oxygen delivery may be increased (or at least better maintained) in the face of modest hemodilution to an Hct of approximately 30% with an improvement in CBF and a reduction in infarction volume. Hemodilution might be beneficial during and immediately after a cerebral focal ischemic event. In spite of this, several clinical trials have failed to demonstrate any benefit from hemodilution in stroke patients [30], except in those who were polycythemic to begin with. Moreover, hemodilution has not been demonstrated to improve survival or functional outcome.

From a theoretical vantage, a hematocrit of 30% to 33% may lead to reduced blood viscosity and improved microcirculation, but this may occur at the expense of reduced blood oxygen-carrying capacity. In the normal brain, the increase in CBF produced by hemodilution is almost certainly an active compensatory response to a decrease in arterial oxygen content; this response is essentially identical to that seen with hypoxia. With a brain injury, however, the normal CBF response to hypoxia and hemodilution is attenuated, and both conditions can contribute to secondary tissue damage. For elective neurosurgical patients and patients suffering from head injuries, hemodilution to a hematocrit below 30% is unlikely to be any more "beneficial" than hypoxia.

V. Water and electrolyte disturbances. Disorders of water balance and electrolytes, especially sodium, are common in critically ill adult neurologic patients [31]. A disruption in the water balance is manifested as an abnormal serum Na^+ concentration, with hypernatremia or hyponatremia [32,33]. Signs and symptoms of hyper/hyponatremia largely reflect CNS dysfunction and are prominent when the increase/decrease in the serum Na^+ concentration is large or occurs rapidly.

Hypernatremia, defined as a rise in the serum Na^+ concentration to a value exceeding 145 mEq/L, is a common electrolyte disorder in neurosurgical patients undergoing surgery in the pituitary and hypothalamic areas. Since sodium is a functionally impermeable solute, hypernatremia invariably denotes hypertonic hyperosmolality and always causes cellular dehydration. Brain shrinkage induced by hypernatremia can cause vascular rupture, with cerebral bleeding, SAH, and the resultant morbidity may be serious, or even life-threatening.

Hyponatremia is defined as a decrease in the serum Na^+ concentration to a level below 136 mEq/L. Whereas hypernatremia always denotes hyperosmolality, hyponatremia can be associated with low, normal, or high plasma osmolality.

Hyponatremia is quite common and the brain is one of the major target organs for hyponatremia-related morbidity. The fact that most cases of hyponatremia are the result of water imbalance rather than sodium imbalance, underscores the role of antidiuretic hormone (ADH) in the pathophysiology. In patients with SAH, it has been demonstrated an increased secretion of a natriuretic factor, the brain natriuretic peptide (BNP), which can explain a defect in the central regulation of renal sodium reabsorption, with natriuresis and hyponatremia [34].

Just as in hypernatremia, the manifestations of hyponatremia are largely related to dysfunction of the CNS and they are more evident when the decrease in the serum Na^+ concentration is large or rapid. Hyponatremia and hypo-osmolality increase brain water content, resulting in cerebral edema and intracranial hypertension with a risk of brain injury.

Postoperative hyponatremic encephalopathy can be difficult to diagnose because the presenting features are nonspecific, and in neurosurgical patients can be confused with other conditions. Headache, nausea, vomiting, lethargy, restlessness, disorientation, and depressed reflexes can be observed. Whereas most patients with a serum Na^+ concentration exceeding 125 mEq/L are asymptomatic, those with lower values may have symptoms, especially if the disorder has developed rapidly. Complications of severe and rapidly evolving hyponatremia include seizures, coma, brain-stem herniation, and death.

Table 3.5 summarizes the principal differences among the commonest water and electrolyte disturbances in patients with intracranial pathology.

A. Diabetes insipidus (DI) is a common sequela of pituitary and hypothalamic lesions. DI can occur also with other cerebral pathology including head trauma, bacterial meningitis, intracranial

TABLE 3.5 Water and electrolyte disturbances in neurosurgical patients

		DI	SIADH	CSWS
Etiology		Reduced secretion of ADH	Excessive release of ADH	Release of BNP
Serum	Sodium	Hypernatremia >145 mEq/L	Hyponatremia <135 mEq/L	Hyponatremia <135 mEq/L
	Osmolality	Hyperosmolality	Hypo-osmolality	Hypo-osmolality
Urine	Output	>30 mL/kg/h	—	—
	Specific gravity	<1.002	—	—
	Sodium	<15 mEq/L	>35 mEq/L	>50 mEq/L
	Urine osmolality versus serum osmolality	Lower <200 mOsm/L	Higher >200 mOsm/L	Higher >200 mOsm/L
Intravascular volume		Reduced	Normal or increased	Reduced

DI, diabetes insipidus; SIADH, syndrome of inappropriate ADH secretion; CSWS, cerebral salt-wasting syndrome; ADH, antidiuretic hormone; BNP, brain natriuretic peptide.

surgery, phenytoin use, and alcohol intoxication. Patients who have markedly elevated ICP and in brain death commonly develop DI [35].

DI is characterized by the production of large volumes of dilute urine in the face of an elevated plasma osmolality caused by the decreased secretion of ADH. This results in failure of the tubular reabsorption of water. Polyuria (>30 mL/kg/h or, in an adult, >200 mL/h), progressive dehydration, and hypernatremia occur subsequently. DI is present when the urine output is excessive, the urine osmolality is inappropriately low relative to serum osmolality (which is above normal because of water loss), and the urine specific gravity is <1.002.

The management of DI requires restoration of normal serum Na$^+$ along with careful balancing of intake and output to avoid fluid overload. The water deficit is replaced over 24 to 48 hours, and the hypernatremia should not be reduced by more than 1 to 2 mEq/L/h, as rapid reduction may cause seizures or cerebral edema. The patient should receive hourly maintenance fluids (Table 3.6) in the form of 0.45% NaCl and free water with appropriate K$^+$ supplementation. Serum Na$^+$, K$^+$, and glucose are checked frequently.

If the urine output is greater than 300 mL/h for two consecutive hours, it is now standard practice to administer aqueous vasopressin, 5 to 10 IU intramuscularly or subcutaneously every 6 hours, or the synthetic analog of ADH, desmopressin acetate, 0.5 to 2 μg in every 8 hours or 10 to 20 μg by nasal inhalation (Table 3.6).

B. Syndrome of inappropriate antidiuretic hormone secretion (SIADH). Postoperative patients are at high risk for developing hyponatremia because they have multiple stimuli for ADH production including pain, stress, nausea and vomiting, positive pressure ventilation, the administration of narcotics, and intravascular volume depletion. The combination of these factors places virtually all postoperative patients at risk for developing hyponatremia. In neurosurgery, however, various cerebral pathologic processes (especially TBI) can cause excessive release of ADH that leads to the SIADH. SIADH is characterized by the presence of hyponatremia, low plasma osmolality without volume depletion or peripheral edema, high urine osmolality (relative to plasma osmolality), continued renal excretion of Na$^+$ (>20 mEq/L) despite

TABLE 3.6 Management of diabetes insipidus

Monitoring	Hourly monitoring of urinary output (UO)
Fluid treatment	Maintenance fluids + 75% of the previous hour's UO or
	Maintenance fluids + the previous hour's UO − 50 mL
Drug treatment if UO > 300 mL/h	Vasopressin: 5–10 IU q6h im or sc
	Desmopressin: 0.5–2 μg IV q8h or 10–20 μg by nasal inhalation

hyponatremia and associated hypo-osmolality, and normal renal, adrenal, thyroid, and cardiac functions. SIADH can also result from the over administration of free water in patients who cannot excrete free water because of excess ADH.

The mainstay of treatment of SIADH is fluid restriction to 1,000 mL/day of an isosmolar solution. If hyponatremia is severe (<110 to 115 mEq/L), the administration of HS (3% to 5%) and furosemide might be appropriate. As rapid correction of hyponatremia has been associated with the occurrence of central pontine myelinolysis, it is advisable to restore serum Na^+ at a rate of about 2 mEq/L/h.

The antagonism of arginine vasopressin (AVP), also known as ADH, represents a new, more direct strategy for the treatment of SIADH [31,36]. Two AVP receptor antagonists, conivaptan and tolvaptan, have been recently approved by the Food and Drug Administration for the treatment of euvolemic and hypervolemic hyponatremia. Vaptans (>V2 antagonists) block the effects of elevated ADH and promote *aquaresis,* the electrolyte-sparing excretion of water, resulting in the correction of serum sodium. Correction of hyponatremia is associated with markedly improved neurologic outcome. Vaptans, however, need to be administered with caution, and serum Na^+ must be carefully monitored during therapy.

C. **Cerebral salt wasting syndrome (CSWS).** CSWS is characterized by excessive natriuresis (urine Na^+ concentration >50 mEq/L), diuresis, hyponatremia, and negative sodium balance (loss of Na^+ in urine is greater than Na^+ intake per day). This syndrome is frequently seen in patients after SAH and the cause seems to be the increased release of BNP from the brain [34]. BNP may be a part of central mechanism for control of blood volume, blood pressure, and electrolyte composition. The intravascular volume status, the key difference to treat neurosurgical patients with hyponatremia, in CSWS is contracted: The increased renal excretion of sodium (150 to 200 mEq/day), which is followed by excretion of water, induces hypovolemia. In patients with SAH and CSWS, the therapy is to re-establish normovolemia with the administration of Na^+ and fluid replacement. HS may be used to increase serum sodium level at a rate less than 0.5 mEq/L.

The identification of the cause of hyponatremia in neurosurgical patients is quite difficult [31]. To distinguish between SIADH and CSWS the key issue is the determination of the intravascular volume status. Identification of hypo- or normovolemia based only on PE findings (mucosal hydration, skin turgor, jugular vein distention), orthostatic changes in pulse (increase of 10% upright compared with supine), and systolic blood pressure (decrease of 10% upright compared with supine) may not be sufficient. Invasive criteria (e.g., central venous pressure) and/or more sophisticated techniques should be used to assess intravascular volume status, since administration of inappropriate treatment can be fatal.

When persistent natriuresis and diuresis occur in the presence of a negative sodium balance, treatment should be fluid and sodium replacement and not fluid restriction. If patients with CSWS are treated by fluid restriction, fatal hypovolemia and cerebral infarction can occur, whereas fluid replacement in patients with SIADH can further reduce the serum Na^+, increasing the risk of cerebral edema and neurologic symptoms.

CLINICAL PEARL Distinction between SIADH and CSWS is very important, because fluid treatment of these two syndromes is quite different: Fluid restriction versus fluid infusion.

In patients who have SAH, in whom normo- to hypervolemia is advocated, fluid restriction (i.e., further volume contraction) might be especially deleterious.

VI. **Conclusion.** As neuroanesthesiologists and neurointensivists, we should always remember that we treat the whole patient, not only the brain. Therefore, with the exception of patients with SIADH, we should abandon the old dogma that patients who have intracranial pathology must be "run dry" and replace it with "run them isovolemic, isotonic, and iso-oncotic."

REFERENCES

1. Tommasino C, Picozzi V. Volume and electrolyte management. *Best Pract Res Clin Anaesthesiol.* 2007;21:497–516.
2. Clifton GL, Miller ER, Choi SC, et al. Fluid thresholds and outcome from severe brain injury. *Crit Care Med.* 2002;30:739–745.
3. Kees MG, Schlotterbeck H, Passemard R, et al. Ringer solution: osmolarity and composition revisited. *Ann Fr Anesth Reanim.* 2005;24:653–655.
4. Vialet R, Leone M, Albanese J, et al. Calculated serum osmolality can lead to systematic bias compared to direct measurement. *J Neurosurg Anesthesiol.* 2005;17:106–109.
5. Tommasino C, Moore S, Todd MM. Cerebral effects of isovolemic hemodilution with crystalloid or colloid solutions. *Crit Care Med.* 1988;16:862–868.
6. Todd MM, Tommasino C, Moore S. Cerebral effects of isovolemic hemodilution with a hypertonic saline solution. *J Neurosurg.* 1985;63:944–948.
7. Drummond JC, Patel PM, Cole DJ, et al. The effect of the reduction of colloid oncotic pressure, with and without reduction of osmolality, on post-traumatic cerebral edema. *Anesthesiology.* 1998;88:993–1002.
8. Zornow MH, Scheller MS, Todd MM, et al. Acute cerebral effects of isotonic crystalloid and colloid solutions following cryogenic brain injury in the rabbit. *Anesthesiology.* 1988;69:180–184.
9. Powell-Tuck J, Gosling P, Lobo DN, et al. *British Consensus Guidelines on Intravenous Fluid Therapy for Adult Surgical Patients (GIFTASUP).* London: NHS National Library of Health; 2009.
10. Rudehill A, Gordon E, Ohman G, et al. Pharmacokinetics and effects of mannitol on hemodynamics, blood and cerebrospinal fluid electrolytes, and osmolality during intracranial surgery. *J Neurosurg Anesthesiol.* 1993;5:4–12.
11. Diringer MN, Scalfani MT, Zazulia AR, et al. Effect of mannitol on cerebral blood volume in patients with head injury. *Neurosurgery.* 2012;70:1215–1219.
12. Todd MM, Cutkomp J, Brian JE. Influence of mannitol and furosemide, alone and in combination, on brain water content after fluid percussion injury. *Anesthesiology.* 2006;105:1176–1181.
13. Tyagi R, Donaldson K, Loftus CM, et al. Hypertonic saline: a clinical review. *Neurosurg Rev.* 2007;30:277–290.
14. Kamel H, Navi BB, Nakagawa K, et al. Hypertonic saline versus mannitol for the treatment of elevated intracranial pressure: a meta-analysis of randomized clinical trials. *Crit Care Med.* 2011;39:554–559.
15. Bulger EM, May S, Brasel KJ, et al., ROC Investigators. Out-of-hospital hypertonic resuscitation following severe traumatic brain injury: A randomized controlled trial. *JAMA.* 2010;304:1455–1464.
16. Khanna S, Davis D, Peterson B, et al. Use of hypertonic saline in the treatment of severe refractory posttraumatic intracranial hypertension in pediatric traumatic brain injury. *Crit Care Med.* 2000;28:1144–1151.
17. Gemma M, Cozzi S, Tommasino C, et al. 7.5% hypertonic saline versus 20% mannitol during elective neurosurgical supratentorial procedures. *J Neurosurg Anesthesiol.* 1997;9:329–334.
18. Wass CT, Lanier WL. Glucose modulation of ischemic brain injury: Review and clinical recommendations. *Mayo Clin Proc.* 1996;71:801–812.
19. Niemi TT, Miyashita R, Yamakage M. Colloid solutions: A clinical update. *J Anesth.* 2010;24:913–925.
20. Myburgh J, Cooper DJ, Finfer S, et al. Saline or albumin for fluid resuscitation in patients with traumatic brain injury. *N Engl J Med.* 2007;357:874–884.
21. Mitra S, Khandelwal P. Are all colloids same? How to select the right colloid? *Indian J Anaesth.* 2009;53:592–607.
22. Westphal M, James MF, Kozek-Langenecker S, et al. Hydroxyethyl starches: Different products–different effects. *Anesthesiology.* 2009;111:187–202.
23. Shenkin HA, Benzier HO, Bouzarth W. Restricted fluid intake: Rational management of the neurosurgical patient. *J Neurosurg.* 1976;45:432–436.
24. Jacob M, Chappell D, Conzen P, et al. Blood volume is normal after preoperative overnight fasting. *Acta Anaesthesiol Scand.* 2008;52:522–529.
25. Chappell D, Jacob M, Hofmann-Kiefer K, et al. A rational approach to perioperative fluid management. *Anesthesiology.* 2008;109:723–740.
26. Wiedemann HP, Wheeler AP, Bernard GR, et al. Comparison of two fluid-management strategies in acute lung injury. *N Engl J Med.* 2006;354:2564–2575.
27. Finfer S, Chittock DR, Su SY, et al. The NICE-SUGAR Study Investigators: Intensive versus conventional glucose control in critically ill patients. *N Engl J Med.* 2009;360:1283–1297.
28. Tiemessen CA, Hoedemaekers CW, van Iersel FM, et al. Intensive insulin therapy increases the risk of hypoglycemia in neurocritical care patients. *J Neurosurg Anesthesiol.* 2011;23:206–214.
29. Thiele RH, Pouratian N, Zuo Z, et al. Strict glucose control does not affect mortality after aneurysmal subarachnoid hemorrhage. *Anesthesiology.* 2009;110:603–610.
30. Kellert L, Martin E, Sykora M, et al. Cerebral oxygen transport failure: Decreasing hemoglobin and hematocrit levels after ischemic stroke predict poor outcome and mortality: Stroke: RelevAnt Impact of hemoGlobin, Hematocrit and Transfusion (STRAIGHT)–an observational study. *Stroke.* 2011;42:2832–2837.
31. Nathan BR. Cerebral correlates of hyponatremia. *Neurocrit Care.* 2007;6:72–78.
32. Adrogué HJ, Madias NE. Hypernatremia. *N Engl J Med.* 2000;342(20):1493–1499.
33. Adrogué HJ, Madias NE. Hyponatremia. *N Engl J Med.* 2000;342(21):1581–1589.
34. Berendes E, Walter M, Cullen P, et al. Secretion of brain natriuretic peptide in patients with aneurysmal subarachnoid haemorrhage. *Lancet.* 1997;349:245–249.
35. Smith M. Physiological changes during brain stem death–lessons for management of the organ donor. *J Heart Lung Transplant.* 2004;23:S217–S222.
36. Murphy T, Rajat Dhar R, Diringer M. Conivaptan bolus dosing for the correction of hyponatremia in the neurointensive care unit. *Neurocrit Care.* 2009;11:14–19.

4

Routine Craniotomy for Supratentorial Masses

Eiman Rahimi and Pirjo H. Manninen

KEY POINTS

General considerations for anesthetic management of craniotomy for supratentorial masses:

1. Appreciate the pathophysiologic changes that may be present such as increased intracranial pressure.
2. Understanding the type, location, size, and vascularity of the mass lesion.
3. A thorough preoperative assessment and optimizing of the medical condition of the patient.
4. Aims of the anesthesia management include the maintenance of adequate cerebral perfusion and provision of excellent operating conditions to prevent neurologic injury.
5. Plan for smooth, controlled, hemodynamically stable induction, maintenance, and emergence, and the ability for neurologic assessment of the patient at the end of the procedure.

I. General considerations

A. Anatomy

1. Supratentorial compartment is the largest component of the craniospinal space.
2. The roof is formed by the calvarium and the floor by the cerebellar tentorium, an extension of the dura mater.
3. The cerebral hemispheres are divided in midline by the falx cerebri.
4. Each hemisphere contains the frontal, parietal, temporal, and occipital lobe.
5. The supratentorial compartment communicates with the infratentorial compartment by an opening in the tentorium.

B. Physiology and pathophysiology

1. **Intracranial pressure (ICP)**
   a. The intracranial contents consist of brain parenchyma, cerebrospinal fluid (CSF), and the cerebral blood volume (CBV). They are confined within the closed space of the skull creating ICP.
   b. An increase in one compartment initially results in compensation by the transfer of intracranial CSF and venous blood to extracranial space, thus maintaining normal ICP.
   c. When this buffering mechanism is exhausted even small increases in volume will lead to large increases in ICP, decreasing cerebral perfusion that results in cerebral ischemia followed by herniation of brain tissue (Fig. 4.1).
   d. Brain tumors that grow slowly will allow for compensation and thus the patient may remain asymptomatic and have a normal ICP.

37

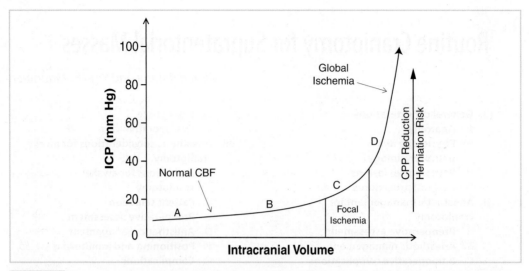

FIGURE 4.1 Schematic diagram of the intracranial pressure (ICP)–volume relationship (elastance). As intracranial volume increases (A to B) compensation occurs resulting in minimal increase in ICP, but as elastance decreases there is a marked increase in ICP (C to D) for even small increases in intracranial volume. Further increases in ICP will result in decrease cerebral perfusion pressure (CPP), global ischemia, and herniation. CBF, cerebral blood flow.

    e. Intracranial volume increases also result from edema surrounding a tumor that responds well to steroid treatment (dexamethasone).

  2. **Blood–brain barrier.** The blood–brain barrier is impermeable to electrolytes; however, water will shift between blood and brain compartments according to osmotic gradients, particularly serum sodium concentrations (see Chapter 3 for details). Intracranial lesions and injury may disrupt the blood–brain barrier allowing water, electrolytes, and osmotic molecules to crossover producing brain edema.

  3. **Cerebral blood flow (CBF)**

    a. CBF is coupled with cerebral metabolic requirement of oxygen ($CMRO_2$) and is controlled by cerebral autoregulation, cerebral perfusion pressure (CPP), cerebrovascular resistance (CVR), and cerebrovascular reactivity to CO_2 (see Chapter 1 for details).

    b. Cerebral autoregulation is the ability of cerebral vessels to provide a constant CBF ($\approx$50 mL/100 g/min of brain weight) over a wide range of mean arterial pressure (MAP). This range is variable among individuals with a lower limit of MAP of approximately 70 mm Hg (Fig. 4.2). In untreated or poorly controlled chronic hypertension, the autoregulation range will shift toward higher values.

    c. CO_2 is a cerebral vasodilator/constrictor. A linear relationship exists between $PaCO_2$ (25 to 80 mm Hg) and CBF. CBF changes from 2% to 4% for each mm Hg change in $PaCO_2$. Excessive hyperventilation may lead to ischemia especially in areas of compromised CBF.

    d. CPP is the difference between MAP and ICP.

    e. Autoregulation and CO_2 reactivity can be disturbed by various pathologic states (injured brain, tumor) and also anesthetic agents [1,2].

CLINICAL PEARL The concept of the range of autoregulation is an evolving concept in which the upper and lower limits are more likely to be a "rounded shoulders" than a "sharp elbows." The lower limits may be as high as a 25% decrease from baseline and cerebral hypoperfusion may occur when the MAP is 40% to 50% of the resting value.

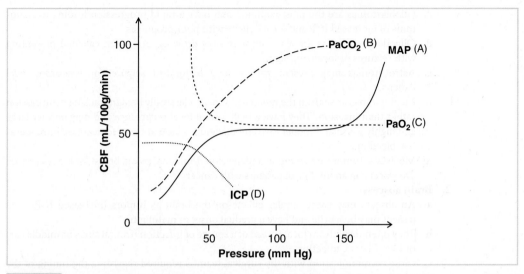

FIGURE 4.2 This is an illustration of the relationships of cerebral blood flow (CBF) to changes in (**A**) mean arterial blood pressure (MAP), known as the cerebral autoregulation curve, (**B**) carbon dioxide ($PaCO_2$), (**C**) oxygen (PaO_2) tensions, and (**D**) intracranial pressure (ICP).

4. **Anesthetic effects**
    a. **Volatile anesthetic agents**
        (1) Volatile anesthetic agents cause cerebral vasodilation (decreased CVR) that increases CBF resulting in increases in CBV and ICP. These agents also have a dose-related decrease in $CMRO_2$ (see Chapter 2 for details).
        (2) Volatile agents should be kept at <1 MAC to maintain CO_2 reactivity and autoregulation in normal brain tissue.
        (3) Nitrous oxide may increase $CMRO_2$ with an increase in CBF and, thus may increase ICP.
    b. **Intravenous anesthetic agents**
        (1) Most intravenous agents (thiopentone, propofol) are potent cerebral vasoconstrictors through their ability to reduce $CMRO_2$. Due to tight coupling of CBF to $CMRO_2$ the decrease in $CMRO_2$ results in an increase in CVR with a reduction in CBF, CBV, and thus ICP.
        (2) Ketamine is the exception as it increases CBF.
        (3) Opioids (fentanyl, remifentanil, sufentanil) cause a modest reduction in $CMRO_2$ but do not affect autoregulation or CO_2 reactivity. However, respiratory depression that results in marked hypercarbia will increase CBF and CBV. In addition, hypotension resulting from large bolus administration of narcotics may cause reflex cerebrovasodilation with an increase in CBV and potentially ICP.
        (4) Neuromuscular blocking agents generally have minimal effect on CBF. However, succinylcholine may cause transient limited increases in ICP under conditions of intracranial hypertension. These ICP changes can be blocked by preadministration of a defasciculating dose of nondepolarizing relaxants, hyperventilation, or an intravenous anesthetic agent.
    C. **Pathology of lesions**
        1. **Tumors**
            a. In adults most primary and metastatic tumors are in the supratentorial compartment (80%); in children they are more frequently infratentorial.
            b. Primary tumors (60% of tumors) range from benign well differentiated to anaplastic. Surgical management usually consists of peritumor edema control (24 to 48 hours of course of corticosteroids) and tumor debulking.

    c. Glioblastomas are the most common and have a rapid progression leading to symptoms of increased ICP and focal deficits with poor prognosis.

    d. Oligodendrogliomas are less common, slow growing, and often calcified presenting with seizures or localizing signs.

    e. Astrocytomas may present with a long history of seizures or late-onset focal deficits.

    f. Meningiomas arise from the meninges and are classically benign, causing compression rather than invasion. They have a high rate of local recurrence and may be very large and highly vascular. Preoperative embolization is used at times to decrease intraoperative bleeding.

    g. Metastatic tumors are common and develop from lung, colon, breast, or kidney cancer. They occur in about 25% of patients with cancer.

2. Brain abscess

    a. An abscess may cause similar effects on the brain as tumors (increased ICP). The patient may be febrile and have a gradual onset of meningitis.

    b. They often result from local spread of a source of infection (frontal sinus or middle ear) or blood-borne infection.

    c. Close communication with the surgical team is required regarding the timing of the administration of antibiotics.

3. Intracranial hematoma

    a. Subdural hematomas

        (1) May present as either an acute, subacute, or chronic hematoma. Symptoms will depend on how quickly they develop. Patient may also have an acute on chronic bleed.

        (2) Chronic subdural hematomas usually affect the elderly. Symptoms (confusion, drowsiness, and fluctuating level of consciousness) may present weeks after the initial injury.

        (3) If acute in nature, there is less time for the brain to accommodate.

        (4) These lesions are treated with burr hole aspiration or minicraniotomy.

    b. Epidural hematoma

        (1) An acute epidural hematoma occurs when blood accumulates between the skull and dura. This usually occurs as the result of a traumatic insult that causes a skull fracture and rupture of the underlying blood vessels (usually an artery).

        (2) Neurologic decompensation occurs rapidly (often within hours) and the patient may be both neurologically and hemodynamically unstable.

        (3) These patients may require rapid treatment of increased ICP, including airway and ventilatory management. Since the brain parenchyma is usually not injured, the prognosis is excellent if the hematoma is rapidly decompressed.

    c. Intracerebral hematoma

        (1) An intracerebral hematoma (hemorrhage) results from bleeding into brain tissue. Etiology is usually related to rupture of normal vessels due to high blood pressure or abnormal blood vessels such as an arteriovenous malformation, an aneurysm, or bleeding into a tumor.

        (2) Symptoms usually are the sudden onset of a stroke.

        (3) Treatment includes management of blood pressure, ICP, and occasional surgical/intra-arterial interventions depending on the primary pathology.

D. Surgical procedures. Patients may undergo a biopsy, curative resection, or debulking of a supratentorial lesion.

    1. Stereotactic surgery

        a. Is a minimally invasive procedure that uses a three-dimensional coordinate system to locate small lesions inside the brain and is often used for obtaining a biopsy.

        b. These procedures may be performed with either general anesthesia or conscious sedation.

            (1) Continuous vigilance is needed to diagnose and treat complications quickly.

       (2) A sudden change in neurologic status or decreased level of consciousness may result from intracranial bleeding or neurologic injury.

       (3) Respiratory changes may occur from oversedation and/or from an intracranial event.

    c. May be "frame-based" which involves the placement of a light-weight headframe with a base that is attached to the cranium with skull pins. Computerized tomography (CT) or magnetic resonance imaging (MRI) then identifies the targeted lesion in relation to reference points on the external frame. Surgical apparatus is attached to the headframe.

       (1) Placement may occur in the operating room or in the imaging suite.

       (2) This can be performed with local anesthesia with or without sedation.

       (3) If general anesthesia is used, then most often the frame is placed after anesthesia induction.

       (4) The headframe may obscure the patient's mouth and/or nose and may limit extension of the neck, making airway manipulation difficult.

       (5) During the procedure, the stereotactic headframe is attached to the operating room table. This results in lack of ability of the patient to move their head and may result in a compromise of the patient's airway.

    d. A "frameless" stereotactic system is now frequently used with placement of external fiducial scalp markers, facial surface features, or a set of marks in the reticule of an optical instrument for points of reference. The use of a head holder frame attached to the operating room table may still be required. If the patient is awake for placement, local anesthesia will be infiltrated at the pin sites.

> **CLINICAL PEARL**   Since stereotactic surgery often relies on precise coordinates from external references, high resolution neuroimaging, and/or advanced computer systems, preventing changes in preoperative brain parenchymal relationships due to changes in $PaCO_2$, or the administration of osmotic diuretics is paramount to the success of these minimally invasive techniques.

   2. Craniotomy

    a. For the excision of a lesion a craniotomy is performed with a lateral pterional, temporal, or frontal surgical approach.

    b. Minimally invasive surgery and endoscopic approaches are also used.

    c. A bifrontal craniotomy increases the risk of venous air embolism (VAE) due to close proximity to the sagittal sinus (see Chapter 22).

    d. Intraoperative MRI is being used to improve patient outcome with better resection of tumors.

 II. Anesthetic management for craniotomy. The overall goals for the anesthetic management begin with full understanding of the patient's neurologic condition and planned procedure (Table 4.1) [3].

TABLE 4.1   Goals of anesthetic management

1. Preservation of uninjured brain by providing brain relaxation for surgery.

2. Treating and/or preventing any increases in ICP and brain edema.

3. Maintaining cerebral homeostasis with adequate cerebral perfusion and appropriate ventilation.

4. Cardiovascular stability throughout whole procedure.

5. Rapid recovery to enable neurologic assessment in the immediate postoperative period.

3

A. Preoperative assessment

1. **Purpose**
   a. Review of patient's medical history and findings.
   b. Optimize patient's overall medical status.
   c. Prepare a plan for the anesthetic management.

2. **Presenting symptoms**
   a. Many tumors grow slowly allowing for adaptive mechanisms before becoming symptomatic.
   b. Symptoms may be generalized with signs and symptoms of increased ICP (headache, nausea, vomiting, and changes in mental status).
   c. Or symptoms may be localized with seizures or focal deficits.
   d. Tumors may be surrounded by edema that responds to corticosteroid treatment. Frequently, at the time of surgery a patient's symptoms may have completely disappeared.

3. **Neurologic assessment**
   a. History of disease including presenting symptoms, and the type, location, and size of lesion.
   b. Neurologic status: Level of consciousness, Glasgow Coma Scale score (GCS), any signs and symptoms of increased ICP.
   c. History of seizures.
   d. Presence of focal deficits (such as hemiparesis).

4. **General medical condition**
   a. Review and optimize cardiac and respiratory systems.
   b. Assessment of other comorbidities such as diabetes, renal impairment, hematology, and allergies.
   c. Malignant tumors may cause coagulation disorders with an increased risk of thromboembolism. Low molecular heparin may be used in these patients postoperatively.
   d. Airway assessment.

5. **Medications**
   a. All routine medications (cardiovascular, respiratory, and gastrointestinal) and especially anticonvulsants, and steroids (dexamethasone) should be continued preoperatively.
   b. Appropriate treatment of diabetic patients.

6. **Laboratory**
   a. Routine blood work including hemoglobin, blood glucose level, and creatinine.
   b. ECG is useful as neurologic diseases can cause a variety of nonspecific ECG changes.
   c. Crossmatched blood (2 to 4 units) should be available if excessive blood loss is anticipated.

7. **Imaging**
   a. **CT and MRI**
      (1) For assessment of type, location, and size of lesion.
      (2) May indicate vascularity of the tumor.
      (3) Proximity of tumor to venous sinuses (risk of VAE).
      (4) Signs of increased ICP such as midline shift, edema, ventricular distortion, or hydrocephalus.
      (5) To determine the ease of surgical access and patient positioning.
   b. **Metabolic imaging.** Positron emission tomography, magnetic resonance spectroscopy, and single photon emission tomography will give more precise information on the size and location of the tumor.
   c. **Chest x-ray.** Assessment of respiratory diseases and of any primary cancer.

4

B. Anesthetic management

1. **Premedication**
   a. Preoperative sedation should be avoided in patients with increased ICP, low GCS, and with large mass lesions.
   b. Sedation may result in depressed respiratory efforts leading to elevated $PaCO_2$ and increase in CBF, CBV, and ICP.

    c. When premedication is used it must be administered with continuous observation and monitoring of the patient.

    d. Particularly anxious patients may be premedicated with a short-acting benzodiazepine with the above precautions.

2. **Monitoring**

    a. All standard monitors should be used. Additional monitoring as indicated by requirements of patient and procedure.

    b. Vascular access for large craniotomy requires two large bore intravenous lines (18G or larger).

    c. **Invasive cardiovascular monitoring**

        (1) Invasive intra-arterial blood pressure for most patients is indicated. In unstable patients, this should be placed preinduction using local anesthesia. Arterial reference should be at the level of the middle ear/circle of Willis.

        (2) Central venous pressure (CVP) monitoring may be useful in procedures with a large estimated blood loss (tumors encroaching venous sinuses, large vascular tumors such as meningioma), possibility of VAE and in procedures or patients with marked fluid shifts, and patients with difficult venous access.

        (3) Pulmonary artery pressure monitoring is rarely required.

    d. Urinary catheter is needed for most procedures, especially when mannitol or diuretics are used or excessive urine output is expected (e.g., diabetes insipidus).

    e. Core temperature monitoring with a nasal-pharyngeal or esophageal probe is indicated.

    f. Warming blankets and blood warmers are useful as indicated to ensure normothermia.

    g. Routine ICP monitoring is rarely used. When the cranium is open, observation of conditions of the surgical field provides useful information (presence or lack of dural bulging). Lumbar CSF drains are rarely used for tumor surgery, but if present may be used to monitor lumbar CSF pressure.

    h. Neurophysiologic monitoring with somatosensory and/or motor evoked potentials, electroencephalography, and electromyography may be used (see Chapter 26).

    i. Other monitors used in specific patients include monitoring neuromuscular blockade, biologic (coagulation, hematology, blood gases, glucose), jugular venous bulb oxygen saturation, transcranial Doppler, transcranial oximetry, precordial Doppler (for VAE), depth of anesthesia, and microvascular ultrasonic blood flow probe.

3. **Induction of anesthesia**

    a. Induction of anesthesia must be smooth and controlled with hemodynamic stability. Adequate depth of anesthesia, particularly at intubation, is important to prevent hypertension. Preventing hypoxemia, hypercarbia, and increases in venous pressure can minimize increases in ICP.

    b. Anesthesia induction can be achieved by using titrated doses of induction agents (midazolam, propofol, thiopentone) and an opioid (fentanyl 2 to 3 μg/kg, sufentanil 0.2 to 0.3 μg/kg, remifentanil 0.5 to 1.0 μg/kg) followed with short-acting nondepolarizing muscle relaxants (rocuronium, vecuronium, cisatracurium). Succinylcholine may be used depending on the risk benefit of rapid airway control versus the small risk of transient increases in ICP.

        (1) Etomidate may be useful in hemodynamically unstable patients.

        (2) Addition of lidocaine 1 to 1.5 mg/kg IV will help to blunt the laryngeal reflex to intubation and reduce ICP by cerebral vasoconstriction.

        (3) Prior to laryngoscopy and intubation, the depth of anesthesia should be deepened with an additional bolus of anesthetic agents (propofol or opioid) or β-blocker (esmolol 0.5 to 1.0 mg/kg) or antihypertensive (labetalol 0.25 to 0.5 mg/kg) to suppress sympathetic response.

    c. Other helpful measures include voluntary hyperventilation by the patient while awake and mild hyperventilation during induction.

4. **Positioning**
   a. Final positioning of the patient must be reviewed by both the surgeon and anesthesiologist.
   b. Supine position with or without a shoulder roll to turn the head away from surgical site is used for most procedures.
   c. For some procedures a full lateral position is used.
   d. The endotracheal tube should be securely placed on the appropriate side. A soft bite block may be useful.
   e. Prior to head fixation with skull pins the depth of anesthesia must be deepened to prevent hypertension. This can be with additional propofol (0.5 mg/kg), fentanyl (2 to 3 μg/kg), or remifentanil (0.5 to 1.0 μg/kg), with or without injection of local anesthesia (lidocaine) at site of pin insertion.
   f. Extreme head rotation and flexion may obstruct internal jugular veins and affect venous drainage causing an increase in ICP.
   g. Slight head up will optimize venous drainage.
   h. Patients' eyes must be securely taped and protected from desiccation or irritation from skin preparation solutions.
   i. Care is needed for all pressure points and the prevention of nerve compression.
   j. Thromboembolism prophylaxis should be considered. Elastic stockings or sequential pneumatic calf compression devices may be used.

5. **Maintenance of anesthesia**
   a. **Pharmacologic management**
      (1) Both total intravenous anesthesia (TIVA) and inhalation techniques have been used. The choice is mostly at the discretion of the anesthesiologist. No major differences in outcome of the patient have been shown between these techniques [4–6].
      (2) **Inhalation-based anesthesia**
         (a) Inhalation anesthesia used in conjunction with opioids is easily controllable and allows for early awakening.
         (b) Inhalation agents (isoflurane, desflurane, and sevoflurane) cause cerebrovasodilation and thus may increase CBF and ICP resulting in brain swelling.
         (c) However at a < 1 MAC CO_2 reactivity remains intact and control of vasodilator effects of volatile agents can be minimized with hypocarbia in normal brain tissue.
         (d) Nitrous oxide (N_2O) increase $CMRO_2$ which may increase CBF and ICP. Hypocapnia and intravenous agents minimize the cerebral vasodilation. N_2O use, though still controversial, is declining [7]. It should not be used in patients with a recent craniotomy as N_2O diffuses into air-containing space leading to pneumocephalus.
      (3) **TIVA**
         (a) The most common TIVA agents used are an opioid and propofol. Propofol reduces $CMRO_2$, CBF, CBV, and ICP, and preserves CO_2 reactivity.
         (b) TIVA may result in prolonged and unpredictable awakening.
         (c) TIVA is indicated in the patient who has high ICP and significant brain swelling.
      (4) **Opioids**
         (a) Opioids (fentanyl, sufentanil, remifentanil) add to hemodynamic stability and reduce the requirement for other anesthetic agents.
         (b) Remifentanil allows more rapid emergence as it is easily titrable, and its metabolism gives it a short context-sensitive half-time.
      (5) **Neuromuscular blockers**
         (a) Muscle relaxation may be used with intermittent bolus or infusion of short- or medium-duration agents: rocuronium, vecuronium, cisatracurium.
         (b) Muscle relaxation should be avoided when neurologic monitoring includes motor evoked potentials or electromyography.

    (c) Higher doses of remifentanil lessen the risk of movement in the absence of muscle relaxants [8].

  (6) Dexmedetomidine (0.2 to 1.0 μg/kg/h)

    (a) An α-2 adrenoreceptor agonist that has sedative, sympatholytic, and analgesic properties [9,10].

    (b) Provides hemodynamic stability during general anesthesia by decreasing hemodynamic responses to noxious stimuli and during surgery and emergence.

  (7) Adjunctive medications

    (a) Administration of antibiotics, steroids (dexamethasone), and antiseizure prophylaxis (levetiracetam, fosphenytoin, phenytoin) is given as indicated and repeated if necessary during prolonged procedures.

    (b) A loading dose of phenytoin (15 mg/kg) must be administered slowly to prevent hemodynamic instability.

    (c) Furosemide (10 to 20 mg), mannitol (0.5 to 1.0 g/kg), or hypertonic saline solutions (3 mL/kg 3% NaCl) may be used to reduce intracranial volume and ICP. With NaCl plasma sodium of up to 160 mmol/L is targeted to control ICP.

    (d) Antiemetics for postoperative nausea and vomiting (PONV) prophylaxis should be given. Most commonly, one of the 5-HT$_3$ receptor antagonists are used (ondansetron, granisetron, dolasetron, tropisetron, or palosetron) [11,12].

b. Ventilation

  (1) Mild to moderate hyperventilation (PaCO$_2$ 25 to 35 mm Hg) results in cerebral vasoconstriction and a reduction in CBF, CBV, and ICP. This is an efficient and rapid means of providing a slack brain and lessening the need for excessive harmful retraction of the brain [13,14].

  (2) A PaCO$_2$ measurement is useful to correlate to end-tidal CO$_2$.

  (3) Changing back to normoventilation should be done with caution as an increase in ICP may occur.

  (4) If required, the use of positive end expiratory pressure (PEEP) must be with caution to prevent decrease in cardiac output and increases in ICP.

c. Optimization of surgical conditions. Anesthetic maneuvers are important in the production of a "slack" brain or to reduce brain bulk to allow for ease of surgical access to the lesion without compromising cerebral perfusion and to prevent ischemic injury (Table 4.2).

d. Fluid management

  (1) Aim is to maintain normovolemia and preserve cerebral perfusion (see Chapter 3 for details).

  (2) Maintenance fluids used are isosmolar, normonatremic crystalloids such as normal saline and plasmalyte. Avoid hypotonic and dextrose-containing solutions as they may result in cerebral edema and hyperglycemia.

TABLE 4.2 Optimization for reduction of brain bulk

1. Head up position and good neck positioning to ensure venous drainage.
2. Mild to moderate hyperventilation (PaCO$_2$ 25–35 mm Hg) with good oxygenation and low intrathoracic pressure.
3. Osmotic diuretics (mannitol 0.5–1.0 g/kg or 3% NaCl 3 mL/kg) 30 min before dural opening.
4. Addition of loop diuretics (furosemide 10–20 mg) if needed.
5. Propofol bolus 0.5–1.0 mg/kg.
6. Ensure adequate cerebral perfusion pressure with near normal blood pressure.
7. Maintain normovolemia and normoglycemia.
8. Appropriate anesthetic technique with either inhalation agents or TIVA.
9. Surgical drainage of cerebral spinal fluid.

(3) Colloid solutions are appropriate to restore intravascular volume following diuresis or moderate blood loss.

e. **Glucose management**

(1) Maintain normoglycemia (80 to 150 mg/dL) and avoid glucose-containing solutions.

(2) Hyperglycemia has been identified as a risk factor for morbidity and mortality in patients at risk of neurologic injury [15].

(3) Blood glucose levels should be monitored continuously in diabetic patients and during prolonged procedures.

(4) Blood glucose levels >180 to 200 mg/dL should be treated with insulin but there is no clear evidence for tight control of intraoperative blood glucose [13].

(5) Steroid (dexamethasone) administration may also produce hyperglycemia [16].

f. **Temperature**

(1) Clinical studies have not shown any benefit to mild intraoperative hypothermia [17].

(2) Hypothermia may impair coagulation, result in wound infection, and prolonged recovery.

(3) Hyperthermia increases brain injury and should be avoided.

g. **Neuroprotection**

(1) There is lack of definitive proof in humans that pharmacologic neuroprotection is useful.

(2) Most anesthetic agents reduce brain metabolic requirements, thus may increase tolerance to ischemia.

(3) Best protection is to ensure good oxygenation, adequate CPP, and to prevent hypo- and hyperglycemia.

C. **Intraoperative complications**

1. **Blood loss and coagulopathy**

a. Vascular tumors (meningiomas) can be associated with rapid blood loss. This may even occur during the opening of the craniotomy.

b. Blood transfusion criteria are conflicting with both advantages and disadvantages of transfusion. An optimal hemoglobin concentration is 8 to 9 g/dL [18].

(1) Brief periods of profound anemia may be associated with inadequate brain perfusion.

(2) In tumor surgery, blood transfusion may impair the body's innate abilities to suppress tumor growth and spread.

c. Coagulopathy may develop during some tumor surgery and is associated with poor outcome.

(1) Fresh frozen plasma may be infused if there is persistent hemorrhage despite adequate surgical hemostasis. The current available data on the use of recombinant factor VIIa for bleeding associated with neurosurgical procedures consist of retrospective studies, expert opinion or isolated case reports. The use of recombinant factor VIIa may provide a cost-effective method of reversing coagulopathy in traumatic brain injured patients [19,20].

2. **Intraoperative bulging (tight) brain.** On removal of bone flap a tight or bulging dura will make surgical access difficult and increases the likelihood of ischemic damage to the brain. Also during resection of the tumor sudden brain swelling may occur from edema or bleeding inside the tumor. Rapid treatment is required as shown in Table 4.3.

3. **Venous air embolism**

a. The incidence is low as the sitting position is rarely used (see Chapter 22 for details).

b. Lesions that encroach on the sagittal venous sinus will be at higher risk.

4. **Hemodynamic instability**

a. Acute hypertensive episodes may occur during painful parts of the procedures such as insertion of headpins, periosteal dissection, and brain manipulation.

TABLE 4.3 Intraoperative treatment of a bulging (tight) brain
1. Place patient in head up position.
2. Increase hyperventilation.
3. Ensure good oxygenation and normal airway pressures.
4. Mannitol (0.5–1.0 g/kg) or 3% NaCl (3 mL/kg) ± furosemide 10–20 mg.
5. Decrease or stop volatile agents and change to TIVA.
6. Surgical drainage of CSF and/or surgical decompression.

    b. Rapid treatment is required, as hypertension (systolic blood pressure >140 to 160 mm Hg as defined by local protocols with neurosurgeons) may result in bleeding and increases in ICP. Treatment can be with increased depth of anesthesia (propofol, opioids) or attenuation of the sympathetic response with esmolol, labetalol, or nicardipine.

    c. Cardiac arrhythmias may also occur such as severe bradycardia from dural or brain tissue traction. The surgeon should be immediately informed and removal of the traction will usually correct the problem. If this is not effective, atropine or glycopyrrolate may be indicated.

D. Emergence. Goals are to have a rapid but smooth, controlled emergence with hemodynamic stability and a patient who is awake for neurologic assessment [21]. A plan for emergence should be formulated for each patient. An undisturbed patient will allow for a smoother emergence.

    1. Planned delayed emergence

        a. Patients with a preoperative impaired level of consciousness, unprotected airway, prolonged or unstable intraoperative course, or with excessive brain swelling at closure may be determined not to be suitable for rapid emergence.

        b. These patients need to be transferred to a neurosurgical intensive care unit with adequate level of sedation and analgesia, support of ventilation, and careful monitoring.

    2. Planned early emergence

        a. Emergence from general anesthesia requires careful titration of anesthetic agents and analgesia until patient is removed from headpins and dressing has been applied.

        b. During application of a full head dressing considerable movement of the head results in movement of the endotracheal tube which may cause coughing and hypertension.

        c. If remifentanil is used, this may be infused to end of head dressing.

        d. Prior to extubation a patient should be able to maintain normal oxygenation and end-tidal CO_2, ideally be awake enough to obey commands, and be neurologically stable (same as preoperative status) (Table 4.4).

TABLE 4.4 Criteria for extubation
1. Stable blood pressure, normothermia, normogylcemia, and normovolemia.
2. Elimination of inhalation (end-tidal near 0) and intravenous agents.
3. Reversal of muscle relaxants (if needed).
4. Adequate spontaneous ventilation with good oxygenation.
5. Pupils equal in size.
6. No gross swelling of face or neck.
7. Ideally, the patient will be arousable and responsive to commands.
8. Neurologic examination shows no new deficits and presence of gag reflex.

e. A plan for analgesic management should be formulated for emergence and the early postoperative period. This may include transitional analgesia (fentanyl, morphine) at closure or after emergence.

f. Intraoperative scalp nerve block or local anesthesia infiltration of wound may help with pain management.

3. **Emergence concerns**

   a. **Hemodynamic instability**

      (1) Cerebral hyperemia and hypertension may occur from the stress of emergence. This may result in bleeding by disrupting the hemostasis state and lead to cerebral edema, increases in ICP, and development of intracranial hematoma [22–24].

      (2) Treatment of hypertension (systolic blood pressure >140 to 160 mm Hg) can be accomplished with intravenous doses of labetalol (10 to 25 mg), esmolol (25 to 50 mg), or nicardipine (5 mg).

   b. Coughing, bucking, and straining increase venous pressure and may result in brain swelling.

   c. Subfrontal, especially bifrontal, surgical approach may result in a delayed emergence or disinhibited activity by the patient.

4. **Failure to emerge from anesthesia**

   a. Management must be implemented early to prevent permanent neurologic deficits.

   b. Discussion with the surgeon is critical.

   c. If anesthesia is a likely explanation, patience in allowing elimination of anesthetic agents (monitoring end-tidal inhaled anesthetics, confirmation of reversal of neuromuscular blockade) is needed.

   d. If there is a possibility that it is attributable to surgery, a brain scan should be performed to rule out hematoma formation.

E. **Postoperative care**

1. **Placement**

   a. Depending on institutional practice, patients will be transferred to a postoperative anesthesia care unit (PACU), a neurosurgical high dependency or neurosurgical critical care unit.

   b. Day surgery may be an option for some patients such as following awake craniotomy or short general anesthesia in a healthy patient.

2. **Assessment on PACU admission**

   a. **Neurologic assessment.** Level of consciousness (GCS), pupil size and light reactivity, neurologic examination and documentation of any deficits.

   b. Cardiovascular and respiratory assessment (blood pressure, heart rate, respiratory rate, SpO_2) and temperature.

   c. Sedation and pain scores

3. **Pain control**

   a. Management must be tailored to the patient's need and will vary greatly [25].

   b. Analgesics used include intravenous fentanyl, morphine, or hydromorphone, and oral agents such as acetaminophen or oxycodone.

   c. The safety of nonsteroidal anti-inflammatory drugs (NSAIDs) is not well documented. There are concerns with antiplatelet effects and the potential for hemostatic complications.

4. **Complications in PACU**

   a. **Neurologic.** The neurosurgery team must be immediately notified of any change or new deficit. Urgent imaging and/or repeat opening may be required to rule out intracranial bleed.

   b. **Hemodynamic instability**

      (1) Immediate recovery from anesthesia may result in increased stress leading to hypertension, tachycardia, and increased catecholamine release. Hypertension may worsen cerebral edema, increase ICP, and disrupt hemostasis resulting in an intracranial bleed.

(2) The exact level of hypertension that needs treatment is not well-defined but systolic blood pressures >140 to 160 mm Hg should be considered based on the development of local treatment protocols.

(3) Treatment may be with esmolol, labetolol, nicardipine, or hydralazine.

c. **Postoperative nausea and vomiting**

(1) The incidence of PONV has been reported to be 44% to 70%.

(2) Harmful effects include hypertension and increased venous pressure.

(3) Patients should receive intraoperative PONV prophylaxis and in PACU. The most commonly used drugs are the $5\text{-}HT_3$ receptor antagonists such as ondansetron and granisetron. Dexamethasone may also help to reduce emesis.

d. **Pneumocephalus**

(1) After a craniotomy most patients will have some subdural free air from head up positioning, extreme brain relaxation, or surgery in the frontal area where large residual airspaces occur.

(2) Tension pneumocephalus may occur when a large volume of air results in mass effect and intracranial hypertension. Patient may have delayed awakening or sudden onset of neurologic deterioration.

e. **Seizures**

(1) Seizures occurring in the PACU may be new onset related to surgery or may occur in patients with preoperative history of seizures.

(2) Rapid treatment with anticonvulsants (midazolam, propofol, phenytoin) is usually effective. Some patients may require protection from injury and full resuscitation.

III. Anesthetic considerations for awake craniotomy. The awake craniotomy is used for resection of tumors located either in or close to areas of eloquent brain function, such as speech, motor, and sensory pathways [26,27].

A. **Indications for awake craniotomy.** Optimal tumor resection and minimization of the risk of neurologic injury is possible with direct electrical mapping of the cortex for accurate localization of eloquent brain function or localization of the motor cortex in an awake patient.

B. **Patient selection**

1. Supratentorial tumors are amenable to awake resection if they have minimal dural involvement. Vascular lesions and tumors in the middle fossa floor, close to tentorium or falx are not suitable, as significant pain will occur with dural manipulation.

2. Patients should be cooperative and alert, able to communicate well, and understand the demands of the procedure. Confused, demented, agitated, or dysphasic patients are poor candidates.

3. Patients who do not speak a language spoken by at least one operating room staff member may also be difficult.

4. Obese patients and patients with a known difficult airway need to be considered individually.

C. **Preoperative assessment**

1. Routine assessment and preparation as for any patient with a brain tumor.

2. Continuation of all preoperative medications including antiseizure and steroids (dexamethasone).

3. Psychological preparation of the patient.

4. Patient informed about the requirements such as brain mapping.

5. The establishment of good rapport with the patient.

D. **Anesthetic management**

1. **Clinical considerations**

a. The goals are to have a comfortable patient who is able to stay immobile on an operating room table for the duration of the procedure and yet be alert and cooperative to comply with cortical mapping (Table 4.5).

b. Have anesthetic drugs and equipment for awake craniotomy, for possible induction of general anesthesia and treatment of complications available.

TABLE 4.5   Success with awake craniotomy
1. Adequate preparation of the patient, both medical and psychological.
2. Provision of a comfortable operating room environment.
3. Appropriate administration of analgesic and sedative medications.
4. Communication, reassurance, and support of the patient.
5. Rapid diagnosis and treatment of complications.

2. **Scalp anesthesia for craniotomy**
   a. Long-acting agents such as bupivacaine with epinephrine are used.
   b. Infiltration of the craniotomy site with a "ring block" or scalp nerve blocks of the auriculotemporal, occipital, zygomaticotemporal, supraorbital, and supratrochlear nerves may be used.
   c. Additional lidocaine may be used for painful areas during surgery.
   d. The total allowable dose of each local anesthetic agent should be calculated for each patient.
3. **Anesthetic techniques.** The decision for the choice of the technique of anesthesia will depend on the preferences of the institutional team including surgeon and anesthesiologist. Two techniques are commonly used.
   a. **Conscious sedation**
      (1) The patient is kept at a level of sedation where they are comfortable, drowsy but easily arousable when spoken to.
      (2) Sedation is stopped just prior to cortical mapping and then resumed for resection and closure.
      (3) There is no manipulation of the airway other than the administration of supplemental oxygen via nasal prongs, cannula, or a face mask.
      (4) Commonly used drugs include midazolam, propofol, fentanyl, and remifentanil. These drugs may be administered as either bolus injections or infusions.
      (5) Dexmedetomidine infusion may be used as an adjunct as it has minimal respiratory depression.
      (6) Nonpharmacologic measures including frequent reassurance, warning the patient in advance about loud noise (drilling bone), and painful areas, and holding the patient's hand.
   b. **Asleep awake asleep**
      (1) General anesthesia is induced at the beginning for the craniotomy, awakened for testing, and then resumed for tumor resection and closure.
      (2) Airway management may be with an endotracheal tube, oral or nasal airway, or, most commonly, the laryngeal mask airway (LMA).
      (3) The patient is fully awake for cortical mapping with removal of airway.
      (4) Either inhalation or intravenous anesthetic agents may be used with or without controlled ventilation.
      (5) Advantages include increased patient comfort and tolerance during craniotomy, especially for longer procedures, and a secured airway with the ability to use hyperventilation.
E. **Positioning and monitoring**
   1. **Positioning**
      a. Extra measures are required for patient comfort such as comfortable table, pillows between the legs, or under the knees.
      b. Patients should be positioned in such a way as to have some freedom of movement of the extremities to allow for intraoperative mapping.
      c. Neuronavigation for imaging is usually used, necessitating rigid fixation of the head. Pins are inserted with the use of local anesthesia under sedation.

    d. The placement of the surgical drapes should allow for maximum visibility of the patient's face by the anesthesiologist and for the patient to see the anesthesiologist.

  2. Monitoring

    a. Monitoring depends on the needs of the patient. Routine invasive monitoring is not required for all patients.

    b. If fluids can be kept to a minimum a urinary catheter is not needed.

  3. Intraoperative cortical mapping

    a. After dural opening, mapping is accomplished by placing a stimulating electrode directly on the cortex.

    b. Most common functions assessed are speech, motor, and sensory.

    c. Some patients may require repeated monitoring and mapping during tumor resection.

F. Complications

  1. Respiratory

    a. Oxygen desaturation and airway obstruction may result from oversedation, seizures, mechanical obstruction, or loss of consciousness from an intracranial event.

    b. Treatment needs to be immediate and can include stopping or decreasing sedation or use of jaw thrust or securing of the airway with an oral or nasal airway, LMA, or endotracheal tube.

  2. Excessive pain or discomfort

    a. Pain may occur during pin fixation, dissection of the temporalis muscle, traction on the dura, and manipulation of the intracerebral blood vessels.

    b. Treatment is with additional analgesia or sedation or infiltration of local anesthesia.

  3. Seizures

    a. May occur in patients who have or have not had preoperative seizures.

    b. Most commonly occurs during cortical stimulation.

    c. Surgeons will treat the seizure by placing cold solution on the cortex.

    d. Additional therapy, if needed, is with small dose of propofol (20 to 30 mg) or midazolam (1 mg).

    e. Some patients may need to be started on fosphenytoin or phenytoin.

  4. Induction of general anesthesia during conscious sedation procedures

    a. This may be required for the management of ongoing complications and catastrophic intracranial events including loss of consciousness and bleeding.

    b. Depending on the patient, the airway may be secured with any technique the anesthesiologist is skilled with. This includes LMA, video laryngoscopy, or fiberoptic bronchoscopy.

  5. Other complications

    a. Less common problems are an uncooperative or disinhibited patient, a tight brain, and nausea and vomiting.

REFERENCES

1. Dagal A, Lam AM. Cerebral autoregulation and anesthesia. *Curr Opin Anaesthesiol.* 2009;22(5):547–552.
2. Sharma D, Bithal PK, Dash HH, et al. Cerebral autoregulation and CO_2 reactivity before and after elective supratentorial tumor resection. *J Neurosurg Anesthesiol.* 2010;22(2):132–137.
3. Sivanaser V, Manninen P. Preoperative assessment of adult patients for intracranial surgery. *Anesthesiol Res Pract.* 2010: 241–307.
4. Hans P, Bonhomme V. Why we still use intravenous drugs as the basic regimen for neurosurgical anaesthesia. *Curr Opin Anaesthesiol.* 2006;19(5):498–503.
5. Engelhard K, Werner C. Inhalational or intravenous anesthetics for craniotomies? Pro inhalational. *Curr Opin Anaesthesiol.* 2006;19(5):504–508.
6. Lauta E, Abbinante C, Del Gaudio A, et al. Emergence times are similar with sevoflurane and total intravenous anesthesia: results of a multicenter RCT of patients scheduled for elective supratentorial craniotomy. *J Neurosurg Anesthesiol.* 2010;22(2):110–118.
7. Pasternak JJ, Lanier WL. Is nitrous oxide use appropriate in neurosurgical and neurologically at-risk patients? *Curr Opin Anaesthesiol.* 2010;23(5):544–550.
8. Maurtua MA, Deogaonkar A, Bakri MH, et al. Dosing of remifentanil to prevent movement during craniotomy in the absence of neuromuscular blockade. *J Neurosurg Anesthesiol.* 2008;20:221–225.

9. Bekker A, Sturaitis M, Bloom M, et al. The effect of dexmedetomidine on perioperative hemodynamics in patients undergoing craniotomy. *Anesth Analg.* 2008;107:1340–1347.

10. Tanskanen PE, Kyttä JV, Randell TT, et al. Dexmedetomidine as an anaesthetic adjuvant in patients undergoing intracranial surgery: a double-blind, randomized and placebo-controlled study. *Br J Anaesth.* 2006;97:658–665.

11. Neufeld SM, Newburn-Cook CV. The efficacy of 5-HT$_3$ receptor antagonists for the prevention of postoperative nausea and vomiting after craniotomy: A meta-analysis. *J Neurosurg Anesthesiol.* 2007;19:10–17.

12. Jain V, Mitra JK, Rath GP, et al. A randomized, double-blinded comparison of ondansetron, granisetron, and placebo for prevention of postoperative nausea and vomiting after supratentorial craniotomy. *J Neurosurg Anesthesiol.* 2009;21:226–230.

13. Randell T, Niskanen M. Management of physiological variables in neuroanaesthesia: maintaining homeostasis during intracranial surgery. *Curr Opin Anaesthesiol.* 2006;19(5):492–497.

14. Gelb AW, Craen RA, Rao GS, et al. Does hyperventilation improve operating condition during supratentorial craniotomy? A multicenter randomized crossover trial. *Anesth Analg.* 2008;106:585–594.

15. Bilotta F, Rosa G. Glucose management in the neurosurgical patient: are we yet any closer? *Curr Opin Anaesthesiol.* 2010;23:539–543.

16. Lukins MB, Manninen PH. Hyperglycemia in patients administered dexamethasone for craniotomy. *Anesth Analg.* 2005; 100:1129–1133.

17. Todd MM, Hindman BJ, Clarke WR, et al. Mild intraoperative hypothermia during surgery for intracranial aneurysm. *N Eng J Med.* 2005;352:135–145.

18. McEwen J, Huttunen KTH. Transfusion practice in neuroanesthesia. *Curr Opin Anaesthesiol.* 2009;22:566–571.

19. Brown CV, Sowery L, Curry E, et al. Recombinant factor VIIa to correct coagulopathy in patients with traumatic brain injury presenting to outlying facilities before transfer to the regional trauma center. *Am Surg.* 2012;78:57–60.

20. Stein DM, Dutton RP, Kramer ME, et al. Reversal of coagulopathy in critically ill patients with traumatic brain injury: recombinant factor VIIa is more cost-effective than plasma. *J Trauma.* 2009;66:63–72.

21. Fàbregas N, Bruder N. Recovery and neurological evaluation. *Best Pract Res Clin Anaesthesiol.* 2007;21:431–447.

22. Basali A, Mascha EJ, Kalfas I, et al. Relation between perioperative hypertension and intracranial hemorrhage after craniotomy. *Anesthesiology.* 2000;93:48–54.

23. Grillo P, Bruder N, Auquier P, et al. Esmolol blunts the cerebral blood flow velocity increase during emergence from anesthesia in neurosurgical patients. *Anesth Analg.* 2003;96:1145–1149.

24. Bruder N, Pellissier D, Grillot P, et al. Cerebral hyperemia during recovery from general anesthesia in neurosurgical patients. *Anesth Analg.* 2002;94:650–654.

25. Flexman AM, Ng JL, Gelb AW. Acute and chronic pain following craniotomy. *Curr Opin Anaesthesiol.* 2010;23:551–557.

26. Manninen PH, Balki M, Lukitto K, et al. Patient satisfaction with awake craniotomy for tumor surgery: a comparison of remifentanil and fentanyl in conjunction with propofol. *Anesth Analg.* 2006;102:237–242.

27. Bilotta F, Rosa G. 'Anesthesia' for awake neurosurgery. *Curr Opin Anaesthesiol.* 2009;22(5):560–565.

5 Emergency Craniotomy

Michael V. Presta and Ricky B. Shah

KEY POINTS

1. Prevention of aggravating factors that worsen secondary injury is the mainstay of perioperative care for patients with traumatic brain injury.
2. Succinylcholine is not contraindicated with patients with intracranial hypertension as human studies have not shown demonstrable increases in ICP, especially if the patient has adequate $PaCO_2$, MAP, and depth of anesthesia.
3. Recommendations by the Brain Trauma Foundation are a cerebral perfusion pressure (MAP – ICP) goals of 50 to 70 mm Hg.
4. Treatment of intracranial hypertension should include enabling venous drainage, diuretic therapy, barbiturates, propofol, and extraventricular drain. Hyperventilation should be used only in short periods of time to quickly and effectively decrease ICP. New data has put decompressive craniectomy into question.
5. Normoglycemia and normothermia should be strived for in caring for these patients in the operating room.

EMERGENCY CRANIOTOMY for neurologic conditions caused by entities such as traumatic brain injury (TBI) and its sequelae involves complex and difficult management decisions. According to the National Center for Injury Prevention and Control, TBI is the leading injury cause of death and permanent disability worldwide. In the United States alone, 1.6 million cases of TBI present to emergency services every year [1]. Many more cases go unreported and untreated. These TBIs lead to more than 250,000 hospitalizations and, ultimately, 50,000 deaths [2]. Treatment of patients with TBI begins at the time of impact. The decision to operate depends mainly on the patient's neurologic status, imaging findings, and extent of cranial injury. Many of these critically ill patients have multiple injuries resulting in significant hemodynamic alterations. As a result, team members from anesthesia play a crucial role throughout the perioperative course and ultimate outcome.

I. **Epidemiology.** TBIs affect all patient populations regardless of race, gender, or age. They occur in a bimodal fashion between the adolescent ages of 15 and 24 and again at age 75 or older. In all age groups, males are affected two times more often than females. The most common causes of TBIs in the United States are motor vehicle collisions, violence, and falls [3–5].

II. **Classification of head injury**
  A. **Primary injury (irreversible impact damage)** manifests within milliseconds and occurs before the patient arrives at the hospital. These include skull fractures, epidural and subdural

hemorrhage, vascular bleeds, subarachnoid bleeds, cortical contusions, bone fragmentations, lacerations, and brainstem contusions. The primary injury may be focal or diffuse. Focal injuries comprise the traumatic intracranial hematomas and contusions; while concussion and diffuse axonal injury are the components of diffuse injury [6,7].

1. **Skull fractures may be of three categories.** Linear fractures, depressed fractures, and penetrating or perforating injuries. This type of injury is related to the nature of the impact. Definite evidence of dural penetration, and/or +/− neurologic deficit usually signals urgent need for craniotomy [8].

2. **Epidural hematomas (EDH)** located between the skull and dura, are almost always caused by skull fractures. Most occur in the temporoparietal region as skull fractures crossing the path of the middle meningeal artery [9].

   a. **Incidence.** 1% of head trauma admissions (≈50% the incidence of acute subdurals) usually occurs in young male adults, and is rare before the age of 2 years or after 60 years.

   b. **Presentation.** Is seen as a "textbook" presentation of a brief posttraumatic loss of consciousness followed by a "lucid interval" for several hours, then obtundation, contralateral hemiparesis, and ipsilateral papillary dilation.

   c. **Emergent treatment.** Emergent craniotomy and surgical evacuation for any symptomatic EDH or any asymptomatic EDH >1 cm in its thickest measurement. Threshold for pediatric patients is even lower as these patients do not have the room adult patients have to reabsorb the blood and for clot to initiate [10,11].

3. **Acute subdural hematomas (ASDHs)** are insidiously developing crescent-shaped focal intracranial lesions frequently caused by the tearing of bridging veins connecting the cerebral cortex and dural sinuses. This is a consequence seen in sudden movements of the head often seen in falls, assaults, and acceleration–deceleration events from sudden motor vehicle collisions. The magnitude of impact damage is usually much higher in ASDHs than in EDHs, which generally makes this lesion more lethal.

   a. **Incidence.** ASDHs have been reported to occur in 5% to 25% of patients with severe head injuries, depending on the study. Chronic SDH has been reported to be 1 to 5.3 cases per 100,000 people per year. Anticoagulation, such as with heparin or warfarin (Coumadin), may be a contributing factor. ASDHs are usually characterized based on their size, location, and age (i.e., whether they are acute, subacute, or chronic). These factors, as well as the neurologic and medical conditions of the patient, determine the course of treatment and may also influence the outcome. ASDHs are usually caused by trauma but can be spontaneous or caused by a procedure, such as a lumbar puncture [12].

   b. **Presentation.** Severe underlying primary brain injury with often no "lucid interval." A host of findings could be associated with these, such as brisk or abnormal reflexes, aphasia (usually with a left-sided hematoma), upper-extremity drift, or impairment of cortical sensory function.

   c. **Emergent treatment.** Rapid surgical evacuation via craniotomy or burr holes should be considered for symptomatic subdurals that are greater than about 1 cm at the thickest point (or >5 mm in peds). Smaller subdurals often do not require evacuation, and surgery may increase the brain injury if there is severe hemispheric swelling with herniation through the craniotomy [13].

4. **Intracerebral hematoma (ICH).** ICH is a common cause of stroke, trailing only embolic infarction and atherosclerotic thrombosis in frequency. When it occurs, ICH is a medical emergency, characterized by high morbidity and mortality, which should be promptly diagnosed and aggressively managed. Hematoma expansion and early deterioration are common within the first few hours after onset. The risk for early neurologic deterioration and the high rate of poor long-term outcomes underscore the need for aggressive early management. Hypertensive hemorrhages occur in the territory of penetrator arteries that branch off major intracerebral arteries, often at 90-degree angles with the parent vessel. The blood vessels that give rise to hypertensive hemorrhage generally are the same as those affected by hypertensive occlusive disease and diabetic vasculopathy. Thus typical locations

of hypertensive ICH are putamen, subcortical cerebral lobe, thalamus, cerebellum, brainstem, and caudate nucleus. Each location may differ in clinical presentation, prognosis, and consideration for surgical treatment. Noncontrast cranial CT is the study of choice to evaluate for the presence of acute ICH, which is evident almost immediately. CT scans define the size and location of the hematoma. They also provide information about extension into the ventricular system, the presence of surrounding edema, and shifts in brain contents (hernia). The decision about whether and when to surgically remove ICH remains controversial. The pathophysiology of brain injury surrounding the hematoma is due to the mechanical effects of the growing mass of blood as well as the subsequent toxic effects of blood in the surrounding brain tissue. Early surgery to limit the mechanical compression of brain and the toxic effects of blood may limit injury, but the surgical risks in a patient with ongoing bleeding may be greater. In addition, operative removal of hemorrhage by craniotomy in all but the most superficial hemorrhages involves cutting through uninjured brain. Even after the International Surgical Trial in Intracerebral Haemorrhage (STICH) published its results from over an 8-year period, drawing firm conclusions from the data is a difficult and daunting task. Among the limitations of ICH surgical trials is that young and middle-aged patients at risk of herniation from large ICHs were unlikely to be randomized for treatment. The American Stroke Association (ASA) 2010 guidelines recommend patients with cerebellar hemorrhage who are deteriorating neurologically or who have brainstem compression and/or hydrocephalus from ventricular obstruction should undergo surgical removal of the hemorrhage as soon as possible. Initial treatment of these patients with ventricular drainage alone rather than surgical evacuation is not recommended. For patients presenting with lobar clots >30 mL and within 1 cm of the surface, evacuation of supratentorial ICH by standard craniotomy might be considered. Although theoretically attractive, no clear evidence at present indicates that ultra-early removal of supratentorial ICH improves functional outcome or mortality rate. Very early craniotomy in these patients may be harmful due to increased risk of recurrent bleeding [14,15].

B. **Secondary injury** develops (minutes to hours) subsequent to the impact damage. It includes a constellation of complicating injuries from the inciting event and consists of intracranial hematomas, edema, hypoxia, ischemia (primarily due to elevated intracranial pressure [ICP]), and/or shock. Prevention of further hypoxemia, hypotension, hypercarbia, anemia, and hyperglycemia are the mainstay of managing further injury.

III. **Preoperative evaluation and preparation**

A. **Neurologic assessment**

1. **The Glasgow coma scale (GCS)** is the most widely used method to assess neurologic status and severity of brain dysfunction following head trauma [16]. The scale, which ranges from 3 to 15 points, is based on evaluating the best motor response, the best verbal response, and eye opening (see table in previous chapter). Of the patients who initially survive TBI, 80% have minor injury (GCS 13 to 15), 10% have moderate injury (GCS 9 to 12), and 10% have severe injury (GCS <9). Serial measurements monitoring the patients status prior to the OR is essential with the knowledge that decreases in the GCS of three or more points are indicative of catastrophic neurologic deterioration. A patient with a GCS of 8 or less is sufficiently depressed that endotracheal intubation is indicated.

2. More complex classification systems, such as the **revised trauma score (RTS)** add physiologic data to the equation in an attempt to more precisely define the severity, which can be useful in triaging casualties as well as in determining medical management and predicting prognosis. It uses three specific physiologic parameters, [1] GCS, [2] systolic blood pressure (SBP), and [3] respiratory rate (RR). The main advantage of the coded RTS is that the weighing of the individual components emphasizes the significant impact of TBI on outcome [17].

B. **Airway**

1. **Intubation.** Given the sensitivity of the brain to hypoxemia and both hyper- and hypocarbia, securing the airway is of utmost importance. Endotracheal intubation not only provides a

secure airway in a patient with an altered ability to protect his airway, but also allows for the ability to hyperventilate the patient, providing a rapid method to lower ICP. Patients with severe TBI usually have several indications for intubation including decreased level of consciousness, increased risk of aspiration, and concern for hypoxemia and hypercarbia.

2. **Cervical spine precautions.** Patients with TBI have up to a 5% to 6% incidence of an unstable cervical spine injury [18,19]. Risk factors include a motor vehicle accident and a GCS less than 8. Therefore, all attempts at intubation should include in-line neck stabilization to decrease the chance of worsening a neurologic injury. This maneuver may worsen the view of the glottis, making intubation more difficult. Therefore, one must always have a backup plan and device in mind when performing an emergency intubation, including but not limited to laryngeal masks and fiberoptic or video laryngoscopy technology. Patients with TBI should generally be intubated orally and not nasally because of the potential risk of intracranial migration of the endotracheal tube through a basal skull fracture defect. A surgical airway remains a viable and appropriate option in the setting of severe facial and neck trauma.

3. **Monitoring.** ASA monitors along with direct intra-arterial pressure monitoring (zeroed at the level of the head to facilitate calculation of cerebral perfusion pressure [CPP]) and bladder catheterization are mandatory.

    a. Rapid changes in hemodynamic parameters during induction, positioning, surgical manipulation, and emergence require invasive monitoring along with large bore IV's and/or central venous access for patients requiring vasoactive drugs.

    b. Subclavian veins are usually preferred as to avoid the jugular vein and the risks of carotid puncture and impaired venous drainage from the brain.

    c. A subdural bolt or ventriculostomy is placed by the neurosurgeons to facilitate perioperative management of ICP.

4. **Induction drugs.** Hypotension is extremely detrimental to the injured brain, as discussed previously, while hypertension may increase ICP, worsening cerebral ischemia and causing cerebral herniation. Therefore, choice of drugs must be tailored to each individual patient.

    a. Sodium thiopental in a dose of 3 to 6 mg/kg is a useful drug in euvolemic hemodynamically stable patients. This drug decreases cerebral blood flow (CBF) through its effect on cerebral metabolic rate of oxygen ($CMRO_2$), thereby decreasing ICP. However, it can cause severe hypotension, particularly in a hypovolemic patient.

    b. Propofol has similar effects as above in doses of 2 to 4 mg/kg; however, the decrease in CBF may exceed that in metabolic rate. Although it has been associated with dystonic and choreiform movements it appears to have an added benefit in its anticonvulsant profile along with a short elimination half-life.

    c. Etomidate can be given in doses of 0.2 to 0.3 mg/kg. This drug also decreases $CMRO_2$ and CBF but has less effect on blood pressure. Care must be taken in the acutely unstable patient with the administration of any potent sedative hypnotic drug, as even etomidate can produce hypotension. Etomidate is associated with a relative high incidence of myoclonic movements and even reports of seizure activity following administration. This may limit its usefulness in patients with a history of epilepsy.

    d. Lidocaine in doses of 1.5 mg/kg may inhibit the effects of laryngoscopy decreasing ICP, CMR, and CBF with minimal hemodynamic effects. The risks of systemic toxicity and seizures, however, limit the usefulness of repeated dosing.

5. **Muscle relaxants.** While muscle relaxants prevent the spikes of ICP associated with coughing, they can be controversial when it comes to TBI. The main choice is between succinylcholine and rocuronium, the two agents with the fastest onset. The main argument against the use of succinylcholine in patients with TBI is the potential transient increase in ICP. Succinylcholine has been shown in animal and human studies to increase ICP through muscle spindle activation with depolarization [20]. This can be eliminated with a small dose of a nondepolarizing drug before administrating succinylcholine. In fact, Kovarik et al. [21] studied the effects of this drug in ventilated neurologically injured patients and observed no increase in ICP or CBF velocity. On the other side, rocuronium, with its

intermediate duration of action, may preclude neurologic examination for the next 60 to 90 minutes. Furthermore, one must be able to manage the airway for that length of time there should be problems with tracheal intubation. The detrimental effects of hypoxemia and hypercarbia are clearly the most important to avoid, often making succinylcholine the preferred agent.

IV. Intraoperative management

    A. Fluids. Crystalloid or colloid resuscitation in TBI remains controversial. Despite the many theoretical benefits of human albumin administration in critically ill patients, there has been little evidence to support its widespread clinical use. Previous systematic reviews have led to conflicting results regarding the safety and efficacy of albumin. The recently reported saline versus albumin evaluation study has provided conclusive evidence that 4% albumin is as safe as saline for resuscitation, although no overall benefit of albumin use was seen [22]. Subgroup analysis of the albumin-treated group revealed a trend toward decreased mortality in patients with septic shock, and a trend toward increased mortality in trauma patients, especially those with TBI. Another commonly used colloid, hydroxyethyl starch, can aggravate coagulopathy, even in small doses, and should be avoided in patients with brain injuries. Thus, hypertonic or isotonic crystalloid is the preferred fluid in patients with TBI, and the most appropriate colloid to be used is blood when indicated [see Chapter 3].

    B. Hemodynamic control. Hypertension and hypotension should both be avoided in emergency craniotomy to maintain adequate CBF.

        1. CBF (normally 45 to 55 mL/100 g brain tissue/min) is regulated by autoregulation.

        2. Autoregulation is the capacity for cerebral vessel resistance to maintain constant CBF over a wide range of mean arterial pressure (MAP). Autoregulation has been shown to be defective in an injured brain, thus protection of constant CBF is lost.

            a. Hypotension—to maintain constant CBF, autoregulation will cause smooth muscle relaxation to cause cerebral vasodilation.

            b. Hypertension—increased cerebral blood pressure could equate to increased CBF. Autoregulation, to maintain constant CBF, will cause contraction of arteriole smooth muscle to cause vasoconstriction.

            c. Cerebral autoregulation—given a wide range of perfusion pressures, will maintain a constant CBF by changing the caliber/diameter of the cerebral vessels.

        3. Hypotension has been shown in clinical surveys to have poor clinical outcomes with TBI.

            a. A sizeable percentage of those who die from TBI, have evidence of ischemia on autopsy.

            b. Recommendations by the Brain Trauma Foundation have stated cerebral perfusion pressure (MAP – ICP) goals of 50 to 70 mm Hg [23].

        4. Uncontrolled hypertension could be harmful as well.

            a. The Lund concept is based on the fact that increased blood pressures equate to high blood volume predisposing to hydrostatic edema.

            b. Increased edema and hyperemia could develop into increased ICP.

            c. Most still agree about a cerebral perfusion pressure of 50 to 70 mm Hg.

    C. Intracranial hypertension. Elevation of pressure in the cranium—normal ICP is defined as 7 to 15 mm Hg.

        1. Monro–Kellie doctrine

            a. The cranium is a fixed-sized cavity which can hold only a specific amount of volume.

            b. The cranium only holds four components. Cerebral spinal fluid (CSF), venous blood, arterial blood, and brain tissue.

            c. Compensation occurs as expansion of one of the component's volume increases (e.g., brain swelling).

                (1) CSF in the brain relocates to spinal CSF space

                (2) Venous blood moves to extracranial veins

                (3) Past a specific volume, compensation is unable to work and pressure increases exponentially causing decreases in CPP (arterial blood) and herniation (brain tissue).

2. **Treatment of intracranial hypertension**
   a. **Hyperventilation**
      (1) Arterial hypercapnia dilates cerebral blood vessels, decreases cerebral vascular resistance, ultimately, increasing CBF.
      (2) Hyperventilation, which does the opposite, is then used to decrease ICP by decreasing cerebral blood volume.
      (3) There is a decrease in CBF without effect on cerebral metabolic oxygen consumption ($CMRO_2$), causing a mismatch.
      (4) Mismatch can cause cerebral ischemia and further neuronal compromise [24]. Only short periods of hyperventilation are recommended to quickly and effectively decrease ICP.
   b. **Diuretic therapy is used to decrease volume (mostly extracelluar)**
      (1) Although osmotic and loop diuretics are used, osmotic diuretics are preferred due to rapid onset.
      (2) Mannitol, possessing an osmotic load, is able to establish a gradient allowing cerebral water to flow from cells across an intact blood–brain barrier.
      (3) Mannitol enters the brain and quickly appears in the CSF space.
      (4) Mannitol's rapid efficacy is probably from the plasma-expanding effect increasing CBF from reduced blood viscosity. This, in turn, causes autoregulatory vasoconstriction.
      (5) Mannitol should be administered as bolus form as infusions may cause interstitial accumulation.
      (6) The dose of mannitol should be 0.25 to 1 g/kg over 10 to 15 minutes (too quick of an administration can cause extreme hyperosmolality causing vasodilatory effect and increased ICP).
      (7) Furosemide removes brain water by acting on aquaporins. Aquaporins are a family of membrane channels that regulate flux of water in and out of cells.
   c. **Enable adequate venous drainage**
      (1) The reverse Trendelenburg position enables good venous drainage.
      (2) If the patient is hypovolemic, decreased venous return caused by this position may inhibit adequate cardiac output and essentially CPP.
      (3) Maintain patient path for venous drainage (e.g., Philadelphia collars, circumferential tracheostomy collar ties).
      (4) Avoid increases in central venous pressure (excessive PEEP or cardiac failure).
      (5) If PEEP is required for improved oxygenation, elevating the head of bed may assist in proper venous drainage.
      (6) Avoid increases in intrathoracic pressure (obstructed endotracheal tubes, Valsalva maneuver, bronchospasm).
      (7) Keeping the head in the neutral position allows for appropriate venous drainage.
   d. **Barbiturates**
      (1) Are used after other modalities have been exhausted and the patient continues to exhibit intracranial hypertension.
      (2) The mechanism is from [1] decreases in $CMRO_2$ and [2] cerebral vasoconstriction causing cerebral blood volume and flow reductions.
      (3) As barbiturates can cause a sudden and dramatic decrease in MAP, adequate fluid resuscitation and possible use of vasopressors may need to be employed.
      (4) There is no evidence that prophylactic barbiturate improves outcomes.
      (5) A slow plasma clearance could delay awakening and thwart a neurologic examination.
   e. **Decompressive craniectomy is performed when all "first-tier" therapies have failed**
      (1) Composes of a large bifrontotemporoparietal craniectomy with bilateral dural opening and storing of excised bone in either the cold (−70°C) or subcutaneous abdominal pouch.

4

        (2) A multicenter-randomized trial was performed comparing standard ICP treatment with decompressive craniectomy as a last resort versus just standard ICP treatment [25].

          (a) Decompressive craniectomy patients had lower ICP, less time on mechanical ventilation, and less time in the ICU.

          (b) They also had a higher amount of unfavorable outcomes (including death, vegetative state, and severe disability) and worse scores on the extended Glasgow outcome scale.

D. Glycemic control

5

    1. Hyperglycemia causing increased morbidity and mortality in TBI has been established by many studies.

    2. The cause of intraoperative hyperglycemia has been postulated to be from the stress response of the injury prior to surgery along with increases in blood glucose values seen under anesthesia in nondiabetic patients.

    3. Hyperglycemia's damage is caused possibly by an increase in brain parenchymal glycolytic rates producing pyruvate and lactate. This induced metabolic acidosis will also produce oxygen-free radicals and ultimately neuronal cell death.

    4. In a recent retrospective study by Pecha et al. [26], it was seen that 95% of patients showed at least one intraoperative glucose value greater than 200 mg/dL.

      a. Moreover, those who had intraoperative hyperglycemia had a mortality of 31% compared to 13% in those without hyperglycemia ($P = 0.02$).

      b. Independent risk factors for hyperglycemia were severe TBI, subdural hematoma, preoperative hyperglycemia, and age >65 years.

E. Temperature control

5

    1. Theoretically, decreasing a patient body temperature should also decrease their cerebral metabolic demand, thus helping with neuroprotection.

    2. Studies on laboratory animals showed a reduction in cerebral edema and death with moderate, systemic hypothermia.

    3. However, The National Acute Brain Injury Study showed different results with hypothermia in human subjects [27].

      a. Randomized, prospective, multicenter study comparing induced hypothermia versus normothermia patients with nonpenetrating head injuries.

      b. There was no significant difference in outcome or mortality between the two.

      c. Significantly higher incidence of critical hypotension causing organ failure and bradycardia causing hypotension in the induced hypothermia patients.

V. Anesthetic agent

A. Induction agents

    1. Barbiturates

      a. Dose-dependent decrease in CBF and $CMRO_2$.

      b. Prolonged use could cause increased context-sensitive half-time.

4

    2. Propofol

      a. Similar reduction in CBF and $CMRO_2$ compared to barbiturates.

      b. Context-sensitive half-life profile better than barbiturates.

    3. Etomidate

      a. Has been shown to decrease CBF similar to barbiturates.

      b. $CMRO_2$ reductions are less pronounced than with barbiturates and are regional (only in forebrain structures).

      c. This mismatch in CBF and $CMRO_2$ could be the reason that more tissue hypoxia and acidosis has been witnessed.

      d. Multiple dosing of this agent has been shown to cause adrenocortical suppression.

    4. Ketamine

      a. Increases both CBF and $CMRO_2$.

      b. Increased ICP has been witnessed in humans after administration.

  c. May be used cautiously in conjunction with other agents (e.g., propofol) and not have such an effect on ICP, CBF, and $CMRO_2$.

B. Volatile anesthetics
 1. Causes a dose-dependent decrease in $CMRO_2$.
 2. Causes a cerebral vasodilation (smooth muscle relaxation) causing increase in CBF.
 3. This mismatch of $CMRO_2$ and CBF is considered "uncoupled" (compared to IV agents which are "coupled").
 4. There are some studies to show that isoflurane has more vasodilatory properties than desflurane or sevoflurane allowing increased CBF [28].

C. Nitrous oxide
 1. Causes an increase in CBF, $CMRO_2$, and ICP.
 2. Increases in CBF and ICP are dramatically seen when administered alone.
 3. When administered with other agents (e.g., propofol) there still is a moderate increase in ICP.
 4. Due to space-occupying property, it should not be used if there is suspicion of pneumocephalus or air embolism.

D. Nondepolarizing muscle relaxants
 1. No effect on CBF or $CMRO_2$.
 2. Possible histamine release after benzoisoquinolones could decrease MAP and ultimately CPP.

E. Opioid
 1. Little intrinsic effect on CBF or $CMRO_2$.
 2. They are useful with analgesia. Especially since pain can cause spikes in ICP.
 3. Decreases MAC.

F. Benzodiazepines
 1. Causes a decrease in both CBF and $CMRO_2$.
 2. May interfere with postoperative neurologic examination if used excessively or over a longer period of time.

REFERENCES

1. National Center for Injury Prevention and Control. Facts about traumatic brain injury. http://www.cdc.gov/TraumaticBrainInjury/index.html.
2. Novack T. TBI inform: introduction to brain injury fact and stats. http://main.uab.edu/tbi/show.asp?durki=27492& site=2988& return=57898.
3. Badjatia N, Carney N, Crocco TJ, et al., Brain Trauma Foundation, BTF Center for Guidelines Management. Guidelines for the prehospital management of traumatic brain injury. 2nd edition. *Prehosp Emerg Care.* 2008;12 suppl 1:S1–S52.
4. NICHCY disability fact sheet: Traumatic brain injury. http://nichcy.org/disability/specific/tbi.
5. Bratton SL, Chestnut RM, Jamshid Ghajar J, et al., Brain Trauma Foundation, American Association of Neurological Surgeons/ College of Neurological Surgeons, Joint Section on Neurotrauma and Critical Care: Guidelines for the management of severe traumatic brain injury, 3rd edition. *J Neurotrauma.* 2007;24 suppl 1:S1–S95.
6. Mendelow AD, Teasdale G, Jennett B, et al. Risks of intracranial haematoma in head injured adults. *Br Med J (Clin Res Ed).* 1983;287(6400):1173–1176.
7. Heary RF, Hunt CD, Krieger AJ, et al. Nonsurgical treatment of compound depressed skull fractures. *J Trauma.* 1993;35(3):441–447.
8. Graham D. Neuropathology of head injury. In: Narayan RK, Wilberger JE, Povlishock JT, eds. *Neurotrauma.* New York, NY: McGraw-Hill; 1996:43–59.
9. Jamieson KG, Yelland JD. Extradural hematoma. Report of 167 cases. *J Neurosurg.* 1968;29(1):13–23.
10. Chen TY, Wong CW, Chang CN, et al. The expectant treatment of "asymptomatic" supratentorial epidural hematomas. *Neurosurgery.* 1993;32(2):176–179; discussion 179.
11. Wong CW. The CT criteria for conservative treatment–but under close clinical observation–of posterior fossa epidural haematomas. *Acta Neurochir (Wien).* 1994;126(2–4):124–127.
12. Wilberger JE, Harris M, Diamond DL. Acute subdural hematoma: morbidity, mortality, and operative timing. *J Neurosurg.* 1991;74(2):212–218.
13. Servadei F. Prognostic factors in severely head injured adult patients with acute subdural haematoma's. *Acta Neurochir (Wien).* 1997;139(4):279–285.
14. Van Loon J, Van Calenbergh F, Goffin J, et al. Controversies in the management of spontaneous cerebellar haemorrhage: a consecutive series of 49 cases and review of the literature. *Acta Neurochir (Wien).* 1993;122(3–4):187–193.

15. Morgenstern LB, Hemphill JC 3rd, Anderson C, et al. Guidelines for the management of spontaneous intracerebral hemorrhage: a guideline for healthcare professionals from the American Heart Association/American Stroke Association. *Stroke.* 2010;41(9):2108–2129.
16. Stein SC. Classification of head injury. In: Narayan RK, Wilberger JE, Povlishock JT, eds. *Neurotrauma.* New York, NY: McGraw-Hill; 1996:31–41.
17. Champion HR, Sacco WJ, Copes WS. A revision of the Trauma Score. *J Trauma.* 1989;29(5):623–629.
18. Alexander RH, Procter HJ, eds. *Advanced Trauma Life Support Program for Physicians.* Chicago, IL: American College of Surgeons; 1993.
19. Davis JW, Parks SN, Detlefs CL, et al. Clearing the cervical spine in obtunded patients: the use of dynamic fluoroscopy. *J Trauma.* 1995;39(3):435–438.
20. Lanier WL, Milde JH, Michenfelder JD. Cerebral stimulation following succinylcholine in dogs. *Anesthesiology.* 1986;64(5):551–559.
21. Kovarik WD, Mayberg TS, Lam AM, et al. Succinylcholine does not change intracranial pressure, cerebral blood flow velocity, or the electroencephalogram in patients with neurologic injury. *Anesth Analg.* 1994;78(3):469–473.
22. Finfer S, Bellomo R, Boyce N, et al; SAFE Study Investigators. A comparison of albumin and saline for fluid resuscitation in the intensive care unit. *N Engl J Med.* 2004;350(22):2247–2256.
23. Bratton SL, Chestnut RM, Jamshid Ghajar J, et al. Guidelines for the management of severe traumatic brain injury. *J Neurotrauma.* 2007;24:S1–S106.
24. Coles JP, Fryer TD, Coleman MR, et al. Hyperventilation following head injury: effect on ischemic burden and cerebral oxidative metabolism. *Crit Care Med.* 2007;35(2):568–578.
25. Mielck F, Stephan H, Weyland A, et al. Effects of one minimum alveolar anesthetic concentration sevoflurane on cerebral metabolism, blood flow, and CO2 reactivity in cardiac patients. *Anesth Analg.* 1999;89(2):364–369.
26. Cooper DJ, Rosenfeld JV, Murray L, et al. Decompressive craniectomy in diffuse traumatic brain injury. *N Engl J Med.* 2011;364(16):1493–1502.
27. Pecha T, Sharma D, Hoffman NG, et al. Hyperglycemia during craniotomy for adult traumatic brain injury. *Anesth Analg.* 2011;113(2):336–342.
28. Clifton GL, Miller ER, Choi SC, et al. Lack of effect of induction of hypothermia after acute brain injury. *N Engl J Med.* 2001;344(8):556–563.

6 Posterior Fossa Tumor Surgery

Audrice Francois

KEY POINTS

1. Most central nervous system tumors in pediatrics are in the posterior fossa.
2. The cerebellum plays a key role in cognition.
3. Central nervous system tumors in young children are diagnosed late in the disease course.
4. When intracardiac right to left shunts are present, the risk of paradoxical air embolism is higher.
5. Posterior fossa syndrome may complicate posterior fossa surgery.

I. Introduction

A. Central nervous system (CNS) tumors are the most common solid cancers in children. They occur almost as often as the leukemias. Although the overall 5-year survival over the past 3 decades has improved significantly, CNS tumors are still the leading cause of childhood cancer deaths [1].

B. The majority of pediatric brain tumors are located in the posterior fossa. The opposite is true in adults, in whom two-thirds of brain tumors are supratentorial with only 15% to 20% of brain tumors in adults occurring in the posterior fossa. Approximately half of these tumors in children are malignant. Children may also have a more favorable outcome than do adults with histologically similar tumors.

CLINICAL PEARL   Most childhood brain tumors are in the posterior fossa, a critical location

II. Neuroanatomy of the posterior fossa

A. The posterior fossa is the largest and deepest of the three cranial fossae. It comprises the cerebellum, the pons, and the medulla oblongata, and lies between the foramen magnum and the tentorium cerebellum. The tentorium cerebellum, an extension of the dura mater, forms a roof or tent over the posterior cranial fossa, separating it from the cerebral hemispheres.

B. The posterior fossa is a critical location for pathology because of the limited space and the potential for involvement of brainstem nuclei. The cerebellum comprises three functionally distinct regions: The vestibulocerebellum, the spinocerebellum, and the cerebrocerebellum which, respectively, control the vestibular system, body and limb movements, and internal feedback, planning, and cognition. The cerebellum has two hemispheres; it also has a narrow, unpaired, midline zone called the vermis.

C. The cerebellum is configured with a large number of tight folds arranged in the style of an accordion, and has numerous, small granule cells. It has a myriad of functions and circuitry loops with the rest of the brain. Its role is not only in motor control and muscle tone, but in cognition, attention, emotion, and speech articulation. Hence, pathology to this region is critical [2]. The cerebellum regulates and coordinates axial and girdle musculature and receives spinal, vestibular and auditory input relayed by the brainstem nuclei. It integrates these various inputs in order to calibrate and fine tune motor activity. The cerebellum also receives and modulates dopaminergic, serotonergic, noradrenergic, and cholinergic inputs. The pons, superior to the medulla, is separated from it by a groove through which the sixth, seventh, and eighth cranial nerves emerge. It is a communication center and relays signals from other parts of the brain to the cerebellum. The pons also has nuclei dealing with a wide range of functions including sleep, respiration, swallowing, bladder control, hearing, equilibrium, and facial expressions. The medulla is the inferior portion of the brainstem and continues on to the spinal cord. The medulla is a highly complex neural structure crowded with cranial nerve nuclei. It contains cardiac, respiratory, vomiting, and vasomotor centers and deals with autonomic functions such as breathing, heart rate, and blood pressure. Therefore, it is not surprising that with all of this neural circuitry, tumors in the posterior fossa present a challenge for the anesthesiologist in the care of these highly vulnerable pediatric patients with such tumors [3].

III. **Types of posterior fossa tumors and associated pathophysiology**

A. Medulloblastomas are the most common pediatric brain tumors [1,2]. They arise from the cerebellar vermis, in the roof of the fourth ventricle and may grow to fill the fourth ventricle. They occur mostly in the first decade of life. These tumors are usually confined to the posterior fossa, but disseminated disease can occur, spreading along the craniospinal axis via the cerebrospinal fluid (CSF) pathways, and may also present with back pain or lower limb weakness. Disseminated disease is a predictor of poor outcome [1,2]. Occasionally, metastatic disease is seen outside of the CNS sometimes with bone or bone marrow disease especially in infants. Typically, medulloblastomas present with signs of increased intracranial pressure (ICP) related to obstructive hydrocephalus due to the growth of the tumor, and obstruction of CSF pathways at the fourth ventricle as well as at the Aqueduct of Sylvius. Since medulloblastomas arise in the cerebellar midline at the vermis, truncal or axial instability is often seen, a common finding in midline tumors. The predominant symptoms are the triad of early morning headache (60%), vomiting (67%), and ataxia or unsteady gait (40%). Nausea (39%) is also significant [4]. The lone presenting symptom in young children may be repeated vomiting which results in failure to thrive. Increased head circumference is seen in children whose cranial sutures are not yet fused; however, in these children, virtually no detectable symptoms develop early [4]. Not until spinal fluid flow becomes markedly compromised and causes rapidly enlarging head circumference, will the intracranial tumor be diagnosed. School-aged children may demonstrate a decline in school performance due to vision changes that may accompany hydrocephalus.

B. Astrocytomas comprise 40% of tumors in the posterior fossa in children. They are cerebellar astrocytomas [2]. They usually occur in the first decade and arise from glial cells, specifically astrocytes, named for their star-like appearance. They have a propensity for midline axial structures such as the brainstem and cerebellar vermis. The low-grade pilocytic astrocytomas, referred to as grade I, are slow-growing tumors that rarely spread and present the best chance for survival [2]. They form inside cysts, hence the term pilocytic. For these tumors, the degree of surgical resection is the single most important factor in determining prognosis [1,2]. After complete resection, the 10-year survival is 70% to 100%. Fibrillary astrocytomas, grade II, usually spread within the cerebellum and tend to recur. Presenting symptoms are produced by raised ICP, including headache made worse with exertion, recumbency, and early morning nausea and lethargy. The patient may also have difficulties with speech, may be confused, disoriented and have ataxic gait. As with medulloblastomas, most astrocytomas develop sporadically; however, in some patients there is a genetic tendency [2,4]. Patients with genetic syndromes including neurofibromatosis type I and tuberous sclerosis are at a higher risk of developing tumors of glial origin.

C. Gliomas are characterized based on their histologic similarity to mature glial cells, which are cells that surround and support the proper functioning of nerve cells. Glial cells include astrocytes and oligodendrocytes. Most gliomas originate from astrocytes; so astrocytomas are also gliomas. Glial cancers, mostly infratentorial in children, consist of many heterogeneous tumors that include pilocytic astrocytomas, fibrillary astrocytomas, ependymomas, and the diffuse, intrinsic pontine gliomas [1]. In the posterior fossa, they can arise from the midbrain, pons, medulla and upper cervical cord. Pontine gliomas are the most common. Ten to twenty percent of posterior fossa neoplasms in children are brainstem gliomas and are seen in the first decade of life [2]. As magnetic resonance imaging (MRI) technology has advanced, several types have been described based on their presenting morphology. They are characterized based on their origin, tendency to remain localized, direction and extent of tumor growth, degree of brainstem enlargement, degree of growth outside of their site of origin, presence or absence of cysts, hemorrhage, and hydrocephalus [1,2]. In 2000, Choux [5] described four types of these tumors using computed tomography (CT) and MRI technology to define them. Intrinsic focal, exophytic focal, and cervicomedullary tumors, which are noninfiltrative, sharply demarcated from the surrounding tissues and are low histologic grade tumors. They also cause less brainstem edema. The intrinsic type lacks visible extension into other areas, while the exophytic type may extend posteriorly in the direction of least resistance. These three are also more amenable to surgical resection followed by radiation treatment and they have a good prognosis. The fourth type is described by Choux [5] as being diffuse and does not have well-demarcated boundaries. Their infiltrative, poorly marginated borders are less amenable to complete surgical resection. They cause diffuse infiltration and swelling in the brainstem and are refractory to treat [2]. Tissue diagnosis may alter treatment regimens.

D. Ependymomas are tumors that arise from cells lining the ventricular system and the central spinal canal [6]. Ependymomas in the posterior fossa begin in the floor of the fourth ventricle and present as a fourth ventricular mass with cerebellopontine angle predilection. They are classified as benign or low-grade ependymoma versus anaplastic ependymoma, malignant or high grade. Half of the cases occur before the age of 5 years. Due to their location in the CSF pathways, they are likely to disseminate via the CSF. Extraneural metastases have been reported in the liver, lungs, peritoneum, pleura, and lymph node with dissemination being more frequent in children younger than 3 years old [2]. This is due to the delay in diagnosis in this age group in whom the subtle symptom presentations of lethargy and irritability are nonspecific and the tumors are, therefore, larger at the time of diagnosis; and there is reluctance to perform radiation therapy in young children due to the potential for radiation-induced neurotoxicity [1]. Since ependymomas arise in the fourth ventricle, they cause symptomatic compromise of the CSF pathway and lead to obstructive hydrocephalus and generalized intracranial hypertension [2]. Their location near the area postrema of the fourth ventricle or near vagal nuclei in the medulla is significant in that they may present with recurrent vomiting [1]. The current standard of therapy for infratentorial ependymomas includes surgical excision, the completeness of surgical excision being the most predictive variable on outcome [2,6]. The majority of complete responders have total tumor removal. However, tumor removal may be incomplete due to location near the brainstem, the worst location. Survival rates for ependymoma therefore depend on age, location, grading, as well as their histologic characteristics [2,6].

IV. Diagnostic tests and neuroimaging

A. CT is usually the first-line neuroimaging modality for patients with posterior fossa tumors [4].

B. Patients can also be diagnosed and followed up with nonenhanced and contrast-enhanced MRI of the brain and spine, an integral part of management. MRI scans have become the preferred diagnostic study for pediatric brain tumors as they avoid radiation and provide better definition of the tumor than CT. With MRI, the tumor can also be studied in multiple planes. Magnetic resonance angiography can aid in showing a better image of tumor vessels if they cannot be adequately seen on a routine MRI. Magnetic resonance spectroscopy is useful in evaluating the biochemical composition of CNS tumors, specifically choline, a marker of biomembranes, n-acetyl aspartate, a neuronal cell marker, taurine and other mobile lipids [4].

C. Single photon emission computed tomography (SPECT) is a clinical aid using radio tracer uptake to differentiate postradiation changes and gliosis from tumor recurrence [4].

V. Surgical interventions and treatment

A. The goal of therapy for all of the posterior fossa tumors is to eradicate the tumor while causing the least morbidity. Circumscribed and well-encapsulated tumors, as demonstrated by neuroimaging, can be surgically resected more completely.

B. Radical resections are especially important for children under 2 years old because of the risks of radiation to the developing brain [2,4]. Maximal tumor resection of pediatric gliomas, though controversial in adults, tend to be more valuable for children [1].

C. Many brainstem gliomas have margins that blend imperceptibly with normal tissue, preventing complete resection of the tumor, so stereotactic biopsies may be the only feasible option.

D. The mainstay of treatment for pilocytic astrocytomas and ependymomas is maximal surgical resection [2]. As many of these tumors produce hydrocephalus by obstructing the flow of CSF, this is occasionally treated by performing an endoscopic third ventriculostomy or an external ventricular drain (EVD) at the time of craniotomy. If the surgical procedure has not reestablished the CSF pathways, a ventriculoperitoneal (VP) shunt may be inserted.

VI. Anesthetic management

A. **Preoperative evaluation.** A baseline neurologic evaluation is essential in order to be able to recognize changes from this baseline when the patient emerges from anesthesia, and to be able to differentiate from possible new neurologic impairments. Postural headaches, or irritability in a young child which worsens in the recumbent position, are suggestive of raised ICP. Full fontanel, widely separated cranial sutures, cranial enlargement, papilledema, and diplopia are also suggestive of raised ICP. If there has been protracted vomiting, the patient may be at risk for pulmonary aspiration as well as electrolyte imbalance. If the patient has any right to left intracardiac shunting due to a patent foramen ovale or ductus arteriosus, the risk of paradoxical air embolization from venous air embolism is higher in the sitting surgical position.

B. **Airway.** Airway evaluation will determine whether special intubating techniques are needed, particularly in the case of distorted airway anatomy.

C. **Neuromuscular blockade.** Although a small and transient increase in ICP has been described with succinylcholine, the benefits of using succinylcholine for rapidly establishing intubation conditions may greatly outweigh the risks of pulmonary aspiration. High-dose rocuronium at 0.8 mg/kg may also be used to rapidly establish intubating conditions, aided by an opioid to blunt the hemodynamic response to laryngoscopy and endotracheal intubation.

D. **Surgical position.** Positioning requires care to pad vulnerable areas including the ulnar nerve at the elbow and peroneal nerve at the knee. The preferred surgical approach to posterior fossa tumor is the prone position, with neck flexion for optimal exposure, and the head of the patient fixed in pins, with the abdomen made free for movement during respiration. Neck flexion can change the location of the tip of the endotracheal tube, or even cause kinking of the small endotracheal tube in the posterior pharynx, so breath sounds should be reassessed after positioning. Lateral or park bench position may also be used. The lateral position may result in decreased compliance of the down-side lung [7]. In this position, a pad should be placed in the axilla to minimize the patient's weight on the lower arm and shoulder, and to avoid brachial plexus injury. In either case, head up tilt is often employed to decrease hemorrhage, but this increases the risk of air embolism. The relatively larger head size in children places them at increased risk for air emboli. If the sitting position is adopted, a precordial Doppler monitor, the most sensitive noninvasive monitoring technique, will be essential to detect air embolism, a potentially catastrophic event. It should be placed in the middle third of the sternum or second to fourth intercostal space, to the right of the sternum, or between the right scapula and the spine in prone infants less than 6 kg [8]. Although a multiorifice, central venous catheter for aspirating any venous air is used in adults, this may not be feasible in infants and small children due to the bore of the catheter and the difficulty of aspirating any embolized air. To test for proper functioning of the Doppler probe, agitated saline may be injected through a right atrial catheter or peripheral line while listening for characteristic Doppler sounds. Doppler combined with end-tidal gas monitoring and arterial blood pressure monitoring is essential in the sitting position. A decrease in end-tidal carbon dioxide, however, is not specific for venous air embolism as a decrease in cardiac output by any cause will have the same effect.

> **CLINICAL PEARL** Positioning plays a critical role in posterior fossa surgery.

E. **Hemodynamic monitoring.** As manipulation of the medulla can cause hypertension as well as cardiac dysrhythmias, the arterial line for blood pressure monitoring will be valuable for permitting strict control of blood pressure perioperatively, and for blood sampling to monitor electrolytes, follow hematocrit, and assess blood gases. The transducer should be zeroed at the level of the external auditory meatus to assess cerebral perfusion pressure as this is accepted as indicating the base of the brain. Surgical manipulation of the medulla can cause hypertension as well as cardiac dysrhythmias. Central venous pressure monitoring may be dictated by cardiac, renal, and pulmonary status of the patient, duration of the procedure, and the anticipation of major hemorrhage. It may be useful also if mannitol is used as the use of urine output as a monitor of intravascular volume status will not be helpful in mannitol therapy.

> **CLINICAL PEARL** Manipulation of the medulla may cause dysrhythmias.

F. **Cranial nerve monitoring.** Because of the risk of injury to the nuclei of cranial nerves V, VII, VIII, XI, and XII during posterior fossa surgery, cranial nerve monitoring is often used. Both nitrous oxide and inhalation agents interfere with motor and somatosensory evoked potential (SSEP) affecting the latency, amplitude, and morphology of the evoked potential waves [9]. Brainstem auditory evoked potential (BAEP) generated in the brainstem also called the auditory brainstem response (ABR) is minimally influenced by anesthetics. Opioids have minimal or no effect on neurophysiologic monitoring. BAEP is useful in posterior fossa procedures to monitor the integrity of the brainstem. The use of muscle relaxants complicates interpretation of electromyogram (EMG). It is therefore essential to communicate with the individual responsible for electrophysiologic (EP) monitoring in order to optimize the information obtainable from the evoked potentials of EP monitoring during surgical procedures on the nervous system.

> **CLINICAL PEARL** Disruption of cerebellar circuitry may lead to postoperative speech and language impairment.

VII. **Postoperative complications**

A. **Tracheal extubation.** Depending on the disease process, postoperative patients may have difficulty swallowing, vocalizing, or protecting their airway and may require ventilator support after surgery. There may be tongue and facial edema due to position-induced venous and lymphatic obstruction, which may compromise the patient's airway.

B. **Posterior fossa syndrome.** A symptom complex that includes cerebellar mutism and absence of vocalization has been observed in 25% of patients after posterior fossa surgery for midline tumors [3,4]. Patients may also exhibit dysarthria, hypotonia, dysphagia, and mood lability, as well as deficiencies in cognition. The onset may be immediate or delayed and may persist. It is thought to result from ischemia and edema due to retracted and manipulated dentate nuclei [3].

VIII. **Conclusion.** Brain tumors in children are more likely to be in the posterior fossa. This is a critical location with many vital structures, injury to which can impact their lives. Although there have been many advances in technology in the past decades which account for a decrease in mortality for these patients, their survival is often marked by severe morbidity and neurocognitive complications.

REFERENCES

1. Pollack IF. Multidisciplinary management of childhood brain tumors: a review of outcomes, recent advances, and challenges. *J Neurosurg Pediatr.* 2011;8(2):135–148.
2. Packer RJ, MacDonald T, Vezina G. Central nervous system tumors. *Pediatr Clin North Am.* 2008;55(1):121–145.
3. Kupeli S, Yalcin B, Binginer B, et al. Posterior fossa syndrome after posterior fossa surgery in children with brain tumors. *Pediatr Blood Cancer.* 2011;56(2):206–210.
4. Crawford JR, MacDonald TJ, Packer RJ. Medulloblastoma in childhood: new biological advances. *Lancet Neurol.* 2007;6(12): 1073–1085.
5. Choux M, DiRocco C, Do L. Brainstem tumors. In: Choux M, DiRocco C, Hackley A, eds. *Pediatric Neurosurgery.* New York, NY: Churchill Livingstone; 2000:471–491.
6. Tamburrini G, D'Ercole M, Pettorini BL, et al. Survival following treatment for intracranial ependymoma: a review. *Childs Nerv Syst.* 2009;25(10):1303–1312.
7. Soriano SG, McCann ME, Laussen PC. Neuroanesthesia.Innovative techniques and monitoring. *Anesthesiol Clin North Am.* 2002;20(1):137–151.
8. Lightburn MH, Gauss CH, Williams DK, et al. Cerebral blood flow velocities in extremely low birth weight infants. *J Pediatr.* 2009;154(6):824–828.
9. Sloan T. Anesthesia and intraoperative neurophysiological monitoring in children. *Childs Nerv Syst.* 2010;26(2):227–235.

7 Carotid Endarterectomy

Chiranjeev Saha

KEY POINTS

1. Carotid stenosis is a manifestation of significant generalized atherosclerosis
2. Carotid bruit is an unreliable clinical sign
3. Type of anesthetic (regional or general) for CEA is practice-based
4. Most strokes associated with CEA occur in the postoperative time frame
5. Maintaining hemodynamic stability is vital to safe perioperative anesthetic management

I. Introduction

A. **Epidemiology.** Carotid artery disease, a manifestation of generalized arteriosclerosis, is commonly asymptomatic but can present with amaurosis fugax, transient ischemic attack (TIA), or a cerebrovascular accident (e.g., stroke) [1,2]. A thromboembolic phenomenon appears to play a key role in the signs and symptoms of this disease more than pure stenosis itself. Stroke is directly related to age and is the leading cause of disability and the third most common cause of death in the United States after heart disease and cancer [3]. The incidence of a new or recurrent stroke is approximately 1:700,000 in the United States with about 150,000 deaths, and the annual cost of treating stroke and its associated disabilities amounts to a staggering $40 billion [4].

B. **Pathophysiology.** Carotid stenosis is narrowing of the internal carotid artery lumen due to atherosclerotic plaque formation in the endothelium, usually at the common carotid bifurcation. The carotid endarterectomy (CEA) procedure involves removal of the atheromatous plaque from the vessel lumen and repairing the wall of the arteries (media and adventitia) through a standardized surgical procedure in the neck. Approximately 140,000 CEA procedures were performed in the United States in 2009 [4].

C. **Clinical evidence.** Two Large Randomized Clinical Trials (RCTs), the European Carotid Surgery Trial (ECST) and the North American Symptomatic Carotid Endarterectomy Trial (NASCET), both reported positive results for symptomatic patients with significant carotid stenosis (70% to 90%) when compared to those who were solely medically managed [5–7]. Patients with symptoms and with moderate to severe carotid stenosis (50% to 99%) should have an "urgent" CEA within 2 weeks as per the National Institutes and Clinical Excellence (NICE) guidelines [8].

D. **Surgical and procedural treatment**

1. The endarterectomy procedure was first developed and performed on the superficial femoral artery by the Portuguese surgeon Joao Cid dos Santos in 1946. However the first CEA recorded in medical literature was in the Lancet in 1954 by Dr. Felix Eastcott, a consultant surgeon and deputy director of the surgical unit at St. Mary's Hospital, London, United Kingdom. In 1953, Dr. Michael DeBakey successfully relieved an atherosclerotic obstruction of the carotid arteries at the Methodist Hospital in Houston, Texas [9,10].

2. CEA is not a benign surgical procedure and is considered prudent only if its own periprocedural risks outweigh the morbidity and mortality events that are associated with the natural course of carotid artery disease. CEA is classified as an intermediate risk surgical procedure (periop cardiac morbidity and mortality 1% to 5%) by the 2007 ACCF/AHA guidelines on perioperative cardiovascular evaluation and care for noncardiac surgery. It has been noted that the last few decades have seen a variation in both the number of CEAs performed as well as wide geographical variations in its use. Prior to the above-mentioned clinical studies, the use of CEA doubled in the early 1980s before dropping in half following reports of frequent complications and a national Medicare study report indicating that a third of CEAs were inappropriate [11].

3. Surgical treatment for asymptomatic carotid artery disease is still controversial but the latest 2011 practice guidelines for CEA by the ACCF/AHA (American College of Cardiology Foundation/American Heart Association Task Force) on the "Management of Patients with Extracranial Carotid and Vertebral Artery Disease" addresses this issue [7]. Two large RCTs have demonstrated that a CEA will benefit asymptomatic patients with ≥60% carotid stenosis who are expected to live for at least 5 years after surgery, when performed in centers with a 30-day stroke and mortality rate of ≤3% [5,6].

4. A more recent procedure, carotid angioplasty and stenting (CAS), is rapidly gaining popularity as an alternative in patients who are deemed "high-risk" for a CEA. The percutaneous procedure of carotid angioplasty and stenting was approved by the FDA in 2004 for clinical application. Since then, numerous carotid stent systems have been approved by the FDA as safe and effective in patients at increased risk of complications for neck surgery.

II. **Pathophysiology**

A. **Cervical and cerebrovascular anatomy**

1. Interpretation of the 20% cardiac output is as follows : The arterial blood supply to the brain accounts for one fifth of the total amount of blood volume that is ejected by the heart in a minute [12]. The right and left common carotid arteries from the brachiocephalic trunk and the aortic arch respectively divide into the internal and external carotid arteries at the level of the upper border of the thyroid cartilage. It is the lateral aspect of this bifurcation that is a common site for atherosclerosis in carotid artery disease, an inflammatory buildup of atherosclerotic plaque causing the luminal narrowing of the internal and common carotid arteries (Figs. 7.1 and 7.2).

2. **Cerebral autoregulation.** In the territory of impending ischemia, autoregulation is disrupted. Cerebral vascular beds subject to relative ischemia are maximally vasodilated and blood flow is dependent on systemic blood pressure. Therefore maintaining hemodynamic stability during a CEA procedure is a paramount goal for optimal perioperative management (Fig. 7.3).

3. Depending on the degree of vessel luminal occlusion by an atherosclerotic plaque, carotid stenosis can be stable and asymptomatic, cause a TIA or be a source of embolization, causing an acute ischemic stroke. The degree and extent of the manifestation of the stroke

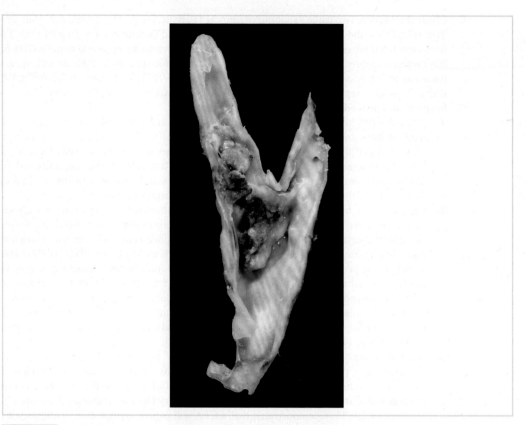

FIGURE 7.1 Carotid plaque. (Courtesy of Dr. Ed. Uthman, MD)

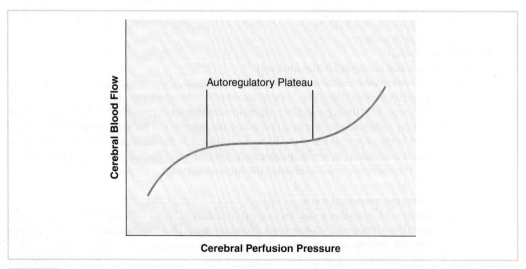

FIGURE 7.2 Cerebral autoregulation. (Reused from Kincaid MS, Lam AM. Anesthesia for neurosurgery. In: Barash PG, Cullen BF, Stoelting RK, Cahalan MK, Stock MC, eds. *Clinical Anesthesia*. 6th ed. Philadelphia, PA: Lippincott Williams & Wilkins; 2009:1008, with permission.)

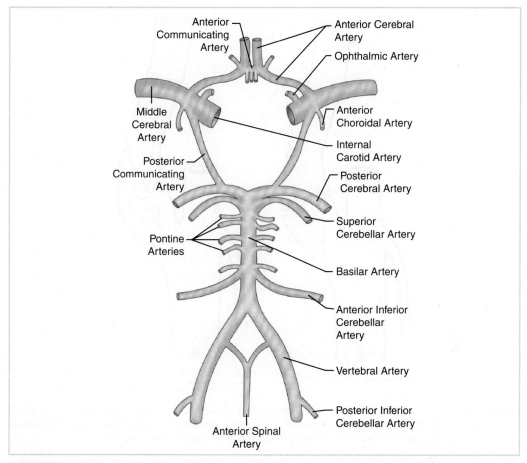

FIGURE 7.3 Circle of Willis. (Reused from Kincaid MS, Lam AM. Anesthesia for neurosurgery. In: Barash PG, Cullen BF, Stoelting RK, Cahalan MK, Stock MC, eds. *Clinical Anesthesia*. 6th ed. Philadelphia, PA: Lippincott Williams & Wilkins; 2009:1006, with permission.)

in the form of a constellation of predictable neurologic deficits in turn depends on where the segment of plaque gets lodged in the arterial vessels supplying the brain. Data acquired from the modality of transcranial Doppler (TCD) along with duplex ultrasonography (USG) suggests that a 70% to 75% carotid artery stenosis correlates with a 1.5 mm residual luminal diameter and comprises a hemodynamically significant stenosis [13]. On the basis of luminal diameter reduction, the severity of stenosis is typically classified into mild (less than 50%), moderate (50% to 69%), and severe (70% to 99%) [1].

  B. **Risk factors [12].** These are the very risk factors for atherosclerosis and include the following:
1. Hypertension (HTN)
2. Cigarette smoking
3. Hyperlipidemia
4. Diabetes mellitus (risk of stroke almost 2.5 times)
5. Excessive alcohol intake (>6 drinks daily)
6. Elevated homocysteine levels

  C. **Natural course of carotid artery disease.** The severity of carotid artery disease parallels the degree of atherosclerosis in other regions of the body. A cerebrovascular accident or stroke is mainly accounted for by a thromboembolic phenomenon as compared to a hemorrhagic one. Usually a stroke is preceded by one or two TIAs in 60% of cases and the highest mortality occurs in

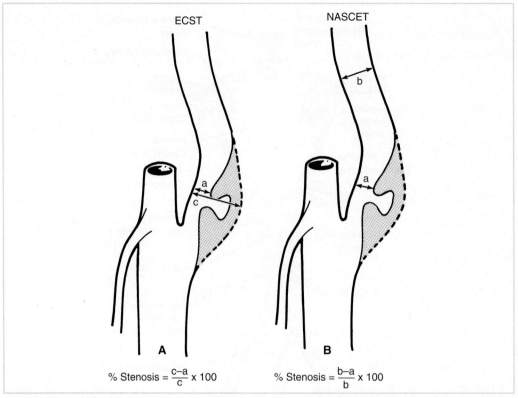

FIGURE 7.4 Commonly used methods for calculating carotid stenosis. **A:** European Carotid Surgery Trial (ECST) method. **B:** North American Symptomatic Carotid Endarterectomy Trial (NASCET) method. (Reused from Osborne AG. *Diagnostic Cerebral Angiography.* 2nd ed. Philadelphia, PA: Lippincott Williams & Wilkins; 1999:373.)

the first 2 years following a TIA [12]. Clinically the risk of stroke from carotid stenosis is evaluated by the absence or presence of symptoms and the degree of stenosis on imaging (e.g., duplex USG).

III. Carotid endarterectomy and carotid angioplasty and stenting

    A. Indications for CEA & CAS. The aim of a CEA is to prevent the adverse sequelae of carotid artery stenosis, e.g., a stroke, which can be devastating for the patient and can even lead to death.

        1. NASCET and ECST Studies (Fig. 7.4)

            a. Both the NASCET and the ECST clinical trials have helped define current guidelines, most notably the 2011 practice guidelines by the ACCF/AHA [7].

            b. Several clinical trials have shown a definite surgical advantage over medical therapy alone especially for symptomatic high grade stenosis [5–7].

            c. The NASCET revealed that one major stroke would be prevented at 2 years for every six patients surgically treated (number needed to treat [NNT] = 6) for symptomatic patients with a 70% to 99% stenosis and the risk of an ipsilateral stroke would be decreased from 26% to 9%.

            d. The European ACST found that a CEA may be of benefit to asymptomatic patients with a high-grade stenosis group (60% or more).

        2. ACCF/AHA class I recommendations

            a. Table 7.1 outlines recommended management guidelines for carotid stenosis. The class I recommendations for carotid revascularization are briefly enumerated below (the author of this chapter strongly advices reviewing the 2011 practice guidelines by the ACCF/AHA) [7].

TABLE 7.1	Summary of recommended treatment guidelines for the management of carotid stenosis

Stenosis

- Symptomatic[a] carotid disease and severe (70%–99%) ipsilateral carotid artery stenosis, CEA is recommended if the estimated perioperative morbidity/mortality risk <6%.
- Asymptomatic patients with severe (70%–99%) ipsilateral carotid disease, CEA is recommended if the estimated perioperative morbidity/mortality risk <6%.
- Symptomatic[a] patients with and moderate (50%–69%) ipsilateral carotid stenosis, CEA is recommended depending on patient-specific factors, if the estimated perioperative morbidity/mortality risk <6%.
- When the degree of stenosis is <50%, there is no indication either CEA or CAS.
- Repeat procedures (CAS or CEA) are indicated for symptomatic carotid disease and recurrent stenosis due to intimal hyperplasia or atherosclerosis progressive restenosis that indicates a threat of complete occlusion.
- All patients should have a life expectancy of at least 5 years to qualify for CEA or CAS in lieu of medical management.

Timing

- After a nondisabling TIA or stroke, CEA within 2 weeks is reasonable if there are no contraindications to early revascularization.

CEA vs. CAS

- CAS is an alternative to CEA for symptomatic[a] patients at average or low risk of complications with stenosis >70% by noninvasive imaging or >50% by catheter angiography.
- CAS is an alternative with symptomatic severe stenosis (>70%) when:
  - Anatomy is unfavorable for CEA intervention[b]
  - Medical conditions greatly increase the risk
- Periprocedural morbidity and mortality rates should be in the range of 4%–6%.

[a]Symptomatic carotid disease is defined as focal neurologic symptoms that are sudden in onset and referable to the carotid artery distribution within the previous 4 to 6 months. These symptoms may be transient ischemic attacks, episodes of transient monocular blindness, or minor (nondisabling) ischemic strokes.
[b]Unfavorable neck anatomy includes arterial stenosis distal to the second cervical vertebra or intrathoracic arterial stenosis, previous ipsilateral CEA, contralateral vocal cord paralysis, open tracheostomy, radical surgery, and irradiation.

      b. **Class I indications.** Patients at average or low surgical risk who experience a nondisabling ischemic stroke or transient cerebral ischemic symptoms, including hemispheric events or amaurosis fugax, within 6 months (symptomatic patients) should undergo CEA if the diameter of the lumen of the ipsilateral internal carotid artery is reduced more than 70% as documented by noninvasive imaging (*Level of Evidence: A*) or more than 50% as documented by catheter angiography (*Level of Evidence: B*), and the anticipated rate of perioperative stroke or mortality is less than 6%.

          Carotid angioplasty and stenting is indicated as an alternative to CEA for symptomatic patients at average or low risk of complications associated with endovascular intervention when the diameter of the lumen of the internal carotid artery is reduced by more than 70% as documented by noninvasive imaging or more than 50% as documented by catheter angiography and the anticipated rate of periprocedural stroke or mortality is less than 6% (*Level of Evidence: B*).

          Selection of asymptomatic patients for carotid revascularization should be guided by an assessment of comorbid conditions, life expectancy, and other individual factors, and should include a thorough discussion of the risks and benefits of the procedure with an understanding of patient preferences (*Level of Evidence: C*).

   B. CEA versus CAS

      1. Carotid angioplasty and stenting technique has gained tremendous momentum in the recent years and is currently the leading alternative to CEA. The Stenting and Angioplasty with Protection in Patients at High Risk for Endarterectomy (SAPPHIRE) trial and the recent Carotid Revascularization Endarterectomy versus Stenting Trial (CREST) have helped shape the latest 2011 ACCF/AHA practice guidelines for extracranial carotid stenosis management [7].

2. In the SAPPHIRE study, Yadav concluded that CAS was noninferior to CEA in regards to total adverse events and lowered event rates for myocardial infarction (MI) and major strokes in high-risk surgical candidates.

3. The most recent clinical trials indicate that CAS may be as safe and effective as the traditional CEA but it must be reiterated that this may hold true for only a small subset of patients, and a generalization must be reserved pending the conduct of further RCTs.

C. **Timing of interventions [5–8,13]**
   1. **Mild stroke or TIA.** Analysis of the NASCET and the ECST trials found that CEA within 2 weeks of a nondisabling stroke or TIA significantly improved the outcomes compared to medical management.
   2. **Moderate to severe stroke.** The benefit of CEA for patients with moderate to severe ischemic stroke has not been evaluated in RCTs. The high perioperative risk in these patients may preclude consideration for an early CEA. Stable neurologic deficits after a moderate to severe stroke probably vary according to clinical and radiologic features.
   3. **Emergent.** Emergent CEA for an evolving stroke or crescendo TIA has a high operative risk. A 2009 systematic review of 47 nonrandomized studies of CEA for recently symptomatic carotid stenosis reported a rate of perioperative stroke or death of 14% versus 4% for emergent versus nonemergent CEA [13].

> **CLINICAL PEARL**   In symptomatic patients with symptoms with moderate to severe carotid stenosis (50% to 99%), an "urgent" CEA should be performed within 2 weeks.

D. **Contraindication to CEA and CAS**
   1. General contraindications
      a. Complete internal carotid artery occlusion
      b. Previous stroke on ipsilateral side with significant sequelae
      c. Significant comorbidities too risky for either CEA or CAS
   2. The major contraindications for CEA are the following:
      a. Tracheostomy
      b. Neck irradiation
      c. Prior neck dissection
      d. Contralateral vocal cord paralysis (from previous CEA)
      e. Atypical lesion surgically inaccessible
      f. Unacceptably high medical risk
   3. CAS contraindications include the following:
      a. Abnormal vessel anatomy (tortuous, ICA < 3 mm)
      b. Diffuse carotid disease
      c. Unacceptably high medical risk—recent stroke, severe renal insufficiency

IV. **Preoperative evaluation**

A. **Carotid imaging**
   1. Patients may or may not be symptomatic from a carotid stenosis and this may have no correlation to the presence of a *carotid bruit*. A positive bruit will however warrant a further investigation by performing a carotid duplex scan. A carotid duplex scan which is a combination of a B-mode USG imaging and a pulse Doppler spectral analyzer for blood flow velocity, is the most common noninvasive investigation.
   2. If the carotid duplex scan results prove inadequate, either a computerized tomography (CT) angiogram, magnetic resonance (MR) angiogram, or a carotid angiogram (gold standard) is sought [12].

B. **Clinical evaluation.** Once it is determined that a carotid lesion is of credible threat to a patient's well-being and is amenable to intervention based on Doppler USG, CT, MRI, or carotid angiogram, the preoperative assessment of the patient's comorbid conditions as well as a discussion of the risks and benefits of the procedure is swiftly and efficiently conducted.

1. **Airway and respiratory system.** Cessation of smoking advice to primarily optimize oxygen-carrying capacity. In addition, other advantages include improved postsurgical site wound healing, decreased airway irritability, and secretions if smoking is stopped 1 to 2 months prior to the date of surgery.

2. **Nervous system.** A careful preoperative neurologic examination must be performed since there is a high incidence of a perioperative stroke. Head position must be checked during the preoperative visit to analyze the cervical range of motion a patient can tolerate when awake, and avoid inadvertent neurovascular and musculoskeletal injuries during general anesthesia.

3. **Cardiovascular system.** A careful review of cardiac symptoms and exercise tolerance is warranted to determine if invasive and/or noninvasive cardiac testing is needed.

   a. Bilateral carotid artery disease significantly increases the perioperative risk of adverse outcomes such that a combined CEA is contraindicated and most surgeons will stage the procedure with a delay of at least 2 weeks in between procedures. The unique dilemma of concomitant significant coronary artery disease (CAD) and carotid stenosis is discussed later in this chapter.

   b. The incidence of perioperative MI is reportedly 0% to 4% during a CEA and therefore a high degree of vigilance of its occurrence is adopted. Baseline and serial electrocardiograms along with troponins may be drawn perioperatively at specific times based on institution protocols [14].

   c. Establish the blood pressure range for a given patient during the preoperative evaluation and if possible review their medical records and previous hospital visits to determine this value to help guide blood pressure control perioperatively.

   d. One should also assess the patient's need for appropriate antianxiety management on the day of surgery. A thorough bedside preoperative evaluation should complement any pharmacologic agent for anxiety, which should be used judiciously.

C. **Perioperative antiplatelet therapy.** The risk of developing a TIA in an asymptomatic carotid artery stenosis patient is approximately 1% to 2% per year for the first few years. A European clinical study demonstrated that a reduction in the incidence of TIA can be achieved with the combined administration of aspirin (ASA) and dipyridamole more so than giving either drug alone [15]. Therefore it has become imperative that during the perioperative period, all patients presenting for CEA be maintained on a regimen of ASA and/or clopidogrel.

CLINICAL PEARL All patients presenting for CEA should be maintained on a regimen of ASA and/or clopidogrel in order to decrease the risk of TIA and stroke.

V. **Intraoperative management**

A. **CEA intraoperative management.** As emphasized throughout this chapter, the main goal of intraoperative management involves employing strategies that protect both the brain and the heart and utilizes techniques that lead to a smooth and expedited awakening of the patient for neurologic examination at the end of the procedure.

CLINICAL PEARL The key to successful management of a CEA is by protecting the heart and brain by preventing ischemic events. This involves maintaining hemodynamic stability with the aid of short-acting vasoactive drugs.

3

1. **Regional versus general anesthesia**
   a. There is currently no scientific evidence to prove that either anesthetic technique (regional vs. general) is superior and thus no corresponding guidelines regarding method of anesthetic management for this procedure exist [16–18].

b. General anesthesia versus awake carotid surgery with local anesthesia (with or without cervical block) is generally decided by surgeon and patient characteristics and preference. A systematic review and meta-analysis of randomized trials comparing local/regional with general anesthesia identified ten trials (4,335 operations) [17]. Of those procedures, 3,526 were from the General Anesthesia versus Local Anesthesia (GALA) trial [18]. In the review and the GALA trial there was no significant difference in outcomes between the local and general anesthesia groups.

> **CLINICAL PEARL** There is no significant difference in outcomes between the local and general anesthesia technique. The choice of anesthetic is institution specific as long as the perioperative goals are met.

2. **General anesthesia.** Volatile anesthetics may provide preconditioning and neuronal protection by inducing nitric oxide synthase [19]. Barbiturates have no proven benefit in CEA. Choice of anesthetic remains institution specific for now with no specific recommendations on drugs as long as the perioperative goals are met.

   a. **Advantages**
      (1) Optimal operating conditions
      (2) Protected airway
      (3) Control of ventilation/oxygenation
      (4) Ability to use Transesophageal echocardiography (TEE) when indicated (rarely)
   b. **Disadvantages**
      (1) Potentially greater challenges with blood pressure control
      (2) Need to secure airway
      (3) Potential need for neurologic monitoring (institution specific)
      (4) Residual sedation can compromise neurologic evaluation
      (5) Smooth emergence can be difficult due to coughing and hemodynamic pertubations
   c. **Monitors**
      (1) Pulse oximetry
      (2) Capnography
      (3) Noninvasive blood pressure (invasive arterial line preferred)
      (4) 5-lead ECG with ST-segment analysis
      (5) Temperature
      (6) Urine output (±, Foley catheter placed at Rush University Medical Center. Duration of procedure is 3 to 4 hours.)
      (7) Rarely central venous pressure (CVP), pulmonary artery catheter (PAC), or TEE for additional hemodynamic monitoring.
         However, in the case of a patient with poor left ventricular function, a central line may be placed in the contralateral internal jugular vein or subclavian vein for tighter hemodynamic control. In addition, a PAC may also be used for the same purpose and in the case of general anesthesia, a TEE probe may be useful in patients with severely compromised cardiac function.
   d. **Induction.** Standard induction techniques are employed with the usual considerations for airway control and careful hemodynamic stability.
   e. **Maintenance**
      (1) **Anesthesia.** Choice of anesthetic remains institution specific for now with no specific recommendations on drugs as long as the perioperative goals are met.
      (2) **Carotid cross clamp**
         (a) **Heparin**
            (i) 5,000 to 7,500 units of intravenous heparin 3 to 5 minutes before arterial occlusion is usually sufficient to increase the activated clotting time (ACT) to 250 to 300 seconds.

        (ii) For patients with heparin-induced thrombocytopenia (HIT), argatroban and bivalirudin have been successfully used for anticoagulation.

    (b) Blood pressure management

        (i) Blood pressure management goals aim at maintaining it at the mid-to-high normal during carotid artery cross clamp and mid-normal at the end of the procedure.

    (c) A few surgeons may infiltrate the carotid sinus at the carotid bifurcation with 1% lidocaine to blunt the baroreceptor reflex and thus achieve hemodynamic parameters with ease.

(3) Ventilation

    (a) Ventilation goals must include normocarbia as both hypo- and hypercapnia can be detrimental.

    (b) Hypoventilation can lead to the patient experiencing an intracerebral steal phenomenon that can potentially worsen impending or ongoing cerebral ischemia.

(4) Temperature and glucose control. Recommendations also involve avoiding hyperthermia and hyperglycemia as poorer outcomes have been documented for patients who have these conditions [20].

(5) Neurologic/perfusion monitoring

    (a) Intraoperative neuromonitoring may play a critical role in the intraoperative management of patients undergoing CEA. Many surgical teams have come to rely on neuromonitoring for improved outcomes of their patients. However, NASCET has reported no decrease in the incidence of stroke with their use. Neuromonitoring requires the presence of neurophysiologists or anesthesiologists in the operating room who are skilled in acquiring and interpreting the responses throughout the procedure.

    (b) The standard electroencephalogram (EEG) is a sensitive indicator of inadequate cerebral perfusion but is limited by the inability to detect subcortical infarcts, has common false-negative results, and is sensitive to depth of anesthesia and arterial carbon dioxide ($PaCO_2$) level (see chapter 26).

    (c) The processed EEG is simpler to employ but only provides regional (right vs. left) information.

    (d) Somatosensory-evoked potential can detect subcortical infarcts, but like the EEG, is also sensitive to anesthetic depth.

    (e) TCD ultrasound is a continuous monitor of blood flow velocity, indicates shunt need and malfunction, detects microemboli, and can be used to manage hyperperfusion syndrome.

    (f) Cerebral oximetry uses near-infrared spectroscopy that can potentially monitor changes in cerebral oxygenation, but at present has limited clinical data regarding its value in correlating with neurologic outcome.

    (g) Stump pressure is considered a poor indicator of the adequacy of cerebral perfusion.

(6) Shunt placement

    (a) The carotid artery opening (arteriotomy) requires temporary occlusion of the proximal common carotid artery, distal internal carotid artery, and external carotid artery. The entire procedure can be achieved under continued occlusion of these vessels if the collateral blood flow to the territory supplied by the occluded internal carotid is deemed adequate (on the basis of intraoperative neurophysiologic and vascular monitoring or clinical neurologic examination, if procedure is done awake). If not, an internal shunt between the proximal common carotid artery and distal internal carotid artery can be placed to minimize the duration of transient interruption in cerebral blood flow during carotid clamping in CEA.

    (b) The use of a shunt, whether routinely or selectively, during a CEA, is another controversial issue that appears to be institution specific or practice specific.

    (c) Shunts tend to be used when cerebral ischemia becomes apparent clinically or with the aid of the above-discussed monitors, on carotid artery cross clamping. A shunt-related adverse event carries an approximate 0.7% embolism-related stroke rate. In NASCET, no increased strokes with shunts were reported in patients undergoing CEA.

    (d) Overall, shunting is probably unnecessary in the majority of patients and may expose them to the following risks:

        (i) Formation of an intimal flap during shunt insertion, resulting in arterial dissection

        (ii) Dislodgement of plaque emboli during vessel manipulation

        (iii) Air embolism due to bubbles in the shunt

    (e) Advocates of routine shunting argue complications may be less because the surgeon and surgical team are familiar with technique. The advantage of routine shunting is that cerebral flow is assured without the need for neurologic monitoring (EEG, stump pressure).

CLINICAL PEARL The use of routine or selective shunting during a CEA is controversial and is institution specific or practice specific.

    f. Emergence

    (1) The goal is for rapid emergence with minimal coughing and straining along with optimal hemodynamic stability.

    (2) Depending on local practice, heparin may be partially reversed after closure of the arteriotomy.

CLINICAL PEARL The goals for emergence from anesthesia focus on minimal coughing and straining along with optimal hemodynamic stability.

  3. Regional with sedation

    a. The awake/sedated state is utilized with regional anesthesia and mild sedation and requires a very cooperative and motivated patient. A potentially difficult airway instrumentation is a relative contraindication and in such cases it is prudent to select general anesthesia instead, securing the airway right at the beginning of the procedure.

    (1) The goals of sedation techniques are to have a cooperative patient who is awake enough for monitoring mental status, speech, and extremity function.

    (2) A neurologic assessment is performed at the beginning of the procedure and repeated every 10 to 15 minutes during carotid dissection, immediately prior to carotid clamping, and continuously during carotid clamping. Agitation, slurred speech, disorientation, and extremity weakness are indications for shunt placement. Shunt placement is usually <5%.

    b. Advantages

    (1) Simplicity, reliability, and cost-effectiveness

    (2) Patient provides functional neurologic monitoring

    (3) Avoidance of airway instrumentation

    (4) Less shunting with decreased potential risks

    (5) Hemodynamic control is easier

    c. Disadvantages

    (1) Potential patient anxiety/restlessness secondary to very light/no sedation

    (2) Intraoperative HTN

    (3) Limited access to airway if necessary

      (4) Risk of seizure, phrenic, or recurrent laryngeal nerve blockade, epidural or total spinal during block if a deep cervical plexus block is employed

      (5) An uncomfortable patient who may necessitate urgent conversion to general anesthesia or urgent shunt placement if neurologic deterioration occurs

    d. Various local or regional techniques can be used ranging from local, superficial cervical with local, and superficial and deep cervical plexus blockade.

      (1) Superficial cervical block. Infiltration of local anesthetic (15 to 20 mL) along the posterior border sternocleidomastoid muscle.

      (2) Deep cervical plexus block. Injection of local anesthetic (4 to 5 mL) at the transverse process of C_2, C_3, and C_4 after negative aspiration for blood. A slight caudal orientation of the needle prevents the inadvertent insertion of the needle in the neural foramina.

    e. Sedation techniques. There is no optimal technique for an "awake" CEA. The goal is a cooperative patient participating in ongoing neurologic evaluation Techniques range from intermittent small doses of fentanyl (25 μg) and midazolam (0.5 to 1 mg) to low-dose infusions of propofol, propofol/remifentanil, or dexmedetomidine.

    f. Conversion from regional to general. The intraoperative conversion rate from local/regional to general anesthesia is about 2%. Depending on the urgency and patient status, rapid airway rescue may consist of either a laryngeal mask airway or tracheal intubation.

B. Carotid angioplasty and stenting (CAS) intraoperative management

    1. The anesthetic management for CAS is similar to that of an awake CEA. Standard monitoring with an arterial line and light sedation is used for the majority of these procedures.

    2. Intraprocedure 5,000 to 7,500 units of intravenous heparin 3 to 5 minutes before arterial occlusion is usually sufficient to increase the ACT to 250 to 300 seconds.

    3. Bradycardia is a common problem during CAS with an up to 60%. Increased age, symptomatic lesions, presence of ulceration and calcification, and carotid bulb lesions have been found to be significant predictors of bradycardia during CAS.

    4. Hypotension immediately following CAS occurs in about 20% of patients but is usually transient and rarely symptomatic.

VI. Postoperative management and complications

  A. Clinical considerations. From the moment the patient is extubated in the operating room, the immediate postoperative period and the following 24 hours will be crucial. During this time period patients are usually closely observed in a critical care unit. Class I recommendations for medical management are outlined in Table 7.2. Specific complications are discussed below.

  B. Neurologic complications

    1. Stroke is the second most common cause of death following CEA. Approximately, 5% of symptomatic and 3% of asymptomatic patients are expected to suffer a stroke or even death due to CEA or CAS.

TABLE 7.2 Summary of recommendations for periprocedural management of patients undergoing carotid endarterectomy (2011 practice guidelines by the ACCF/AHA) [7]

Class I

1. Aspirin (81–325 mg daily) is recommended before CEA and may be continued indefinitely postoperatively (*Level of Evidence: A*).

2. Beyond the first month after CEA, aspirin (75–325 mg daily), clopidogrel (75 mg daily), or the combination of low-dose aspirin plus extended-release dipyridamole (25 and 200 mg twice daily, respectively) should be administered for long-term prophylaxis against ischemic cardiovascular events (*Level of Evidence: B*).

3. Administration of antihypertensive medication is recommended as needed to control blood pressure before and after CEA (*Level of Evidence: C*).

4. The findings on clinical neurologic examination should be documented within 24 hours before and after CEA (*Level of Evidence: C*).

    a. Multiple factors can contribute to postoperative stroke in patients who have undergone CEA. However, neurologic changes secondary to thrombosis and technical errors must be ruled out.

    b. Evaluation and management may include an ultrasound, angiogram, or cervical re-exploration under anesthesia for direct inspection.

    c. Systemic heparinization is controversial as is intra-arterial thrombolytic therapy.

  2. Cranial nerve injury and dysfunction can occur during CEA. These injuries usually resolve after a few months with the risk of permanent cranial being very low. Cranial nerves potentially at risk are the following:

    a. Vagus nerve

    b. Recurrent laryngeal nerve

    c. Marginal mandibular branch of the facial nerve

    d. Hypoglossal nerve

    e. Branches of the trigeminal nerve

    f. Superior laryngeal nerve

C. Cardiovascular complications

  1. Myocardial infarction. The risk of a MI after CAS or CEA is 1% to 3%.

  2. HTN and hypotension are the most common cardiovascular events experienced during CEA and CAS.

    a. In general, the postoperative systolic blood pressure should be maintained between 100 and 150 mm Hg. HTN may increase the likelihood of neck hematoma or suture line disruption, while relative hypotension may result in inadequate cerebral perfusion and potential thrombosis of the endarterectomy site. Patients may require either vasopressor or antihypertensive drips to maintain the target blood pressure.

    b. HTN is more frequent with awake procedures and on emergence from general anesthesia, small doses of rapid-acting antihypertensive medications are sufficient for treatment.

    c. Hypotension is common with the maintenance of general anesthesia and CAS, and can be managed with intravenous doses of phenylephrine or ephedrine.

    d. Carotid bulb stimulation during CEA can cause hypotension both during the procedure and in the early postoperative period. Adequate cerebral perfusion pressure should be maintained during periods of hemodynamic instability to avoid low cerebral blood flow and cerebral ischemia.

  3. Hyperperfusion syndrome. While the clinical manifestations of hyperperfusion occurs in only a small percentage of patients after carotid revascularization (1% to 3%), the cerebral hyperperfusion syndrome is probably the cause of most intracerebral hemorrhages and seizures in the first 2 weeks after CEA.

    a. After correction of the carotid stenosis, blood flow is restored to a normal or elevated perfusion pressure and the distal arteries are unable to vasoconstrict due to a chronic change in cerebral blood flow autoregulation. The consequences of the increased perfusion pressure and blood flow are edema and possibly vessel rupture.

    b. The clinical characteristics of the hyperperfusion syndrome are as follows:

      (1) Ipsilateral headache that may be improved by an upright posture

      (2) Focal motor seizures are common

      (3) Intracerebral hemorrhage is the most feared complication, occurring in about 0.5% of patients within 2 weeks after surgery.

      (4) More frequent with revascularization of a high-grade stenosis especially after a recent cerebral infarction.

      (5) Neuroimaging studies such as CT or MRI with T_2 sequences frequently reveal cerebral edema, petechial hemorrhages, or intracerebral hemorrhage.

    c. Treatment for cerebral hyperperfusion is prevention through control of postoperative blood pressure (systolic blood pressure <150 mm Hg) with judicious use of intravenous and then oral antihypertensive agents (labetalol, nitroprusside, nicardipine).

    d. Seizures related to hyperperfusion are usually successfully treated with standard anti-epileptic drugs such as levetiracetam (Keppra), fosphenytoin, or phenytoin.

CLINICAL PEARL   Cerebral hyperperfusion occurs in only a small percentage of patients after carotid revascularization (1% to 3%) and is probably the cause of most intracerebral hemorrhages and seizures in the first 2 weeks. Cerebral hyperperfusion is prevented through control of postoperative blood pressure (systolic blood pressure <150 mm Hg) with judicious use of intravenous and then oral antihypertensive agents (labetalol, nitroprusside, nicardipine).

    D. **Airway and respiratory complications**
        1. Airway compromise can be secondary to a hematoma, soft tissue edema, or loss of airway reflexes from neurologic injuries.
        2. Postoperative bleeding, resulting in neck hematoma, occasionally occurs after CEA and patients can rapidly suffer from a compromised airway. If there is any airway concern the patient should be returned to the OR for exploration.
        3. Since intraoral swelling can be significant, topicalization with local anesthesia and awake/sedated intubation techniques may be warranted.
        4. Loss of ipsilateral carotid body function occurs in most patients after CEA that could lead to decreased ventilatory and circulatory response to hypoxia and an elevated resting $PaCO_2$ level. Adequate ventilation and oxygenation should thus be carefully assessed and supplemental oxygen administered to the patient in the postoperative period.

CLINICAL PEARL   Hematoma formation and airway compromise after CEA is a life-threatening complication. Mucosal edema, swelling, and distortion can greatly compromise the ability for successful direct laryngoscopy and intubation after the induction of general anesthesia. Topicalization with local anesthesia and an awake/sedated intubation technique may represent the safest method of airway management.

  VII. **Combined carotid endarterectomy and coronary artery bypass graft**
    A. The incidence of a stroke in the perioperative period during open-heart surgery is 2% to 6%. Studies have indicated that the etiology of the stroke is primarily embolic in nature. Patients with CAD likely have carotid artery disease with clinically significant stenosis (2% and 16% in those presenting for CABG). Patients with concomitant symptomatic CAD and carotid disease belong to a higher risk cohort than either group alone [21,22]. In comparison, the incidence of stroke in general surgical procedures is less than 0.5%.
    B. Centers performing combined CABG and CEA procedures have reported conflicting outcomes and recommendations. The stroke rate for the combined CEA and CABG was approximately double that of either procedure alone and on the contrary, none suffered a MI. When a staged operation is performed, cardiac morbidity can reach 20% if a CEA is done prior to a CABG. The risk of stroke can be as high as 14% when the order is reversed. At Rush University Medical Center, the order of the above-staged surgery is primarily determined and prioritized by the organ system that is the most symptomatic.
    C. No RCTs have been conducted so far to determine the benefit of staged versus combined procedures, and at present, the management of such an individual warrants an individualized approach.
  VIII. **Conclusion.** As long as man ages, the innate process of atherosclerosis will guarantee the existence of carotid artery disease. CEA will remain a gold standard against which future minimally invasive procedures aimed at subduing carotid stenosis will be compared. With the aging population, the management of carotid stenosis will continue to challenge the anesthesiologist while the

cardiovascular, neurosurgical, and the interventional radiologists engage themselves in a turf war with guidelines incorporating both open and percutaneous procedures.

ACKNOWLEDGMENT

The author would like to thank Dr. K.J. Tuman, M.D., Chairman, Department of Anesthesiology, Rush University Medical Center, Chicago 60612.

REFERENCES

1. Brunicardi F, Andersen D, Billiar T, et al. *Schwartz Principles of Surgery.* 9th ed. New York, NY: McGraw-Hill; 2009.
2. Kasper DL, Braunwald E, Hauser S, et al. *Harrison's Principles of Internal Medicine.* 16th ed. New York, NY: McGraw-Hill; 2005.
3. Minino AM, Smith BL. Deaths: preliminary data for 2000. *Natl Vital Stat Rep.* 2001;49(12):1–40. (http://www.cdc.gov/nchs/data/nvsr/nvsr49/nvsr49_12.pdf)
4. National Institute of Neurological Disorders and Stroke (NIH) National Hospital Discharge Survey 2009
5. European Carotid Surgery Trialists Collaborative Group. Randomised trial of endarterectomy for recently symptomatic carotid stenosis: final results of the MRC European Carotid Surgery Trial (ECST). *Lancet.* 1998;351:1379–1387.
6. North American Symptomatic Carotid Endarterectomy Trial Collaborators. Beneficial effect of carotid endarterectomy in symptomatic patients with high-grade carotid stenosis. *N Engl J Med.* 1991;325:445–453.
7. Brott TG, Halperin JL, Abbara S, et al. 2011 ASA/ACCF/AHA/AANN/AANS/ACR/ASNR/CNS/SAIP/SCAI/SIR/SNIS/SVM/SVS Guideline on the Management of Patients With Extracranial Carotid and Vertebral Artery Disease: A Report of the American College of Cardiology Foundation/American Heart Association Task Force on Practice Guidelines, and the American Stroke Association, American Association of Neuroscience Nurses, American Association of Neurological Surgeons, American College of Radiology, American Society of Neuroradiology, Congress of Neurological Surgeons, Society of Atherosclerosis Imaging and Prevention, Society for Cardiovascular Angiography and Interventions, Society of Interventional Radiology, Society of NeuroInterventional Surgery, Society for Vascular Medicine, and Society for Vascular Surgery Developed in Collaboration With the American Academy of Neurology and Society of Cardiovascular Computed Tomography. *J Am Coll Cardiol.* 2011;57(8):e16–e94.
8. Swain S, Turner C, Tyrrell P, et al. on behalf of the Guideline Development Group. Diagnosis and initial management of acute stroke and transient ischaemic attack: summary of NICE guidance. *BMJ.* 2008;337:a786.
9. Eastcott HHG, Pinching GW, Rob CG. Reconstruction of internal carotid artery in a patient with intermittent attacks of hemiplegia. *Lancet.* 1954;2:994–996.
10. "Felix Eastcott arterial surgeon." The Times (London). 2009;12–31.
11. Halm EA. The good, the bad, and the about-to-get ugly: national trends in carotid revascularization: comment on "Geographic variation in carotid revascularization among Medicare beneficiaries, 2003–2006". *Arch Intern Med.* 2010;170(14):1225–1227.
12. Rerkasem K, Rothwell PM. Systematic review of the operative risks of carotid endarterectomy for recently symptomatic stenosis in relation to the timing of surgery. *Stroke.* 2009;40(10):e564.
13. Hines RL, Marschall K. *Stoelting's Anesthesia and Coexisting Disease.* 6th ed. Philadelphia, PA: Saunders; 2012.
14. Diener HC, Cunha L, Forbes C, et al. European Stroke Prevention Study 2. Dipyridamole and acetylsalicylic acid in the secondary prevention of stroke. *J Neurol Sci.* 1996;143:1–13.
15. Guay J. Regional or general anesthesia for carotid endarterectomy? Evidence from published prospective and retrospective studies. *J Cardiothorac Vasc Anesth.* 2007;21:127–132.
16. Rerkasem K, Rothwell PM. Local versus general anaesthesia for carotid endarterectomy. *Cochrane Database Syst Rev.* 2008;(4):CD000126. doi: 10.1002/14651858.CD000126.pub3.
17. GALA Trial Collaborative Group; Lewis SC, Warlow CP, Bodenham AR, et al. General anaesthesia versus local anaesthesia for carotid surgery (GALA): a multicentre, randomised controlled trial. *Lancet.* 2008;372(9656):2132–2142.
18. Kapinya KJ, Löwl D, Fütterer C, et al. Tolerance against ischemic neuronal injury can be induced by volatile anesthetics and is inducible NO synthase dependent. *Stroke.* 2002;33:1889–1898.
19. McGirt MJ, Woodworth GF, Brooke BS, et al. Hyperglycemia independently increases the risk of perioperative stroke, myocardial infarction, and death after carotid endarterectomy. *Neurosurgery.* 2006;58:1066–1073.
20. Kaplan NM. Meta-analysis of hypertension treatment trials. *Lancet.* 1990;335:1092–1094.
21. Howard G, Manolio TA, Burke GL, et al. Does the association of risk factors and atherosclerosis change with age? An analysis of the combined ARIC and CHS cohorts. The Atherosclerosis Risk in Communities (ARIC) and Cardiovascular Health Study (CHS) Investigators. *Stroke.* 1997;28:1693–1701.
22. Wilson PW, Hoeg JM, D'Agostino RB, et al. Cumulative effects of high cholesterol levels, high blood pressure, and cigarette smoking on carotid stenosis. *N Engl J Med.* 1997;337:516–522.

8

The Pituitary Gland—Considerations in the Adult

Jeffrey J. Pasternak

KEY POINTS

1. Eighty-five percent of all pituitary tumors are adenomas. Most functional tumors secrete a specific hormone and are microadenomas. Nonfunctional tumors are often identified by signs and symptoms related to compression of adjacent structures.
2. Hormonal aberrations can occur following pituitary tumor resection and include hypopituitarism, diabetes insipidus, or the syndrome of inappropriate antidiuretic hormone. Urine output should be monitored postoperatively to assess for diabetes insipidus or less likely the syndrome of inappropriate antidiuretic hormone.
3. Cushing's disease results from excessive production of ACTH. Preoperative management of blood pressure, serum glucose concentration, electrolyte abnormalities, and the presence of fluid retention should be assessed, optimized, and managed.
4. Acromegaly results from growth hormone excess and can result in obstructive sleep apnea, hypertension, cardiac hypertrophy with diastolic dysfunction or coronary insufficiency, and glucose intolerance.
5. Signs and symptoms of hyperprolactinemia are more distinct in females and include galactorrhea, amenorrhea, and infertility. It can also include adverse effects associated with drugs used to treat hyperprolactinemia.

(continued)

6. Pituitary hyperthyroidism results from excess thyroid-stimulating hormone (TSH) with symptoms of anxiety, weight loss, heat intolerance, tachycardia, hypertension, and cardiac dysrhythmia (e.g., atrial fibrillation).
7. Diseases of the posterior pituitary gland include problems with the secretion of oxytocin and vasopressin. Common problems include the syndrome of inappropriate ADH (SIADH) and diabetes insipidus (DI).
8. Pituitary apoplexy results from sudden hemorrhage within the pituitary gland with the abrupt onset of headache, visual disturbances, ophthalmoplegia, and altered mental status (hydrocephalus and coma may occur). Patients may develop vasopressor-resistant hypotension due to acute cortisol deficiency.

I. Anatomic relationships and physiology
   A. Anatomy. The pituitary gland resides within the sella turcica, an invagination of the sphenoid bone (Fig. 8.1). The hypothalamus is located superior to the gland and these structures are separated by dura mater, also known as the diaphragm sella. The hypothalamus and pituitary gland remain connected via the pituitary stalk and blood vessels. Lateral to the sella turcica are the cavernous sinuses. In addition to a venous plexus, each cavernous sinus contains a carotid artery and an oculomotor (III), trochlear (IV), abducens (VI), and ophthalmic (V_1) and maxillary (V_2) branches of the trigeminal nerves which traverse each cavernous sinus. Inferior and anterior to the sella turcica are the sphenoid sinuses.

   Structurally and functionally, the pituitary gland is divided into two separate regions: The anterior pituitary gland (adenohypophysis) and posterior pituitary gland (neurohypophysis).
   B. Physiology of the adenohypophysis. The adenohypophysis consists of both secretory and nonsecretory cells (i.e., null cells). Each secretory cell synthesizes, stores, and secretes a specific hormone in response to hormones secreted by the hypothalamus. Hypothalamic hormones are secreted into a capillary bed within the hypothalamus that then travel via portal vessels to

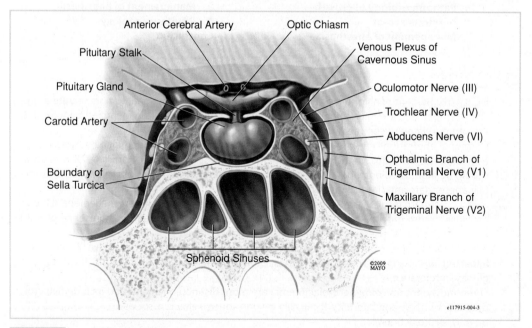

FIGURE 8.1 Coronal section of the sella turcica demonstrating the anatomic relationship between the pituitary gland and cranial nerves, carotid arteries, and the cavernous and sphenoid sinuses. (By permission of Mayo Foundation for Medical Education and Research. All rights reserved.)

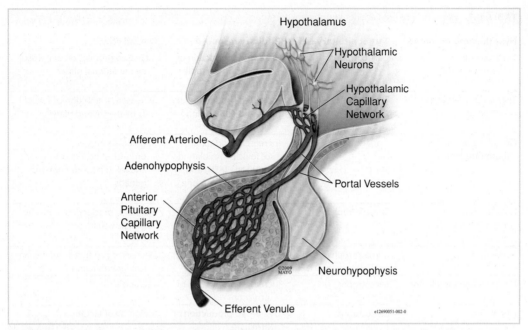

FIGURE 8.2 Physiology of the adenohypophysis. Afferent arterioles enter the hypothalamus where hypothalamic neurons secrete hormone into the circulation. Blood then leaves the hypothalamus via portal vessels and enters the adenohypophysis (i.e., anterior pituitary gland) where the hypothalamic hormones enter a second capillary network and act upon adenohypophyseal cells thus regulating the secretion of hormones. Hormones produced by the adenohypophysis enter the capillary network and enter the systemic circulation by the efferent venule. The advantage of a portal system allows for low volumes of hypothalamic hormones to be secreted since their concentration will be much higher in the portal vessels than in the systemic circulation also allowing rapid regulation of hormone secretion by the adenohypophysis. (By permission of Mayo Foundation for Medical Education and Research. All rights reserved.)

a secondary capillary bed located within the adenohypophysis (Fig. 8.2). These hypothalamic hormones will either stimulate or inhibit the release of hormones by cells of the adenohypophysis (Table 8.1).

C. **Physiology of the neurohypophysis.** A direct extension of the brain, the neurohypophysis contains the terminal axons of neurons located in the supraoptic and paraventricular nuclei (Fig. 8.3). Thus the pituitary stalk contains axons of the hypothalamo-hypophyseal tract. These neurons synthesize, store, and secrete into capillaries located within the neurohypophysis, both oxytocin and antidiuretic hormone (ADH) (i.e., vasopressin).

CLINICAL PEARL   Nonfunctional pituitary tumors often become symptomatic due to growth and compression of surrounding structures, thus are often larger and more locally invasive at resection than functional tumors.

II. **Pituitary tumors.** Tumors of the pituitary gland are the most common cause of pituitary dysfunction in adults. Eighty-five percent of all pituitary tumors are adenomas; however, other tumors such as craniopharyngiomas, meningiomas, primary carcinomas, metastatic tumors, astrocytomas, hemangiomas, and hamartomas can also occur [1]. Most adenomas consist of a single cell type and are generally classified into two categories based on whether or not the tumor cells secrete a specific hormone which results in clinical manifestations of hormone excess.

A. **Functional tumors.** These tumors will manifest as clinical signs and symptoms of excess production of one or more specific hormones. These specific clinical scenarios are addressed in section III of this chapter. As functional tumors often produce clinical signs and symptoms

TABLE 8.1   Hypothalamic and adenohypophyseal hormones

Hypothalamic hormone	Target pituitary cell	Pituitary response	Overall effect
Corticotropin-releasing hormone (CRH)	Corticotrophs	Increased production of adrenocorticotropic hormone (ACTH)	Increased production of cortisol by the adrenal gland
Thyrotropin-releasing hormone (TRH)	Thyrotrophs	Increased production of thyroid-stimulating hormone (TSH)	Increased production of T_3 and T_4 by the thyroid gland
Gonadotropin-releasing hormone (GnRH)	Gonadotrophs	Increased production of follicle-stimulating hormone (FSH) and luteinizing hormone (LH)	Regulates estrogen, progesterone, testosterone, and inhibin production by gonads
Growth hormone-releasing hormone (GHRH)	Somatotrophs	Increased production of growth hormone	Increased production of insulin-like growth factor
Somatostatin	Somatotrophs	Decreased production of growth hormone	Decreased production of insulin-like growth factor
Prolactin-releasing factor	Lactotrophs	Increased production of prolactin	Lactation
Dopamine	Lactotrophs	Decreased production of prolactin	Inhibition of lactation

related to hormone overproduction prior to those related to compression of structures adjacent to the sella turcica, they are often smaller at the time of diagnosis. Hence, most functional tumors are microadenomas or <1 cm in diameter at diagnosis.

   B.   Nonfunctional tumors. Adenomas may also be derived from either nonfunctional cell lines or from hormone-producing cell lines in which hormonal overproduction does not lead to overt

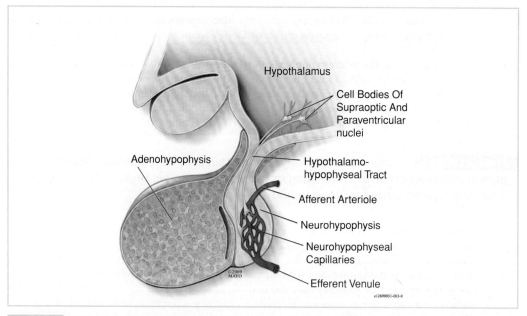

FIGURE 8.3 Physiology of the neurohypophysis. The axons of neurons located in the supraoptic and paraventricular nuclei of the hypothalamus extend via the hypothalamo-hypophyseal tract to the neurohypophysis. When stimulated, these neurons secrete either oxytocin or vasopressin into the capillary network of the neurohypophysis. (By permission of Mayo Foundation for Medical Education and Research. All rights reserved.)

clinical manifestations. In the latter scenario, adenomas derived from gonadotropin-producing cell lines (e.g., follicle-stimulating hormone, luteinizing hormone) or prolactin-secreting cell lines may produce very nonspecific clinical signs and symptoms, or no symptoms related to excessive hormone production. Nonfunctional tumors are often identified either by signs and symptoms related to compression of structures within the confines of the sella turcica or may extend to impinge on surrounding structures. Increased pressure from the tumor within the sella may produce headache or hypopituitarism. Superior extension may result in compression of the optic chiasm which contains the axons of afferent neurons from the medial retina. As these neurons relay information from the lateral visual fields, early inferior compression from a tumor results in bitemporal superior quadrantanopia whereas later, more severe compression results in bitemporal hemianopsia or complete loss of lateral visual fields. (Fig. 8.4). Further rostral tumor grown may result in hypothalamic dysfunction or obstructive hydrocephalus. Lateral extension can lead to dysfunction of cranial nerves that traverse the cavernous sinus causing dysfunction of extraocular muscles and diplopia or sensory disturbances of the face. In

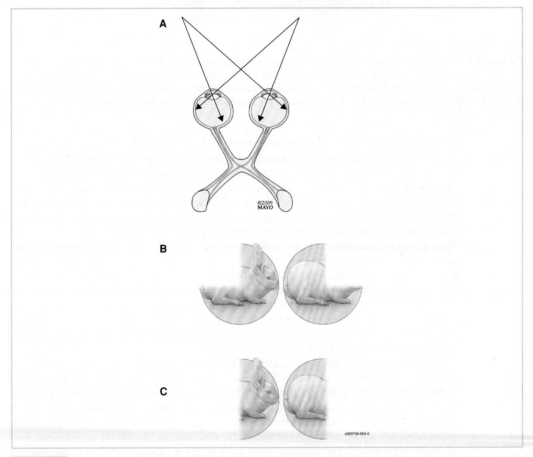

FIGURE 8.4 Visual fields. **A:** Light from the left and right lateral (or temporal) visual fields strikes the left and right medial regions of the retina, respectively. Afferent neurons originating from the medial regions of the retina cross in the optic chiasm. Injury to the optic chiasm results in dysfunction of these neurons thus loss of the lateral visual fields. Early in the course of enlargement of the contents of the sella turcica, axons located within the inferior portion of the optic chiasm are compressed. These axons carry information from the inferiomedial bilateral retinas and visual information from the superiolateral visual fields resulting in loss of the superiolateral quadrants of the visual field (i.e., bitemporal superior quadrantanopia **(B)**). As tumor growth continues, as all axons within the optic chiasm can become compressed, full loss of the lateral visual fields occurs (i.e., bitemporal hemianopsia **(C)**). (By permission of Mayo Foundation for Medical Education and Research. All rights reserved.)

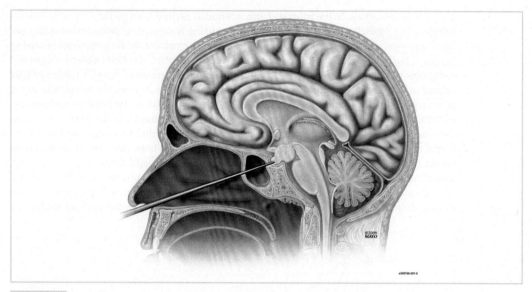

FIGURE 8.5 The transsphenoidal route is the most common approach for the resection of pituitary tumors in adults. Usually with the aid of an operating microscope, instruments are advanced through the nasal cavity. The sphenoid sinus is entered after which the roof of the sphenoid sinus is opened and the pituitary gland is approached through the floor of the sella turcica. (By permission of Mayo Foundation for Medical Education and Research. All rights reserved.)

addition, compression of the carotid artery may occur. As nonfunctional tumors need to grow in order to produce clinical manifestations, they are usually larger than functional tumors at the time of diagnosis; hence they are often referred to as macroadenomas (>1 cm diameter).

C. Treatment. Treatment of pituitary tumors depends on multiple factors such as patient age, tumor type, size, invasiveness, hormonal aberrations, and comorbidities. Patients may undergo medical therapy for specific tumor pathologies, radiation therapy, or surgical resection. Medical therapy will be discussed later in this chapter in the context of specific tumor pathologies.

D. Management of anesthesia. In the majority of cases, surgical resection of a pituitary tumor is accomplished via the transsphenoidal route (Fig. 8.5) whereas other approaches, such as translabial or craniotomy, are often reserved for patients requiring increased tumor exposure due to size or invasiveness, or in children in whom the size of the nares and nasal cavity may not permit the introduction of necessary surgical instruments. Transsphenoidal resection of a pituitary mass is performed via general anesthesia. The sphenoid sinus is entered endoscopically and the posterior/superior wall of the sphenoid sinus is traversed to enter the sella turcica. The tumor is then resected with the aid of microscope.

Airway management, specific drug choices, and the need for invasive monitoring and large-bore intravenous access are typically determined based on the size and degree of invasiveness of the tumor, stigmata of endocrinopathy, and the presence of comorbid conditions. Significant bleeding may occur during the resection of large invasive tumors. Pharyngeal packing should be considered to limit gastric accumulation of blood. As vasoconstrictors, such as cocaine or epinephrine, are usually administered within the nasal mucosa, significant hypertension may occur. Patient movement should be avoided given the close proximity of the carotid artery to the sella. In addition, the surgeon may request placement of a lumbar drainage catheter. This will allow indirect manipulation of the tumor via the withdrawal of cerebrospinal fluid (to elevate the tumor by reducing intracranial pressure) or instillation of either air or sterile saline to displace the tumor caudally. If air is injected, nitrous oxide, if used, should be either discontinued or reduced in concentration.

Hormonal aberrations can occur following pituitary tumor resection and include hypopituitarism, diabetes insipidus (DI), or syndrome of inappropriate antidiuretic hormone (SIADH).

Generally, a serum cortisol concentration is obtained the day following surgery as changes in hormonal concentrations of the pituitary–adrenal axis are most sensitive to acute pituitary insufficiency as the serum half-lives of adrenocorticotropic hormone (ACTH) and cortisol are short (10 minutes and 70 to 120 minutes respectively). If serum cortisol is >10 μg/dL, the patient is unlikely to develop hypopituitarism [2,3]. Urine output should be monitored postoperatively to assess for DI, or less likely the SIADH. Patients developing DI may require treatment with desmopressin acetate (DDAVP). Persistent cerebrospinal fluid leak occurs in approximately 2% of cases and is evident by rhinorrhea with symptoms of low cerebrospinal fluid pressure (e.g., headache occurring in the sitting or standing position) [4]. The presence of β_2-transferrin in the rhinorrhea fluid is diagnostic. Other complications include postoperative nausea and vomiting, bleeding, infection, and injury to nearby neurologic structures (e.g., cranial nerves, optic chiasm).

CLINICAL PEARL Postoperative complications of pituitary tumor resection include nausea and vomiting, bleeding, hypopituitarism, infection, cerebrospinal fluid leak, and although rare, injury to local neurologic and vascular structures.

III. Cushing's disease

    A. Physiology of the hypothalamic–hypophyseal–adrenal axis. Cortisol is the primary glucocorticoid produced in humans. Production of cortisol by the adrenal gland is regulated by a negative feedback loop that also involves the hypothalamus and adenohypophysis (Fig. 8.6). Secretion of corticotropin-releasing hormone (CRH) by the hypothalamus stimulates

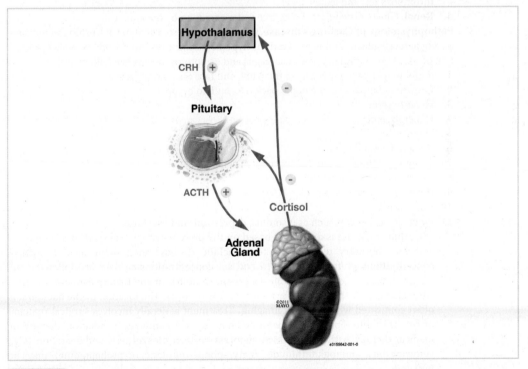

FIGURE 8.6 Cortisol production by the adrenal gland is regulated via a feedback loop involving both the hypothalamus and adenohypophysis. Corticotropin-releasing hormone (CRH) stimulates the production of adrenocorticotropic hormone (ACTH) by the adenohypophysis. ACTH stimulates production of cortisol by the adrenal glands which suppresses further production of both CRH and ACTH. (By permission of Mayo Foundation for Medical Education and Research. All rights reserved.)

the production of ACTH by the adenohypophysis. In turn, ACTH enters the systemic circulation and stimulates the secretion of cortisol by the adrenal cortex. Cortisol production then inhibits production of CRH and ACTH by the hypothalamus and adenohypophysis, respectively, thus reducing further stimulus for cortisol production. Of note, central nervous system-mediated changes in cortisol production (e.g., during times of stress, diurnal variation) are likely mediated by the hypothalamus as changes in CRH production.

B. **Physiologic role of cortisol.** Although named for their role in modulating glucose metabolism, glucocorticoids have wide physiologic effects.

1. **Metabolism.** Cortisol stimulates both gluconeogenesis and glycogen synthesis by the liver. Cortisol also decreases the sensitivity of tissues to the effect of insulin by decreasing the expression of glucose transporters on cell membranes. As such, cortisol increases serum glucose concentration and facilitates the storage of glycogen. Cortisol also increases energy substrate availability by stimulating protein degradation in muscle and increasing lipolysis in adipose tissue.

2. **Vasculature.** Cortisol is critical to maintaining the sensitivity of the vasculature to the vasoconstrictive effects of catecholamines, specifically epinephrine and norepinephrine.

3. **Immune system.** The anti-inflammatory and immune system suppressive effects of cortisol and other glucocorticoids are well known. These effects are likely mediated by diverse actions of glucocorticoids on many different pathways responsible for the inflammatory and immune responses. Glucocorticoids inhibit the release and antagonize the actions of interleukin-1, a cytokine that is pivotal in mediating the immune response via promoting leukocyte chemotaxis and lymphocyte proliferation. Degranulation of leukocytes, mast cells, and macrophages is inhibited by the glucocorticoids. Glucocorticoids also interfere with the metabolism of arachidonic acid thus reducing the synthesis of prostaglandins, thromboxanes, and leukotrienes.

4. **Renal.** Glucocorticoids facilitate free water excretion by the kidney.

C. **Pathophysiology of Cushing's disease.** Cushing's disease is a subtype of Cushing's syndrome (i.e., hypercortisolism) and is reserved for hypercortisolism resulting from excessive production of ACTH by a pituitary adenoma. Signs and symptoms include the following:

1. Rapid weight gain, especially in the trunk and face (i.e., moon facies)
2. Growth of fat pads on the upper back (i.e., buffalo hump)
3. Hypertension
4. Hyperglycemia
5. Hypokalemic alkalosis
6. Impaired wound healing
7. Thinning of the skin and development of acne
8. Development of purple striae
9. Proximal muscle weakness
10. Osteoporosis
11. Psychological effects such as insomnia, depression, and psychosis

Cushing's disease is diagnosed based on the presence of clinical signs and symptoms and via laboratory tests. These tests include increase in 24-hour urinary cortisol concentrations or failure of serum cortisol concentrations to decrease following the administration of dexamethasone—a potent inhibitor of the hypothalamic–pituitary–adrenal axis (i.e., the dexamethasone suppression test). The location of the adenoma is often confirmed with pituitary imaging. Treatment generally involves surgical removal of the adenoma. For patients who are not surgical candidates, radiation therapy or medical therapy with drugs which suppress cortisol biosynthesis and secretion (e.g., ketoconazole, aminoglutethimide, metyrapone, mitotane, cyproheptadine) may be initiated.

D. **Management of anesthesia.** Preoperative management of blood pressure, serum glucose concentration, electrolyte abnormalities, and the presence of fluid retention should be assessed, optimized, and managed. Obesity, moon facies, and buffalo hump may theoretically predispose to a challenge with mask ventilation and laryngoscopy; however, data suggest that Cushing's disease itself does impair airway management [5]. Careful attention should be paid to positioning and placement of adhesive dressings as skin damage can easily occur. The specific choice of anesthetic agents is not influenced by hypercortisolemia. However, etomidate may transiently decrease secretion of cortisol by the adrenal gland; it is unknown if this effect has clinical relevance. The presence of pre-existing muscle weakness may increase sensitivity to nondepolarizing muscle relaxants.

IV. Acromegaly

  A. Physiology and regulation of growth hormone. Growth hormone is a peptide hormone secreted by the somatotropic cells of the anterior pituitary gland. Secretion is regulated by the hypothalamus via the secretion of both growth hormone–releasing hormone (GHRH) and somatostatin, that respectively stimulate or inhibit secretion of growth hormone by the adenohypophysis. Once in the systemic circulation, the effects of growth hormone are mediated either directly via its action at growth hormone receptors or via hepatic production of insulin-like growth factor (ILGF, also known as somatomedin C). Together, the actions of growth hormone and ILGF include the following:

  1. Stimulation of cell growth and proliferation within all major organ systems except the central nervous system
  2. Stimulation of muscle protein synthesis and sarcomere hyperplasia
  3. Chondrocyte proliferation
  4. Increased bone ossification
  5. Effects on metabolism
      a. Increased hepatic gluconeogenesis
      b. Lipolysis
      c. Increased protein synthesis
  6. Immune system stimulation

  B. Pathophysiology of growth hormone excess. Although both manifestations of the same disorder, pituitary gigantism occurs when growth hormone excess occurs prior to ossification of the epiphyseal cartilage and acromegaly results when the onset of growth hormone excess occurs following epiphyseal ossification. Despite the difference in stature, pituitary gigantism and acromegaly share many features. Bone and soft tissue growth results in enlargement of the hands and feet, coarse facial features, and jaw hypertrophy leading to prognathism and malocclusion. Other airway manifestations include enlargement of the tongue, tonsils, epiglottis, and larynx. As such, patients often develop obstructive sleep apnea. Vocal cord dysfunction can occur due to stretching of the recurrent laryngeal nerves and impaired mobility of the cricoarytenoid joints. Cardiovascular system effects account for most deaths from untreated acromegaly. Hypertension is common. Cardiac hypertrophy is due to direct effects of growth hormone on cardiac muscle and secondary to increased afterload from hypertension and often leads to diastolic dysfunction [6,7]. The combination of increased cardiac mass (hence increased oxygen requirements) and diastolic dysfunction predisposes to coronary insufficiency. Patients can also exhibit dysrhythmias and electrocardiographic abnormalities [8]. Peripheral neuropathies are common and are due to demyelination and perineural edema [9]. Metabolic abnormalities include glucose intolerance or frank diabetes mellitus secondary to increased gluconeogenesis.

  Diagnosis is often based on the presence of signs and symptoms in addition to laboratory tests. As growth hormone is secreted in a pulsatile fashion, single random serum growth hormone values are often not helpful in establishing the diagnosis. Serum concentrations of ILGF in fasting patients are more reliable as normal values are 0.3 to 1.4 U/mL whereas those found in patients with acromegaly are 2.6 to 21.7 U/mL [10]. The diagnosis of a tumor is then confirmed via radiologic imaging of the sella.

  Treatment usually involves surgical resection of the adenoma. For patients who are not candidates for surgery, or in whom surgery has failed, radiation or medical therapy with either octreotide (a somatostatin analog) or dopamine agonists (e.g., bromocriptine, cabergoline, pergolide, lisuride) may be beneficial at preventing further progression.

  C. Management of anesthesia. Hypertrophy of the mandible and enlargement of the tongue and other soft tissues in the mouth and airway, including glottic structures, can not only increase

4

the difficulty of laryngoscopy, but may make mask fit and mask ventilation difficult [5]. The most conservative means to secure an airway in an acromegalic patient is via awake fiberoptic bronchoscope. If the decision is made to induce general anesthesia prior to laryngoscopy, the clinician should have appropriate back-up equipment readily available in the event that either mask ventilation or direct laryngoscopy is difficult or impossible. This may include oral or nasal airways, an assistant to help with two-person bag-mask ventilation, and various airway devices (e.g., laryngeal mask airway, video laryngoscope). As mandibular hypertrophy can increase the distance between the mouth and glottis, and glottic narrowing may be present, a full-length endotracheal tube with a smaller diameter should be available. Hypertrophy of the costal cartilage can lead to restrictive pulmonary mechanics. As hypertension, diastolic dysfunction, coronary insufficiency, and dysrhythmias may be present or occur, direct arterial blood pressure monitoring may be warranted. Despite beliefs to the contrary, hypertrophy of the transverse carpal ligament does not increase the risk of ischemic complications of the hand with radial artery cannulation [11].

CLINICAL PEARL Clinical manifestations of acromegaly are likely to impact mask ventilation and laryngoscopy as standard preoperative airway assessment may not reliably predict ease of mask ventilation and laryngoscopy.

V. Hyperprolactinemia

A. Physiology and regulation of prolactin. Prolactin is a peptide hormone produced by the mammotropic cells of the adenohypophysis and secretion is regulated by hypothalamic hormones. Although the hypothalamus produces a prolactin-releasing hormone, the regulation of prolactin secretion is largely inhibitory and mediated by hypothalamic dopamine. In addition to a prolactin-secreting pituitary adenoma, there are multiple other causes of hyperprolactinemia:

1. Pregnancy and lactation
2. Sleep
3. Exercise
4. Compression of the pituitary stalk by other pituitary pathology (thus preventing hypothalamic dopamine from reaching the mammotrophs)
5. Decreased clearance of prolactin (e.g., renal failure, hypothyroidism)
6. Diseases leading to decreased hypothalamic dopamine production (e.g., histiocytosis X, sarcoidosis, gliomas)
7. Drugs that decrease dopamine synthesis or antagonize its action (e.g., α-methyldopa, phenothiazine)

Prolactin has multiple physiologic effects. Although not responsible for breast development, it is the primary hormone responsible for regulating lactation. Elevated serum prolactin concentrations can suppress sex steroid (i.e., estrogen and testosterone) secretion.

B. Pathophysiology of hyperprolactinemia. Typical signs and symptoms of elevated serum prolactin concentrations are more distinct in females and include galactorrhea, amenorrhea, and infertility. Males will often complain of nonspecific symptoms such as loss of libido. As such, prolactin-producing adenomas tend to present earlier (and are thus smaller at the time of diagnosis) in women. In males, a pituitary prolactinoma may not come to attention until it has grown enough to produce compression of surrounding structures causing headache and visual changes such as diplopia or visual field deficits.

Diagnosis should begin with a history and physical examination, and determination of serum prolactin concentrations. Normal serum prolactin is <25 ng/mL. In general, prolactin-secreting adenomas are usually associated with higher prolactin concentrations (i.e., >150 ng/mL) whereas other causes of hyperprolactinemia (e.g., stalk compression, decreased clearance, drug effect) generally cause only mild-to-moderate elevations in prolactin (25 to

150 ng/mL) [12]. Workup for hyperprolactinemia involves ruling out nonpituitary causes (e.g., drugs, hypothalamic dysfunction) and imaging of the sella turcica.

In patients with a prolactinoma and a serum prolactin >500 ng/mL, medical therapy with dopamine agonists (e.g., bromocriptine, pergolide, cabergoline) is often preferred. In those with a serum prolactin <500 ng/mL or those refractory to medical therapy, surgical resection is considered.

C. Management of anesthesia. In general, hyperprolactinemia has no direct influence on the management of anesthesia. However, the clinician should be aware of the consequences of tumor size and invasiveness (i.e., increased risk for pre-existing elevated intracranial pressure and intraoperative bleeding during resection in larger tumors) and adverse effects associated with drugs used to medically manage hyperprolactinemia. The latter point is important as many patients undergo chronic medical management and may undergo surgery unrelated to their prolactinoma. Common side effects of dopamine agonists include nausea and orthostatic hypotension that can be exacerbated by anesthesia. Pergolide and cabergoline possess serotonin agonist properties and are associated with cardiac valvulopathies similar to carcinoid syndrome [13,14].

VI. Pituitary hyperthyroidism

A. Regulation of thyroid-stimulating hormone secretion. Secretion of thyroid-stimulating hormone (TSH) by the adenohypophysis is stimulated by thyrotropin-release hormone (TRH), secreted by the hypothalamus. TSH then stimulates the thyroid gland to secrete T_3 and T_4 which subsequently inhibit further release of TRH and TSH.

B. Pathophysiology of increased TSH production. Initially, patients will present with symptoms of hyperthyroidism including anxiety, weight loss, heat intolerance, tachycardia, hypertension, cardiac dysrhythmia (e.g., atrial fibrillation). Diagnostic workup may reveal elevated serum concentrations of TSH and thyroid hormones suggesting a secondary cause of hyperthyroidism as TSH levels are often reduced in the setting of primary hyperthyroidism. As TSH-secreting adenomas are rare, some patients may undergo treatment for primary hyperthyroidism (i.e., Graves disease). In this circumstance, loss of negative feedback from reductions in serum concentrations of circulating thyroid hormone following treatment results in increased TRH production and further stimulation of the pituitary tumor, leading to further tumor growth.

C. Management of anesthesia. Unless vision is acutely threatened, patients should be medically optimized prior to surgery and rendered euthyroid. Octreotide reduces TSH production by adenomas and is often first-line therapy [15]. Control of tachycardia is a useful endpoint and may require institution of β-adrenergic receptor antagonists. Patients who have undergone thyroid ablation for suspected Graves disease may be hypothyroid and should also be rendered euthyroid with thyroid hormone supplementation. For large invasive tumors, large-bore intravenous access should be obtained due to increased risk of bleeding. Invasive arterial blood pressure monitoring should be considered, especially in patients who remain hyperthyroid at the time of surgery or in those with large tumors.

VII. Diseases of the posterior pituitary gland

A. Physiology of the posterior pituitary gland. The primary secretory units of the posterior pituitary gland are the distal axons of neurons with cell bodies located in the hypothalamus. The octapeptide hormones, oxytocin and vasopressin, are synthesized within the hypothalamus and transported to and stored within the neurohypophysis. Upon stimulation, these hormones are then released into the systemic circulation.

The primary stimulus for the release of vasopressin, also known as ADH, is an increase in serum osmolarity (normal is approximately 285 mOsm/L). Osmoreceptors within the organum vasculosum, a structure located anterior to the hypothalamus, mediate this effect via initiating a cascade that results in the release of vasopressin by the neurohypophysis. Likewise, a decrease in serum osmolarity causes a reduction in the output of vasopressin. An increase in the secretion of vasopressin can also occur in response to a reduction in blood pressure and blood volume that is mediated by arterial baroreceptors in the aortic arch and carotid sinus and by venous baroreceptors in the atrial and pulmonary venous system. The secretion of vasopressin is less sensitive to changes in blood pressure and volume than to changes in serum osmolarity because sympathetic reflexes will often initially compensate for mild-to-moderate changes in blood pressure and volume. It is when these reflexes are exhausted that an increase in vasopressin secretion occurs. The actions of vasopressin are mediated via specific receptors located on vascular smooth muscle (V_1 receptors) causing vasoconstriction and in the renal collecting duct (V_2 receptors) increasing water reabsorption in the kidney.

B.   Syndrome of inappropriate ADH. The hallmark finding in SIADH is hyposmolarity due to inappropriately elevated serum concentrations of ADH. SIADH is the most common cause of euvolemic hyposmolarity [16]. Causes of SIADH include the following:

1.   **Malignancy.** Especially bronchogenic carcinoma, mesothelioma
2.   **Central nervous system disorders.** Traumatic head injury, postcraniotomy, meningitis, encephalitis, subarachnoid hemorrhage, tumors, Guillain–Barré syndrome, elevated intracranial pressure, pituitary stalk transection
3.   **Drugs**
     a.   Stimulation of ADH release: Nicotine, tricyclic antidepressants, phenothiazine
     b.   Potentiation of the renal effects of ADH: DDAVP, oxytocin, chlorpropamide
     c.   Other: Thiazide diuretics, serotonin reuptake inhibitors, angiotensin-converting enzyme inhibitors, chemotherapeutic agents
     d.   Nonmalignant pulmonary disorders: Pneumonia, tuberculosis, chronic obstructive pulmonary disease, acute respiratory failure, positive-pressure ventilation
     e.   Physiologic stress: Exercise, anemia, pain

     The diagnosis of SIADH requires hyponatremia, inappropriately concentrated urine, and no evidence of renal, adrenal, or thyroid dysfunction. Typically, serum sodium concentration is less than 134 mEq/L and serum osmolarity is less than 275 mOsm/L. In addition, urine sodium is increased (i.e., >18 mEq/L). Patients with mild SIADH are often asymptomatic but as serum sodium decreases, especially if this occurs acutely, confusion, lethargy, nausea, vomiting, seizures, and finally coma can develop.

     The treatment of SIADH usually begins with identifying and treating the cause, if possible. Patients with mild or asymptomatic SIADH usually respond to fluid restriction (<1 L/day in adults). The addition of a loop diuretic will aid in the excretion of water, especially if combined with sodium supplementation (e.g., high-sodium diet). The use of vasopressin-receptor antagonists, such as conivaptan or satavaptan, are under investigation for the treatment of chronic SIADH [17,18]. In cases of SIADH with moderate or severe symptomatic hyponatremia, treatment with hypertonic saline should be considered. Serum sodium should increase by no more than 0.5 to 2 mEq/L/h, depending on severity. An initial infusion rate of hypertonic saline (3%) can be estimated using the following equation:

     Rate of 3% NaCl (mL/h) = patient weight (kg) × expected hourly change in serum sodium concentration (mEq/L).

     Treatment with hypertonic saline should be terminated when any of the following occur:

     (1) The patient is asymptomatic.
     (2) A safe serum sodium is achieved (>120 mEq/L).
     (3) A total magnitude of correction of 20 mEq/L is achieved.

CLINICAL PEARL   In patients with moderate-to-severe symptomatic SIADH, hyponatremia should be corrected slowly (0.5 to 2 mEq/L/h) until either the patient is asymptomatic, safe serum sodium is achieved (>120 mEq/L), or total magnitude of correction of 20 mEq/L is achieved.

C.   Diabetes Insipidus. The hallmark finding in DI is the inappropriate production of dilute urine not due to the use of a diuretic agent. Two major mechanisms that produce DI are reduced production of ADH by the neurohypophysis (i.e., central DI) and failure of the kidney to appropriately respond to ADH (i.e., nephrogenic DI). Specific causes of DI include the following:

1. Traumatic or anoxic brain injury or brain death
2. Surgical hypophysectomy
3. Hypothalamic or pituitary pathology
4. Meningitis, encephalitis
5. Granulomatous disease
6. Congenital mutations of the ADH receptor
7. Polycystic kidney disease
8. Renal infarcts
9. Sickle-cell disease
10. Drugs such as lithium carbonate or demecycline

Signs and symptoms include excessive urination, thirst, and evidence of dehydration (e.g., loss of skin turgor, hypotension, tachycardia, lethargy). A urine specific gravity of <1.005 or a urine osmolarity <300 mOsm/L despite serum hypertonicity (serum osmolarity >295 mOsm/L) and in the absence of diuretic drugs is diagnostic for DI. To distinguish between central and nephrogenic DI, 5 U of subcutaneous vasopressin should reduce urine output in those with central, but not nephrogenic DI.

Treatment goals in patients with DI are to correct the fluid deficit and to stop ongoing renal fluid loss. Oral free water replacement is preferred. For patients not able to tolerate oral intake or for symptomatic patients, intravenous fluid replacement should be initiated. Free water deficit can be estimated by the following equation:

$$\text{Free water deficit (L)} = ((\text{serum } [Na^+] - 140)/140) \times \text{total body water (L)}$$

For those with DI existing for >24 hours the free water deficit should be corrected over 48 to 72 hours and plasma sodium concentrations should not decrease by >1 mEq/L every 2 hours as rapid correction can lead to cerebral edema. Hyposmolar solutions, such as 0.45% sodium chloride or lactated Ringer's solution, are suitable options. In patients with severe dehydration and organ hypoperfusion, expansion of the intravascular volume with administration of 0.9% sodium chloride solution should be instituted prior to correction of the free water deficit.

In patients with central DI, ongoing water loss can be treated by the administration of vasopressin or DDAVP. For those with nephrogenic DI, no specific treatment exists; however, salt restriction and thiazide diuretics, may be helpful. Thiazide diuretics enhance water reabsorption in the distal nephron independent of the action of a vasopressin.

D. Oxytocin. Oxytocin is best known for its role in childbirth. During labor, oxytocin is a potent stimulator of cervical dilation and uterine contraction. In addition, oxytocin is released in response to suckling and mediates the let-down reflex where milk is expelled from the mammary gland into the subareolar sinuses. Oxytocin also plays a role in the human sexual response and modulates human behaviors.

VIII. Hypopituitarism

A. Pathophysiology. Hypopituitarism, or pituitary failure, refers to the condition when the pituitary gland production of at least one hormone fails to meet the physiologic requirements of the body. Common causes of hypopituitarism are the following:

1. Pituitary tumors: Tumor growth, apoplexy
2. Pituitary surgery
3. Traumatic head injury
4. Infections: Meningitis, encephalitis
5. Genetic disorders: Prader–Willi syndrome, Kallmann syndrome
6. Vascular disorders: Sickle cell disease, Sheehan's syndrome, apoplexy
7. Inflammatory disorders: Sarcoidosis, Wegener's granulomatosis, hypophysitis, histiocytosis X

Signs and symptoms of hypothyroidism can be diverse and are dependent on the hormones that are deficient and the degree of their deficiencies. Growth hormone deficiency results in nonspecific symptoms such as fatigue, reduced exercise tolerance, metabolic changes such as reduced muscle mass, increased central fat, and hyperlipidemia. If growth hormone deficiency occurs in childhood, short stature will result. Hypocortisolism results in fatigue, hypoglycemia, hyponatremia, and hypotension. A deficiency in gonadotropins such as follicle-stimulating hormone and luteinizing hormone can result in amenorrhea, infertility, decreased libido, loss of body hair, and decreased muscle mass. Finally, decreased TSH production results in fatigue, cold intolerance, weight gain, and bradycardia. Prolactin deficiency is exceedingly rare in the setting of hypopituitarism given that prolactin secretion is predominantly under inhibitory control by the hypothalamus. As such, patients with hypopituitarism may have hyperprolactinemia. Deficiencies of hormones produced by the neurohypophysis can also occur.

In acute pituitary failure, the hypophyseal–adrenal axis is usually the first to be affected as the serum half-lives of ACTH and cortisol are shorter than the hormones involved in the other pituitary axes. Symptoms of acute hypocortisolism include nausea, dilutional hyponatremia, and profound hypotension. Treatment with corticosteroids can be life-saving as it re-establishes vascular responsiveness to vasoconstrictors.

The diagnosis of hypopituitarism is generally based on signs and symptoms and demonstrating reduced serum concentrations of one or more pituitary hormones. Further, there is often a blunted response to stimulating agents such as CRH, GHRH, or TRH. Imaging of the sella may help establish the cause if not clear from other clinical clues. Treatment involves treating the cause and hormonal supplementation as appropriate.

B. **Management of anesthesia.** In general, the goal of perioperative management of patients with hypopituitarism is replacement of deficient hormones, if necessary. This must be made on a case-by-case basis. Factors affecting the perioperative management of hypopituitarism are: (1) whether the disease is acute or chronic, (2) the nature and degree of each hormone deficiency, and (3) whether the physiologic stress of surgery or critical illness will result in increased hormonal requirements.

Hypofunctioning of the hypophyseal–adrenal axis generally requires the most attention in the perioperative period as glucocorticoid requirements increase during surgery and physiologic stress and glucocorticoid deficiencies can lead the significant and potentially life-threatening physiologic aberrations. In acute hypopituitarism, as may occur with pituitary apoplexy (see following section), corticosteroid supplementation can be lifesaving as patients may demonstrate severe and vasoconstrictor-resistant hypotension as corticosteroids are required to maintain vascular tone [19]. In patients with hypopituitarism, the increase in corticosteroid requirements associated with surgery may stress this axis even if patients are not requiring corticosteroid supplementation on a daily basis. Patients should receive their usual morning dose of glucocorticoid (if they take steroid supplements) and additional steroids should be considered based on the expected surgical stress as shown in Table 8.2 [20].

TSH and thyroid hormones have relatively long half-lives. As such, clinically significant hypothyroidism rarely occurs in acute hypopituitarism. In patients with chronic hypopituitarism, serum thyroid hormones should be assessed and adjusted if necessary prior to surgery. Of note, because of reduced production of TSH in hypothyroidism, serum TSH concentrations should not be relied upon to guide management of thyroid hormone concentrations. Patients may also demonstrate evidence of DI if ADH production is inadequate and may require DDAVP supplementation and close attention to fluid and electrolyte management perioperatively. Abnormalities in growth hormone, prolactin, oxytocin, and gonadotropins rarely impact perioperative management.

C. **Pituitary apoplexy.** Apoplexy refers to sudden hemorrhage within the pituitary gland. In the majority of cases, bleeding is associated with the presence of a pre-existing pituitary mass, commonly either an adenoma or Rathke's cleft cyst, but may also occur in a normal pituitary gland. The exact mechanism accounting for apoplexy is not well understood. Signs and symptoms include the abrupt onset of headache, visual disturbances, ophthalmoplegia, and altered

TABLE 8.2 Guidelines for perioperative supplementation of glucocorticoids. Patients taking <5 mg/day of prednisone should receive their usual dose of prednisone but may not need additional supplementation

	Administer usual daily steroid dose	Preoperative supplementation
Minor surgical stress Colonoscopy Inguinal hernia repair Local anesthesia only	Yes	25 mg IV hydrocortisone or 5 mg IV methylprednisolone on day of procedure only
Moderate surgical stress Open cholecystectomy Hemicolectomy	Yes	50–75 mg IV hydrocortisone or 10–15 mg IV methylprednisolone on day of procedure and tapered over 1–2 days following procedure to usual dose
Major surgical stress Cardiac surgery Liver resection	Yes	100–150 mg IV hydrocortisone or 20–30 mg IV methylprednisolone on day of procedure and tapered over 1–2 days following procedure to usual dose
Major critical illness Septic shock	Yes	50–100 mg IV hydrocortisone every 6–8 h plus 50 μg/day fludrocortisone until shock resolved, then gradually taper following vital signs and serum sodium concentration

From Coursin DB, Wood KE. Corticosteroid supplementation for adrenal insufficiency. *JAMA*. 2002;287:236–240 modified with permission [20].

mental status. With rostral extension of the hemorrhage, hydrocephalus and coma may occur. Patients may also develop vasopressor-resistant hypotension due to acute cortisol deficiency. Diagnosis is confirmed by imaging the contents of the sella turcica and demonstrating a hemorrhagic mass. Treatment consists of emergent surgical decompression, rapid administration of corticosteroid, treatment of hypotension, management of hydrocephalus via ventricular drainage, and assessment and management of dysfunction in hormonal axes. An initial dose of 100 mg of hydrocortisone followed by 50 mg every 6 hours for the first 24 hours should be considered.

CLINICAL PEARL   In patients with acute hypopituitarism, such as in the setting of apoplexy, glucocorticoid supplementation is critical. An initial dose of 100 mg IV hydrocortisone (or equivalent dose of an alternate glucocorticoid) should be considered.

IX. Conclusion. Disorders of the pituitary gland and associated endocrinologic axes can have a broad impact on a host of biologic functions. Further, these effects can often have a significant impact on perioperative management. As such, awareness of both the local and systemic effects of pituitary pathology is critical for effective and safe perioperative patient management.

REFERENCES

1. Saeger W, Ludecke DK, Buchfelder M, et al. Pathohistological classification of pituitary tumors: 10 years of experience with the German Pituitary Tumor Registry. *Eur J Endocrinol*. 2007;156:203–216.
2. Jane JA Jr, Thapar K, Kaptain GJ, et al. Pituitary surgery: transsphenoidal approach. *Neurosurgery*. 2002;51:435–442.
3. Vance ML. Perioperative management of patients undergoing pituitary surgery. *Endocrinol Metab Clin North Am*. 2003;32:355–365.
4. Esposito F, Dusick JR, Fatemi N, et al. Graded repair of cranial base defects and cerebrospinal fluid leaks in transsphenoidal surgery. *Neurosurgery*. 2007;60:295–303.
5. Nemergut EC, Zuo Z. Airway management in patients with pituitary disease: a review of 746 patients. *J Neurosurg Anesthesiol*. 2006;18:73–77.
6. Fazio S, Cittadini A, Cuocolo A, et al. Impaired cardiac performance is a distinct feature of uncomplicated acromegaly. *J Clin Endocrinol Metab*. 1994;79:441–446.

7. Lopez-Velasco R, Escobar-Morreale HF, Vega B, et al. Cardiac involvement in acromegaly: specific myocardiopathy or consequence of systemic hypertension? *J Clin Endocrinol Metab.* 1997;82:1047–1053.

8. Kahaly G, Olshausen KV, Mohr-Kahaly S, et al. Arrhythmia profile in acromegaly. *Eur Heart J.* 1992;13:51–56.

9. Jenkins PJ, Sohaib SA, Akker S, et al. The pathology of median neuropathy in acromegaly. *Ann Int Med.* 2000;133:197–201.

10. Clemmons DR, Van Wyk JJ, Ridgway EC, et al. Evaluation of acromegaly by radioimmunoassay of somatomedin-C. *N Engl J Med.* 1979;301:1138–1142.

11. Losasso T, Dietz NM, Muzzi DA. Acromegaly and radial artery cannulation. *Anesth Analg.* 1990;71:204.

12. Randall RV, Scheithauer BW, Laws ER Jr, et al. Pituitary adenomas associated with hyperprolactinemia: a clinical and immunohistochemical study of 97 patients operated on transsphenoidally. *Mayo Clin Proc.* 1985;60:753–762.

13. Horvath J, Fross RD, Kleiner-Fisman G, et al. Severe multivalvular heart disease: a new complication of the ergot derivative dopamine agonists. *Mov Disord.* 2004;19:656–662.

14. Pritchett AM, Morrison JF, Edwards WD, et al. Valvular heart disease in patients taking pergolide. *Mayo Clin Proc.* 2002; 77:1280–1286.

15. Chanson P, Weintraub BD, Harris AG. Octreotide therapy for thyroid-stimulating hormone-secreting pituitary adenomas. A follow-up of 52 patients. *Ann Int Med.* 1993;119:236–240.

16. Anderson RJ, Chung HM, Kluge R, et al. Hyponatremia: a prospective analysis of its epidemiology and the pathogenetic role of vasopressin. *Ann Int Med.* 1985;102:164–168.

17. Decaux G. Long-term treatment of patients with inappropriate secretion of antidiuretic hormone by the vasopressin receptor antagonist conivaptan, urea, or furosemide. *Am J Med.* 2001;110:582–584.

18. Soupart A, Gross P, Legros JJ, et al. Successful long-term treatment of hyponatremia in syndrome of inappropriate antidiuretic hormone secretion with satavaptan (SR121463B), an orally active nonpeptide vasopressin V2-receptor antagonist. *Clin J Am Soc Nephrol.* 2006;1:1154–1160.

19. Grunfeld JP, Eloy L. Glucocorticoids modulate vascular reactivity in the rat. *Hypertension.* 1987;10:608–618.

20. Coursin DB, Wood KE. Corticosteroid supplementation for adrenal insufficiency. *JAMA.* 2002;287:236–240.

9

Intracranial Aneurysms

Leslie Jameson

KEY POINTS

1. Cardiac arrhythmias, impaired cardiac function, impaired oxygenation, hypovolemia, hyperglycemia, and electrolyte abnormalities are common and their severity parallels the patient's initial Hunt and Hess grade.
2. Prophylactic treatment for vasospasm and hyperglycemia should be immediately instituted and maintained during all anesthetics.
3. Hypervolemia, hypertension, hemodilution (triple H therapy) is no longer recommended as prophylactic therapy for vasospasm and delayed cerebral ischemia.
4. Blood pressure should be maintained at 130 to 160 mm Hg systolic, 70 to 110 mm Hg mean, or at agreed values while securing the aneurysm and allowed to increase after securing the aneurysm.
5. Patients have abrupt and severe increases in ICP after SAH, thus anesthetic drug management should be designed to decrease ICP (e.g., TIVA) and not increase it (e.g., volatile anesthetic).
6. Patient risk in interventional radiology includes vessel rupture and cerebral ischemia from errant embolic materials.

ALTHOUGH RARE, SUBARACHNOID HEMORRHAGE (SAH) from a cerebral aneurysm or an arteriovenous malformation (AVM) is one of the most immediately catastrophic neurologic illnesses. An anesthesiologist's initial encounter with a patient suspected or diagnosed as having a SAH maybe either the interventional radiology (IR) suite or the operating room (OR) and the patient may have few neurologic symptoms or be comatose. Management of a patient with a SAH requires recognition that not only must the anesthesiologist manage the acute intracranial hypertension and the risk of aneurysmal rupture or bleeding but that these patients also have a high incidence of cardiac, pulmonary, and metabolic derangements. Abnormal autoregulation will make blood pressure (BP), intracranial pressure (ICP), and anesthetic choices critical to patient outcome.

I. Characteristics of patients with SAH

    A. Demographics. Aneurysmal SAH accounts for 10% to 30% of all strokes in the adult population. Overall incidence is about 8.8 to 9.5/100,000 patients in both the United States and Europe. The incidence is significantly greater in people of Japanese (21.9 to 23.5/100,000) and Finnish (18.1 to 21.3/100,000) descent while people from South and Central America have a significantly lower risk (3.1 to 5.7/100,000) [1]. Increasing age is a strong risk factor with the peak prevalence during the individual's fifth decade of life. When considering all the patients with the diagnosis of SAH, the age distribution is approximately [2]:

        1. 5% <20 years

        2. 15% between 20 and 40 years

        3. 75% between 41 and 65 years

        4. 5% >65 years.

        Women by a 3:2 ratio are more likely to have a SAH than men [3].

    B. Outcome. Approximately 15% of patients with acute SAH do not survive to hospital admission. Of those who do, 25% will die within the first 24 hours, 40% by day 7, and 50% by 1 year. Only 20% of those who survive to hospital discharge will be able to return to their previous lifestyle and 25% will have significant cognitive deficits that require assistance to perform some daily tasks [1,4,5]. Forty percent of these patients will have major neurologic deficits that require continuing medical care in a long-term care facility [1]. Prognostic factors for an unfavorable outcome are increasing age, worsening neurologic grade (Tables 9.2 and 9.3), ruptured posterior circulation aneurysm, increasing aneurysm size, increased hemorrhage size and systolic hypertension on admission. Medical conditions associated with a less favorable outcome include hypertension, myocardial infarction, liver disease, or SAH [6,7].

    C. Patient characteristics

        1. Risk factors. Risk factors for SAH are determined by genetics, lifestyle, and aneurysm size.

            a. Genetic factors. Genetic factors influence the location of the aneurysm. However, the strongest determinant of risk is familial. The relative risk of having a cerebral aneurysm is 2.15 (CI 1.77 to 2.59) when one first-degree relative and 51.0 (8.56 to 1,117) when two first-degree relatives have an aneurysm [8]. This association has led to public health organization providing voluntary screening of all first-degree relatives of patients who have had a SAH. Other genetic diseases such as polycystic kidney disease, Ehlers–Danlos type IV, Moyamoya disease, all heritable connective tissue disorders, and any heritable coagulopathies are associated with an increased risk of cerebral aneurysm [2].

            b. Lifestyle. Lifestyle choices, smoking, use of cocaine or amphetamines and frequent, significant alcohol use are all associated with increased risk of SAH. In patients under the age of 30 years, the most common cause of SAH is cocaine and amphetamine use although there have been reports of excessive use of cold medicine containing phenylephrine or derivatives leading to hypertension and eventual SAH. The most common associated medical condition is poorly controlled or uncontrolled hypertension. This constitutes a very large risk group, since according to the Centers for Disease Control (CDC) approximately 31% of the population over 20 years has hypertension.

            c. Risk of rupture. In a patient with an aneurysm, the risk of rupture depends on the size and location. Aneurysms in the anterior circulation make up 97% of most aneurysms and they are distributed in the following manner (approximate values): Ophthalmic (1%), posterior communicating (25%), internal carotid (5%), anterior communicating artery (ACOA [41%]), A2 segment of the anterior cerebral artery (2%), and middle cerebral artery (24%). The posterior circulation has only 3% to 4% of all aneurysms; they occur on the basilar (30%) and posterior inferior cerebellar artery (70%) [9]. The location and size of the aneurysm is important for anesthesia management because it will determine the patient's position and the risk of rupture during intraoperative or neurointerventional treatment. The risk of rebleeding is approximately proportional to the aneurysm size and location and is similar to the risk of spontaneous rupture [9,10].

TABLE 9.1   Hunt and Hess grade of patient status after SAH

Grade	Criteria[a]
I	Asymptomatic or minimal headache with mild nuchal rigidity
II	Moderate-to-severe headache, nuchal rigidity, but not neurologic deficits other than a cranial nerve palsy
III	Drowsiness, confusion, mild focal deficit (usually motor)
IV	Stupor, hemiparesis (mild to severe), possible early decerebrate rigidity and vegetative disturbances
V	Deep coma, decerebrate rigidity, moribund appearance

[a]With serious pre-existing systemic disease or severe vasospasm on arteriography place patient in the next less favorable category.

II. Medical presentation

A. **Presenting symptoms.** The classic description of a SAH is the patient's statement "the worst headache of my life." This statement may or may not be accompanied by focal neurologic symptoms. Symptoms that typically accompany SAH are [2,11]:

1. nausea and vomiting
2. meningismus
3. decreased level of consciousness
4. focal neurologic signs

Atypical presentations include seizure, confusion, and a fall which can confuse the diagnosis since it suggests head trauma rather than SAH. In about 20% of patients the only symptom is an atypical or mild prodromal headache and half of these patients (10%) will be misdiagnosed as migraine or tension headache. Patients with a missed diagnosis have much poorer overall outcome as they usually have a major rebleed shortly after the prodromal event. All patients with a "thunderclap headache" or other unusual neurologic complaints need an immediate CT scan. Patients with a prodromal headache that is misdiagnosed are a major concern for the anesthesiologist. When this patient population has subsequent SAH, they are likely to have vasospasm at the time of diagnosis. BP management of possible vasospasm and an unsecured leaking aneurysm requires precise control [2,12,13].

B. **Severity of hemorrhage.** SAH grading scales provide accurate prognostic information to assist in decision making by the patients, their family, and the physicians providing care. Hunt and Hess Classification of Status (Table 9.1) and the World Federation of Neurosurgeons (WFNS) SAH scale (Table 9.2) are the current standard assessment tools. It is not possible to assign the ASA physical status classification without an understanding of these evaluation tools. The Hunt and Hess (H&H) grade is unique in that it incorporates the pre-existing medical conditions into the scoring. Patients with serious systemic disease (e.g., hypertension, diabetes, chronic pulmonary disease, cardiac disease) or with vasospasm on angiogram will be moved to the next less favorable score (e.g., from II to III). The WFNS SAH scale utilizes the Glasgow coma scale (GCS) to assess neurologic status.

TABLE 9.2   World federation of neurosurgeons (WFNS) SAH scale

WFNS grade	Glasgow coma score	Motor deficit
I	15	Absent
II	14–13	Absent
III	14–13	Present
IV	12–7	Present or absent
V	6–3	Present or absent

TABLE 9.3 Fisher grades for computed tomography (CT) findings in SAH

Grade	CT findings
1	No blood detected
2	Diffuse thin layer of subarachnoid blood (vertical layers <1 mm thick)
3	Localized clot or thick layer of subarachnoid blood (vertical layers >1 mm thick)
4	Intracerebral or intraventricular blood with or without diffuse subarachnoid blood

Although often under recognized by anesthesiologist, the Fisher Grade for SAH (Table 9.3) classifies the amount of blood seen on computerized axial tomography (CT) scan of the brain. It is very useful in assessing the risk of vasospasm and delayed ischemic neurologic deficit (DIND) [11,14,15]. This knowledge is very important for the immediate medical and anesthesic management.

III. Associated physiologic complications. Many severe and minor medical complications are associated with the severity of the SAH. While much is made of the morbidity and mortality caused by vasospasm and delayed cerebral ischemia (DCI), the associated medical complications are the causative factors in mortality and morbidity. The conditions that have the highest association with severe morbidity and mortality occur as an immediate and direct consequence of SAH and are present often on admission. Many problems are correctable (e.g., hyperglycemia, fever) and although evidence is lacking that correction of these issues will unequivocally prevent poor outcome, there is strong evidence that it will improve outcome [16]. The proportional contributions to mortality and significant morbidity are medical complications (23%), vasospasm and DCI (23%), rebleeding (22%), multiple factors (34%) [15]. Knowledge and appropriate management of medical complications associated with SAH by the anesthesiologist will contribute to better outcomes and make planning and management decisions more effective. The extent and consequences of the medical complications are found in Figure 9.1. High-risk, high-frequency physiologic perturbations that have recognized impact on anesthesia management are discussed. Anesthetic management will extend past the initial securing of the aneurysm either in IR or OR as follow up procedures for treatment for vasospasm and high ICP (ventriculoperitoneal shunt, decompressive craniectomy) [17] and on rare occasions clipping of additional aneurysms [5,11].

CLINICAL PEARL **Intraventional radiology (IR) procedures:** Fluid overload and renal injury due to the volume of dye administered can be managed by monitoring urine output and administering N-acetylcysteine and $NaHCO_3$.

A. Cerebral. Cerebral autoregulation, the ability to maintain a stable cerebral perfusion or cerebral blood flow (CBF) relatively constant over a range of BP, is dependent on the size of the hemorrhage, the ICP, and the time since the SAH. The basic principles of autoregulation are discussed elsewhere (Chapter 1). Immediately after SAH, impairment is directly related to the degree of injury determined by the H&H grade [5]. Immediately after rupture, patients with an H&H grade of I and II would be expected to have normal autoregulation in areas of their brain that are not directly affected by the SAH. In patients with an H&H grade of III or more, the lower limit where autoregulation fails (hypotension) is significantly higher. Failures of autoregulation during relative hypo- or hypertension increase cerebral blood volume, ICP, and impair perfusion causing cerebral ischemia. The vascular response to changing CO_2 and hypoxia remains normal immediately after injury when H&H grade is less than III. Cerebrovascular reactivity impairment is seen in all patients with vasospasm and this impairment begins prior to development of vasospasm. An entirely normal response to changing

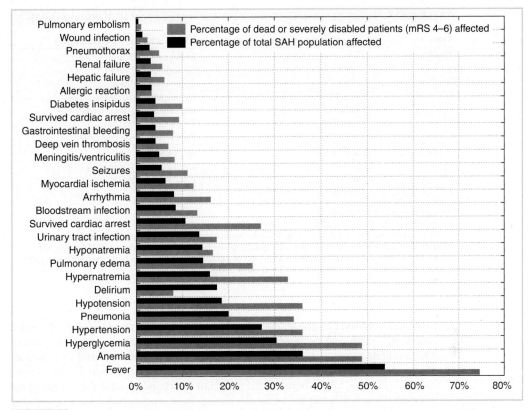

FIGURE 9.1 A comparison of the complication profiles of 576 patients with the subgroup of patients (220). Source: Wartenberg KE, Schmidt JM, Claassen J, et al. Impact of medical complications on outcome after subarachnoid hemorrhage. *Crit Care Med.* 2006;34:617–623.

PaCO$_2$ or PaO$_2$ is unlikely to be present >24 hours after rupture [18]. The principles regarding elevation in ICP due to the sudden increase in intracranial volume are the same as covered in Chapter 27.

B. **Cardiac.** Cardiac abnormalities are the most commonly seen associated injury and occur immediately after SAH. They fall into two categories: Those that produce cardiac arrhythmias and those that decrease myocardial contractility. The etiology of these effects is believed to be the sudden catecholamine surge that accompanies the SAH. Catecholamines produce marked vasoconstriction and an accompanying increase in systemic and pulmonary BP. Autopsy findings in previously healthy patients describe diffuse microinfarctions distributed throughout the myocardium. This effect exacerbates underlying cardiac disease seen in the fifties and older age groups [11,14,19]. Some cardiac findings predict poor-quality outcomes.

1. **Arrhythmias.** Between 60% and 100% of patients will have ECG conduction abnormalities after SAH. Most are not indicators of eminent cardiac catastrophe and will resolve spontaneously within 3 days. Arrhythmias linked to ischemic myocardial injury are associated with increased relative risk of death and DCI. The most commonly seen ECG changes are listed in Table 9.4.

   Considering the percent of patients who experience cardiac arrhythmias, they represent a fairly benign finding that can serve as an alert to examine the patient carefully for other signs of cardiac injury [11,14,19].

TABLE 9.4 Compilation of common cardiac rhythm and conduction abnormalities seen in SAH

Type	Description of change (percent of patients who have ECG changes)	
Conduction	ST segment (27%)	ST depression[a,b] (8%)
		ST depression[a,b] (8%)
		ST elevation (19%)
	Any T-wave changes[a] (39%)	T-wave inversion (18%)
	Other	U waves and Q wave (26%)[a]
		T-wave inversion (18%)
		Prolonged QT interval (34%)
Arrhythmias	Ventricular	AV or BB block (7%)
		Ventricular tachycardia (4%–8%)
	Atrial	Atrial flutter/fibrillation[a] (4%–78%)
	Arrest	

[a]Increased relative risk of death.
[b]Increased relative risk of delayed cerebral ischemia (DCI).
Source: Extracted from Rose MJ. Aneurysmal subarachnoid hemorrhage: an update on the medical complications and treatments strategies seen in these patients. *Curr Opin Anaesthesiol.* 2011;24:500–507; van der Bilt IAC, Hasan D, Vandertop WP, et al. Impact of cardiac complications on outcome after aneurysmal subarachnoid hemorrhage: a meta-analysis. *Neurology.* 2009;72:635–642.

2. **Myocardial injury.** Catecholamine release is believed to cause the decreased myocardial contractility producing decreased cardiac output [20]. Elevations in troponins (35% to 83%) and brain nauretic protein (BNP) (45% to 92%) are frequently seen and are indicators of considerable increased relative risk of death and morbidity and predict vasospasm and DCI [11,16,19]. Transthoracic echo is used to detect and monitor the severity of the myocardial injury. This may not be possible during the emergency period immediately after the SAH. Thus, identifying the clinical syndrome of neurogenic stress cardiomyopathy or "stunned myocardium" is important for anesthesia management. It presents with chest pain, dyspnea, hypoxia, and often cardiogenic shock and appears within hours of the SAH. It usually lasts up to 3 days. It is believed to be the cause of sudden death in up to 12% of patients. Medical management is supportive; the most important components are maintaining euvolemia, catecholamine support when needed, and BP control. Monitoring of cardiac output is recommended using transthoracic (TTE) or transesophageal echocardiography (TEE) when available and appropriate [16]. The indicators of increased relative risk of death and DCI are [19].
   a. Elevated BNP—Death: 11.1 (CI 4.7 to 26.0), DCI: 4.5 (CI 1.8 to 11.4)
   b. Elevated troponins—Death: 2.0 (CI 1.2 to 3.4), DCI: 3.2 (CI 2.3 to 4.4)
   c. Wall motion abnormalities—Death: 1.9 (CI 1.2 to 2.9), DCI: 2.1 (CI 1.2 to 3.8)
   d. Selected rhythm abnormalities (see Table 9.4)

CLINICAL PEARL **Cardiac risk:** While arrhythmias are usually a benign finding, cardiogenic shock associated with SAH is best managed in the OR with euvolemia and appropriate catecholamine support (e.g., dobutamine, norepinephrine).

3. **Blood volume.** Patients experience a diuresis and are hypovolemic *prior* to administration of loop and osmotic diuretics [16]. Hypovolemia contributes to the secondary hypoperfusion brain injury. The Neurocritical Care Society Multidisciplinary Consensus Conference recommended goals should be euvolemia, *not* hypervolemia as was previously recommended. Hypervolemia even when used after securing the aneurysm is associated

with significant patient harm. Fluid replacement with an isotonic crystalloid has moderate consensus support [16]. Anesthetic management goals should be consistent with these recommendations.

CLINICAL PEARL **Hypovolemia:** Most patients are hypovolemic prior to the medically induced diuresis, consequently maintaining intravascular volume with normal to hyperosmotic solutions like balanced salt or normal saline solutions, 5% albumin or in some organizations, hetastarch is appropriate.

1

C. Pulmonary. Pulmonary symptoms occur in about 20% of patients after SAH but there is evidence of impaired oxygenation in about 80% [16]. Immediately postSAH, the most likely cause is neurogenic or cardiogenic pulmonary edema while later in the patient's course aspiration pneumonitis, acute respiratory distress syndrome, and transfusion-related acute lung injury (TRALI) becomes more likely [21]. Impaired oxygenation may manifest as lower than expected SpO_2. The proposed mechanism is direct lung injury due the catecholamine storm at the time of SAH or acute right-sided failure from myocardial injury. Immediately postSAH, apneic oxygen reserve is likely to be significantly decreased and the oxygen reserve decreases as the H&H grade increases [16]. About 14% of patients with SAH will have pulmonary edema [14]. This lack of oxygen reserve must be anticipated when planning the most appropriate method to secure the airway.

1

D. Glucose metabolism. Abnormal glucose metabolism, hypo- and hyperglycemia are predictive of outcome with hyperglycemia being one of three independent medical management predictors of mortality and morbidity [14]. Patients with admission serum glucose values below 160 mg/dL had a 33% mortality whereas glucose values above 160 mg/dL and above 230 mg/dL increased mortality to 71% and 95%, respectively [22]. Hyperglycemia has also been identified as an independent predictor of symptomatic vasospasm, permanent neurologic disability, and death within 3 months [23–25]. Most studies suggested that glucose value of greater than 140 mg/dL is associated with increased neurologic complications. Glucose control also decreases nonneurologic medical problems, for example, infection, pneumonia, and sepsis [15]. Identifying the ideal glucose values is complex since some research studies utilizing microdialysis catheters in patients after SAH found tissue glucose was significantly lower

2

than serum glucose values [26]. Recommendations from the Neurocritical Care Society's Multidisciplinary Consensus Conference suggests maintaining serum glucose between 80 mg/dL and 200 mg/dL and carefully avoiding hypoglycemia, considered serum glucose <70 mg/dL [16,26]. American Diabetes Association recommends use of an insulin infusion for maintenance of serum glucose between 140 mg/dL and 180 mg/dL in critically ill patients [27].

1

E. Electrolytes. Electrolyte abnormalities are common postSAH. They are exacerbated by therapeutic interventions like osmotic diuresis with mannitol, loop diuretic, and contrast dye.

1. Sodium. Hyponatremia, serum Na <130 mEq/L, occurs in about 30% of patients after a SAH and is the most common electrolyte imbalance in patients with SAH. It is associated with an inappropriate loss of Na triggered by the release of either natriuretic peptide (cerebral salt wasting syndrome [CSWS]) or antidiuretic hormone (syndrome of inappropriate antidiuretic hormone [SIADH]). CSWS causes a hypovolemic hyponatremia by increasing renal Na loss in excess of water. It is treated by carefully administering hypertonic saline; usually 0.9% NaCl is adequate to replace volume and Na losses although hypertonic saline can be used. Volume replacement is a critical factor in therapy for CSWS. SIADH causes a euvolemic hyponatremia from water retention in excess of Na loss. It is treated by administration of small doses of a loop diuretic with fluid replacement to maintain euvolemia. Hyponatremia has not been associated with poor outcomes [11,13,15]. Hypernatremia, serum Na >150 mEq/L, is an iatrogenic disease caused by the use of osmotic and renal loop diuretics. It has not been associated with poor outcomes [16].

2. **Calcium, magnesium, potassium.** Hypocalcemia occurs in about 41% to 74% of all patients after SAH and is assumed to be associated with the diuresis caused by the SAH, administration of contrast and diuretics. It is not associated with documented neurologic complication but may contribute to hypotension when combined with calcium-channel blockers. Although not frequently measured, low serum Mg concentrations are assumed to accompany hypocalcemia. Many organizations have elected to preemptively treat vasospasm or DCI with $MgSO_4$ infusion making hypermagnesiumemia more likely. Mg counteracts Ca effects and can further decrease cardiac contractility, BP, and potentiate nondepolarizing muscle relaxants. Hypokalemia is usually a complication of diuretic therapy. The usual considerations of arrhythmogenesis apply.

F. **Pituitary hormones.** Hypopituitarism occurs in 37% to 55% of patients who survive the initial illness. Deficiencies of growth hormone and adrenocorticotropic hormone are the most commonly reported. Patient quality of life rather than outcome is affected by these deficiencies. Anesthesiologists are most likely to encounter this problem when this population returns for shunt revisions or elective ablation of additional aneurysms. Primary operative concerns would be inadequate cortisol, inadequate steroid response to surgical stress, and increased possibility of hypoglycemia. Both can be managed with the preemptive use of steroids. Diabetes insipidus, deficiency of antidiuretic hormone, presents prior to initial hospital discharge and is relatively rare [28,29].

IV. **Vasospasm and delayed cerebral ischemia.** Cerebral vasospasm and DCI occur in 70% of patients who survive the initial hemorrhage and 20% to 40% of this group becomes symptomatic. Symptoms usually begin by 72 hours after the *initial* hemorrhage. Early in the recovery period, vasospasm and the ischemic consequences remain the most common cause of death and severe disability.

A. **Diagnosis.** While the gold standard for the diagnosis of vasospasm is an arteriogram, most clinicians use a combination of transcranial doppler (TCD) and neurologic signs as the trigger for initiating an arteriogram [30]. TCD uses ultrasound to evaluate arterial blood flow in the anterior and posterior circulation. Multiple daily examinations evaluate the vasculature for an increase in arterial flow velocity. Increasing velocity is diagnostic of vasospasm. Common neurologic symptoms include altered level of consciousness and new focal neurologic finding, although recognized risk factors play a role. Some organizations perform a "screening" arteriogram based on risk alone [5,16,18]. Using the Fischer scale, the odds ratio (OR) for developing systematic vasospasm when compared to Fischer grade 0 to 1 patients is grade 2 and 3— OR 1.6, and grade 4—2.2 OR [18]. The decision to proceed to IR for assessment and treatment is organization dependent [16] and varies from routine time intervals to only with severe neurologic deterioration (see Chapter 28).

B. **Preemptive treatment.** Causation of vasospasm and DCI is not entirely clear. Accepted knowledge suggests the hemoglobin molecule disrupts the balance between endothelin, a vasoconstrictor, and nitric oxide, a vasodilator, but this does not explain the wide variation in severity, response to therapy, and outcome. Research into genetic mechanisms may produce major changes in management [32,33]. Preemptive treatment of vasospasm and DCI is a priority and may need to be initiated by the anesthesia team in the OR. It should be continued during all subsequent anesthetics until therapy has been discontinued. Meta-analysis strongly supports that preemptive therapy decreases the incidence of vasospasm and DCI but treatment does not change outcomes [31].

1. **Calcium-channel blockers.** Nimodipine is the only drug with a clearly demonstrated benefit in reducing the incidence and severity of vasospasm. Nicardipine, an intravenous substitute, does not have the same demonstrable benefits [25,32]. Nonetheless, most patients will receive one of these drugs. Nicardipine is an effective antihypertensive and is very useful in controlling hypertension immediately post SAH and before securing the aneurysm. Nicardipine can lead to significant hypotension during anesthesia induction and maintenance. There are no clear guidelines defining whether to continue nicardipine

during general anesthesia. Since hypotension should be studiously avoided, management is up to the individual practitioner with the consensus goal to continue nicardipine whenever possible.

> **CLINICAL PEARL** **Vasospasm:** Preemptive treatment and therapeutic control of vasospasm is based on intravenous infusion of nicardipine between 2.5 mg/h and 10 mg/h. Hypertension, hypervolemia, and hemodilution (triple H or HHH) therapy has been replaced by normovolemia, maintaining hemoglobin between 10 g/dL and 11 g/dL and selective use of hypertension in patients with neurologic changes due to vasospasm.

    2. **MgSO$_4$.** The use of Mg has become common before securing the aneurysm. In animal models, magnesium reduces vasospasm by blocking calcium from entering the neuron, thereby preventing disruption of mitochondrial and other cellular functions. The most recent randomized control trials [11,25] and meta-analysis [25] have not found a reduction in vasospasm but observational studies have suggested efficacy [11,25,32,33]. Due to the modest risk, many centers continue to administer MgSO$_4$. Mg will contribute to hypotension during anesthesia and will potentiate the effects of nondepolarizing muscle relaxants.

    3. **Statins.** Statins are continued when patients are already taking this class of drug and are often immediately administered to drug-naive patients. Results are mixed regarding the long-term outcome after statin administration. Three systematic reviews found reduced delayed neurologic injury (DNI) and infarcts in patients receiving statins, however, only one found an effect on outcome [25,34,35]. These drugs have no adverse interactions with general anesthesia.

C. **Symptomatic treatment.**

    1. **Hypervolemic, hypertensive, hemodilution (HHH) therapy.** A mainstay of therapy and prophylaxis for symptomatic vasospasm has been HHH therapy due to the belief that it increased cerebral perfusion pressure and blood flow in critical area. Suggested therapeutic goals were systolic BP 160 to 180 for clipped and 120 to 150 for embolized aneurysm, central venous pressure 8 to 12 mm Hg, and hematocrit of 30 to 35 [36]. Complications associated with HHH included pulmonary edema, congestive heart failure, myocardial ischemia, and death. Taken together these complications eliminated survival gains [5,16]. Anesthesia risk for these patients receiving HHH is considerable. Systematic reviews and meta-analysis have found that in controlled trials there was no long-term improvement in outcome and in longitudinal studies only hypertension had an effect on perfusion or outcome [5,16,36]. Current recommendations are to maintain BP between 140 mm Hg and 160 mm Hg, treat hypovolemia with a goal of euvolemia, and keep hemoglobin/HCT at appropriate levels considering the patients comorbid conditions [16,37,38]. These objectives should be continued in the OR.

    2. **Interventional radiology therapy.** IR procedures have become the mainstay therapy for vasospasm and consequently often require a critically ill patient undergo multiple anesthetics. During the treatment of vasospasm, anesthesia management must avoid hypotension, avoid hyper- or hypoglycemia, and prevent increases in ICP. Wide swings in BP have been implicated in worse outcomes [11,16]. Intra-arterial infusion of vasodilator drugs into the offending artery is often the initial therapeutic intervention. These drugs include papaverine, verapamil, milrinone, and nicardipine. Papaverine has a dramatic but short-lived vasodilator effect and has been associated with sudden increases in ICP, rebound vasospasm, seizures, and arrhythmias. Verapamil is currently considered the best intra-arterial drug therapy and does carry the risk of increased ICP. Balloon angioplasty and stent placement are gaining in popularity due to their long-term effects. Both carry an increased risk of vessel perforation and dissection requiring immediate intervention. Effectiveness of BP reduction, a suggested management technique, is not known [5,11,13,39].

V. Anesthetic management unique to SAH. The anesthetic management of aneurysm care has two scenarios:

1.   Before securing the aneurysm and before the development of vasospasm or DCI.
2.   Immediately after securing the aneurysm and until symptomatic vasospasm or DCI occurs.
3.   During treatment of symptomatic vasospasm or DCI.

Elective treatment of unruptured or asymptomatic aneurysm

A. With SAH. Critical events occur primarily associated with SAH and dictate management of rapid increase in intracranial volume, rapid uncompensated increase in ICP, regional and global hypoperfusion/ischemia (DIND or DCI), and direct compression of critical neurologic tissue including brain herniation. All anesthetic management coalesces around maintaining adequate brain perfusion since ultimately brain ischemia is the cause of death. This is accomplished by reducing ICP and brain bulk and maintaining enough but not too much BP to provide adequate perfusion.

> **CLINICAL PEARL**   **Anesthetic management:** Immediately after SAH all patients have increased ICP, thus anesthetic management strategies that reduce ICP such as propofol-based TIVA plus appropriate BP support to minimize hypotension or hypertension are recommended.

1.   **Drug management.** Patients with a presumptive diagnosis of SAH who present for anesthesia will be receiving a calcium-channel blocker, nifedipine or nicardipine, possibly intravenous magnesium for preemptive management of vasospasm. There are many suggested protocols for the conduct of an anesthetic. Currently there are no large studies, meta-analysis, or population studies that support one technique over another in terms of short- or long-term outcomes. Consequently, decisions are based on general principles outlined previously in this chapter and in other chapters, the skill of the clinicians involved, and the drugs available. Table 9.5 presents an outline of a frequently used protocol. Some aspects of anesthetic management differ depending on whether the intervention is a neuroradiology procedure [40,41] or a craniotomy [42–45] (Table 9.5). Due to the different levels of patient stimulation, the primary issues during IR procedures are managing ICP and maintaining BP, while during a surgical procedure are maintaining stable BP and managing brain perfusion during placement of proximal clip, permanent clip, and aneurysm rupture.

2.   **Important physiologic management issues**

     a.   **Blood pressure.** Before securing the aneurysm, the management goal is to keep the systolic or mean BP at values that allow adequate brain perfusion while avoiding an aneurysmal rebleed (Table 9.6). The BP value selected depends on the patient's BP prior to the SAH and their overall medical condition. In the adult population, this usually is a value between 130 mm Hg and 150 mm Hg systolic or a mean of 80 to 110 mm Hg. Hypoperfusion can be detected in patients with H&H grade of I, II, and occasionally III, by changes in their neurologic examination. Principles of maintaining cerebral perfusion pressure apply (Chapter 1). During anesthesia BP is maintained ±20% of the patient's normal value, the preinduction value, or the agreed to goals, and it is maintained within this range throughout the anesthetic. After surgical clip placement, many neurovascular surgeons will allow higher BP since the aneurysm is isolated from the circulation. An embolized aneurysm is still subject to shear stress from hypertension, thus, BP may be controlled at lower values. In patients who require anesthesia for ventriculoperitoneal shunt placement and IR treatment of vasospasm or DCI, BP should be maintained at ±20% of preinduction ICU values. A vasopressor, if necessary, should be chosen based on the patient's cardiac status with the most commonly used infusions, phenylephrine, norepinephrine,

5 **TABLE 9.5** Anesthetic management protocol for patients with acute SAH

Management	Suggested therapeutic management
Evaluation	Emphasis on neurologic, cardiac, and pulmonary status
Monitors	Required: ASA Standard, urine output, arterial catheter Optional: ICP, CVP (dependent on patient condition)
Induction drugs	Hypnotic: Propofol–stable or high ICP, Etomidate–unstable; Narcotic: infusion; no recommendation (NR) for drug Muscle relaxant: For rapid sequence induction rocuronium (>0.6 mg/kg) or succinylcholine; standard induction: NR
Maintenance	High ICP, large hemorrhage: TIVA with propofol, narcotic, muscle relaxant Normal ICP: Volatile of choice, TIVA, dexmedetomidine Narcotic, muscle relaxant: NR
Ventilation	Moderate hyperventilation—PaCO$_2$: 25–32 mm Hg Minimize peak and mean airway pressure, increase minute ventilation using rate
Intravenous fluids	Maintain euvolemia; fluid choices: NR; choices: balanced salt solutions, 0.9% normal saline (NS), 5% albumin (in 0.9% NS), and Hetastarch (6%); hetastarch may be associated with coagulopathy
BP control	See Table 9.6
BP drugs	Increase: Dependent on cardiac condition with infusion recommended; frequency of use: Phenylephrine, norepinephrine, dopamine Decrease (order of preference): Nicardipine, labetolol, esmolol, hydralazine, nitroprusside (risk of metabolic acidosis)
ICP control	Goal: Below 20 mm Hg, treat above 20 mm Hg. Keep cerebral perfusion pressure above 50 mm Hg Treatment: Mannitol, furosemide, hyperventilation, CSF drainage, elevate head of bed, propofol/narcotic; consider hypertonic saline as a substitute for mannitol particularly with refractory elevations of ICP
Proximal clip placement	Collateral flow present: Most common bolus of propofol but NR No collateral flow: Bolus of propofol, report time every 3 min
Aneurysm clipping	Institutional preferences
Rupture	IR: Occlude vessel with balloon proceed to OR OR: Proximal or temporary aneurysm clip, manage cardiac and blood loss conditions Institutional variations: Decrease BP, compress carotid, and administer adenosine
Extubation	Dependent on preoperative neurologic condition and procedural events

TABLE 9.6 Principles of blood pressure control in patients with acute SAH

Event	Management
Preoperative	IR and OR: Maintain BP within agreed range; patient's normal or mean BP: 70–80 mm Hg, systolic BP >140 mm Hg; patients with prodromal bleed or neurologic symptoms BP goal may be different
During initial anesthetic	
Prior to occlusion	IR and OR: Maintain BP within agreed range; patient's normal or mean BP: 70–80 mm Hg, systolic BP >140 mm Hg
During occlusion	IR: Unchanged, occasional decrease in BP OR-proximal clip: Unchanged OR-permanent clip: Institutional variation from decreased BP to no change
After occlusion	IR: Maintain BP within agreed range; patient's normal or mean BP: 70–80 mm Hg, systolic BP >140 mm Hg OR: Return to patient's preoperative values, generally a systolic BP ≤160 mm Hg, mean ≤110 mm Hg allowed
During therapy for vasospasm	
Therapeutic arteriogram	Maintain at ICU pressure goals: mean BP >80 mm Hg or where neurologic symptoms decrease

Note: Operating room (OR) or intervention radiology (IR) procedures indicated only if there are management differences.

Note: Standard points where therapeutic interventions may be required. Specific management relies on institutional best practices with the personnel involved. Only strong recommendation is to maintain mean BP at or above 70 mm Hg in adults.

and dopamine; unwanted hypertension is usually managed with calcium-channel blockers or β-blockers (esmolol, labetolol). This choice is largely an institutional preference [5,11,46].

CLINICAL PEARL **Control of BP:** Before securing the aneurysm, ideally an adult BP should be maintained within approximately 20% of the patient's normal BP. When BP is unknown, a mean of 70 to 80 mm Hg and systolic ≥140 mm Hg is usually recommended. Acceptable BP after embolization remains unchanged but after clipping may be allowed to increase to mean BP as high as 110 mm Hg.

---

3. **Fluid and glucose management.** Maintenance of euvolemia is recommended. Glucose management is the same as in the critical care unit (III. D).

4. **Anemia.** Anemia (Hb below 10 g/dL) occurs in about 50% of patients, and about 80% of patients will have Hb values below 11 g/dL. Decrease in Hb occurs over 3 to 4 days and is not associated with blood loss. In theory, low Hb reduces oxygen-carrying capacity and increases risks of DCI. Anemia and transfusion is associated with death, severe disability, or DNI; current consensus is that anemia is an indicator rather than a cause of these outcomes. There is very little if any literature examining the effect of transfusion on outcome in patients with SAH but in critical care literature, transfusion is clearly associated with immunosuppression, postoperative infections, and pneumonia. Better long-term outcomes are reported in patients with Hb values between 10 mg/dL and 12 mg/dL but the studies are of low quality [37,47]. Consensus opinion is to maintain Hb between 10 mg/dL and 11 mg/dL [11,48]. The decision to transfuse remains the judgment of the anesthesiologists and their assessment of what action will benefit the patient when considering the patient's overall medical condition [15,16,37,38,48].

B. **Elective treatment of unruptured aneurysm.** There is an ever-increasing group of patients that undergoes elective aneurysm clipping. Some cerebral aneurysms are genetic disorders and are discovered during routine screening of first-degree relatives who have experienced a SAH. These individuals then can elect to do nothing, undergo an arteriogram with embolization, or have a surgical intervention [49]. Anesthetic management for embolization differs very little from a standard arteriogram or during embolization of a ruptured aneurysm. These patients do not have elevations in ICP or any neurologic deficits. The basic principle of a balanced general anesthetic for a neurosurgical procedure is the standard approach. In some centers the interventionalist may occasionally request brief reductions in BP which can usually be accomplished with esmolol or a bolus of propofol. There is no evidence supporting one technique over another. Anesthesia for the craniotomy is the same as that administered for any aneurysm. Very tight BP control, treatment for intracranial hypertension, and treatment of vasospasm is not necessary but usually practiced. BP should be maintained with a mean of at least 70 mm Hg or within 20% of the patient's normal BP. Chance of rupture is small but not zero; standard anesthetic neuroanesthesia preparation and care is adequate. As is routine in craniotomy for a vascular lesion, most surgeons will request osmotic diuretics, generally mannitol 0.5 g/kg or 50 g and furosemide.

C. **Special considerations.**

1. **IR procedures.** The diagnosis and possible treatment of the aneurysm responsible for the SAH will occur as quickly as possible after the CT scan or clinical diagnosis is made. There are three types of materials used to occlude the aneurysm: Coils with thrombus inducing coat, particles in a variety of solvents, and cyanoacrylate glue. Each has a slightly different risk profile [49]. Complications from the interventional procedure include hemorrhage, vessel occlusion, and medical complications (Table 9.7). Renal injury, due to the large volume of contrast administered, is managed with intravenous administration of

TABLE 9.7   Interventional radiographic procedures—complications and treatment

Category	Complication	Therapy	Anesthesia
Hemorrhage	Aneurysm rupture or perforation Vessel dissection	Surgical intervention	Anesthetic plan for acute aneurysm clipping
Occlusive	Thromboembolic event (particulate, coil) Vasospasm	Variable Standard therapy	Normalize ET CO_2, elevate BP Treat hypotension, initiate therapy for vasospasm
Systemic	Renal insufficiency Contrast reaction or anaphylaxis	Administer N-acetylcysteine, $NaHCO_3$ Stop administration Change drug or discontinue procedure	Maintain intravascular volume Consider fenoldopam, dopamine Administer diphenhydramine, steroid Initiate anaphylaxis therapy

Source: Varma MK, Price K, Jayakrishnan V, et al. Anaesthetic considerations for interventional neuroradiology. *Br J Anaesth.* 2007;99:75–85.

N-acetylcysteine and $NaHCO_3$ [40]. The large volume of contrast dye can initially cause fluid overload in a patient potentially vulnerable to heart failure followed by a diuresis. Attention to fluid management is important aspect of anesthetic management. Anesthetic planning should consider the risks for rapid conversion to a craniotomy and these patients may have severe cardiovascular and pulmonary injury with ongoing neurologic damage [2,5,11,40].

2. **Surgery.** The primary goal of anesthesia for an aneurysm clipping is to maintain adequate cerebral perfusion and reduce intracranial volume.

   a. **Surgical details.** Aneurysm "clipping" is attempted as soon as possible after the diagnosis is made to reduce the probability of rebleeding and allow better treatment of vasospasm [10]. To reduce the risk of bleeding during clip placement, most surgeons will place a proximal clip, a clip placed prior to the aneurysm. When an aneurysm has perfusion from two sources, for example, the ACOA, the aneurysm is "trapped" by placing a clip on both sources of blood flow. With this technique, tissue perfusion distal to the proximal clip(s) is dependent on collateral blood flow, a situation with potential for hypoperfusion. If the placement of the aneurysm clip will take more than 1 to 3 minutes, the surgeon will often request a bolus of propofol since thiopental is currently unavailable in the United States to reduce neuronal metabolic rate and ischemic injury. BP should be maintained at normal values or slightly higher to improve collateral flow. When a proximal clip is used to allow completion of the dissection, removal and reperfusion should occur every 10 to 15 minutes with propofol administration during the reperfusion period. Monitoring and informing the surgeon of the proximal clip time should reduce likelihood of ischemic injury [5,11]. Intraoperative hypotension is not routinely used during aneurysm clipping.

   b. **Intraoperative rupture.** Current practice would be to place a proximal clip to control blood loss. Some centers advocate use of propofol-based TIVA in this situation since it decreases metabolic activity and does not cause arterial vasodilation. There is no evidence to support or refute this technique. Transfusion should be decided based on cardiovascular stability. Best evidence for a transfusion trigger comes from the neuro-critical care literature.

   c. **Unique operative anesthetic management techniques.** Intraoperative and postoperative hypothermia have been advocated for improving long-term outcomes in SAH. Mild intraoperative hypothermia (33°C) has not been found to alter outcome in WFNS SAH score I, II, and III patients [51,52]. Hypothermia in WFNS IV, V patients and all patients in the critical care unit has not been shown to have benefit. Deep hypothermia for giant aneurysm, usually in the posterior circulation, has been reported to have good long-term outcomes. This technique requires cardiopulmonary bypass and the expertise of cardiac anesthesiologist, it should be approached cautiously in primarily elective situations [53,54]. There has been resurgence in interest in use of adenosine to cause brief cardiac arrest. Previous case reports from the late 1980s to 1990 [55] were restricted to a few locations. Similarly, recent case reports or case series discuss the use of adenosine in difficult-to-clip aneurysms that are not amenable to IR therapy [56–58]. These are primarily large basilar aneurysm or aneurysm where proximal clip placement is difficult. There are no outcome comparisons for this technique. Developing guidelines for this technique is advised to assure best outcomes. This is an off-label use of the drug. Since large studies have found angiographic interventions to be safe, these very specialized techniques are applicable in uncommon circumstances and may be best performed by teams experienced in their use [59].

    d. Intraoperative neurophysiologic monitoring. When the circulation at risk involves components of the motor or sensory cortex or tracts, somatosensory evoked potentials (SEPs) and motor evoked potentials (MEPs) may be requested by the surgeon (Chapter 26). Anesthesia techniques need to be adjusted to provide ideal conditions for monitoring. The modalities used are electroencephalography (EEG), SEPs, and MEPs [57].

VI. **Summary.** The physiologic perturbations that occur in patients who experience an SAH include cardiac rhythm changes, myocardial injury, hypertension decreased pulmonary reserve, abnormal electrolytes, and glucose homeostasis. Those who survive often have permanent cognitive and other devastating neurologic changes. These difficulties make anesthesia care especially challenging. Nonetheless, anesthesia management that incorporates neurocritical care principles can make a significant contribution to improving patient outcome.

REFERENCES

1. de Rooij NK, Linn FH, van der Plas JA, et al. Incidence of subarachnoid haemorrhage: a systematic review with emphasis on region, age, gender and time trends. *J Neurol Neurosurg Psychiatry.* 2007;78:1365–1372.
2. Suarez JI, Tarr RW, Selman WR. Aneurysmal subarachnoid hemorrhage. *N Engl J Med.* 2006;354(4):387–396.
3. Eden SV, Meurer WJ, Sanchez BN, et al. Gender and ethnic differences in subarachnoid hemorrhage. *Neurology.* 2008;71: 731–735.
4. Suarez JI. Outcome in neurocritical care: advances in monitoring and treatment and effect of a specialized neurocritical care team. *Crit Care Med.* 2006;34:S232–S238.
5. Priebe HJ. Aneurysmal subarachnoid haemorrhage and the anaesthetist. *Br J Anaesth.* 2007;99:102–118.
6. Rosengart AJ, Schultheiss KE, Tolentino J, et al. Prognostic factors for outcome in patients with aneurysmal subarachnoid hemorrhage. [see comment]. *Stroke.* 2007;38(8):2315–2321.
7. Soehle M, Chatfield DA, Czosnyka M, et al. Predictive value of initial clinical status, intracranial pressure and transcranial Doppler pulsatility after subarachnoid haemorrhage. *Acta Neurochir (Wien).* 2007;149:575–583.
8. Bor ASE, Rinkel GJE, Adami J, et al. Risk of subarachnoid haemorrhage according to number of affected relatives: a population based case-control study. *Brain.* 2008;131:2662–2665.
9. Bulters DO, Santarius T, Chia HL, et al. Causes of neurological deficits following clipping of 200 consecutive ruptured aneurysms in patients with good-grade aneurysmal subarachnoid haemorrhage. *Acta Neurochir (Wien).* 2011;153:295–303.
10. Starke RM, Connolly ES, Jr. Participants in the International Multi-Disciplinary Consensus Conference on the Critical Care Management of Subarachnoid H. Rebleeding after aneurysmal subarachnoid hemorrhage. *Neurocrit Care.* 2011;15(2): 241–246.
11. Rose MJ. Aneurysmal subarachnoid hemorrhage: an update on the medical complications and treatments strategies seen in these patients. *Curr Opin Anaesthesiol.* 2011;24:500–507.
12. Randell T. Principles of neuroanesthesia in stroke surgery. *Acta Neurochir Suppl.* 2010;107:111–113.
13. Diringer MN. Management of aneurysmal subarachnoid hemorrhage. *Crit Care Med.* 2009;37:432–440.
14. Wartenberg KE, Mayer SA. Medical complications after subarachnoid hemorrhage: new strategies for prevention and management. *Curr Opin Crit Care.* 2006;12:78–84.
15. Wartenberg KE, Schmidt JM, Claassen J, et al. Impact of medical complications on outcome after subarachnoid hemorrhage. *Crit Care Med.* 2006;34:617–623; quiz 24.
16. Diringer MN, Bleck TP, Claude Hemphill J, 3rd, et al. Critical care management of patients following aneurysmal subarachnoid hemorrhage: recommendations from the Neurocritical Care Society's Multidisciplinary Consensus Conference. *Neurocrit Care.* 2011;15:211–240.
17. Hellingman CA, van den Bergh WM, Beijer IS, et al. Risk of rebleeding after treatment of acute hydrocephalus in patients with aneurysmal subarachnoid hemorrhage. *Stroke.* 2007;38:96–99.

18. Frontera JA, Claassen J, Schmidt JM, et al. Prediction of symptomatic vasospasm after subarachnoid hemorrhage: the modified fisher scale. *Neurosurgery.* 2006;59(1):21–27; discussion 21–27.

19. van der Bilt IAC, Hasan D, Vandertop WP, et al. Impact of cardiac complications on outcome after aneurysmal subarachnoid hemorrhage: a meta-analysis. *Neurology.* 2009;72:635–642.

20. Lee VH, Oh JK, Mulvagh SL, et al. Mechanisms in neurogenic stress cardiomyopathy after aneurysmal subarachnoid hemorrhage. *Neurocrit Care.* 2006;5:243–239.

21. de Chazal I, Parham WM 3rd, Liopyris P, et al. Delayed cardiogenic shock and acute lung injury after aneurysmal subarachnoid hemorrhage. *Anesth Analg.* 2005;100:1147–1149.

22. Alberti O, Becker R, Benes L, et al. Initial hyperglycemia as an indicator of severity of the ictus in poor-grade patients with spontaneous subarachnoid hemorrhage. *Clin Neurol Neurosurg.* 2000;102:78–83.

23. Kruyt ND, Roos YW, Dorhout Mees SM, et al. High mean fasting glucose levels independently predict poor outcome and delayed cerebral ischaemia after aneurysmal subarachnoid haemorrhage. *J Neurol Neurosurg Psychiatry.* 2008;79(12):1382–1385.

24. Pasternak JJ, McGregor DG, Schroeder DR, et al. Hyperglycemia in patients undergoing cerebral aneurysm surgery: its association with long-term gross neurologic and neuropsychological function. *Mayo Clin Proc.* 2008;83:406–417.

25. Velat GJ, Kimball MM, Mocco JD, et al. Vasospasm after aneurysmal subarachnoid hemorrhage: review of randomized controlled trials and meta-analyses in the literature. *World Neurosurg.* 2011;76:446–454.

26. Prakash A, Matta BF. Hyperglycaemia and neurological injury. *Curr Opin Anaesthesiol.* 2008;21(5):565–569.

27. American Diabetes Association. Standards of medical care in diabetes–2011. *Diabetes Care.* 2011;34 Suppl 1:S11–61.

28. Schneider HJ, Kreitschmann-Andermahr I, Ghigo E, et al. Hypothalamopituitary dysfunction following traumatic brain injury and aneurysmal subarachnoid hemorrhage: a systematic review. *JAMA.* 2007;298:1429–1438.

29. Vespa P. Participants in the International Multi-Disciplinary Consensus Conference on the Critical Care Management of Subarachnoid H. SAH pituitary adrenal dysfunction. *Neurocrit Care.* 2011;15:365–368.

30. Rasulo FA, De Peri E, Lavinio A. Transcranial Doppler ultrasonography in intensive care. *Eur J Anaesthesiol Suppl.* 2008;42:167–173.

31. Etminan N, Vergouwen MDI, Ilodigwe D, et al. Effect of pharmaceutical treatment on vasospasm, delayed cerebral ischemia, and clinical outcome in patients with aneurysmal subarachnoid hemorrhage: a systematic review and meta-analysis. *J Cereb Blood Flow Metab.* 2011;31:1443–1451.

32. Dorhout Mees SM, Rinkel GJ, Feigin VL, et al. Calcium antagonists for aneurysmal subarachnoid haemorrhage. *Cochrane Database Syst Rev.* 2007:CD000277.

33. Wong GKC, Boet R, Poon WS, et al. Intravenous magnesium sulphate for aneurysmal subarachnoid hemorrhage: an updated systemic review and meta-analysis. *Crit Care.* 2011;15:R52.

34. Tseng MY. Participants in the International Multidisciplinary Consensus Conference on the Critical Care Management of Subarachnoid H. Summary of evidence on immediate statins therapy following aneurysmal subarachnoid hemorrhage. *Neurocrit Care.* 2011;15:298–301.

35. Kramer AH. Statins in the management of aneurysmal subarachnoid hemorrhage: an overview of animal research, observational studies, randomized controlled trials and meta-analyses. *Acta Neurochir Suppl.* 2011;110:193–201.

36. Dankbaar JW, Slooter AJ, Rinkel GJ, et al. Effect of different components of triple-H therapy on cerebral perfusion in patients with aneurysmal subarachnoid haemorrhage: a systematic review. *Crit Care.* 2010;14:R23.

37. Le Roux PD. Participants in the International Multi-disciplinary Consensus Conference on the Critical Care Management of Subarachnoid H. Anemia and transfusion after subarachnoid hemorrhage. *Neurocrit Care.* 2011;15:342–353.

38. Kramer AH, Gurka MJ, Nathan B, et al. Complications associated with anemia and blood transfusion in patients with aneurysmal subarachnoid hemorrhage. *Crit Care Med.* 2008;36:2070–2075.

39. Jun P, Ko NU, English JD, et al. Endovascular treatment of medically refractory cerebral vasospasm following aneurysmal subarachnoid hemorrhage. *Am J Neuroradiol.* 2010;31:1911–1916.

40. Varma MK, Price K, Jayakrishnan V, et al. Anaesthetic considerations for interventional neuroradiology. *Br J Anaesth.* 2007;99:75–85.

41. Lakhani S, Guha A, Nahser HC. Anaesthesia for endovascular management of cerebral aneurysms. *Eur J Anaesthesiol.* 2006;23:902–913.

42. Randell T, Niskanen M. Management of physiological variables in neuroanaesthesia: maintaining homeostasis during intracranial surgery. *Curr Opin Anaesthesiol.* 2006;19:492–497.

43. Randell T, Niemela M, Kytta J, et al. Principles of neuroanesthesia in aneurysmal subarachnoid hemorrhage: The Helsinki experience. *Surg Neurol.* 2006;66:382–388; discussion 388.

44. Pasternak JJ, Lanier WL. Neuroanesthesiology update 2010. *J Neurosurg Anesthesiol.* 2011;23:67–99.

45. Pasternak JJ, Lanier WL. Neuroanesthesiology update. *J Neurosurg Anesthesiol.* 2010;22:86–109.

46. Warner DS, Laskowitz DT. Changing outcome from aneurysmal subarachnoid hemorrhage: another step closer. [comment]. *Anesthesiology.* 2006;104:629–630.

47. Naidech AM, Jovanovic B, Wartenberg KE, et al. Higher hemoglobin is associated with improved outcome after subarachnoid hemorrhage. [see comment]. *Crit Care Med.* 2007;35:2383–2389.

48. Kurtz P, Schmidt JM, Claassen J, et al. Anemia is associated with metabolic distress and brain tissue hypoxia after subarachnoid hemorrhage. *Neurocrit Care.* 2010;13:10–16.

49. Pierot L, Spelle L, Vitry F, et al. Immediate clinical outcome of patients harboring unruptured intracranial aneurysms treated by endovascular approach: results of the ATENA study. *Stroke.* 2008;39:2497–2504.

50. Johnston SC, Dowd CF, Higashida RT, et al. Predictors of rehemorrhage after treatment of ruptured intracranial aneurysms: the Cerebral Aneurysm Rerupture After Treatment (CARAT) study. [see comment]. *Stroke.* 2008;39:120–125.

51. Todd MM, Hindman BJ, Clarke WR, et al. Mild intraoperative hypothermia during surgery for intracranial aneurysm. [see comment]. *N Engl J Med.* 2005;352:135–145.

52. Li LR, You C, Chaudhary B. Intraoperative mild hypothermia for postoperative neurological deficits in intracranial aneurysm patients. *Cochrane Database Syst Rev.* 2012;2:CD008445.

53. Levati A, Tommasino C, Moretti MP, et al. Giant intracranial aneurysms treated with deep hypothermia and circulatory arrest. *J Neurosurg Anesthesiol.* 2007;19:25–30.

54. Colby GP, Coon AL, Tamargo RJ. Surgical management of aneurysmal subarachnoid hemorrhage. *Neurosurg Clin N Am.* 2010;21:247–261.

55. Sollevi A, Lagerkranser M, Irestedt L, et al. Controlled hypotension with adenosine in cerebral aneurysm surgery. *Anesthesiology.* 1984;61:400–405.

56. Bebawy JF, Gupta DK, Bendok BR, et al. Adenosine-induced flow arrest to facilitate intracranial aneurysm clip ligation: dose-response data and safety profile. *Anesth Analg.* 2010;110:1406–1411.

57. Bendok BR, Gupta DK, Rahme RJ, et al. Adenosine for temporary flow arrest during intracranial aneurysm surgery: a single-center retrospective review. *Neurosurgery.* 2011;69:815–820; discussion 820–821.

58. Guinn NR, McDonagh DL, Borel CO, et al. Adenosine-induced transient asystole for intracranial aneurysm surgery: a retrospective review. *J Neurosurg Anesthesiol.* 2011;23:35–40.

59. Peluso JP, van Rooij WJ, Sluzewski M, et al. Coiling of basilar tip aneurysms: results in 154 consecutive patients with emphasis on recurrent haemorrhage and re-treatment during mid- and long-term follow-up. *J Neurol Neurosurg Psychiatry.* 2008; 79:706–711.

10

Intracranial Arteriovenous Malformations (AVMs)

Sabin Caius Oana and N. Kurt Baker-Watson

KEY POINTS

1. AVMs are abnormal vascular structures with a central nidus and one or several feeding arteries and draining veins.
2. AVMs are associated with chronic intracerebral hypoxia of varying degrees.
3. Most common clinical presentations are intracerebral hemorrhages, seizures, and mass effects.
4. AVM treatment is multimodal involving a coordinated multidisciplinary team approach.
5. Treatment options include observation, microsurgery, neuroendovascular embolization, and radiosurgery.
6. The general principles of neuroanesthesia apply to the management of AVMs.
7. The typical modern neuroanesthetic regimen uses volatile or intravenous agents plus a narcotic.
8. Blood loss is highly variable and can be massive.
9. Intraprocedural complications can be obstructive or hemorrhagic.
10. Special techniques employed include induced hypertension, controlled hypotension, and/or flow arrest as well as cerebral protection.
11. Most feared postoperative AVM complication is a state of generalized brain hyperemia.

I. General considerations

A. Introduction

1. **Epidemiology**

   a. Much of the evidenced, definitive science and clinical management of AVMs remain to be elucidated by both research and medical practice. The exact prevalence of AVMs in any particular population is evasive as many individuals have undeclared lesions, even with subclinical microhemorrhages, that are serendipitously discovered during unrelated medical evaluations or autopsy studies.

   b. Approximately 1 case per 100,000 patient-years (cumulative disease-free years of the pool of individuals under consideration) is a reasonable estimation of annual incidence for adults within the United States. Occurrence in young children is rare [1].

2. **Etiology**

   a. The exact etiology of intracranial AVMs has not been known historically. Considered to be causally related to multifactorial intrauterine issues that result in a congenital vascular structure with pathology of both anatomy and physiology, they were known to present in association with congenital syndromes such as craniofacial arteriovenous metameric syndrome and simply assumed to be another presentation of inborn errors of structure or function.

   b. These lesions have now been increasingly described however as part of several autosomal dominantly inherited syndromes such as Parkes Weber syndrome due to genetic mutations. There are also indications of intracerebral AVMs originating later in life and reoccurring after being obliterated or excised.

B. Anatomy and physiology

   1. Angioarchitecture

     a. AVMs can be conceptually defined as a focus of abnormal vascular structures, referred to as a nidus, which is an interface between the arterial and vascular systems in lieu of a capillary bed. Its infrastructure can be composed of multiple subunits supplied by feeding arteries that can vary in number and origin.

     b. Histologic examination of the wall of a typical large-caliber nidal vessel demonstrates a thickened intimal layer with a paucity of smooth muscle within the media [2]. It is relatively fragile and prone to both edema formation and hemorrhage as only this structure and the intraparenchymal pressure act to maintain its integrity.

     c. As it does not perform the metabolic functions of a capillary bed there is no neuronal tissue within the confines of the usual compact (glomerular) nidus. A diffuse (proliferative) nidus with incorporated islands of neuronal tissue is rare [3].

     d. An individual feeding artery may terminate within the nidus or may supply the nidus "en passage" to its termination in neuronal tissue distal to the nidus.

     e. Aneurysms within the nidus or feeding arteries have also been described and add to the complexity of treatment.

     f. Draining veins can be grossly ectatic and torturous due to exposure to arterial pressure.

     g. The majority of AVMs (70% or more) are supratentorial in location. Most of these are superficially located in pericortical areas whose blood supply can be traced from the Circle of Willis to superficial (pial) arteries. Venous drainage is common to pericortical external cerebral veins but can also involve the internal venous system located deep to the corpus callosum.

     h. A subset of supratentorial AVMs can be deeply located near the ventricles or midbrain with consequential deep central arterial supply from the Circle and internal venous drainage.

     i. The remainder (up to 30%) of AVMs are infratentorial with a corresponding vertebrobasilar arterial supply and venous drainage.

     j. Due to the typical intraparenchymal location of AVMs, hemorrhages too are usually intraparenchymal rather than subarachnoid as with aneurysms.

   2. Pathophysiology

     a. The physiologic interactions between intracranial AVMs and parenchymal brain tissue are known to be exquisitely intricate and increasingly delicate in the event that compensatory reserve mechanisms are exhausted by hemodynamic stressors.

     b. It should be understood that AVMs impart chronic hypoxic stress on the brain, with localized or generalized effects, by a multitude of methods that reduce blood supply in aggregate.

       (1) As they lack capillary function, AVMs do not support perfusion within their confines.

       (2) A local mass effect can be established due to size or hemorrhage.

       (3) To a greater extent, AVMs act as low-resistance arteriovenous shunts to varying degrees, which steal perfusion from neighboring neuronal tissue. Decreased resistance to blood flow afforded by reflexive vasodilation within the vascular beds of ischemic neuronal tissue is only partially corrective and may be limited by mass effect.

       (4) Large AVMs can have a global effect on brain perfusion as can be seen in children with malformations involving the deep central arterial supply and internal venous system. In reference to the internal central vein (of Galen) these lesions are referred to as vein of Galen malformations which is usually a misnomer as the nidus typically involves the median prosencephalic vein of Markowski in actuality.

       (5) The arterial pressure traversing AVMs can increase the pressure within the corresponding draining venous system. Parenchymal regions that share venous drainage with AVMs typically have decreased perfusion pressure owing to this phenomenon ($\downarrow$perfusion pressure = mean arterial pressure $- \uparrow$venous pressure).

  c. AVMs lack barrier functions and represent a breach in the blood–brain barrier.

  d. Adjacent neuronal regions are typically atrophic and can be infiltrated by reactive glial cells and scar tissue in response to ongoing hypoxic neuronal injury and necrosis.

  e. Gliotic regions of the brain, through excessive production of the excitatory neurotransmitter glutamate, can develop into putative epileptic foci.

  f. It should be recognized that AVMs are not static structures. They have been known to both dilate, such as under the influence of vasodilatory progesterone that is increased during pregnancy, and contract. Research is ongoing concerning the role vascular remodeling and angiogenesis have in their generation and maintenance. Alterations in expression and concentration of biomarkers are known to exist.

> **CLINICAL PEARL**   AVMs lack the functions of the blood–brain barrier.

  C. Clinical aspects

    1. Presentation. Most common clinical presentations are intracerebral hemorrhages, seizures, and mass effects.

      a. The causality of intracerebral hemorrhages varies with the population considered. In the United States, although AVMs represent the minority of these hemorrhages (aneurysms being the primary reason), they are the most common manner (42% to 70%) [4] in which AVMs present with morbidity and mortality associated with the neurologic site and degree of the particular bleed. This represents an annual incidence of 0.51 cases per 100,000 patient-years usually within the second to fourth decade of life.

      b. Risk of primary hemorrhage is 2% to 4% per year with a percentage lifetime risk equal to 105 − patient's age (in years) [5]. Risk factors include deep and infratentorial position, small size less than 3 cm, a single feeding artery or draining vein, deep venous drainage, venous varicies, and associated aneurysms. Associated aneurysms occur in 10% to 23% of patients [2].

      c. Risk of rebleeding is highest within the first year (4.5% to 34%) but decreases to primary-hemorrhage rates afterward [6]. Associated factors include previous hemorrhage, deep location, older age, and exclusively deep venous drainage [7].

> **CLINICAL PEARL**   The risk of rebleeding is highest within the first year of the initial bleed.

      d. Neurologic morbidity (20% to 30%) rather than mortality (10% risk) [8] is the usual result of initial hemorrhages which can arise from the vessels of the nidus or an aneurysm associated with the nidus or a feeding artery.

      e. The next most frequent presentation (16% to 53%) [4] is seizures which can be resultant of the gliotic areas adjacent to AVMs as previously mentioned.

      f. Less common manifestations are due to the mass and/or cardiovascular effects of lesions. Headache (7% to 48%) [4], hydrocephaly, and elevated intracranial pressure can follow from obstruction of cerebrospinal fluid circulation by the nidal volume. Malformations with large shunt components can result in syncope due to acute episodes of increased cerebral hypoxia, impaired mental functioning or dementia due to chronically progressive cerebral hypoxia, and a bruit audible to the patient. Neonates can present with congestive heart failure from vein of Galen malformations that are large enough to impart an overwhelming cardiovascular shunt.

> **CLINICAL PEARL**   An aneurysm associated with an AVM adds to the complexity of treatment.

2. **Evaluation**

   a. As most AVMs present posthemorrhage, at least for the immediate future, the gold standard technique for emergent evaluation of patients with symptoms and signs of a cerebrovascular accident continues to be a computed tomography (CT) scan without contrast.

   b. Preponderant benefits in the critical hours of initial presentation are that extravasated blood is clearly visible in differentiating an ischemic versus a hemorrhagic stroke, the dilated vasculature of the nidus or associated vessels can identify a causal AVM, and CT machines are logistically available.

   c. The assessment should include the size and location of the hematoma, the development and degree of hydrocephaly from obstruction of cerebrospinal fluid flow, and whether there is mass effect of significance to require an emergent craniotomy for hematoma evacuation as a life-saving measure. CT angiography using the latest multidetector row machines is an adjunctive technique that can subsequently be used to generate a 3-D image of the intracerebral vasculature in studying an AVM.

   d. Although the sensitivity of diagnosing a hemorrhagic stroke with magnetic resonance imaging (MRI) is similar to that of CT, it will not supplant CT as the primary evaluation strategy until MRI machines are more plentiful and more closely located to emergent care facilities to render their utilization practical. With this technique AVMs are represented as dark, nonenhancing "flow voids" of the nidus and associated vessels within the region of hemorrhage. MRI imagery can deliver higher tissue resolution with T 2 star weighted and gradient echo techniques useful in distinguishing chronic hemorrhage. Functional MRI can investigate the interaction between lesions and eloquent, commissioned neuronal centers. Magnetic resonance angiography can also be used to render a 3-D image of an AVM's architecture while highlighting relationships with intracerebral anatomy which is superior to that of CT angiography in planning follow-up treatment.

   e. Follow-up studies include angiography which is the gold standard for evaluating the angioarchitecture of AVMs. Superselective digital subtraction angiography which highlights contrast-enhanced vasculature by subtracting the signals of other tissues has the additional benefit of delineating perinidal vascular physiology and is used in neurointerventional procedures.

   f. Transcranial Doppler ultrasonography can detect AVMs through identifying the rapid, turbulent flow through them.

   g. Each of these techniques can be employed toward clinical decision-making with regard to unruptured AVMs as well of course.

   h. Establishing the perinidal architecture is critical in clinical decision-making. Clinical symptomatology finds correlation with distinct structures which are therefore candidates to be targeted for intervention (Table 10.1).

3. **Indications for intervention**

   a. Both the decision to intervene and the manner of intervention are dependent upon the degree of impairment the patient is experiencing as well as the future hazards posed by the AVM and the plan of intervention. Therapeutic plans must have a reasonable chance of success in eradicating the lesion or to cure or stabilize deficits.

   b. Beyond the dangers of a particular therapy there is evidence within the literature that incompletely treated AVMs and intervention itself may increase risk of rupture [8]. Posited mechanisms include detrimental alteration of the hemodynamics within the AVM and loss of fragile vascular integrity as an ischemic nidus necroses or attempts anastomosis with immature vasculature recruited through angiogenesis.

   c. Again the chance of hemorrhage mostly dictates the need for intervention. The risk of hemorrhage without therapy must be higher than that posed by undergoing the therapy. This can be estimated by aspects of the AVM identified through radiologic assessment that are associated with hemorrhage as described previously.

   d. Special populations include children, in whom intervention is typically pursued; the elderly, in whom intervention is less aggressive; and pregnant patients, in whom

TABLE 10.1   Clinical correlation of AVM anatomy [1,3]

Aspect	Clinical correlate	Pathophysiology
Small (<3 cm)	Hemorrhage	Nidal rupture from high wall stress
Intranidal aneurysm	Hemorrhage	Aneurysmal rupture
Venous stenosis or ectasia	Hemorrhage	Venous rupture from high wall stress
Deep or single venous drainage	Hemorrhage	Nidal rupture from limited outflow
Deep or posterior fossa location	Hemorrhage	Nidal rupture from limited outflow
High flow shunt	Deficits of psychomotor function, epilepsy	Hypoxia from decreased perfusion pressure, regional or global
Venous congestion or outflow obstruction	Deficits of psychomotor function, epilepsy	Hypoxia from decreased perfusion pressure, regional or global
Mass effect, hydrocephalus	Deficits of psychomotor function, epilepsy	Hypoxia from decreased perfusion pressure, regional or global
Gliosis, perifocal, or perinidal	Epilepsy	Glutamate from glial cells
Long pial course of draining vein	Epilepsy	Regional hypoxia from decreased perfusion pressure
Arterial steal	Migraines, transient focal signs	Regional hypoxia

intervention depends upon the assessment of hemorrhage risk for a particular patient versus risks to the fetus [5].

  e. Other plausible indications for intervention include intractable seizures and impaired psychomotor function from ischemia or mass effect, cardiovascular failure from severe shunting, and quality of life issues such as anticipated childbirth.

D. Management

  1. **Clinical considerations**

   a. Detailing the intensive care of ruptured AVMs is part of the consideration of intracerebral hemorrhage therapy in general and will not be highlighted here apart from the radiologic assessment and craniotomy for life-threatening hematoma evacuation as discussed. Insight into the controversial points of deliberation concerning the non-emergent, subsequent management of AVMs including the advantages and liabilities of treatment courses will instead be evaluated (Tables 10.2 and 10.3).

   b. Contemporary AVM treatment is multimodal and founded upon a coordinated multidisciplinary team approach including medical professionals in intensive medicine, neurology, neurosurgery, and radiology (Fig. 10.1A–C). There are four treatment options: observation, surgery, neuroendovascular intervention, and radiosurgery.

   c. Upon full assessment of prospective management strategies with respect to a particular patient's concept of personal integrity, psychological well-being, quality of life, and life expectancy, patients should be advised of risk management during their clinical course. This may entail a sequential intervention where a less definitive therapy is initially pursued due to its lower risk. This acts as a catalyst by lowering the otherwise unacceptable risk of a more definitive therapy to succeed it. For example, an interventional neuroradiologist may embolize feeding arteries to an AVM which are situated in deep, eloquent areas of the brain preoperatively in order to facilitate a less traumatic

TABLE 10.2   Summary of rates per hundred patient years [6]

Result	Overall	Neuroendovascular	Microsurgery	Radiosurgery
Case fatality[a]	0.68	0.96	1.1	0.5
Long-term hemorrhage[b]	1.4	1.7	0.18	1.7

[a]Less than 30 days posttherapy.
[b]After 30 days posttherapy.

TABLE 10.3   Summary of rates in median percentages [6]

Result	Neuroendovascular	Microsurgery	Radiosurgery
Complication[a]	6.6	7.4	5.1
	Range (0–28)	Range (0–40)	Range (0–21)
Successful obliteration	13	96	38
	Range (0–94)	Range (0–100)	Range (0–75)

[a]Leading to death or permanent neurologic deficit.

and hemorrhagic operation. The overall risk of the entire treatment plan is therefore reduced through the employment of a catalytic therapy initially. The treatment plan of a patient is determined through application of the Spetzler–Martin scale (Table 10.4) which recently has proposed revisions (Table 10.5). Each major therapeutic modality will be highlighted within a cumulative algorithm (Fig. 10.2).

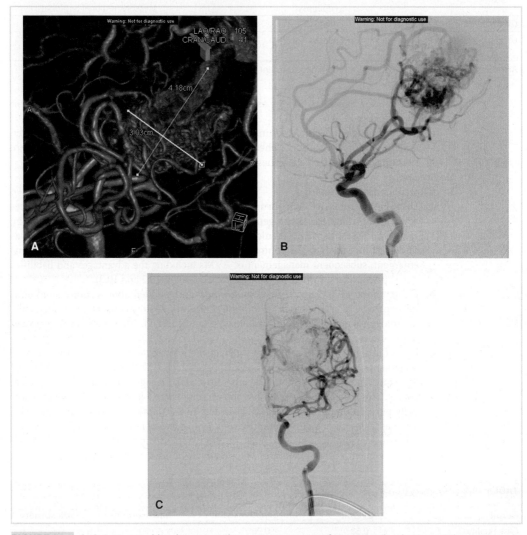

FIGURE 10.1 A–C: A 41-year-old male presented to emergency room after a generalized seizure. Subsequent investigations revealed large temporoparietal AVM. Patient underwent successful two-stage embolization (afferents of middle cerebral artery and then of anterior cerebral artery) followed by radiosurgery. (Courtesy of John Whapham, M.D., Assistant Professor, Director Neurointerventional Program, Loyola University Medical Center.)

TABLE 10.4 Spetzler–Martin AVM grading scale [46]

Aspect	Point score (1–5)
Maximum diameter size	
Small <3 cm	1
Medium 3–6 cm	2
Large >6 cm	3
Location to eloquent regions of brain	
None	0
In or contiguous	1
Venous drainage	
Exclusively superficial	0
Any deep	1

CLINICAL PEARL   The definitive procedure can be somewhat temporized until the patient stabilizes.

2. **Monitoring**
   a. The most conservative care plan is one of monitoring with serial neurologic and radiologic evaluations including CT and MRI. This would seem to be most prudent for asymptomatic patients but can be utilized even for patients with declared AVMs who, following assessment, are estimated to be at greater risk for morbidity and mortality from intervention.
   b. There are few prospective trials comparing treatment to monitoring for unruptured AVMs but one expected study finalizing in 2017 is a randomized trial of unruptured brain AVMs (ARUBA) [9].
   c. While "to do no harm" in the spirit of the Hippocratic oath and potentially less cost are the most obvious benefits, the specter of hemorrhage is the most ominous risk of monitoring.
3. **Microsurgery**
   a. This can be utilized as monotherapy with permissive AVM anatomy and location or as a succeeding therapy in a sequential intervention.
   b. The intraoperative course involves dissection of arterial vasculature on course to the lesion with temporary clipping to maintain hemostasis, definitive transection of feeding arteries as they are identified, dissection of the nidus, and dissection and transection of venous drainage.
   c. Operative management has the primary advantage of excising AVMs at once that either cannot be treated effectively by embolization or radiosurgery or can only be treated by these means in stages.
   d. Surgical patients tend to have longer hospital courses, can have higher rates of neurologic dysfunction, and are under threat from normal perfusion pressure hemorrhage in the acute postoperative period.

TABLE 10.5 Spetzler–Martin AVM grading scale comparison [46]

Established five-tier classification Total point score	Proposed three-tier classification
I–II	A
II–III	B
IV–V	C

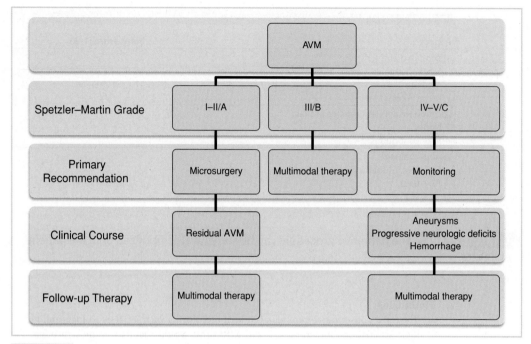

FIGURE 10.2 Treatment algorithm [5,46–48].

4. **Neuroendovascular embolization**
   a. First, this can be used as monotherapy to obliterate a small AVM in its entirety at once or in a staged procedure with a larger lesion to avoid acute destabilization of the AVM's hemodynamics leading to rupture.
   b. Second, as a catalyst for neurosurgery or radiosurgery. Compartments of the nidus, aneurysms of the nidus or feeding arteries, and feeding arteries deemed operatively inaccessible are targeted. Also, often in conjunction with coiling, high-flow nidal fistulas can be preoperatively diminished.
   c. Lastly, partial embolization can be used as palliative therapy for debilitating symptoms from large, inoperable AVMs due to intracerebral edema or shunt. This is usually not permanent as the residual nidus, now ischemic, will act to revascularize and reconstitute itself [10].

CLINICAL PEARL   Partially obliterated AVMs can reconstitute and are at higher risk of rupture.

   d. Once arterial access has been obtained, routinely through the femoral vasculature but also via the brachial or carotid vasculature as necessary, the cerebral circulation is acquired by either of two delivery systems: Smaller, flexible, flow-directed microcatheters; or larger, more rigid catheters directed over less-compliant guidewires. The latter system assumes an increased risk of vascular trauma and perforation.
   e. Two liquid polymer embolic substances used are n-butyl cyanoacrylate (commercially known as Trufill®) and ethylene-vinyl alcohol (commercially known as Onyx®) which act to acutely obliterate the vascular lumen while initiating an inflammatory reaction toward fibrosis and induration chronically.
   f. Factors such as solution viscosity, polymerization rate, and injection rate can be chosen toward optimal penetration of the nidus while minimizing the possibility of

extension to the venous system with threatened pulmonary embolization or reflux of these compounds out of the AVM to the arterial circulation with unintentional embolization of perinidal neural sites. The premature occlusion of venous drainage should also be avoided to prevent distension of the AVM with impending rupture [10].

   g. Primarily, use of the cyanoacrylate polymer is advantageous in that it is administered through the compliant flow-directed microcatheter. However, with extended injection times the threat of catheter retention increases because this substance is adhesive and risks bonding to the catheter within the vasculature.

   h. While the ethylene-vinyl alcohol product is not adhesive and can facilitate a more controlled, measured, and extensive embolization, it is deployed using catheters over guidewires.

   i. Coils also can be delivered by either system with the particular advantage of reducing flow through intranidal fistulas so that liquid polymers can subsequently be employed under reduced risk of crossing into venous outflow.

   j. There is no formal consensus as to whether deep sedation or general anesthesia with complete muscle relaxation is best for patients undergoing endovascular therapy, but logic directs that general anesthesia would at least be more appropriate for the use of wire-guided systems to obviate the hazard of vascular perforation from patient motion.

   k. Overall, neuroendovascular interventions decrease the time of hospitalization for patients but have limits to the size of the lesions that are treatable.

   5. Radiosurgery

   a. Radiation therapy can be considered as monotherapy in the treatment of small lesions that are not candidates for other methods and in Spetzler–Martin grade three or greater lesions with the goal of cure rather than palliation.

   b. Radiosurgery is noninvasive, does not require lengthy hospitalization, and can be combined with embolization and or microsurgery. While there are some reports that prior embolization reduces the efficacy of radiosurgery, it is possible that all three techniques are employed in a scenario such as embolization prior to microsurgery with radiotherapy for any residual lesion. By definition however, radiosurgery is a staged process that can take up to 3 years to obliterate the AVM during which time there is continued risk for rupture. In addition, intracerebral edema, necrosis, cyst formation, and malignant tumors can result from this technique.

E. Radiation safety. As anesthesiology practitioners are increasingly consulted for patient care in interventional radiologic procedures, it should be remembered that precautions against radiation exposure should be maintained just as universal precautions. Protective eyewear, thyroid shields, and gowns should be worn as well as a dosimeter to monitor the cumulative exposure with extensive duty in a radiology suite. Using a mobile shield or exiting the room entirely during periods of intense radiation should be utilized.

II. Anesthetic management

A. General considerations

   1. The indications, timing, and succession for various interventions are still in flux [9] but overall the anesthesiologist can encounter AVMs in the interventional radiology suite, in the operating room, or in the radiosurgery center. We elected to present their management together because in the modern era of the "hybrid operating room" the physiologic principles are the main guide to the management independent of the place of intervention.

   2. The procedures are done on an elective or emergent basis. Fortunately, AVMs have a lower chance of rebleeding, so the definitive procedure can be somewhat temporized until the patient stabilizes. A common indication for emergent treatment is decompression of a large hematoma after an initial bleed. The caveats of emergent cases are well known to any practicing anesthesiologist. We recommend establishing institutional-based protocols and clinical pathways ahead of time that delineate various team member responsibilities. We should remember that often speed is essential. In cases of neurologic deterioration, either spontaneous or iatrogenic, prompt evacuation of hematoma (within 30 minutes if possible) is associated with better outcomes [11].

TABLE 10.6 Common neurophysiologic targets and neuroanesthetic interventions

Targets	Interventions
• Oxygen	• Oxygen supply manipulation
• Carbon dioxide →	• Ventilation changes
• Arterial pressure	• Normal saline, colloid administration
• Venous pressure	• Reverse trendelenburg, head positioning
• Temperature	• Insulin
• Blood volume	• Barbiturates, propofol
• Glucose	• Pressors or hypotensive agents (adenosine, rapid cardiac pacing)
• Sodium	• Cerebrospinal fluid drainage
• Potassium	• Mannitol, furosemide
• Osmolarity	• Hemotherapy
• Hemoglobin	• Heparin and protamine
• Coagulation	• Neuromuscular blockers
• Immobility	
• Urine output	

3. Anesthesiologists need to have a deep understanding of the current and rapidly changing physiopathologic principles that govern the interactions between AVMs and the surrounding brain. We can be called to action to either strictly enforce normal homeostatic variables and/or create controlled disturbances intended to facilitate the operative correction and/or to compensate for various abnormalities present or iatrogenically created.

4. The general principles of neuroanesthesia apply to the management of AVMs (Table 10.6). We will especially try to make recommendations following an evidence-based approach.

5. Providing anesthesia care in the interventional neuroradiology or radiosurgery suites invokes the general precautions necessary at remote locations, including but not limited to the unavailability of specialized help in case of emergency, decreased lighting, decreased mobility of the operating table, unusual configurations for the position of the anesthesia machine and cart, decreased direct access to the patient (increased distance and interposition of imaging tools).

B. Preoperative considerations

1. Most of preoperative anesthetic considerations are common to all surgical patients, however the presence of specific comorbidities should be actively sought.

2. All patients should have a preoperative anesthesia evaluation performed before the beginning of the procedure, including all emergent and monitored anesthesia care cases:

   a. **Cardiac history,** including the presence of coronary disease and myocardium at risk, heart systolic or diastolic dysfunction (reports of ejection fraction percentage), intra-cardiac shunts (for sitting position procedures), and neurogenic pulmonary edema. Recent cardiac stents are associated with a higher risk of in-stent thrombosis if anti-platelet medications are to be stopped prematurely. Risks and benefits of open versus neuroradiologic procedures should be analyzed carefully in these cases.

   b. **Arterial hypertensive history** predisposes the patient to wider fluctuations in blood pressure. While these are generally of reduced significance in the general surgical population, it might be different for the patient with an AVM that has regions of the brain chronically exposed to disparities in perfusion. However, in population studies, the relationship between hypertension and AVM progression and hemorrhage is not proven definitively.

   c. **Lung diseases.** Chronic obstructive pulmonary disease or asthma can influence our ability to ventilate the patient or extubate at the end of the procedure.

   d. **Obstructive sleep apnea** has a close association with neurologic disorders, especially after acute events. The disorder is often underdiagnosed or patients are not using their prescribed devices. Close observation in monitored units is usually warranted after anesthesia.

e. **Renal insufficiency.** Neurosurgical patients are often exposed to large volume challenges that can either overload or severely dehydrate them. Therefore, baseline renal function plays an important role.

   (1) Contrast media are an important cause of renal deterioration. Risk factors include pre-existing renal disease, diabetes, heart failure, presence of hypotension or pressors, old age, anemia, and volume of contrast used. Proven preventing methods include generous hydration and use of low-osmolality contrast media. There is evidence for administration of steroids, N-acetylcysteine, and sodium bicarbonate but efficacy is still to be determined. Mannitol and furosemide should be avoided [12].

f. Patients with **diabetes mellitus** are to be instructed to continue all long-acting insulins and stop the oral agents the morning of surgery. Close monitoring is warranted throughout the perioperative period.

g. **Vascular diseases.** Presence of femoral, aortic or carotid disease or grafts has obvious implications for the interventional radiologist as well as for the anesthesiologist in obtaining adequate venous or arterial access.

h. **History of seizures and associated medications.** Anticonvulsants interact with cytochrome enzymatic systems. They can induce (fosphenytoin), have no effect (levtiracetam), or inhibit (valproate) them. In general, enzyme-inducing medications will show resistance to neuromuscular blockers and opioids. Preoperative adherence to regimens should be reinforced and drug levels sometimes are warranted.

i. **Coagulation disorders.** Baseline coagulation tests are usually ordered in all cases, despite problematic evidence, usually because patients will require anticoagulation and because any amount of abnormal bleeding in the tight space of the brain can be disastrous.

j. **Medication reconciliation**

   (1) Day-of-surgery status of β-blockers, antiseizure medications, and antibiotics.

   (2) Narcotic or drug history indicates a patient tolerant to opioids. Increased doses of medication are necessary in order to obtain the same clinical effects. Conversions to different opioid medications, nonopioid adjuvants, and nerve blocks can be helpful. Caution is warranted since these patients do not exhibit the same degree of tolerance to the adverse respiratory effects of opioids.

k. **Nothing per mouth status** is relative and might be hard to elicit, especially in cases of emergencies, for patients with decreased awareness, immobile in bed for various periods of time, or actively vomiting. We recommend a conservative approach geared toward an expeditious protection of the airway.

l. **Allergy history.** Especially important are:

   (1) History of heparin-induced thrombocytopenia (thrombosis and thrombocytopenia in relation with heparin administration) should be elicited. Confirmatory tests usually performed in association are antigen tests (ELISA) and functional assays (serotonin). Alternatives to heparin like direct thrombin inhibitors (hirudins) exist but they are harder to dose, monitor, and reverse.

   (2) Iodinated agent allergy (shellfish, internal vs. external). Considering that a true allergy to iodine is technically impossible (vital body constituent) and most common shellfish allergies are in fact directed against a protein, it is at least as important to enquire about other food allergies or asthma [13].

   (3) Protamine, derived from salmon, has also been linked with a higher incidence of hypersensitivity reactions, especially in patients with histories of fish allergy, exposure to neutral protamine hagedorn insulin or vasectomy.

3. Any anesthesiologic interaction should include a physical examination with emphasis on:

a. **The possibility of difficult airway.** Depending on the neurologic status, sometimes the only information that can be obtained is about the external appearance of the face (retrognathic mandible), neck (thickness, length), and dentition (missing or loose teeth, presence of prosthesis).

   b. Rapid, focused neurologic examination. We can encounter a wide range of presentations, from quasinormal ambulatory patient to the unconscious, critically ill after a possibly fatal hemorrhage. In the former, the primary provider has already performed a thorough neurologic examination, which is present in the medical chart and should be reviewed. The anesthesiologist's examination should document significant findings (signs and symptoms of increased intracranial pressure or the presence of lateralization syndromes) and alert of any interval changes. In the latter, unconscious patient, we should review the size of pupils and response to light, response to noxious stimuli, presence of abnormal reflexes, and if possible rough motor and sensory examination.

   c. While the primary provider is very likely focused on the neurologic aspects of the patient, we should not forget about the rest of the body. Cardiac examination (murmurs and arrhythmias, neck bruits), pulmonary examination (wheezes and rales), presence of scars, to cite just a few, are key findings.

C. Intraoperative considerations

  1. Monitoring

    a. All patients undergoing anesthesia care should be monitored according to the standards of basic anesthesia monitoring of the American Society of Anesthesiologists. While for patients undergoing general anesthesia, compliance is generally very good, every effort should be undertaken to extend similar care to the patients scheduled for monitored anesthesia care.

    b. Cardiovascular monitors

     (1) In addition to the standard monitors, intracranial procedures necessitate an invasive arterial line in order to facilitate

      (a) beat-to-beat blood pressure monitoring during rapid intraoperative changing conditions of high stimulation (induction of anesthesia, head pinning, incision, sudden blood loss, emergence) interspersed with lower-intensity periods (angiography, lesion exposure, closure);

      (b) frequent arterial blood gases and point-of-care hemoglobin and electrolyte checks;

      (c) the necessity to place an arterial line before induction is usually directly proportional to general physical status of the patient.

     (2) Central venous catheters are encouraged for hemodynamic monitoring and administration of medications especially for larger AVMs. When performed, ultrasound guidance, maximal sterile conditions, and Seldinger technique with pressure transduction are recommended.

    c. Precordial Doppler is used for craniotomies in sitting position (for AVMs of the posterior fossa) to monitor for a venous air embolism. See Chapter 26 for details on venous air embolism.

    d. Cerebral and neurophysiologic monitors

     (1) Bispectral index monitoring or full-standard electroencephalogram is sometimes employed in relation to total intravenous anesthesia or institution of burst suppression.

     (2) Jugular venous oxymetry is an invasive measure of jugular bulb blood saturation, intermittent or continuous with oxymetric catheters. Generally physicians are concerned with low values, lower than 55% that signal insufficient oxygen delivery. In the case of AVMs, due to the presence of shunt, the values are actually excessively high, 80% to 90%. One can monitor in real time the success of embolization or resection by observing the decrease in the abnormally high values. It has also been used to monitor the limit of safely induced hypotension (see chapter 28).

     (3) Transcranial Doppler demonstrates higher flow velocity and decreased pulsatility in the feeding arteries of medium and large AVMs. The method has diagnostic and monitoring value but is less sensitive for small lesions. Post treatment, whether surgical or embolization, the flows are reliably decreased and pulsatility index increases, resembling normal arteries. Intraoperative uses are usually harder to implement due to logistical reasons (see chapter 28).

(4) Awake testing and neurophysiologic monitoring (somatosensory, motor, auditory-evoked potentials, or electromyographic recordings). In cases of AVMs located in language, motor, or sensory areas, precise dissection will offer a better chance at preserving function. In awake patients, intracarotid (Wada test) or superselective injection of amobarbital (inhibits grey matter), lidocaine (inhibits white matter), and even propofol (5 to 10 mg doses) permits testing of any deficits that may appear. For patients under general anesthesia, one has to employ various neurophysiologic monitors to obtain the same results. Before resection or embolization, electrical stimulation or provocative medication is administered and the neural pathways are monitored for significant changes. The anesthesiologist has to be vigilant because occasionally intraoperative seizing can be triggered. Treatment is propofol 1 mg/kg and flooding the area with sterile cold saline [14,15] (see chapter 26).

(5) Cerebral oxymetry values can be skewed by the presence of AVMs. After careful baseline calibrations, it can be used to detect vascular complications related to catheter manipulation during neuroendovascular procedures or for monitoring of cerebral oxygenation during induced hypotension.

2. **Anesthetic regimen** [16]. The typical modern neuroanesthetic regimen uses volatile or intravenous agents plus a narcotic. By and large, for the average patient, both regimens are similar in regards to the main characteristics of an ideal neuroanesthetic: amnesia, cardiovascular stability, rapid emergence, good operating conditions. More important is the practitioner's familiarity with a specific one. There might be subtle differences in regards to a specific patient with a specific abnormality but definitive studies are lacking. Some of their pros and cons are listed below:

a. Inhalation agents' advantages include ease of titration, long track record, lower cost, and fast emergence. The main disadvantage is the direct cerebral vasodilation that offsets the decrease in flow associated with decreased cerebral metabolism.

b. Intravenous anesthetic are beneficial because they provide cerebral vasoconstriction, less postoperative nausea and vomiting, and less interference with neurophysiologic monitoring. They have more unpredictable pharmacokinetics so there is potential for longer emergence due to overdosage and the opposite of intraoperative awareness due to underdosage. Also, there can be severe acidosis from the propofol-infusion syndrome and shift of structures during stereotactic surgery due to decreased cerebral blood volume.

c. In one of the very few studies that compared patients with AVMs, isoflurane versus propofol-based anesthesia groups did not differ in terms of awakening times and early recovery of motor and respiratory functions. In the same note, both groups had impairment of higher cognitive functions for up to 24 hours after anesthesia [17].

d. In analyzing a subgroup of patients that had total intravenous anesthesia for their craniotomies, those with intravascular disorders (including AVMs) still had the highest rates of early postoperative complications, for an aggregate of 76.5% when adding postoperative shivering, hypertension, nausea, and vomiting [18].

CLINICAL PEARL For AVMs, hypertension on induction is less likely to cause rupture and hemorrhage than for an aneurysm.

3. **Induction and positioning**

a. Typical neuroanesthetic induction stresses the importance of strict blood pressure and heart rate control. This is usually achieved with a slow controlled drug titration (vs. a rapid sequence induction) complemented with interventions (narcotic, β/α blockers, vasopressors) to maintain hemodynamic stability.

(1) There is evidence that for AVMs hypertension is less likely to cause rupture and hemorrhage that is in the case for aneurysms [19]. The results were obtained in the

context of awake patients that underwent placement of stereotactic frames. It is our interpretation that blood pressure variations still need to be fairly limited especially for patients that have associated aneurysms, hemorrhagic, or ischemic phenomena.

(2) Induction of the general anesthesia in the adult patient is typically accomplished with a rapid acting intravenous agent (propofol or thiopental most commonly, etomidate in case of cardiovascular compromise) titrated to effect.

(3) Profound neuromuscular blockade confirmed by a twitch monitor has to be present at the time of the laryngoscopy and is usually achieved with succinylcholine or a nondepolarizing agent. Among the latter, rocuronium is an attractive choice because it has a faster onset of action. Both are acceptable choices that always put the neuroanesthesiologist in a classical dilemma. Succinylcholine is short acting but may increase the increased intracranial pressure and rocuronium administration is accompanied by prolonged paralysis that is undesirable in the face of a difficult airway. The decision is usually made based on patient-specific considerations.

(4) Direct laryngoscopy is usually first choice because of the availability and familiarity with the technique. Videolaryngoscopes are also very popular devices used in neuroanesthesia. They might provide a shortened intubation time, but not necessarily attenuation of hemodynamic responses to intubation. The explanation for this phenomenon might be that even if the response to pharyngeal stimulation might be diminished, the tracheal response to tube passage is still present [20]. While the combination of direct laryngoscopy and videolaryngoscopy is hugely effective, familiarity with awake intubation techniques, stylets, and supraglottic devices might prove life-saving especially in remote locations.

(5) Narcotics are administered liberally to blunt hemodynamic responses. For optimal results, the provider has to account for the agent-specific delay between administration and effect. Alfentanil and remifentanil have blood–brain equilibration half times of approximately 1 minute and sufentanil and fentanyl of around 6 minutes.

(6) Lidocaine, administered intravenously or tracheally, is widely used in order to blunt tachycardia or hypertension in response to intubation, despite minimal proven benefit.

b. During time-out confirm the status of antibiotics, β-blockers, and venous thromboembolism prophylaxis according to the local safety checklist (surgical or specific to interventional radiology).

c. Final positioning of the patient provides surgical comfort and is a multistep process:

(1) 90- to 180-degree table rotation should be accompanied by minimal interruption in monitoring;

(2) body positioning with care to padding all pressure points and avoiding peripheral nerve injuries;

(3) placement of pin holders represents a period of maximal stimulation that should be preemptively treated by deepening the anesthetic;

(4) final position of the head and neck should avoid extremes of flexion or rotation.

4. **Anesthetic maintenance**

a. Usual neuroanesthetic maintenance is low-dose volatile anesthetic and/or propofol plus an opioid infusion.

b. Fentanyl, sufetanil, or alfentanil infusions have been used successfully. Their pharmacokinetic profile involves a context-sensitive half time (that is proportional with the duration of infusion). The practitioner should monitor the total administered dose and allow for sufficient time before the end of the procedure for their metabolism (see chapter 13).

c. Fast-track neuroanesthesia usually involves remifentanil. It can be used for induction (1 to 2 μg/kg), maintenance (0.125 to 0.375 μg/kg/min), and emergence (0.0125 to 0.0375 μg/kg/min). In general it might be associated with deeper levels of anesthesia, less postoperative respiratory depression, same amount of muscle rigidity, and nausea and vomiting, but more incidences of bradycardia and hypotension, more requirements for rescue analgesia, and more shivering [21]. Brain-related effects include stable electroencephalogram with high-amplitude, low-frequency waves, decrease in intracranial pressure with maintenance of cerebral perfusion pressure, minimal interference with neurophysiologic monitoring, and creation of a "low-flow state" with extended autoregulatory values [22].

d. Dexmedetomidine is an attractive new addition to the neuroanesthesiologist's arsenal. It is an α-2 agonist that provides sedation, analgesia, and sympatholytic effects with minimal respiratory depression. Dexmedetomidine decreases cerebral blood flow without decreasing cerebral metabolic rate for oxygen and intracranial pressure.

(1) For monitored anesthesia care purposes during awake craniotomies and interventional neuroradiologic procedures, patients are in a state of "cooperative sedation" with a bispectral index around 60, can be very quickly aroused and are able to follow simple commands, then they return to sleep. It is administered as a loading dose of 0.5 to 1 μg/kg, with an infusion of 0.2 to 0.7 μg/kg/h and stopped 10 minutes before desired testing. There are reports that suggest that it interferes with cognitive testing for up to 1 hour after administration [23].

(2) For general anesthesia techniques, it is started 20 minutes before induction and occasionally is continued in recovery room, as an adjuvant to various regimens of balanced anesthesia. It has an opioid sparing effect and blunts hypertensive responses especially during induction and emergence [24].

e. Repeated arterial blood gas and electrolyte checks permit tight control of physiologic variables.

5. Fluid, electrolyte and transfusion management. Normal blood–brain barrier is composed of endothelial cells with few transporting vesicles tightly connected together. Electron microscopy studies of AVM differentiate two zones. Somewhat surprisingly, there is an intranidal portion that has preserved tight junctions and a perinidal component where endothelial cells have fenestrated surfaces, an abundance of vesicles and large gaps in the junctions between them [25]. This could play a role in the edema/hemorrhage after the surgery, recurrence of AVM after resection, but could also influence the intravascular behavior of fluids administered during surgery (see chapter 3).

a. Current dogma in neuroanesthesia demands for isovolemic, isoosmotic, isotonic fluid management [26].

(1) Isosmolar crystalloids like 0.9% normal saline are preferred and administration of free water should be avoided. The amount of fluid should match the urine output, insensible losses, and blood loss and should be adjusted based on the full array of hemodynamic data available at our disposition.

(2) There might be a merit in maintaining oncotic pressure near normal values by administering colloids [27]. The purported benefits are noted especially when the injury is milder, so it does not totally disrupt the blood–brain barrier.

b. Electrolyte abnormalities are frequent in patients with intracranial pathology, due to the disease itself, lack of oral intake, various intravenous fluid regimens, and diuretic/osmotic treatments.

(1) Hyponatremia can be caused by cerebral salt wasting syndrome or syndrome of inappropriate antidiuretic hormone secretion and hypernatremia by diabetes insipidus. Treatment has to be instituted immediately but in a gentle manner because rapid corrections are associated with neurologic sequelae.

c. Blood loss and transfusion therapy [28,29]:

(1) The overall goal is to provide optimal oxygen delivery and clot formation to the brain while minimizing the risks of blood and blood product transfusions.

(2) Hemodilution to a hemoglobin around 10 g/dL decreases blood oxygen content and carrying capacity but is thought to improve blood rheology and therefore assists in cerebral oxygenation.

(3) Different types of brain injury might need different approaches (traumatic brain injury might be more permissive to anemia than subarachnoid hemorrhage).

(4) We lack definitive evidence to address these issues for patients with AVMs. One can only postulate that decreased hemoglobin and the hyperdynamic state of circulation that accompanies hemodilution could be deleterious to rapid flowing arteriovenous shunts and to the breakthrough phenomena that accompanies their treatment. Also surrounding areas, chronically hypoperfused, might be excessively sensitive to decreased oxygen-carrying capacity.

(5) Magnitude of blood loss is proportional with the malformation size and grade, and preoperative embolization reduces intraoperative blood loss. Significant intraoperative hemorrhage is generally rare, but when it occurs it is rather extensive. In a large series of patients only approximately one-third of patients required a blood transfusion. However, those that did, received up to 18 units of packed red blood cells [30].

(6) Most institutions obtain type and cross in all patients; however, this approach is associated with a low crossmatch-to-transfusion ratio.

(7) In case of hemorrhage, activation of massive "trauma-type" transfusion protocol might be appropriate. In principle, such a protocol follows the ratios found in whole blood, providing adequate amounts of coagulation factors (specifically fibrinogen) and platelets.

(8) Monitoring the transfusion needs is a complex task that always starts with observing the surgical field, checking frequent blood counts, and standard coagulation tests like prothrombin time, activated thromboplastin time, and fibrinogen. We recommend incorporating real-time input from various neurophysiologic monitors (cerebral oxygen tension, microdialysis) and especially point of care testing like thromboelastometry. Such an approach should permit individualization of dose and type of hemotherapy.

CLINICAL PEARL   Transfusion therapy should be patient specific and goal directed.

(9) In conclusion, we should be prepared to massively transfuse on a moment's notice with specific goal therapy.

6. **Anticoagulation and reversal**

   a. The presence of foreign material (intravascular sheaths, catheters, and embolization agents) creates a thromboembolic environment.

   b. Initial anticoagulation is obtained by giving a bolus of heparin of 60 to 80 mg/kg or 3,000 to 5,000 U, followed either by boluses every 45 to 60 minutes or an infusion.

   c. There is substantial variability in the individual response to a certain dose of heparin, so monitoring of anticoagulation is recommended. Activated clotting time is employed, because when compared with activated thromboplastin time, it provides rapid, point-of-care results and also has a linear response to a wider range of doses of heparin, providing ease of titration. Different machines give different activated clotting time results, so calibration and baseline results are mandatory. Tests should be repeated every 30 to 60 minutes during the procedure, the goal being to maintain an activated clotting time of 2 to 2.5 times the baseline.

   d. At the end or in the event of a hemorrhagic emergency, protamine can be administered in the dose of 1 mg/100 U of heparin given, depending on the time elapsed from the last administration.

7. **Emergencies/surgical requests**

   a. Generally speaking, there are two types of intraprocedural crises: Obstructive or hemorrhagic [31].

(1) For obstructive events deliberate hypertension and cerebral protection might be necessary. Induced hypertension is accomplished by establishing a lighter plane of anesthesia and supplementing with an α-1 adrenergic agent, like phenylephrine, norepinephrine, or epinephrine. Associated bradycardia might necessitate concomitant atropine administration.

(2) Hemorrhagic occurrences prompt immediate heparin reversal if present, induced hypotension and cerebral protection.

b. Cerebral protective strategies [32]:

(1) During the perioperative period, due to local causes or general hemodynamic disturbances, brain can be exposed to ischemia and hypoxia that cause either:

(a) immediate cessation of any metabolic processes or

(b) secondary insults after restoration of flow: apoptosis, inflammation, oxidative stress, excitotoxicity, degeneration

(2) Strategies to decrease those risks can be employed

(a) Preemptively (cerebral protection per se) when there might be a foreseeable insult, in order to decrease brain susceptibility to ischemia.

(b) As soon as possible after the insult has occurred (cerebral resuscitation) to minimize the secondary injury and to enhance the restorative processes.

(3) Hypothermia proportionally decreases metabolic rate. While it is useful after resuscitation of cardiac arrest patients, but no benefit has bee found for traumatic brain injury, aneurysm surgery, and subarachnoid hemorrhage.

(4) Barbiturates decrease cerebral metabolism, cerebral blood volume, and intracranial pressure. Results in diffuse traumatic brain injury have been less than stellar but there are better results when ischemia is milder and temporary. Barbiturates have been used successfully in the treatment of hemorrhage associated with AVM resection. Anesthetic doses are usually employed and those are associated with delayed emergence [33].

(5) Propofol in burst suppression doses and volatile anesthetics could provide the same benefits as thiopental but human outcome trials are missing. The overall opinion is that the protection they provide is weaker and it may fade over time. There is insufficient data regarding nitrous oxide and hyperoxia.

(6) More clearly, we know what to avoid: Hyperthermia and hyperglycemia. Both are associated with worsened neurologic outcomes.

c. Deliberate hypotension and/or flow arrest [34]:

(1) The concept behind induced hypotension it is that a lower blood pressure will provide a better operating field, and lessen the blood loss while maintaining safe tissue perfusion and oxygenation. Common targets are systolic blood pressure less than 100 mm Hg and mean blood pressure around 50 to 60 mm Hg. A careful risk/benefit analysis needs to be done in the presence of specific comorbidities (cerebral, carotid, cardiac, renal disease).

(2) Hypertensive patients, especially untreated or poorly treated ones, have an autoregulatory curve that is displaced to the right, that is, toward higher values. For these patients, the limits of safe hypotension also need to be adjusted toward higher values. In addition, the presence of increased peripheral vasoconstriction of sympathetic origin is exposed during general anesthesia and results in a higher incidence of hypotension. While the exact correlation of these perturbations with postoperative morbidity is less clear, the overall management of blood pressure in hypertensive patients undergoing intracranial procedures can be quite challenging, especially in the presence of induced hypotension.

(3) For a list of most commonly used agents and their side effects please refer to Table 10.7. A clinical dilemma is due to the fact that while targeting sympathetic outflow, several agents also produce cerebral vasodilation that can cause increases in cerebral blood flow, intracranial pressure, and overall hyperemic conditions especially when dura is closed.

TABLE 10.7 Common agents used for induced hypotension

Pharmacologic class	Agents	Side effects
Inhaled anesthetics	Isoflurane, sevoflurane	Cerebral vasodilation, prolonged emergence
β-adrenergic blockers	Esmolol, labetalol	Bradycardia, bronchospasm, myocardial depression
Direct vasodilators	Nitroprusside	Cerebral vasodilation, tachyphylaxis, cyanide toxicity, reflex tachycardia
Calcium-channel blockers	Nicardipine, clevidipine	Atrioventricular block, cerebral autoregulation impairment
Dopamine-receptor agonist	Fenoldopam	Atrial fibrillation, heart failure
Opioids	Remifentanil	Profound bradycardia, nausea
Purine analogue	Adenosine	Bradycardia, myocardial ischemia, bronchospasm
Secondary agents (used only in association)	Angiotensin-converting enzyme inhibitors, clonidine	—

(4) Nitroprusside, isoflurane, and esmolol had been used successfully for induced hypotension during AVM surgery. Pulmonary artery catheter measurements show a decreased systemic vascular resistance for nitroprusside and isoflurane versus a decreased cardiac output for esmolol as primary mechanisms for the hypotensive effects [35].

(5) Nicardipine produces a dose-dependent decrease in blood pressure in about 15 minutes, but can last for a longer time than desired after infusion is stopped and it may impair cerebral autoregulation.

(6) Fenoldopam produces peripheral vasodilation and cerebral vasoconstriction (α-2 mediated similar to dexmedetomidine), concomitantly reducing cerebral blood flow.

(7) In selected patients, under a low-dose volatile anesthetic – remifentanil – propofol regimen, adenosine in a dose of 0.3 to 0.4 mg/kg will provide 45 seconds of mean blood pressure less than 60 mm Hg with minimal side effects. Subsequent doses, if necessary, might need to be reduced due to a carryover effect. Other anesthetic regimens and especially the combination with nitroprusside might necessitate higher doses. Intraoperative pacing pads placement and postoperative troponin checks are indicated. Adenosine is contraindicated in patients with extensive coronary and reactive airways diseases. Potential side effects are prolonged bradycardia, atrial fibrillation, and bronchospasm [36].

(8) Rapid right ventricular pacing, a method borrowed from interventional cardiology, with rates of 180 bpm, produces drops of at least 50% in blood pressures. The pacing rate can be titrated to effect and the duration is decided by the operator according to the needs. The special pacing wire is threaded through a central line introducer and is positioned in the right ventricle with the aid of fluoroscopy and by demonstrating a low threshold for ventricular capture. Complications consist of ventricular tachyarrhythmias and mechanical (cardiac perforation, associated with central line placement). Defibrillator pads and cardiac surgery capabilities are recommended [37].

8. **Emergence [38]**

    a. Rapid is the preferred method since it permits neurologic examination – in case of good neurologic status preoperative, no major complications intraoperative, and no significant morbidity expected postoperative.

    b. Delayed—in all other cases. Common indications for the decision not to extubate to include: airway protection from aspiration and/or secretion, necessity of ventilatory support because of respiratory abnormalities, hemodynamic instability or administration of vasopressors, ability to control intracranial pressure through hyperventilation, barbiturates, and paralysis.

   c. In general, hypertension during emergence is related with a higher incidence of intracranial hemorrhage [39] so aggressive control is suggested. Authors usually employ an escalating algorithm using esmolol (if deemed to be extremely time limited), labetalol (for longer occurrences), and nicardipine (when previous measures fail).

   d. Be prepared to transport patient to the imaging scanner when there is a delayed emergence or otherwise directly to the intensive care unit (provide enough time for bed and ventilator availability).

   e. If remifentanil is employed, please do not forget supplemental long-term analgesia before discontinuation of the infusion.

> **CLINICAL PEARL** AVMs have high postoperative rates of shivering, hypertension, and nausea or vomiting.

  D. **Postoperative considerations**

    1. **Location.** Most patients are cared for in neurocritical care units by a specialized intensivist. There is a wide range of physical statuses for such patients, from unstable and critically ill to relatively uncomplicated "admissions for observation" after uneventful neuroradiologic procedures. We recommend full attention in these cases too, because complications can happen very fast and patients enter a vicious downward spiral. Consideration should be given at direct postoperative admission to neurosciences intensive care units, bypassing traditional postanesthesia care units, for intubated and also for freshly extubated patients.

    2. **Frequent neurologic examinations are essential**

      a. Intracranial pathology is unique in the fact that it is rapidly manifested in changes from baseline clinical examination. These changes are frequently nonspecific and point toward intracranial hematoma, generalized hyperemia, increased intracranial pressure, sodium abnormalities, or hypercapnia. More localized signs suggest more discrete abnormalities.

      b. A clinical change usually prompts an imagistic examination, either CT or MRI in order to define the underlying process. However, despite generally viewed as necessary, the number of examinations that herald a change in management is rather rare.

    3. **Monitors:**

      a. heart rate and rhythm in a 3 or 5 lead system;

      b. blood pressure is usually monitored invasively (radial arterial line or femoral sheaths left in place after procedure);

      c. central venous and pulmonary artery catheters for specific indications.

      d. There is also a plethora of neuromonitors being employed, very much institution dependent.

    4. **Postoperative complications**

      a. Most feared specific AVM complication is a state of brain hyperemia that can manifest as edema or hemorrhage, with varying degrees of severity and extension relative to the initial location of the malformation.

        (1) Preoperatively, the AVM is characterized by high flow and low resistance. Feeding artery pressure is approximately 60% of the systemic pressure and draining vein pressure is about 10 mm Hg above central venous pressure. A phenylephrine challenge (increasing blood pressure) and Valsalva maneuver (increasing venous pressure) are only partially transmitted to the draining vein, determining a buffering capacity of the malformation [40]. The tissues surrounding the lesion are chronically hypoperfused, with a left shifted autoregulatory curve [41].

11

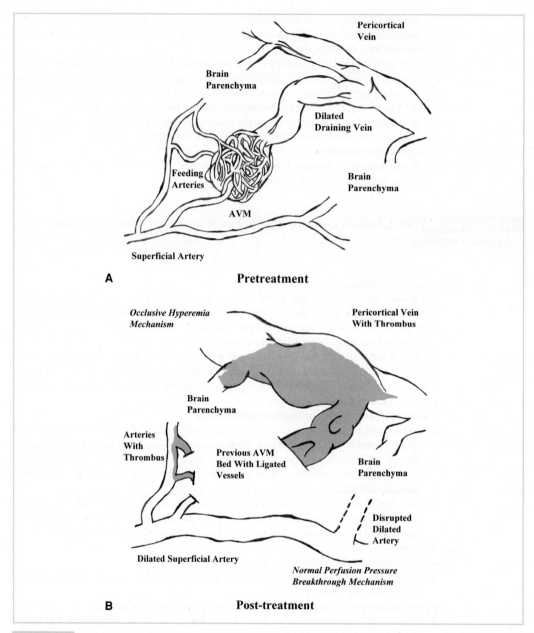

FIGURE 10.3 A,B: Diagrams showing the dynamics of the "normal perfusion pressure breakthrough" and "occlusive hyperemia" mechanisms. Pretreatment, the AVM has several feeding arteries and draining veins with luxurious perfusion in contrast with chronic hypoperfused areas in the adjacent brain. Posttreatment, exclusion of the AVM has significant effects on the arterial and venous sides of the brain circulation, overwhelming cerebral autoregulation, and promoting creation of brain edema.

(2) Postoperatively, the exclusion of the low-resistance malformation re-establishes normal pressures in the surrounding regions. There are also some patients with generalized increases in cerebral blood flows after resection. Such increases in pressures and flows overwhelm local autoregulation with ensuing edema and hemorrhage, a phenomenon called normal perfusion pressure breakthrough [42] (see Fig. 10.3A,B). There are several important corollaries to this theory. First, a staged approach to treatment might diminish the impact of these hemodynamic changes. Second, a **complete control** of the blood pressure remains the most logic treatment. To further illustrate the degree of regulation required, we would mention that there have been reports where "minimal" increases of blood pressure to 140 to 160 mm Hg up to 8 days after surgery precipitated such complications [43].

(3) After treatment there is obstruction in the venous system that promotes passive occlusive hyperemia in the adjacent regions and stagnation of arterial blood with worsening ischemia, thrombosis, and edema [44] (see Fig. 10.3A,B). Subsequently, one should avoid hypotension that can be a compounding factor and employ thromboprophylaxis with aspirin and/or heparin.

(4) The above two theories can be encompassed in one term of arterial–capillary–venous hypertensive syndrome and are not mutually exclusive. The needs of each patient have to be assessed independently and therapeutic decisions are made based on clinical, neuromonitoring, and neuroimaging grounds.

(5) On a practical note, blood pressure control, surgical reintervention, and cerebral protection strategies are mainstays of therapy.

b. Postoperative seizures are another feared complication. Most patients receive prophylactic medications for some duration after treatment, especially when epileptic activity was present pretreatment. Motivations for this approach include acknowledgement that nonconvulsive epilepsy is more frequent than we suspect and delays in diagnosis and treatment are common when seizures occur.

c. There is increased recognition of the negative role of pain, shivering, and nausea and vomiting after neurosurgical procedures. In addition, respiratory care, glycemic and electrolyte control, nutritional and hydration stratus, and thromboprophylaxis are important issues that should be included in a more general approach to postoperative care.

E. **Anesthesia for stereotactic surgery and radiosurgery** usually involves monitored anesthesia care for an awake patient. The stereotactic frame is applied after generous local anesthesia. Immobility is essential. The procedures can be long, involving multiple locations. For young or uncooperative patients, general anesthesia may be necessary. Therefore, the anesthesiologist must accompany the patient during transport in the hospital. Full monitoring, emergency airway equipment, emergency drugs, full tank of oxygen, total intravenous anesthesia delivered with continuous pumps, and enough help are necessary. Despite the apparent minimalistic approach, complications can be devastating, including brain hemorrhage, seizures, venous air embolism, and arrhythmias, necessitating rapid escalation of care [45].

REFERENCES

1. Al-Shahi R, Warlow C. A systematic review of the frequency and prognosis of arteriovenous malformations of the brain in adults. *Brain.* 2001;124:1900–1926.
2. Choi JH, Mohr JP. Brain arteriovenous malformations in adults. *Lancet Neurol.* 2005;4:299–308.
3. Geibprasert S, Pongpech S, Jiarakongmun P, et al. Radiologic assessment of brain arteriovenous malformations: what clinicians need to know. *Radiographics.* 2010;30:483–501.
4. Hartmann A, Mast H, Choi JH, et al. Treatment of arteriovenous malformations of the brain. *Curr Neurol Neurosci Rep.* 2007;7:28–34.
5. Ogilvy CS, Stieg PE, Awad I, et al. Recommendations for the management of intracranial arteriovenous malformations: a statement for healthcare professionals from a special writing group of the Stroke Council, American Stroke Association. *Circulation.* 2001;103:2644–2657.

6. van Beijnum J, van der Worp HB, Buis DR, et al. Treatment of brain arteriovenous malformations. *JAMA*. 2011;306: 2011–2019.

7. Stapf C, Mast H, Sciacca RR, et al. Predictors of hemorrhage in patients with untreated brain arteriovenous malformation. *Neurology*. 2006;66:1350–1355.

8. Weerakkody RA, Trivedi R, Santarius T, et al. Arteriovenous malformations. *Br J Neurosurg*. 2009;23:494–498.

9. Mohr JP, Moskowitz AJ, Stapf C, et al. The ARUBA trial: current status, future hopes. *Stroke*. 2010;41:e537–e540.

10. Fiorella D, Albuquerque FC, Woo HH, et al. The role of neuroendovascular therapy for the treatment of brain arteriovenous malformations. *Neurosurgery*. 2006;59:S163–S177; discussion S3–13.

11. Jafar JJ, Rezai AR. Acute surgical management of intracranial arteriovenous malformations. *Neurosurgery*. 1994;34:8–12; discussion 12–13.

12. Barrett BJ, Parfrey PS. Preventing nephropathy induced by contrast medium. *N Engl J Med*. 2006;354:379–386.

13. Schabelman E, Witting M. The relationship of radiocontrast, iodine, and seafood allergies: a medical myth exposed. *J Emerg Med*. 2010;39:701–707.

14. Gabarros A, Young WL, McDermott MW, et al. Language and motor mapping during resection of brain arteriovenous malformations: indications, feasibility, and utility. *Neurosurgery*. 2011;68:744–752.

15. Fitzsimmons B-FM, Marshall RS, Pile-Spellman J, et al. Neurobehavioral differences in superselective wada testing with amobarbital versus lidocaine. *Am J Neuroradiol*. 2003;24:1456–1460.

16. Cole CD, Gottfried ON, Gupta DK, et al. Total intravenous anesthesia: advantages for intracranial surgery. *Neurosurgery*. 2007;61:369–377; discussion 377–378.

17. Munte S, Munte TF, Kuche H, et al. General anesthesia for interventional neuroradiology: propofol versus isoflurane. *J Clin Anesth*. 2001;13:186–192.

18. Wong AY, O'Regan AM, Irwin MG. Total intravenous anaesthesia with propofol and remifentanil for elective neurosurgical procedures: an audit of early postoperative complications. *Eur J Anaesthesiol*. 2006;23:586–590.

19. Szabo MD, Crosby G, Sundaram P, et al. Hypertension does not cause spontaneous hemorrhage of intracranial arteriovenous malformations. *Anesthesiology*. 1989;70:761–763.

20. Xue FS, Zhang GH, Li XY, et al. Comparison of hemodynamic responses to orotracheal intubation with the GlideScope videolaryngoscope and the Macintosh direct laryngoscope. *J Clin Anesth*. 2007;19:245–250.

21. Komatsu R, Turan AM, Orhan-Sungur M, et al. Remifentanil for general anaesthesia: a systematic review. *Anaesthesia*. 2007;62:1266–1280.

22. Fodale V, Schifilliti D, Pratico C, et al. Remifentanil and the brain. *Acta Anaesthesiol Scand*. 2008;52:319–326.

23. Bustillo MA, Lazar RM, Finck AD, et al. Dexmedetomidine may impair cognitive testing during endovascular embolization of cerebral arteriovenous malformations: a retrospective case report series. *J Neurosurg Anesthesiol*. 2002;14:209–212.

24. Bekker A, Sturaitis M, Bloom M, et al. The effect of dexmedetomidine on perioperative hemodynamics in patients undergoing craniotomy. *Anesth Analg*. 2008;107:1340–1347.

25. Tu J, Stoodley MA, Morgan MK, et al. Ultrastructure of perinidal capillaries in cerebral arteriovenous malformations. *Neurosurgery*. 2006;58:961–970; discussion 961–970.

26. Tommasino C. Fluids and the neurosurgical patient. *Anesthesiol Clin North Am*. 2002;20:329–346, vi.

27. Drummond JC. Colloid osmotic pressure and the formation of posttraumatic cerebral edema. *Anesthesiology*. 2010;112: 1079–1081.

28. McEwen J, Huttunen KH. Transfusion practice in neuroanesthesia. *Curr Opin Anaesthesiol*. 2009;22:566–571.

29. Gerlach R, Krause M, Seifert V, et al. Hemostatic and hemorrhagic problems in neurosurgical patients. *Acta Neurochir (Wien)*. 2009;151:873–900.

30. Ledezma CJ, Hoh BL, Carter BS, et al. Complications of cerebral arteriovenous malformation embolization: multivariate analysis of predictive factors. *Neurosurgery*. 2006;58:602–611; discussion 602–611.

31. Young WL, Dowd CF. Chapter 14. Interventional neuroradiology: anesthetic management. In: Young WL, Cottrell JE, eds. *Cottrell and Young's Neuroanesthesia*. Philadelphia, PA: Mosby/Elsevier; 2010:247–263.

32. Fukuda S, Warner DS. Cerebral protection. *Br J Anaesth*. 2007;99:10–17.

33. Cordato DJ, Herkes GK, Mather LE, et al. Barbiturates for acute neurological and neurosurgical emergencies—do they still have a role?. *J Clin Neurosci*. 2003;10:283–288.

34. Degoute CS. Controlled hypotension: a guide to drug choice. *Drugs*. 2007;67:1053–1076.

35. Ornstein E, Young WL, Ostapkovich N, et al. Deliberate hypotension in patients with intracranial arteriovenous malformations: esmolol compared with isoflurane and sodium nitroprusside. *Anesth Analg*. 1991;72:639–644.

36. Bebawy JF, Gupta DK, Bendok BR, et al. Adenosine-induced flow arrest to facilitate intracranial aneurysm clip ligation: dose-response data and safety profile. *Anesth Analg*. 2010;110:1406–1411.

37. Saldien V, Menovsky T, Rommens M, et al. Rapid ventricular pacing for flow arrest during cerebrovascular surgery: revival of an old concept. *Neurosurgery*. 2011;70:270–275.

38. Bruder N, Ravussin P. Recovery from anesthesia and postoperative extubation of neurosurgical patients: a review. *J Neurosurg Anesthesiol*. 1999;11:282–293.

39. Basali A, Mascha EJ, Kalfas I, et al. Relation between perioperative hypertension and intracranial hemorrhage after craniotomy. *Anesthesiology*. 2000;93:48–54.

40. Young WL, Kader A, Pile-Spellman J, et al. Arteriovenous malformation draining vein physiology and determinants of transnidal pressure gradients. The Columbia University AVM Study Project. *Neurosurgery*. 1994;35:389–395; discussion 395–396.

41. Young WL, Pile-Spellman J, Prohovnik I, et al. Evidence for adaptive autoregulatory displacement in hypotensive cortical territories adjacent to arteriovenous malformations. Columbia University AVM Study Project. *Neurosurgery*. 1994;34:601–610; discussion 610–611.

42. Spetzler RF, Wilson CB, Weinstein P, et al. Normal perfusion pressure breakthrough theory. *Clin Neurosurg.* 1978;25:651–672.

43. Morgan MK, Sekhon LH, Finfer S, et al. Delayed neurological deterioration following resection of arteriovenous malformations of the brain. *J Neurosurg.* 1999;90:695–701.

44. al-Rodhan NR, Sundt TM Jr, Piepgras DG, et al. Occlusive hyperemia: a theory for the hemodynamic complications following resection of intracerebral arteriovenous malformations. *J Neurosurg.* 1993;78:167–175.

45. Edler A. Special anesthetic considerations for stereotactic radiosurgery in children. *J Clin Anesth.* 2007;19:616–618.

46. Spetzler RF, Ponce FA. A 3-tier classification of cerebral arteriovenous malformations. Clinical article. *J Neurosurg.* 2011;114:842–849.

47. Starke RM, Komotar RJ, Hwang BY, et al. Treatment guidelines for cerebral arteriovenous malformation microsurgery. *Br J Neurosurg.* 2009;23:376–386.

48. International RadioSurgery Association. Stereotactic radiosurgery for patients with intracranial arteriovenous malformations (AVM). 2009. Available at: http://www.irsa.org/AVM%20Guideline.pdf. Accessed January 10, 2012.

11

Neurosurgical Procedures and Chronic Pain

Cuong Vu, Joseph Salama-Hanna, and Grace Chen

KEY POINTS

1. Compression on a peripheral nerve results in axonal degeneration and ischemic changes that may result in pain and motor weakness. The goal of surgical decompression is to relieve the compression.

2. In some pain disorders, the sympathetic nervous system may contribute to the maintenance of the painful sensory input. In this sympathetically maintained pain, a sympathectomy may help provide pain relief.

3. Trigeminal neuralgia is associated with compression of the trigeminal nerve by another nerve or an artery, and is commonly treated with microvascular decompression surgery.

4. Deep brain stimulation for pain control is thought to work through a number of mechanisms including enabling the release of endogenous opioids and increasing descending inhibition.

5. Spinal cord stimulation is postulated to work by stimulating nonpainful nerves in the dorsal columns to inhibit painful nerve signals. This utilizes the Gate Control Theory of Pain.

6. Peripheral nerve stimulation activates large fiber nerves which may close the gate for painful small fiber nerve transmission.

7. Drug pumps are most commonly placed to deliver medications to the intrathecal space. The most widely used medications are opioids and anti-spasmotics.

8. Ziconotide is a snail toxin that is a calcium channel blocker and can block nociceptive input intrathecally by its actions on the dorsal horn. It has significant side effects including nystagmus and psychosis.

I. **Introduction.** Neuropathic pain is a common disease that all anesthesiologists will encounter throughout their careers. Neuropathic pain encompasses a wide range of nerve disorders from disorders of small and large fiber peripheral nerves, like those seen in diabetic neuropathy, to disorders of the central nervous system as seen in central post-stroke pain.

These conditions can be difficult to treat and after extensive conservative treatments, including medication management and minimally invasive interventions, these patients may present to the

TABLE 11.1 Neuropathic pain disorders and their surgical management

Neurosurgical techniques	Objective	Examples of applicable clinical condition
Peripheral nerve decompression	Releases peripheral nerve entrapments or compressions	Carpal tunnel syndrome, cubital tunnel syndrome, suprascapular nerve entrapment, piriformis syndrome, thoracic outlet syndrome
Neurectomy	Resects prior nerve injury, surgery, or trauma	Intercostal neuralgia, meralgia paresthetica, Morton's neuroma, cancer pain, neuroma excision
Dorsal rhizotomy	Dorsal root and dorsal root ganglion resection to denervate a sensory dermatome	Targets specific damaged and painful nerves in spastic conditions as in cerebral palsy
Sympathectomy	Reserved for sympathetically maintained pain, refractory to other treatments	Sympathetic ganglia resection for medically refractor hyperhidrosis and ischemic rest pain when vascular surgery fails.
Microvascular decompression	Trigeminal nerve compression; treated with microvascular decompression surgery primarily	Craniotomy with incision retroauricular at the mastoid process, using a lateral park bench position; goal is dissection of the compressing nerve or vessel
Ablative therapy	Targets the spinal thalamic tract and its projections; reserved for intractable pain, significant comorbidities, and shortened life expectancies	For intractable cancer related pain Locations: Anterior cingulate cortex, thalamus and spinal cord—cordotomies and cordectomies
Deep brain stimulation	Tremors treatment resistent depression central pain syndromes pystonia epilepsy	Stimulates: Thalamus periaqueductal/periventricular gray matter
Motor cortex stimulation	Unknown mechanism of relief.	Phantom limb pain, anesthesia dolorosa, pain from MS, and post-stroke pain.
Neurostimulation	"Utilize gate control theory": Thought to stimulate nonpainful nerves in the dorsal columns to inhibit painful nerve signals	Neuropathic pain from failed back surgical syndrome; also for complex regional pain syndrome, ischemic and visceral pain, including refractory angina and interstitial cystitis; causes vasodilation, bronchodilation, and may decrease bladder spasticity

operating room for surgical treatment of their pain disorder. The procedures include implantable pumps, stimulation devices, ablations, excisions, and decompressions of the offending nerves.

Perioperative care can be fraught with difficulty due to multiple comorbidities of these patients. They may be severely deconditioned with a poor functional status. They may have a high opioid tolerance and be on multiple centrally acting medications that have synergistic side effects. All these considerations make it important to be knowledgeable about neuropathic pain disorders and their management (see summary in Table 11.1).

II. **Peripheral nervous system.** The peripheral nervous system (PNS) encompasses all nerves outside of the brain and spinal cord. The locations of these nerves, as well as their extensive number, make them particularly prone to injury by surgery, trauma, or entrapment. Peripheral nerves have the benefit of regeneration and regrowth, but this is not always perfect and may result in neuropathic pain. Surgical treatment ranges from decompression to excision [1].

A. Peripheral nerve decompression

1. **Indications.** Surgical decompressions are used to treat peripheral nerve entrapments. Where nerves are usually compressed in areas where they rest in superficial locations or are confined in small anatomic spaces. The pressure from the compression results in axonal degeneration and ischemic changes that may result in pain and motor weakness. The goal of surgery is to relieve the compression [2].

2. **Common nerve entrapments**

   a. **Carpal tunnel syndrome.** Carpal tunnel syndrome is the most common nerve entrapment and results from compression of the median nerves between the bones of the wrist and the flexor retinaculum that make up the carpal tunnel. Symptoms include pain in the first three fingers of the hand that is often worse at night, with weakness in the thumb [3].

   b. **Cubital tunnel syndrome.** Cubital tunnel syndrome is the second most common nerve entrapment and results from entrapment of the ulnar nerve at the elbow. Patients may have symptoms of pain in the last two digits of their hand and weakness in their intrinsic hand muscles [4].

   c. **Suprascapular nerve entrapment.** The suprascapular nerve travels through the suprascapular notch beneath the suprascapular ligament. Compression of this nerve by the ligament can result in shoulder pain with radiation to the shoulder blades as well as weakness in abduction and external rotation of the shoulder [5].

   d. **Piriformis syndrome.** The sciatic nerve travels anterior to the piriformis muscle but can travel posterior, or even through this muscle, that can result in entrapment of the sciatic nerve. Entrapment can also be caused by muscular hypertrophy or repeated trauma [6]. Symptoms include buttock pain that radiates down the back of their leg [7]. Patients may also have knee weakness. Piriformis syndrome can be hard to differentiate from a lumbar radiculopathy.

   e. **Thoracic outlet syndrome.** Thoracic outlet syndrome can also be difficult to diagnose. This syndrome involves compression at the thoracic inlet of the neurovascular bundle that consists of the brachial plexus, subclavian vein, and artery [8]. Compression may be of any of these structures with the most common compression being of the brachial plexus. This compression can occur in multiple areas including the interscalene triangle, between the clavicle and first rib, or at the attachment of the pectoralis minor [9]. Some patients also have a cervical first rib which may also cause compression of the neurovascular bundle.

      (1) Surgical approach toward thoracic outlet syndrome depends on the structures involved in the entrapment. These may include resection of the first rib or cervical rib, anterior scalene muscle, or resection of the costoclavicular ligament [10]. This procedure can be done by either a transaxillary or supraclavicular approach.

3. **Anesthetic considerations.** Nerve entrapments are associated with a higher incidence of endocrine diseases. Approximately 15% of these patients may have diabetes [1]. Acromegaly is associated with nerve entrapment as well as obesity and pregnancy [11,12]. Other comorbid conditions associated with nerve entrapments include rheumatoid arthritis, gout, amyloidosis, and carcinomatosis.

CLINICAL PEARL   Neuropathies are associated with a higher incidence of endocrine diseases including diabetes, in addition to other comorbid conditions like acromegaly, obesity, rheumatoid arthritis, gout, amyloidosis, and carcinomatosis.

---

   a. Many different anesthetic techniques have been used successfully. It is presently controversial to perform a regional or neuraxial technique in patients who may have pre-existing nerve injury. A thorough physical examination and documentation of pre-existing nerve injury should be done prior to any anesthetic and the risks and benefits of each technique should be weighed.

    b. With any pain in patients, postoperative pain management can be a challenge. This is particularly so in patients receiving rib resections for their thoracic outlet syndrome since this can be a painful procedure. Paravertebral blocks for postoperative pain control in first rib resections have been successful and may be considered [13]. Other anesthetic concerns include the potential for rapid blood loss as well as the inability to trust or use the affected limb for blood pressure or IV access.

B. **Neurectomy.** A neurectomy may be performed to treat a number of conditions. One intention is to denervate a painful area, providing symptomatic relief to the patient. Another may be to remove an aberrantly firing nerve that is thought to be the pain generator. This may be a previously injured nerve that has formed a painful neuroma and excision allows the nerve to heal, forming a new neuroma that may not be as painful [14].

    1. **Patient characteristics.** Patients presenting for a neurectomy may have a prior history of nerve injury, surgery, or trauma that resulted in nerve injury. They may present with symptoms of burning, shooting pain in the distribution of a peripheral nerve or in the area of a neuroma with signs of allodynia, dysesthesia, or hypoesthesia. These patients may have undergone conservative treatment with neuropathic pain medications or diagnostic procedures including nerve blocks to help identify the abnormal nerve [1].

        a. Another type of patient undergoing a neurectomy is one with localized disease, either joint disease from osteoarthritis or visceral disease from a malignancy that results in severe pain. The goal of the neurectomy is to denervate the sensory input from the painful areas.

    2. **Common indications**

        a. **Intercostal neuralgia.** This may be caused by chest trauma or a prior thoracotomy. A neurectomy can be performed through a video-assisted thorascopic (VATS) procedure or through an open procedure [15].

        b. **Meralgia paresthetica.** This is the result of either entrapment or injury to the lateral femoral cutaneous nerve, and the nerve can be transected surgically if decompression is not helpful [16].

        c. **Morton's neuroma.** This is compression of a digital nerve in the foot causing swelling of the digital nerve resulting in pain with walking and wearing shoes. Though not a true neuroma, surgical excision may provide pain relief [17].

        d. **Cancer pain.** Neurolysis of the celiac plexus is commonly performed for treatment of painful upper abdominal malignancies. The superior hypogastric plexus can also be neurolysed for pelvic malignancies, either percutaneously or through an open procedure with direct visualization of the nerves.

        e. **Neuroma excision.** Painful neuromas can be excised and while they may grow back, relocation may provide pain relief. One of the most common areas for this is in amputation stumps which may contain multiple neuromas causing stump pain.

C. **Dorsal rhizotomy.** This procedure involves surgical resection of the dorsal root and the dorsal root ganglion to denervate a painful sensory dermatome [18].

    1. **Indications.** This procedure is no longer commonly performed, but has been used to treat intercostal neuralgia, angina, and visceral pain. It is generally reserved for individuals with pain in an area corresponding to one dermatome. There may be a high recurrence rate for pain which may not have been seen in the studies that examined cancer pain treatment [19].

    2. **Technique.** This procedure is performed either through a laminectomy, intradurally, or by resecting a facet and approaching the nerve through an extradural approach. Multiple levels may need resecting due to the dermatome overlap since multiple nerve roots provide small contributions to each dermatome [20].

D. **Sympathectomy.** The sympathetic nervous system has multiple connections with sensory afferents and in some pain disorders it may contribute to the maintenance of the painful sensory input. In this sympathetically maintained pain, a sympathectomy may help provide pain relief [21].

    1. **Indications.** A surgical sympathectomy for pain is reserved for sympathetically maintained pain syndromes that are refractory to nonsurgical treatments. Patients may show signs of

2

sympathetic nervous system involvement including vasomotor and pseudomotor changes in the affected area. They are usually diagnosed with a sympathetic blockade which provides significant pain relief.

2. **Surgical approach.** The surgical approach is highly dependent on the area of the sympathetically maintained pain. For treatment of the upper extremity, the upper thoracic sympathetic ganglia need to be removed. This is most commonly done thorascopically, but can also be done through a superclavicular transaxillary or posterior costotransversectomy approach. The lumbar sympathetic chain can be accessed with an anterolateral retroperitoneal approach [22].

3. **Anesthetic considerations.** The surgical approach should be discussed with the surgeon given the possible need for one-lung ventilation to gain access to the thoracic sympathetic chain. Patients may develop hypotension that is generally transient. They may also have transiently increased gastrointestinal motility and may develop postsympathectomy pain characterized by burning or deep aching pain with hyperalgesia, though the onset does not usually occur for a few weeks postoperatively [23].

CLINICAL PEARL   After sympathectomy, patients may develop transient hypotension, increased gastrointestinal motility, and postsympathectomy pain.

3   E. **Trigeminal neuralgia.** This is a disorder of the trigeminal nerve that results in paroxysmal lancinating pain in the trigeminal nerve distribution that lasts a few seconds to minutes and is precipitated usually by a tactile stimulus. It is associated with compression of the trigeminal nerve by another nerve or an artery, and is commonly treated with microvascular decompression surgery.

1. **Surgical technique.** This procedure is done as a craniotomy with the incision located retroauricular at the mastoid process. Patients are generally positioned in a lateral park bench position. The goal of surgery is to dissect the compressing vessel off the trigeminal nerve [24].

2. **Anesthetic considerations.** Patients may be on multiple antiepileptic or neuropathic medications that may have significant side effects and drug interactions (see Table 11.2). Operative location is in close proximity to a transverse sinus putting these patients at higher risk for massive blood loss or an air embolus.

III. **Central nervous system**

A. **Anatomy.** The spinal thalamic tract is the main nociceptive pain pathway. Painful stimulus is carried along a peripheral nerve where it enters the spinal cord in the dorsalateral fasciculus and ascends several levels before synapsing onto second-order neurons in the substantia gelatinosa that cross over and ascend through the medulla and pons to the ventroposteriorlateral nucleus of the thalamus. From here connections ramify throughout the brain, including connections to the somatosensory cortex as well as the limbic forebrain system. It is along this tract and its connections where it may be targeted for surgery [25].

B. **Ablative therapy.** Though not as commonly done anymore, any part along the spinal thalamic tract and its projections can be targeted for ablative therapy. This is reserved for patients with significant comorbidities and shortened life expectancies with intractable pain. It can provide symptomatic relief, but can also produce significant numbness and possible motor and cognitive impairment. A feared complication is deafferentation pain where patients may develop worse pain that is difficult to treat.

CLINICAL PEARL   A potentially devastating complication of ablative therapy is deafferentation pain where patients may develop worse pain than prior to surgery. A classic example of deafferentation pain is anesthesia dolorosa from trigeminal ablation.

TABLE 11.2 Commonly used neuropathic pain medications and their side effects

Class	Medication	Common or special side effect
NSAIDS	Naproxen	GI upset
	Ketorolac	Anaphylactoid reactions, asthma, bronchospasm, Steven–Johonson syndrome
	Piroxicam	Tinnitus, dizziness, headache, rash, and pruritus
	Celecoxib	Possible increased risks of stroke and heart attack in people who are predisposed to it
Opioids	Morphine	Nausea, addiction, sphincter of Oddi spasms, histamine release, constipation, urinary retention
	Hydromorphone Oxycodone	Nausea, addiction, constipation, urinary retention
	Codeine	10% of Caucasian population do not metabolize this into morphine (active metabolite) and thus not effective for them as analgesic
	Methadone	Long half-life and shorter analgesic effectiveness make it dangerous to take as needed
Antidepressants	Amitriptyline	Anticholinergic effects SVT Sedation
	Nortriptyline	Sedation, less anticholinergic effect than Amitriptyline
	Venlafaxine	Common serotonergic effects and norepinephrine effects, such as sedation or GI upset
	Duloxetine	Nausea, activation in some cases and sedation in others, hypertension
Anticonvulsants	Gabapentin	Sleepiness, dizziness, myoclonus, mood effects
	Pregabalin	Sleepiness, dizziness, myoclonus, mood effects
	Carbamazepine	Coordination difficulties, aplastic anemia, exacerbate hypothyroidism, terotogenic
	Oxcarbazepine	Dizziness, hyponatremia, teratogenic
	Topiramate	Paresthesia, URI, GI upset, kidney stones

1. **Locations for ablative therapy**
   a. **Anterior cingulate cortex.** This structure is involved in emotional expression and affective experience. Ablative therapy in this area is used for cancer pain. In the past it has also been used to treat anxiety, depression, and obsessive compulsive disorder [26].
   b. **Thalamus.** The thalamus is involved in the processing of painful stimulus. This is usually reserved for severe cancer pain with poor response to opioid therapy, or patients with central pain syndromes including post-stroke pain or central pain from a spinal cord injury [27].
   c. **Spinal cord.** Cordotomies and cordectomies are used to treat unilateral intractable pain and result in unilateral deafferentation below the lesion [22]. It can be done percutaneously or through an open procedure. This is reserved for intractable pain syndromes including central pain from spinal cord injury or cancer pain.
C. **Deep brain stimulation.** With the large number of complications and side effects from ablative lesions in deep brain structures, there has been a move toward neuromodulation therapies instead of destructive lesioning. Deep brain stimulation is thought to work through a number of mechanisms including enabling the release of endogenous opioids and increasing descending inhibition for treatment of intractable pain.
   1. **Locations for deep brain stimulation**
      a. **Thalamus.** Patients with neuropathic pain may undergo somatotopic alterations to their sensory thalamus. This area has been successfully treated with stimulation for a number of conditions including refractory trigeminal pain, peripheral neuropathy, and phantom limb pain [28].

b. **Periaqueductal/periventricular gray matter.** This has been used to treat severe pain with cancer, and chronic low back pain. The mechanism is thought to be due to promoting the endogenous release of opioids.

IV. Motor cortex stimulation. It is unknown why motor cortex stimulation provides pain relief in some patients. It has been used for a number of pain conditions [29]. It is currently not commonly used has been used in the past to treat: Phantom limb pain, anesthesia dolorosa, pain from multiple sclerosis, and post-stroke pain [30].

A. **Operative technique.** Both ablative therapies as well as deep brain stimulation are usually done through a stereotactic technique involving either a frame or rigidly attached skull markers. A frame can be affixed under local anesthesia prior to the mapping procedure [31]. These cases are done through a burr hole under local sedation to allow for communication with the patient during stimulation.

After the stimulator leads are placed, an implantable pulse generator is also placed, usually in the infraclavicular location.

B. **Anesthetic considerations.** These procedures require a very cooperative patient. Short-acting sedatives should be used, as patient communication is necessary during the electrophysiologic mapping. Blood pressure control is important since elevated blood pressures can lead to intracranial hemorrhage during lead placement. Steoreotactic frame may make airway access difficult. General anesthesia may be used for generator placement if done at a subsequent procedure.

V. Spinal cord stimulators. The theory behind the mechanism of spinal cord stimulation (SCS) for the treatment of pain is that there is a balance between large and small nerve fibers in the PNS and when one of the fibers is dominant it works to inhibit the signals of the other fibers. This is called the "Gate Control Theory" [32]. SCS is postulated to work by stimulating nonpainful nerves in the dorsal columns to inhibit painful nerve signals [33].

This procedure is one of the more common surgical procedures done for chronic pain.

A. **Indications.** The most common indication for SCS is neuropathic pain from failed back surgical syndrome or chronic pain that develops or persists after back surgery. It is also commonly used to treat pain from complex regional pain syndrome. SCS causes vasodilation, bronchodilation, and can decrease bladder spasticity. It has been also used to treat ischemic and visceral pain including refractory angina and interstitial cystitis [34–36].

CLINICAL PEARL The most common indications for SCS is neuropathic pain from postlaminectomy syndrome and complex regional pain syndrome. It has been also used to treat ischemic and visceral pain including refractory angina and interstitial cystitis.

B. **Operative technique.** This is generally a two-step procedure. Patients first receive trial leads placed percutaneously through a loss of resistance technique. The patients evaluate the effect of stimulation on their pain and then may proceed with a permanent implant.

Permanent implants are done either through a midline incision with a loss of resistance technique or they are done with a midline incision with a laminotomy. The leads are tunneled and an implantable pulse generator is placed subcutaneously, usually in the posterior flank or buttock area.

C. **Anesthetic considerations.** Patients are often on multiple pain medications with very high opioid tolerances. In addition, prior back surgery can make access difficult. These cases are usually done as a MAC since the patient may be required to communicate to help sensory mapping. Laminotomy leads are usually placed under general anesthesia, but occasionally are placed under a deep sedation with a wake up for sensory mapping.

Patients are positioned prone, making airway access more difficult. A cervical positioner to maintain their neck in a midline position may be necessary for cervical leads.

Spinal cord stimulators are not an absolute contraindication to neuraxial anesthesia, but radiographic imaging should be obtained to determine where the leads are placed and any local anesthetic solution in the epidural space may affect stimulation. Commonly, patients have had previous back surgery as well that may also make epidural placement more difficult.

VI. Peripheral nerve stimulation. The exact mechanism of peripheral nerve stimulation's ability to relieve pain is unknown [1]. It is thought to be similar to SCS and the Gate Control Theory of pain. Peripheral nerve stimulation activates large fiber nerves which may close the gate for painful small fiber nerve transmission [32].

A. **Indications.** This procedure is not as commonly done as SCS. It is reserved for patients with pain that is refractory to treatment through conservative means. Patients should have pain in a single nerve distribution that is relieved by local anesthetic blockade of this nerve. The nerve should also not have a surgically correctable entrapment.

Peripheral nerve stimulations have been done for multiple different painful nerve conditions with one of the most common being the occipital nerve for occipital neuralgia [37]. It has also been used to treat trigeminal neuralgia and painful mononeuropathies [38,39].

> **CLINICAL PEARL** Peripheral nerve stimulations have been done for multiple different painful conditions. One of the most common is for occipital neuralgia. It has also been used to treat trigeminal neuralgia and painful mononeuropathies.

B. **Technique.** Similar to SCS, patients generally undergo a trial procedure with a temporary implant, prior to permanent implantation. Temporary peripheral stimulation leads are placed on top of the offending nerve and connected to an external generator and the patient is sent home to evaluate the device's effectiveness [1].

For permanent implantation, the nerve is exposed and the permanent leads are placed on top of the nerve and anchored to the overlying muscle or fascia. The leads are then tunneled to an implantable pulse generator that is placed subcutaneously in a different location.

VII. Implantable drug delivery systems. Drug pumps are most commonly placed to deliver medications to the intrathecal space. The most widely used medications are opioids. Due to their lack of long term efficacy in some non-malignant pain patients and due to the risk of catheter tip granulomas [40] the number of new implantable pumps has decreased over time, but this still remains a common procedure. Intrathecal opioids are more potent because it bypasses the blood brain barrier and allows patients the freedom of not having to take frequent oral doses of opioids.

> **CLINICAL PEARL** Due to their risk of catheter tip granulomas, possible opioid-induced hyperalgesia, and lack of consistent functional improvement in nonmalignant chronic pain patients, the number of new implantable intrathecal pumps has decreased over time. But it is still considered effective for cancer pain.

A. **Indications.** Implantable intrathecal pumps are generally used for refractory cancer pain with a prognosis of greater than 3 months. They are commonly used for patients who are responsive to opioids, but who suffer significant side effects from them. Delivering the drug intrathecally, allows for direct action on spinal opioid receptors and enables a reduced dose, in the hope of reducing side effects [41]. The pumps are also placed for other chronic pain conditions that have been refractory to conventional treatments.

B. **Medications**
1. **Opioids.** Opioids are the most commonly used drugs in the intrathecal delivery system. Many different opioids have been used with the most common being morphine and hydromorphone. The biggest concern is respiratory depression from brainstem migration of the medication.

2. **Local anesthetics.** These drugs can be added to intrathecal pumps at very low doses, to act synergistically with opioids. Higher doses can result in significant motor and sympathetic nervous system blockade and are reserved for terminally ill, bed-bound patients.

3. **Ziconotide.** This is a snail toxin that is a calcium channel blocker and can block nociceptive input intrathecally by its actions on the dorsal horn [42]. It has significant side effects including psychiatric disease and cognitive impairment [43].

4. **Clonidine.** This is an α-2 receptor agonist that modulates inhibitory pathways, working to inhibit painful sensory pathways. Side effects include hypotension and sedation.

C. **Surgical technique.** Patients are generally placed in the lateral decubitus position. The procedure is best tolerated under general anesthesia due to the required positioning and the long route required for tunneling. The catheter is placed in the lower lumbar level through a needle after a midline incision. It is then tunneled across the flank and connected to the pump that is placed in the lateral abdomen.

D. **Anesthetic considerations.** Patients are often on very high doses of opioids and may potentially be severely deconditioned with a low functional status. Positioning is important since the surgical field consists of both the midline back as well as the abdomen.

REFERENCES

1. Fishman S, Ballantyne J, Rathmell JP, et al. *Bonica's Management of Pain.* 4th ed. Philadelphia, PA: Lippincott Williams & Wilkins; 2010.
2. Omer GE, Spinner M, Van Beek A. *Management of Peripheral Nerve Problems.* 2nd ed. Philadelphia, PA: Saunders; 1998.
3. Phalen GS. The carpal-tunnel syndrome. Clinical evaluation of 598 hands. *Clin Orthop Relat Res.* 1972;83:29–40.
4. Spinner M, Spencer PS. Nerve compression lesions of the upper extremity. A clinical and experimental review. *Clin Orthop Relat Res.* 1974;(104):46–67.
5. Post M, Grinblat E. Nerve entrapment about the shoulder girdle. *Hand Clin.* 1992;8(2):299–306.
6. Papadopoulos SM, McGillicuddy JE, Albers JW. Unusual cause of 'piriformis muscle syndrome'. *Arch Neurol.* 1990;47(10): 1144–1146.
7. Pecina M. Contribution to the etiological explanation of the piriformis syndrome. *Acta Anatomica.* 1979;105(2):181–187.
8. Novak CB. Thoracic outlet syndrome. *Clin Plast Surg.* 2003;30(2):175–188.
9. Atasoy E. Thoracic outlet syndrome: anatomy. *Hand Clin.* 2004;20(1):7–14.
10. Sheth RN, Campbell JN. Surgical treatment of thoracic outlet syndrome: a randomized trial comparing two operations. *J Neurosurg Spine.* 2005;3(5):355–363.
11. O'Duffy JD, Randall RV, MacCarty CS. Median neuropathy (carpal-tunnel syndrome) in acromegaly. A sign of endocrine overactivity. *Ann Intern Med.* 1973;78(3):379–383.
12. Weimer LH, Yin J, Lovelace RE, et al. Serial studies of carpal tunnel syndrome during and after pregnancy. *Muscle Nerve.* 2002;25(6):914–917.
13. Patel AN, Finlay KU, Schyra KC, et al. Use of general anesthetic only vs general anesthetic combined with paravertebral block for perioperative pain management after first rib resection. *Proc (Bayl Univ Med Cent).* 2002;15(4):374–375.
14. Dellon AL, Mackinnon SE. Treatment of the painful neuroma by neuroma resection and muscle implantation. *Plastic Reconstr Surg.* 1986;77(3):427–438.
15. Lai YY, Chen SC, Chien NC. Video-assisted thoracoscopic neurectomy of intercostal nerves in a patient with intractable cancer pain. *Am J Hosp Palliat Care.* 2006;23(6):475–478.
16. Alberti O, Wickboldt J, Becker R. Suprainguinal retroperitoneal approach for the successful surgical treatment of meralgia paresthetica. *J Neurosurg.* 2009;110(4):768–774.
17. Johnson JE, Johnson KA, Unni KK. Persistent pain after excision of an interdigital neuroma. Results of reoperation. *J Bone Joint Surg.* 1988;70(5):651–657.
18. Abbott R. Sensory rhizotomy for the treatment of childhood spasticity. *J Child Neurol.* 1996;11(1)Suppl:S36–S42.
19. Barrash JM, Leavens ME. Dorsal rhizotomy for the relief of intractable pain of malignant tumor origin. *J Neurosurg.* 1973;38(6):755–757.
20. White JC. Posterior rhizotomy: a possible substitute for cordotomy in otherwise intractable neuralgias of the trunk and extremities of nonmalignant origin. *Clin Neurosurg.* 1965;13:20–41.
21. Roberts WJ. A hypothesis on the physiological basis for causalgia and related pains. *Pain.* 1986;24(3):297–311.
22. Winn HR, Youmans JR. *Youmans Neurological Surgery.* 5th ed. Philadelphia, PA: Saunders; 2004.
23. Kramis RC, Roberts WJ, Gillette RG. Post-sympathectomy neuralgia: hypotheses on peripheral and central neuronal mechanisms. *Pain.* 1996;64(1):1–9.
24. Teo C, Nakaji P, Mobbs RJ. Endoscope-assisted microvascular decompression for trigeminal neuralgia: technical case report. *Neurosurgery.* 2006;59(4 Suppl 2):ONSE489–490; discussion ONSE490.
25. Willis WD, Westlund KN. Neuroanatomy of the pain system and of the pathways that modulate pain. *J Clin Neurophysiol.* 1997;14(1):2–31.
26. Foltz EL, White LE Jr. Pain "relief" by frontal cingulumotomy. *J Neurosurg.* 1962;19:89–100.

27. Ohye C. Stereotactic treatment of central pain. *Stereotact Funct Neurosurg.* 1998;70(2–4):71–76.

28. Levy RM. Deep brain stimulation for the treatment of intractable pain. *Neurosurg Clin North Am.* 2003;14(3):389–399, vi.

29. Tsubokawa T, Katayama Y, Yamamoto T, et al. Treatment of thalamic pain by chronic motor cortex stimulation. *Pacing Clin Electrophys.* 1991;14(1):131–134.

30. Brown JA, Barbaro NM. Motor cortex stimulation for central and neuropathic pain: current status. *Pain.* 2003;104(3):431–435.

31. Schulder M. *Handbook of Stereotactic and Functional Neurosurgery.* New York, NY: Marcel Dekker; 2003.

32. Melzack R, Wall PD. Pain mechanisms: a new theory. *Science.* 1965;150(3699):971–979.

33. Shealy CN, Mortimer JT, Reswick JB. Electrical inhibition of pain by stimulation of the dorsal columns: preliminary clinical report. *Anesth Analg.* 1967;46(4):489–491.

34. Wu M, Linderoth B, Foreman RD. Putative mechanisms behind effects of spinal cord stimulation on vascular diseases: a review of experimental studies. *Auton Neurosci.* 2008;138(1–2):9–23.

35. Sanderson JE. Electrical neurostimulators for pain relief in angina. *Br Heart J.* 1990;63(3):141–143.

36. Peters KM. Neuromodulation for the treatment of refractory interstitial cystitis. *Rev Urol.* 2002;4(Suppl 1):S36–S43.

37. Weiner RL, Reed KL. Peripheral neurostimulation for control of intractable occipital neuralgia. *Neuromodulation.* 1999;2(3):217–221.

38. Slavin KV, Colpan ME, Munawar N, et al. Trigeminal and occipital peripheral nerve stimulation for craniofacial pain: a single-institution experience and review of the literature. *Neurosurg Focus.* 2006;21(6):E5.

39. Strege DW, Cooney WP, Wood MB, et al. Chronic peripheral nerve pain treated with direct electrical nerve stimulation. *J Hand Surg.* 1994;19(6):931–939.

40. Bejjani GK, Karim NO, Tzortzidis F. Intrathecal granuloma after implantation of a morphine pump: case report and review of the literature. *Surg Neurol.* 1997;48(3):288–291.

41. Smith TJ, Staats PS, Deer T, et al. Randomized clinical trial of an implantable drug delivery system compared with comprehensive medical management for refractory cancer pain: impact on pain, drug-related toxicity, and survival. *J Clin Oncol.* 2002;20(19):4040–4049.

42. Rauck RL, Wallace MS, Leong MS, et al. A randomized, double-blind, placebo-controlled study of intrathecal ziconotide in adults with severe chronic pain. *J Pain Symptom Manage.* 2006;31(5):393–406.

43. Thompson JC, Dunbar E, Laye RR. Treatment challenges and complications with ziconotide monotherapy in established pump patients. *Pain Phys.* 2006;9(2):147–152.

12

Anesthesia for Spinal Cord Injury Surgery

Katherine S.L. Gil

KEY POINTS

1. **Preoperative workup.** In urgent situations, routine history and physical examinations need to be hastened. The most important points to elicit include altered states of consciousness, circumstances of SCI, neurologic signs and symptoms, severity of other injuries or illnesses (particularly those that might mask SCI complaints), and pertinent laboratory, spinal, and/or other radiographic results.

2. **Autonomic dysreflexia or hyperreflexia.** Patients having T6–T7 or higher SCI may have autonomic dysreflexia. Noxious stimulation below the injury level may result in the thoracolumbar sympathetic nerve transmission of a strong afferent impulse to the spinal cord with the development of vasoconstriction below the SCI level and systemic hypertension. Inhibitory signals from the carotid sinus reflexes are unable to traverse the injured area to reach lower sympathetic outflow segments, but cause symptoms above the SCI level, including reflex bradycardia, vasodilation, headache, and profuse sweating. Inadequacy to overcome the precipitous hypertension may cause seizures, stroke, myocardial infarction, neurogenic edema, and death unless treatment with rapid-onset vasodilators is administered.

3. **Fluid therapy, hemodynamic care, and oxygenation in complete SCI patients.** Patients who have acute complete SCI are more susceptible to cardiovascular abnormalities such as early hypotension from neurogenic shock and/or concomitant organ injury. Treatment goals include limiting crystalloids to 2,000 mL to prevent pulmonary edema and acute respiratory distress syndrome, using fluid plus vasoactive therapy to maintain perfusion with a goal of systolic blood pressure (BP) level ≥90 to 100 mm Hg and heart rates 40 to 100 beats per minute, maintaining oxygenation, and keeping urine output at ≥0.5 mL/kg/h.

4. **Indications for CT or MRI prior to surgery.** A Glasgow Coma Score <15, acute paralysis, history of spinal disease/surgery, vital sign instability, and at-risk suspicion in minors (depending on the mechanism) indicate a need for computed tomography (CT) or magnetic resonance

(continued)

imaging (MRI). Indicators for radiologic study in awake, mobile patients include injury associated with a dangerous mechanism, extremity paresthesias, age ≥65 years, or inability to rotate the neck 45 degrees to the left or right beyond the acute phase of neck pain.

5. **Association of concomitant SCI and bodily trauma.** The incidence of concomitant spinal cord injury (SCI) involved with any major blunt "head-trauma" patient is in the range of 5% to 8%, while for those suffering multiple, blunt bodily injuries it is almost 8%. Older patients have a 10-fold greater chance of simultaneous cervical SCI in comparison to children. Conversely, of patients admitted with known cervical SCI, approximately 33% have head injury. Approximately 20% of patients with SCI have multiple spinal levels of damage.

6. **Factors associated with vision loss following spinal cord surgery.** Age 50 years ±14, male gender, morbid obesity, tobacco intake, hypertension, diabetes mellitus, hyperlipidemia, coronary artery disease or cerebrovascular disease, pre-existing anemia, glaucoma, and carotid artery disease in patients undergoing spinal surgery are risk factors for visual loss. Highly significant procedure-related risk factors include surgical duration >6 hours, blood loss >1,000 mL, and prone positioning with head down.

I. Spinal column anatomy

A. Structural anatomy

1. **Bone, cartilage, ligaments.** The protective skeletal spine anatomy has 33 vertebrae: 7 cervical, 12 thoracic, 5 lumbar, 5 fused sacral, and 4 fused coccygeal elements [1]. Each individual vertebra is designated in a numbered nomenclature such that the first cervical, thoracic, lumbar, and sacral elements are defined as C1, T1, L1, and S1, respectively.

Posteriorly, each vertebra has a spinous process attached to bilateral laminae to form an arch. The laminae connect to bilateral transverse processes and then the pedicles, until finally fusing with the anterior vertebral body. This forms a central opening, the vertebral foramen or spinal canal, wherein the spinal cord resides. Between the spinous and transverse processes are two sets of paired superior and inferior facets, or articulating processes, that allow vertical, forward, backward, and twisting motion and assist with anterior vertebral column stabilization.

Intervertebral disks (IVDs) act as resilient, vertical cushions between vertebral bodies. Disks are composed of circumferential fibrocartilaginous material, the annulus fibrosus, and a central gelatinous material, the nucleus pulposus.

The atlas or C1 is a ring-like formation with no spinous process, vertebral body, or inferiorly located IVD. Its superior facets articulate with a connection of alar ligaments to the occipital skull condyles bilaterally. It forms a unique joint able to swivel up to 50% around the cone-like dens or odontoid process protruding from the superior aspect of C2, the axis. The spinal cord passes through the canal next to this process as an extension from the brainstem through the foramen magnum of the skull.

The transverse atlantal ligament attaches between the medial tubercles of the superior facets bilaterally, crossing the vertebral column to provide odontoid stability anteriorly and free spinal cord motion posteriorly. Atlantoaxial instability (AAI) can develop from transverse atlantal ligament laxity, odontoid hypoplasia, or other boney abnormality. Transverse ligament laxity can drive the dens into the spinal cord as C1 subluxates anteriorly. On the other hand, if the dens is hypoplastic, C1 can subluxate posteriorly. AAI is associated with a number of syndromes and pathologic states such as trauma, oropharyngeal infection, Pierre Robin syndrome, Ehlers–Danlos syndrome, Marfan's syndrome, hypermobility syndrome, nonachondroplastic dwarfism, and Morquio syndrome, but its greatest incidence is in patients with Down's syndrome and rheumatoid arthritis (RA) [2]. Although 10% to 20% of patients with Down's syndrome have AAI, only 1% to 2% are symptomatic, making it vital that airway management specialists be alert to this possibility. Degenerative changes may also develop secondary to fibrocartilage within the ligament, as found in RA patients, who have a 12% to 25% incidence of AAI.

Normal spinal curvatures include an anterior cervical convexity between the odontoid apex and mid-T2 vertebra, posterior thoracic convexity from mid-T2–T12, and an anteriorly directed lumbar convexity from mid-T12 until the sacral bone. Multiple ligaments maintain the S-shaped spinal integrity by preventing excessive motion. The anterior longitudinal ligament traverses the length of the spinal columns from the axis, along the anterior surface contiguously with the vertebrae and IVDs. Meanwhile, the posterior longitudinal ligament courses down the posterior surface of the vertebral bodies within the spinal canal. Posteriorly within the spinal canal, the ligamentum flavum lies opposite to the posterior longitudinal ligament, while connecting vertebral laminae. Lastly, the interspinous ligament joins the ligamentum flavum anteriorly. Below C7, it is joined by the supraspinous ligament, which connects the spinous processes.

Ligamentous disruption, or laxity, has a greater propensity for cervical instability, in contrast to C1 or C2 fracture with intact ligaments. Instability in the former situation demands surgical repair, while the latter pathologic state usually heals spontaneously. Magnetic resonance imaging (MRI) best detects ligamentous instability. In these instances, particularly with spinal cord injury (SCI), airway management specialists must take precautions to prevent excessive cervical motion and secondary neurologic damage.

2. **Spinal cord and nervous tissue.** The spinal cord extends downward from the medulla oblongata toward the L1–L2 vertebrae in adults, where it forms the conus medullaris [1]. Nearby, its nerve roots combine to form the cauda equina, and it finishes in the filum terminale between S2/S3 and the coccyx. It is surrounded by the meninges and spinal fluid. Excepting C1 and C2, 31 pairs of segmental nerves take off through the intervertebral foramina. Eight are cervical, while the three coccygeal elements form a single pair that exits through the sacral hiatus.

Examination of a transverse plane through the spinal cord reveals peripheral sensory and motor neurons in the white matter surrounding a central butterfly-shaped area of nerve cell bodies in the gray matter. The spinal cord is surrounded by the very thin pia mater with dentate ligaments serving to secure it. Cerebrospinal fluid (CSF) freely communicates between the cerebral ventricular system and the most caudal regions of the spinal subarachnoid space, between the pia mater and the arachnoid membrane. External to this lies the subdural space occupying an area between the arachnoid membrane and the dura mater. The dura is an extension from the brain that narrows near S2 and ends in the filum terminale.

The autonomic nervous system consists of complementary functioning sympathetic, parasympathetic, and nonadrenergic/noncholinergic-mediated divisions [3]. The sympathetic division encompasses preganglionic synapsing neurons between T1–L2, with cell bodies in the lateral gray horns on both sides of the spinal cord. The parasympathetic division consists of preganglionic synapsing neurons, with cell bodies in the nuclei of the brainstem (cranial nerves III, VII, IX, and X) and the lateral gray horns of S2–S4.

3. **Blood supply to the spinal cord**
   a. **Arterial supply.** Similar to the cerebral circulation, spinal circulation supplies its gray matter with 3 to 4 times more blood flow than its white matter. Two vertebral artery branches originate from the aorta. Next, near the base of their confluence and before the formation of the basilar artery, a single anterior spinal artery is formed [1]. Constituting 75% of spinal circulation, this artery exits at the level of the foramen magnum to accompany the spinal cord while supplying the anterior surface and most of the lateral areas down to the level of the filum terminale.

   Two posterior spinal arteries also arise to complete the supply, mainly serving the posterior spinal columns and horns. Considerable branching and plexus formations of arterioles and capillaries from these vessels develop in the cervical, thoracic, and lumbar regions. They anastomose with intercostal and lumbar arteries comprised of 4 to 10 radicular branches, thus permitting additional arteriolar sources of blood. Frequently, at the level of T8–T11, a left branch from the aorta supplies an important vessel, which may be the main source for the upper lumbar regions and often the lower thoracic spine, called the arteria radicularis magna or artery of Adamkiewicz [4]. Serious damage to the spinal cord may occur as a result of significant compromise of this artery from trauma, abdominal/thoracic aortic surgery, and so forth.

During spinal surgery, awareness of this blood supply has prompted anesthesia providers to avoid SCI by maintaining spinal cord perfusion pressure >60–70 mm Hg. SCI patients undergoing spinal surgeries require maintenance of perfusion pressures at or significantly above normal, depending on the amount of pre-existing neurologic damage. Of course, the possibility of greater blood loss is an ongoing concern. Maintaining perfusion can be accomplished by standard hemodynamic methods and for some surgeries, assisted with the use of a spinal drain to maintain CSF pressure <10 mm Hg. Occasionally attempts for draining ≤10 to 15 mL/h are undertaken to increase the arterial/spinal fluid gradient. Pre-existing SCI is very susceptible to vascular insufficiency. The use of mild hypothermia and mannitol may assist by decreasing metabolic demand and tissue edema, respectively.

   b. **Venous drainage.** Venous outflow from the spinal cord is accomplished by up to six anterior and posterior superficial vessels draining into plexes or veins entering the internal epidural venous system [1]. From there, blood can escape cephalad into the basivertebral vein, terminal veins, or dural sinuses. Further drainage takes place via vertebral veins and inferior vena cava conduits. The valveless nature of this system makes it prone to reverse flow characteristics following elevations in intrathoracic or intra-abdominal pressure, due to coughing, pregnancy, Valsalva maneuvers, or obesity. This can result in symptoms such as headache, but even worse, the entrance of systemically carried neoplastic or infective cells into the central nervous system (CNS).

   For spine surgery, anesthesia providers can employ techniques to avert conditions that promote higher venous pressure. Diligent attention to preventing excessive fluid load and minimizing intra-abdominal pressure is particularly important while prone. This optimizes visualization in the surgical field and diminishes blood loss.

B. **Functional anatomy**
   1. **Motor system.** Cerebral cortical signals and brainstem motor nuclei impulses travel along motor neuron pathways [5] (Fig. 12.1). In the spinal cord, these are primarily divided among (1) pyramidal tracts (upper motor neurons in the lateral and anterior corticospinal tracts) and (2) extrapyramidal tracts (vestibulospinal, reticulospinal, olivospinal, and rubrospinal). In the anterior medulla, 90% of spinal motor neurons cross to the contralateral side at the decussation of the pyramids.
   2. **Sensory system.** The sensory system has three major pathways. The dorsal column medial lemniscus transports signals for fine touch, conscious proprioception, and vibration. It decussates in the medulla on the way to the cortex (Fig. 12.1). The spinocerebellar tracts transmit signals for proprioception and terminate in the ipsilateral cerebellum. Lastly, the anterolateral system, within the anterior and lateral spinothalamic tracts, relays impulses for pain, temperature, and gross touch, ascends one or two levels, synapses, and decussates in the substantia gelatinosa on the way to the brain.
   3. **Spinal cord autoregulation.** Research on human spinal cord blood flow (SCBF) is not as extensive in comparison to cerebral blood flow investigations [6]. Nevertheless, SCBF in multiple animal studies (rats, dogs, cats, and primates) have shown consistent homeostatic flow of approximately 55 to 60 mL/100g/min. Autoregulatory control is similar to the brain, in response to alterations in mean arterial pressure (MAP) between 40–70 and 120 mm Hg, arterial partial pressure of carbon dioxide ($PaCO_2$) between 20 and 80 mm Hg, and arterial partial pressure of oxygen (PaO_2) under 60 mm Hg. The concept of spinal cord autoregulation motivates caregivers to consider maneuvers or drugs applied to SCI patients in a mode parallel to that of brain injury cases.

II. **Preoperative assessment of spinal cord injury.** In urgent situations, routine history and physical examinations need to be hastened and perhaps abbreviated. The most important points to elicit include states of consciousness before and during examination, circumstances of SCI, neurologic signs and symptoms, severity of other injuries or illnesses (particularly those that might mask SCI complaints), and laboratory, spinal, and/or other radiographic results.

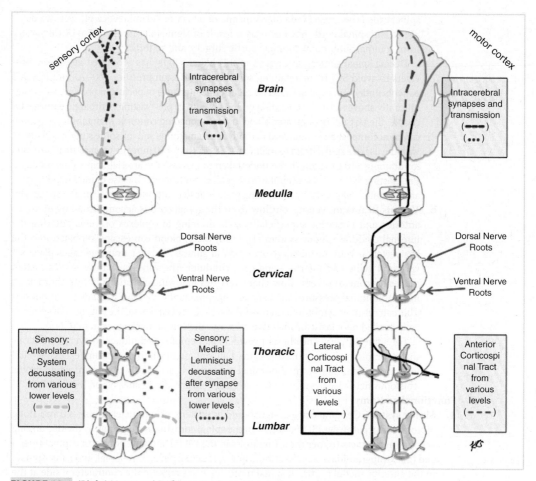

FIGURE 12.1 (**Right**) Motor and (**Left**) sensory branching and crossovers in the spine.

A. History and physical examinations. Whenever feasible, documentation is needed concerning prior anesthetic, surgical, and familial anesthetic history, airway history, allergies, medications, social history of tobacco, alcohol, or illicit drug consumption, recent oral intake, height, weight, airway and physical examination, neurologic assessment, and appropriate studies.

B. Neurologic assessment and clinical consequences of SCI. The American Spinal Injury Association (ASIA) dermatome chart is used for recording the extent and site of neurologic injury [7]. A 28-dermatome sensory section is used for recording "pinprick and light touch stimuli" sensory levels. Three scores are available: "0" (no sensation), "1" (impaired sensation), and "2" (normal sensation). A 0- to 5-point motor scale allows recording of specific muscle groups for strength, where "0" represents complete paralysis, and "5" is normal. It also permits documentation of proprioception, external anal sphincter tone/contraction, perirectal sensation, bulbocavernosus reflex, and anal-cutaneous reflex.

Symptoms of SCI are frequently characterized by complete or incomplete losses of neurologic function below the point of damage in any of the three main nervous system tracts—motor, sensory, and autonomic. While motor injury involves a degree of paralysis, and somatosensory injury causes losses in touch, pain, temperature, vibration, and/or proprioception, autonomic deficits are evident by alterations in hemodynamic, respiratory, gastrointestinal, urinary, piloerective, and/or sexual function. The ASIA Impairment Scale is a classification meant to differentiate a patient's SCI into one of the five categories (Table 12.1).

TABLE 12.1 ASIA Impairment scale

A. *Complete:* No sensory or motor function is preserved in sacral segments S4–S5.
B. *Sensory incomplete:* Sensory, but not motor, function is preserved below the neurologic level and includes sacral segments S4–S5.
C. *Motor incomplete:* Motor function is preserved below the neurologic level, and more than half of key muscles below the neurologic level have a muscle grade <3.
D. *Motor incomplete:* Motor function is preserved below the neurologic level, and at least half of key muscles below the neurologic level have a muscle grade ≥3.
E. *Normal:* Sensory and motor functions are normal.

As discussed, complete SCI is indicative of <5% chance for recovery if no improvement transpires within 24 hours. An incomplete lesion is defined by ASIA when there is at least sacral or segmental sparing, even if only to pinprick, and has up to a 50% probability of functional return [7,8].

1. **Spinal shock.** Spinal shock includes sensory and motor neurologic reflex changes from sudden traumatic SCI or infrequently, injury developing over several hours. Simultaneously, neurogenic shock or hemodynamic changes caused by autonomic dysfunction may be present [8]. A review by Ditunno et al. [9] depicts four time frames correlating with presenting signs and symptoms of ongoing pathophysiologic changes.

   Phase 1 of spinal shock is usually immediate, developing within 24 hours. Reflex loss below or possibly immediately above the level of SCI results in flaccid paralysis, arreflexia, and loss of descending facilitation due to hyperpolarized neurons. Hypotension results from muscular atony and loss of vascular tone below the SCI.

   Over the next 1 to 3 days, the second phase involves returning reflexes, denervation supersensitivity, after upregulation of receptors within muscle groups. Consequently, polysynaptic reflexes reappear before the return of more rapid monosynaptic reflexes, such as deep tendon reflexes or aversion responses.

   Within 1 to 4 weeks and lasting up to 6 months, the third phase is associated with hyperreflexia as interneurons and lower motor neuron axonal-supported synapses proliferate or "sprout" and the tempering effects from higher centers is absent.

   During the fourth phase, over a period of 1 week to 12 months, an imbalance occurs between the alpha and gamma motor neurons with alpha neurons sending fewer or alternatively, more signals, resulting in either a weak or excessive contracture.

   For anesthesia and other caregivers, post-SCI spasm is treated with baclofen, benzodiazepines, or other medications. Note that other influences such as hyperventilation can alter the motor neuronal receptors' co-dependent action, but SCI spasms are unlikely to be relieved by hypoventilation or breathing CO_2.

2. **Neurogenic shock.** Neurogenic shock results in a constellation of hemodynamic consequences from disrupted sympathetic pathways [8]. SCI above T6 precipitates decreased vasomotor input, systemic vascular resistance, and cardiac output resulting in hypotension and hypothermia. Injury including T1 will block cardiac accelerators (T1–T4), causing bradycardia due to unopposed parasympathetic activity.

   Thus, it is important to be aware that SCI patients may be in spinal shock, neurogenic shock, and/or hypovolemic shock, in order to differentiate and administer appropriate treatments. Hypovolemic shock is usually characterized by hypotension, tachycardia, and a narrowed pulse pressure, requiring fluid administration therapy. On the other hand, pure fluid administration for spinal or neurogenic shock may result in symptomatic fluid overload. Bilello et al. [10] noted that vasopressors and chronotropic agents were required in 24% of high (C1–C5) versus 5% of low (C6–C7) cervical SCI patients. Of the high cervical injury group, 3% required a pacemaker.

3. **Autonomic dysreflexia or hyperreflexia.** Autonomic dysreflexia can occur in patients with an SCI T6–T7 or higher [11]. Following a noxious stimulus below that level (often of hollow viscous organs), the thoracolumbar sympathetic nerves transmit a strong afferent

impulse to the spinal cord with the development of vasoconstriction below the SCI level and systemic hypertension. Normally, hypertensive carotid sinus activation (vasovagal) ceases sympathetic firing by sending inhibitory signals down the spinal cord. But, because of the SCI, inhibition does not reach the lower sympathetic outflow segments. Inhibition above the SCI level provokes reflex bradycardia, vasodilation, headache, and profuse sweating. Frequently, this rostral bradycardia and vasodilation are inadequate to overcome the severe, precipitous rise in blood pressure (BP), which may cause seizures, stroke, myocardial infarction, neurogenic edema, and death.

In anticipation of noxious stimuli below the level of SCI, even a full bladder during surgery, anesthesia providers must try to elicit a history of autonomic dysreflexia, sometimes using descriptive lay terminology. Spinal or epidural anesthetics completely block this reflex. General or monitored care anesthetics are often less effective because of the hit-or-miss nature of drug dosages. Very frequent BP monitoring while having immediate availability of rapid-onset, vasodilating agents such as sodium nitroprusside, is strongly advised with these techniques.

4. **Cervicomedullary syndrome.** The cervicomedullary syndrome is very similar to the central cord syndrome with the caveat that it is characterized by loss of facial sensation, starting from the mouth to the nose and extending outwardly to the chin, eyes, and forehead in a Dejerine or "onion peel pattern" [12,13]. Pathologic changes involve the nucleus or fibers in the descending spinal tracts of the trigeminal nerve. Upper extremity sensory loss and weakness is typically greater than that in the lower extremity, in a similar fashion to the anterior cord syndrome.

   Inciting factors frequently include disk pathology or spondylosis in the cervicomedullary region down to C4. This may be worsened by cervical hyperextension or trauma. Compression due to atlas–axis dislocation, excessive traction, odontoid fracture, or anterior–posterior complications from a burst fracture or atlantal ligament disruption may be involved. Vascular injury to the vertebral artery is also a possibility.

   These patients need close monitoring to detect hemodynamic or respiratory compromise, and anesthesia or other caregivers must be prepared to institute immediate management.

5. **Central cord syndrome.** Hyperextensive compression mechanisms involving the ligamentum flavum, syringomyelia, and tumors causing violation of the integrity of the mid to lower cervical spine can result in the central cord syndrome. Symptoms are typical for more significant upper extremity loss of motor function, with variable sensory deficit due to centrally crossing, corticospinal tracts carrying pain, fine touch, temperature, and proprioception information [13]. Often patients have a good recovery even without surgery, but hemodynamic and respiratory monitoring is important.

6. **Anterior cord syndrome.** The anterior cord syndrome is usually brought on by flexion injuries, disk pathology, or anterior spinal artery disruption [13]. Damaged corticospinal and/or spinothalamic tracts result in deficits in motor, pain, and temperature conduction below the SCI. Sacral sparing and autonomic dysfunction can occur only if cervical lesions are involved. Prognosis for complete recovery has been reported to be as high as 50%.

   Anesthesia and other caregivers particularly monitor these patients for hemodynamic and respiratory functions if cervical injury is suspected.

7. **Posterior cord syndrome.** Vascular compromise of the posterior spinal arteries may be responsible for the rare occurrence of the posterior cord syndrome. Patients lose ipsilateral fine touch, vibration, and proprioception sense, resulting in ataxia and a faltering gait [13].

8. **Brown-Séquard syndrome.** This syndrome is a rarity due to a hemisection type of SCI from tumor, penetrating wound, vascular obstruction, infection, myelitis, multiple sclerosis, or trauma [13]. Injury to the dorsal medial lemniscus, decussating at the medulla, results in ipsilateral motor, fine touch, vibration, and proprioception losses. Uniquely, damage to contralateral corticospinal tracts and spinothalamic tracts, decussating in the substantia gelatinosa, results in pain, coarse touch, and temperature sensation losses on the opposite side of the body.

9. **Conus medullaris syndrome.** The conus medullaris syndrome can be incurred following injury at T12–L1 from intrinsic cord compression. Consequences include perianal analgesia, bladder and bowel areflexia, impotence, and disordered ankle reflex and lower limb motor function. Knee reflexes are intact because the cauda equina is unaffected [12].

10. **Cauda equina syndrome.** Lastly, the cauda equina syndrome often develops from spinal, disk, ligament, or tumor pathology at L1–L5 [13]. Although appearing similar to peripheral nerves, the proximity of these nerve roots to their spinal cord motor neurons where axonal growth inhibitors reside, may prevent axon regrowth, causing permanent damage. Patients exhibit signs of bladder dysfunction, sensory and motor dysfunctions involving L4–S3 with asymmetric paraplegia, anal dysfunction, sciatica, unilateral or bilateral saddle anesthesia, pubic anesthesia, and lower extremity numbness.

C. **Neurologic effects on other systems**

1. **Respiratory system.** Compete SCI at C3 or higher is a leading cause of prehospital deaths from total diaphragmatic paralysis. Lesions below C5 provoke paradoxical breathing with 33% to 50% of normal vital capacity, due to decreased functional residual capacity as well as maximal inspiratory and particularly, expiratory volumes [14]. Any SCI above T6 with loss of abdominal muscle strength may result in difficulty with coughing, atelectasis, pneumonia (≤50% incidence, particularly the left lung), and respiratory failure. Recovery is only weakly predicted by the lesion level, whereas spontaneous recovery and motivation to improve recovery are important factors.

   Since SCI may lead to acute respiratory failure, hypoxemia, or hypercarbia, close monitoring is essential. Critical levels of $PaO_2 \leq 50$ mm Hg, $PaCO_2 \geq 50$ mm Hg, or vital capacity <10 mL/kg are indications for proactive support by caregivers, assuming no preexisting chronic changes due to obstructive pulmonary or other disease.

2. **Gastrointestinal system.** Paralytic ileus is more likely in tetraplegics than paraplegics. Pulmonary aspiration is more likely, particularly after heightened vomiting episodes, hypokalemia, and hypovolemia. Abdominal distension can impede adequate inspiration. Constipation and pseudo-obstruction may occur. In addition, unopposed vagal efferents may lead the way to the development of gastric stress ulcers and bleeding.

3. **Genitourinary system.** Two types of bladder dysfunction can result from SCI. A spastic or reflex bladder may develop from injury above T12. When the bladder fills, it reflexively empties without the patient's awareness. Bladder contraction with an unrelaxed sphincter raises pressure, making ureteral reflux likely, and increases the possibility of bladder infection spread to the kidneys. In contrast, a flaccid bladder and overdistension problems may develop from SCI below T12/L1. Both problems have attendant requirements for frequent catheterization, danger of infection, and potential for kidney dysfunction, damage, failure, and hypertension.

4. **Thermoregulatory system.** With high SCI, sympathectomy, vasodilation, and lack of piloerection may result in a partial poikilothermic-type situation, resulting in significant temperature loss in cold environments. Whether conversely, an inability to perspire below the level of damage may prevent cooling in hot environments is somewhat controversial. It may be that at higher environmental temperatures the thermoregulatory set point is increased, while the opposite may result at lower environmental temperature conditions.

5. **Thrombogenesis.** Historically, vasodilation and immobility with venous pooling, low blood flow, and increased blood viscosity were associated with increased risk of deep vein thrombosis (DVT) in SCI patients, particularly 3 days post injury. The result was a DVT rate of 48% to 100% and chances of pulmonary embolism were 8% to 25%. With the advent of prophylactic anticoagulants, patients treated with low molecular weight heparin (LMWH) and a targeted international normalized ratio (INR) of 2 to 3 resulted in reductions in DVT rates to 5.4%.

   Some SCI patients presenting for surgery have a history of, or need for, anticoagulant therapy. Discontinuation of warfarin 5 days prior to surgery is a common goal. For urgent surgeries where blood loss is unlikely, the Australian Society of Thrombosis and Hemostasis consensus guidelines recommended reversal with injectable vitamin K to achieve an acceptable INR above the subtherapeutic range so that postoperative return to warfarin therapy may be seamless [15]. If bleeding is more probable the most desirable INR value should approach normal. Since fresh frozen plasma (FFP) has an INR of 1.6, it cannot be the sole treatment. FFP, recombinant factor VIIa, and prothrombin complex concentrates are alternative "anti-warfarin effect" therapies.

For patients receiving heparin, careful protamine titration can easily reverse its effect. At this time LMWH reversal is uncertain. Protamine binds preferentially to larger weight molecular heparin but not as well to LMWH, with the result that reversal success rate approaches only 85%.

Direct thrombin inhibitors (DTI) used for DVT prophylaxis are also difficult to reverse. Attempts with plasma complex concentrates and recombinant factor VIIa have had varying success depending on the DTI and dosages.

D. **Preoperative testing.** Radiologic testing, evoked potential (EP) analysis, electromyography (EMG), ultrasonography, urologic incontinence studies, and spinal fluid analysis can demonstrate sites, types, and degrees of SCI to formulate therapeutic courses and prevent deterioration.

1. **Radiologic studies of the spine**

   a. **Diagnostic radiologic studies**

      (1) **Plain radiographs.** In trauma cases, the triple view series visualizing all seven cervical vertebrae to the C7–T1 junction with a "swimmer's view" is important if CT or MRI is unavailable. Particularly lateral images can reveal fractures of the odontoid, vertebral bodies, and spinous processes. Anterior–posterior and oblique images are best to locate pedicle, lamina, or facet damage and lateral mass vertebral body detection, especially at C1. Flexion/extension films can be judiciously used to assist in determinations of ligamentous injury by looking for increased dens and C1 arch distance, abnormally spread apart posterior elements or kyphosis in flexion, or vertebral subluxation. Care must be taken not to worsen an unstable spine with flexion/extension movements, which should only be allowed in conscious and cooperative patients so that they can vocalize discomfort if pain occurs. Plain radiographs elsewhere along the spinal column can also be used to detect boney changes, including prevertebral soft tissue swelling.

      Plain x-ray criteria for lower cervical spine instability include the presence of greater than 11 degrees and 3.5 mm of sagittal plane translation. Interspinous widening, absence of the cervical lordotic curve or facet joint correspondence, and vertebral body compression greater than 50% are diagnostic of spinal pathology.

      (2) **Computed tomography.** Although clinical judgment to predict diagnostic SCI may be inadequate, plain x-ray studies may be woefully worse [16]. Among symptomatic SCI patients, the correct diagnosis after plain radiographic study may be missed in ~5% of patients and 30% of those may develop permanent sequelae. In contrast, SCI is identified in 95% to 100% of patients by cervical spine computed tomography (CT scan) in comparison to less than 50% by cervical spine plain radiographs. Thus, many investigators and clinicians view CT scans as the definitive study for acute SCI suspicions for boney structure and spinal canal diameter to detect impingement. Neuroforaminal distances and facet joints can be examined for ligamentous instability. Intrathecal contrast can help somewhat to visualize neural elements.

      (3) **Magnetic resonance imaging.** MRI is superior for soft tissue visualization, including the spinal cord, myelomalacia, nerve roots, cauda equina, epidural and subarachnoid spaces, hematoma, edema, syringomyelia, IVDs, ligaments, and compression in any of these areas. SCI without radiographic abnormality (SCIWORA) occurring particularly in children and the elderly is diagnosed by MRI only. Although not as sensitive in detection as CT, MRI can demonstrate boney changes, including fractures, fragmentation, and osteophytes.

   b. **Criteria for radiologic studies for acute cervical spine injury.** How can clinicians decide on which type of radiologic examination is best? While less accurate, plain x-rays have minimal radiation exposure and are much cheaper than CT or MRI. Clinicians worry about missing critical SCI, particularly in blunt trauma patients known to

TABLE 12.2 Alert-patient criteria to determine if radiography is needed to rule out cervical SCI (Glasgow Coma Scale score ≥ 14–15)

Canadian C-spine rule: Criteria mandating radiography	NEXUS low-risk criteria: Indicating no need for radiography
I. Dangerous mechanism[a]	I. No painful, distracting injury[a]
II. Paresthesias in extremities	II. No midline cervical tenderness
III. Unable to rotate neck 45 degrees left/right[b]	III. No focal neurologic deficit
IV. Age ≥65 yrs	IV. Normal alertness[b]
	V. No intoxication[c]

[a]Motorized vehicle (60 mph/100 km/h), bicycle, fall (≥3 ft/0.91 m), rollover, ejection, hit by high-speed or large vehicle, axial load to the head such as diving.
[b]If sitting or ambulatory, and beyond any initial period of possible acute neck pain, neck motion can be tested as long as it will cease if symptoms occur.

[a]Any significant condition thought to be producing distracting pain that directs attention away from cervical injury.
[b]Glasgow Coma Scale score ≥14, unable to remember three objects in 5 min, disoriented, delayed responses, and so forth.
[c]If patient/observer reports intoxication or alcohol odor, slurred speech, ataxia, dysmetria, and so forth.

have risks for SCI [17]. Fear has prompted anywhere from 15.6% to 91.5% of clinicians to order radiographic studies on most, if not all, of their patients. Attempts were made to develop clinical criteria to determine the following: Which patients would benefit from radiologic studies, such that no clinically important SCI would be missed and fewer patients would receive needless irradiation or incur excessive expenditures?

Two sets of criteria were developed to decrease the inappropriateness of radiologic testing for alert patients: The National Emergency X-Radiography Utilization Study (NEXUS), Low-Risk Criteria (NLC) study, and the Canadian C-Spine Rule study. Their salient points are summarized (see Table 12.2). In general a Glasgow Coma Score <15, acute paralysis, history of spinal disease/surgery, vital sign instability, and at-risk suspicion in minors (depending on the mechanism) indicate a need for computed axial tomography (CT) or magnetic resonance imaging (MRI). Indicators for radiologic study in awake, mobile patients include injury associated with a dangerous mechanism, extremity paresthesias, age ≥65 years, or inability to rotate the neck 45 degrees to the left or right beyond the acute phase of neck pain.

The comparative values of the two sets of criteria showed that the sensitivity (99.4% vs. 90.7%) and specificity (45.1% vs. 36.8%) were significantly higher when using the Canadian C-Spine Rule versus the NEXUS criteria, respectively [17]. Note that acute paralysis, age of minors, changes in consciousness, vital sign instability, and/or history of spinal disease or surgery are also likely to make patients candidates for radiographic studies. In 45 clinically unimportant cases, the sensitivity was 97.8% using the Canadian C-Spine Rule versus 80% with the NEXUS criteria.

2. **Additional diagnostic techniques.**

   a. **Cortical somatosensory evoked potentials.** Cortical somatosensory evoked potentials (SSEPs) generated by electrical square wave stimulation of peripheral nerves can identify the location and extent of sensory radiculopathy or other pathology [18]. Recording electrodes, located proximally along the spine and/or on the scalp in a similar pattern to the international EEG 10–20 system, detect recordable computer-averaged waveforms with specific amplitudes and poststimulus latencies. Even though only sensory tract EPs are monitored, mixed nerves (median, posterior tibial, and so forth) are chosen for stimulation with surface electrodes or needles, so that a visible twitch gives assurance that the nerve is in fact being targeted correctly. In the event of SCI, EP waveforms demonstrate decreased polarity amplitudes and delayed latencies (assuming intact peripheral nerves) (see Chapter 26).

   Successful preoperative use of intraoperative neurophysiologic monitoring techniques (IOM) has translated to the surgical suite with a presence in approximately 75% of major spinal surgeries and an incidence of SSEP abnormalities approaching 2% to 65%. Preoperatively, SSEPs are also useful in uncooperative patients unable to undergo CT or MRI or for patients needing better detection of the extent of damage.

If preoperative SSEPs show extensive pre-existing SCI, anesthesia providers may change plans to include total intravenous anesthesia (TIVA) instead of inhalation anesthetics to avoid injury-mimicking effects on SSEP waveforms.

b. **Cortical motor evoked potentials.** Transcranial motor evoked potentials (MEPs) can be generated by electrical stimulation while observing for neuroelectrical signals at Recording electrodes in epidural space or muscle responses in peripheral muscles. Magnetic transcortical stimulation is another possibility in awake patients with the advantage of being less painful. Coiled magnets generate ≥5,000 A of current (2,800 V) to produce magnetic field strengths of 2.5 T with a 1-millisecond pulse duration. SCI is more easily detected by cortical MEPs in comparison to SSEPs.

c. **Electromyography.** Preoperatively, EMG may be valuable to differentiate neurologic damage from peripheral nerve pathology versus SCI and as a diagnostic tool for determining and differentiating the site of functional impairment following SCI.

d. **Ultrasonography.** Ultrasonography can be utilized if MRI or CT is contraindicated, unavailable, cost-prohibitive, or more difficult to obtain as in the neonatal or infant period. Diagnostic criteria for use include enthesitis in ankylosing spondylitis (AS), syringomyelia, meningomyeloceles, other myeloceles, and congenital malformations such as spina bifida occulta, tight filum terminale, spinal soft tissue mass, dorsal dermal sinus, and misshapen coccyx.

3. **Urologic incontinence studies.** EMG, cystometrography, postvoid residual urine measurement, and videourodynamic studies are used to determine the likelihood and degree of urinary incontinence impairment secondary to SCI for preoperative testing prior to or during surgeries.

4. **Cerebrospinal fluid testing.** Detection of increased CSF pressure and abnormalities in chemistries or cell count related to tumor, infection, or syringomyelia may be important in determining potential outcomes.

III. **Disorders with potential for spinal cord injury.** More common causes for SCI and treatments are presented in two broad groupings: Nontraumatic or traumatic. Nontraumatic entities include noninflammatory disorders, inflammatory disorders, or infectious diseases, and mixed origin demyelinating diseases or upper neuron disorders. Traumatic SCI is further grouped as either cervical SCI or thoracic/lumbar/sacral SCI.

A. **Nontraumatic spinal cord disorders**

1. **Noninflammatory disorders**

a. **Spondylosis.** Cervical spondylosis is a degenerative spinal disease found in 90% of patients ≥65 years of age, but rarely at other ages. No gender inequality exists. Spondylosis results in osteoarthritis of facet joints and vertebral bodies with osteophyte formation, spinal stenosis, foraminal narrowing, associated IVD herniation, and ossification of the longitudinal ligament and ligamentum flavum. Patients may develop radiculopathy due to cervical spine nerve root and/or nerve damage or myelopathy from SCI. Symptoms include suboccipital headache, cervical pain, and radiculopathic and/or myelopathic symptoms.

Cervical spondylosis with myelopathy is a very commonly surgically treated spinal disorder in the elderly, usually by anterior cervical fusion (ACF), anterior cervical diskectomy with fusion (ACDF), posterior decompression and fusion, or cervical laminoplasty. Indications for surgery include failed medical/physical therapy, intractable pain, progressive neurologic deficits, and/or progressive painful or deficit-associated spinal cord or nerve root/nerve compression.

Thoracolumbar spondylosis is usually asymptomatic but can progress to the point of spinal stenosis, instability, and spondylolisthesis (subluxation of one vertebra in relation to another). Lumbar spondylosis, particularly at L3, has a far higher rate of occurrence (80%) and younger age of onset (40 years). There is an association of this spondylosis and osteophytosis with transforming growth factor $\beta 1$ genotype in some populations.

Anesthesia providers often employ arterial lines for hemodynamic control if specific BP ranges are necessary for perfusion. Vasoactive agents, fluids, colloids, blood products, laboratory testing, and adequate intravascular access with volume or venous air embolism (VAE) monitoring may be required. Airway management may be undertaken with minimal or no neck motion in patients suffering from cervical spine instability or myelopathy, often using awake-fiberoptic intubation (awake-FOI) techniques. Endotracheal tube (ETT) cuff pressures must be minimized for ACF/ACDF during instrumentation to prevent recurrent laryngeal nerve (RLN) injury. Vigilance is required for possible caudad displacement of ETT resulting from neck flexion in sitting, prone, and other abnormal positions.

b. Disk herniation. IVD herniation is more frequent in patients over 40 years of age due to degenerative changes from dehydration and tears or crack formation in the annulus fibrosus; or, it may present at any age from lifting or other trauma. The net result is that the nucleus pulposus extrudes beyond its normal limits causing compression of the spinal cord or nerve roots.

In the cervical region, degenerative disc pathology occurs most frequently at C5–C6, then at C6–C7, and less commonly at C4–C5. Symptomatology often includes cervical pain, radicular dysfunction, and if located centrally, myelopathy.

Rarely in occurrence, thoracic disk herniations usually develop at T8–T12. In contrast, lumbar disk herniation occurs in up to 2% of the overall population. L4–S1 is most often affected, usually posterolaterally, while higher lumbar levels are more involved in older patients. Symptomatology may vary from transient sciatica to radiculopathy, which normally resolves with conservative medical therapy. Significant SCI, such as cauda equina syndrome from central involvement, is indicative for immediate surgical therapy. Other surgical criteria include pain that does not resolve after 6 to 12 weeks or large disk herniation.

Anterior cervical and lumbar diskectomy are preferentially selected surgical techniques. Fusion, hemilaminotomy, and/or laminectomy may also be required.

Anesthesia provider concerns are similar to those for spondylosis surgery, although blood loss and invasive monitoring are less common.

c. Spinal stenosis. Spinal stenosis in any spinal region develops in 0.5% to 1% of the population. Congenital stenosis predisposes to worsening conditions as the body ages. Acquired causes include osteoarthritis, disk degeneration, ligament flavum thickening, neoplasm, trauma, infection, boney inflammatory disease such as AS, and bony metabolic disorders such as Paget's disease. Most etiologies result in slow central canal or lateral recess stenosis with dysfunction that rarely goes on to major significant SCI. Trauma and other more rapidly evolving etiologies can be much more injurious.

Cervical spine stenosis typically develops from arthritis, AS, or posterior longitudinal ligament calcification. Here and in the thoracic areas, radiculopathy has a greater incidence because of the higher likelihood of cord compression.

Lumbosacral stenosis is more associated with radicular pain and painful cramping, tingling, or weakness in the legs. The lowest levels, particularly L4–L5, are most likely to be affected because of the larger dorsal root ganglia diameter in the face of foraminal stenosis and other stenotic disorders that come with aging. Medical management of underlying causes and their resultant SCI tends to be effective. Otherwise, decompression and perhaps fusion surgery may be necessary. Long-term benefits show greater improvement in symptoms and quality of life after surgery.

Anesthetic management is dependent upon the cause, specific anatomical areas involved, extent of SCI, risk of blood loss, or intraoperative risk of new SCI.

d. Spondylolisthesis. Spondylolisthesis can precipitate SCI when IVD degeneration narrows the disk space, causing buckling of the ligamentum flavum and slippage of one vertebra over another in an anterior–posterior direction. Mild rotational effects from segmental instability often coincide and degenerative scoliosis may complicate the condition. Sagitally remodeled arthritic facet joints and multiparity might be a risk factor for the development of this disease. Congenital dysplasia, which is fortunately rather rare, tends to cause more extensive SCI due to rapid progression. Its concomitant poorly developed posterior elements and transverse processes make attempts at surgical fusion quite difficult. The form that is most frequent is isthmic spondylolisthesis. It is associated with a defective neural arch developing in mid-childhood and is estimated to occur in 5% to 7% of the population over 40 years of age with a 4:1 male:female ratio. Traumatic spondylolisthesis can result from facet skipping, damage to articular processes, and/or laminal fractures. Infection, and rare boney tumor or boney metabolic disease with posterior element compromise, can also result in pathologic spondylolisthesis.

The lumbar area, especially L5–S1, is a prime site for this entity, which is rare in other spinal regions. Mild or no symptomatology is common but rare severe SCI can develop, especially with more extensive subluxation. The Meyerding classification of anterior–posterior slippage grades illustrates the percent of subluxation based on lateral x-rays measuring distances from posterior edges of adjoining vertebrae [19].

Conservative therapy is often successful, with up to 70% of Meyerding Class 1 and 2 patients (<50% subluxation) improving quite well. In a minority, signs for surgical intervention include Meyerding Class 3 or 4 (50% to 100% subluxation), progressive subluxation beyond 30%, and perhaps cosmetic or gait deformity. Outcomes are often good with a variety of procedures such as decompression, posterior fusion, pedicle screw fixation devices, anterior interbody fusion, and prosthetic facet joint replacement, but almost 20% of the more complex techniques result in neuronal deficits.

Anesthetic requirements are similar to those previously discussed, with possibly more blood loss depending on the extent of surgery.

e. **Osteoporosis.** Osteoporosis is a generalized skeletal boney disorder found in 10% of the population in the United States, characterized by reductions in bone mineral density with altered microarchitecture leading to fractures. Spinal fractures are rather numerous, particularly compression fractures of the thoracic or lumbar vertebrae. Primary osteoporosis includes type I (postmenopausal) and type II (senile osteoporosis) found mostly in over 70 years of age population. Secondary osteoporosis is related to genetics, endocrine disease, inflammatory disease, hypogonadal syndromes, calcium balance disorders, and chronic steroid use.

Anterior compression is most likely in the thoracic spine and kyphosis may develop. Pain amenable to conservative therapy is the commonest result. When indicated, vertebroplasty or kyphoplasty is a suitable surgical alternative.

For anesthesia providers, vertebroplasty and kyphoplasty are frequently performed under monitored anesthesia care. Layton et al's [20] study on 552 patients undergoing 1,000 fracture vertebroplasties documented a drop in the general anesthesia rate from 96% to 3%.

f. **Scoliosis.** Scoliosis or spinal curvature greater than 10 degrees is of three types: Congenital (~15%), idiopathic (~65%), or neuromuscular (~10%). Up to 5% of pediatric populations have some scoliosis, especially in females and increasing with age. Neuromuscular causes include degenerative disease, osteoporosis, infection, and trauma.

Curvatures are most prevalent in lower thoracolumbar and upper lumbar regions.

Backache is most common, but progression to radiculopathy, fatigue, and respiratory compromise may also occur. Uniquely, thoracic scoliosis may develop restrictive pulmonary disorders correlating directly to the degree of deviation as the spinal column angle worsens from 60% to 100%. Patients may experience dyspnea and should undergo periodic pulmonary function studies to monitor progression.

Conservative therapy is normally sufficient but surgical criteria uniquely include cosmetic appearance and respiratory insufficiency.

Anesthetic providers are mindful that major corrective, fusion surgery for scoliosis is often extensive enough to require two stages to complete. Awareness of preoperative status permits detailed preoperative planning to encompass possibilities of external obstructive pressures on the airway system, pre-existing restrictive respiratory effects, IOM use, and large-scale blood loss. Anesthetic choices might include ≤0.5 minimum alveolar concentration (MAC) adaptations to volatile anesthetics with supplemental intravenous propofol and narcotic to prevent IOM effects and "deliberate hypotension" methods to reduce blood losses, provided that SCI and other comorbidities are minimal. Preoperatively, awareness heightens regarding greater rates of respiratory, hemodynamic, and coagulation complications, particularly in older patients. In McDonnell et al.'s [21] retrospective analysis on 447 patients undergoing anterior procedures on the thoracic, thoracolumbar, or lumbar spine, 11% had at least one major complication (most commonly pulmonary) and 24% had at least one minor one (frequently, genitourinary). Preoperative awareness of these factors advocates for patient preparation regarding invasive lines, a "wake-up test" (because of the potential for anterior spinal artery or the artery of Adamkiewicz injuries with anterior surgical approaches), and chances of postoperative intubation.

g. **Spinal dysraphism.** Spinal dysraphism involves defects resulting from incomplete fusion of the neural tube during fetal development. This relatively common occurrence, one in 1,000 live births, is more frequent in the presence of maternal folic acid or vitamin B deficiency. Open neural tube defects have coexisting vertebral abnormalities, including various forms of spina bifida or myelomeningocele. When the defect fills with mesenchyme, it can evolve into fat or a spinal lipoma and often present with a tethered, "dorsally-cleft" cord (see Chapter 16).

Syringomyelia entails progressively elongating and expanding fluid-filled cavities or cysts formed within the spinal cord. CSF obstruction or spinal cord damage from multiple sources, Arnold–Chiari malformation, arachnoiditis, trauma, hemorrhage, radiation necrosis, tumors, meningitis, and idiopathic origins, can develop a syrinx.

The average age at diagnosis is 30 years, after a slow course of minor symptoms such as back pain, upper body numbness, painless hand ulcers, loss of temperature sensation, and autonomic changes. The syrinx location dictates the symptomatology and can lead to severe SCI, scoliosis, or even cranial nerve and cerebral signs. Rarely, syringomyelia patients may experience singular manifestations such as RLN dysfunction, obstructive sleep apnea (OSA), or attention deficit syndrome. Depending on the cause, CSF pressure, protein, or red cell counts may be elevated or abnormal cells may be found.

Chronic, stable syringomyelia patients, who are accurately diagnosed with nonurgent etiologies, need periodic monitoring even if placed on analgesics or physical rehabilitation. Percutaneous aspiration can temporize acute decompensation or SCI. Surgical therapy includes removal of known causes, decompression, laminectomy, duraplasty, shunting, syrinx excision, or even suboccipital craniotomy.

Avoidance of excessive neck movement and attention to rising intracranial pressure (ICP) are among major concerns for anesthetic providers.

h. **Spinal neoplasm.** Spinal neoplasms can be benign or malignant, but most are metastatic from prostate, breast, renal, pulmonary, or gastric primaries. Absence of valves in the spinal venous architecture predisposes to metastatic invasion. Anatomic pathologic locations correlate with diagnoses and treatment. See Chapter 13: Anesthesia for Intramedullary Spinal Cord Tumors for further details. They are classified into three groups:

(1) Intramedullary tumors (10%) reside in the interstitium of the spinal cord and are usually malignant. They may originate from glial, ependymal, or metastatic sources (ependymoma, astrocytoma, ganglioblastoma, hemangioblastoma, lymphoma).

(2) Intradural/extramedullary tumors (40%) lie within the subarachnoid space, often arising from meningeal cells or metastases (schwannoma, neurofibroma, meningioma, paraganglioma).

(3) Extradural tumors (50%) often remain outside the dura in the vertebral body or epidural space, but can extend into the spinal cord through the intervertebral foramina in a "dumbbell shape." They may be benign, developing from cells near nerve roots (hemangioma, osteoma, bone cyst, giant cell tumor, osteochondroma). However, most are malignant (multiple myeloma, chordoma, chondrosarcoma, osteosarcoma, Ewing sarcoma, metastasis).

Symptomatology depends on the mechanism of pathologic development, causing nerve root or spinal cord impingement, stretching and erosion of neural tissues, collapse of IVDs, boney erosion, or blockage of CSF migration. An indolent course of pain (usually thoracic), fractures, deformity, radiculopathy, or cord compression may result.

Treatment varies according to the type of tumor, size, site, symptoms, concomitant disease, or even predicted life span, where palliative therapy may play an important role. Benign, intradural/extramedullary, and intramedullary tumors are more amenable to surgical excision and radiotherapy. Radiotherapy and high-dose steroid therapy to diminish vasogenic edema are temporizing measures. Chemotherapy is less successful due to difficulties in crossing the blood–brain barrier. Anesthetic planning hinges on effects of tumor location and surgical approaches as described previously. Bleeding is much more likely with neoplastic lesions but can be preempted by interventional radiologic embolization.

2. **Inflammatory/infectious disorders**

   a. **Rheumatoid arthritis.** RA is an inflammatory autoimmune disorder prevalent in 1% of the general population with a threefold incidence in women. Synovial joints may produce an antigen that stimulates rheumatoid factor (RF) production. RF is an "anti" immunoglobulin that attacks autologous glycoproteins, resulting in increased inflammatory responses, polymorphonuclear leukocyte infiltration, and cytotoxic enzymes, which destroy ligaments, tendons, cartilage, and bone.

   In the cervical region, RA affects C2–C4 almost exclusively. Subsequently, progression may extend to AAI (49% rate of occurrence), odontoid process migration upward (38%), and anterior subluxation of the first cervical spine.

   Patients may exhibit neck pain, headache, radiculopathy, myelopathy, vertebrobasilar insufficiency (vertigo, imbalance, dysphagia, cranial nerve disorder, and so forth), and rarely, brainstem compression.

   Analgesics, physical rehabilitation, and single/combination drug therapy to retard progression and induce remissions are popular. Medicines include disease-modifying antirheumatic drugs (DMARDs) including immunosuppressants such as methotrexate, antimalarial drugs such as hydroxychloroquine, tumor necrosis factor (TNF)-α antagonists such as etanercept, corticosteroids, and nonsteroidal anti-inflammatory drugs (NSAIDs).

   Anterior decompression ± corpectomy with fusion or posterior decompression and fusion are favored approaches. C1–C2 subluxation may precipitate the need for emergency surgery including use of stabilizing hardware and/or bone grafting.

   Anesthesia providers must ensure that airway management produces little cervical motion. Hypoperfusion should be prevented in vertebrobasilar insufficiency cases. Concern is often directed toward the interactions and effects of pre-existing drug therapy.

   b. **Ankylosing spondylitis.** The diagnosis of AS is carried by 0.02% to 0.20% of the population. Of this population, 80% have an onset before 30 years of age while 10% to 20% become symptomatic before 16 years of age. The male to female ratio is 2 or 3 to 1 with greater severity of radiologic evidence of disease in men, but better functional capacity than women. Caucasians (90% to 95%) and African-Americans (50%) can express the HLA-B27 genotype, a class I surface antigen on B chromosome that is associated with seronegative spondyloarthropathies and autoimmune disease.

   This chronic, progressive inflammatory disease is characterized by enthesitis or inflammation of skeletal ligamentous boney insertion foci, especially in vertebral and sacroiliac articular/para-articular structures. Osseous excrescence or syndesmophytes form and attach to ligaments, bridging across calcified IVDs. An ingrowth of synovial material into joints, myxoid bone marrow, and superficial cartilage results in destruction with joint fusion. Paradoxical osteopenia may develop secondary to decreased joint motion, increased osteoclasis, and degenerative erosion by inflammatory cells. In the cervicothoracic area, where 75% of AS fractures occur, the disease may progress to severe kyphotic deformity, accompanied by a myriad of health and psychosocial problems.

   Related comorbidities include peripheral polyarthritis (40%), aortic valve thickening (42% to 82%), aortic regurgitation (45%), aortitis (5%), restrictive lung disease (42%), renal amyloidosis (15%), and uveitis or iritis (30% to 50%).

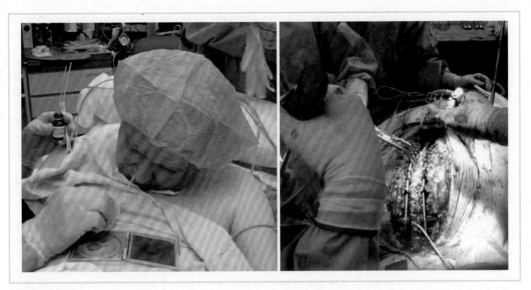

FIGURE 12.2 Surgery in a patient with severe ankylosing spondylitis: Nasal local anesthesia in a patient who uses a mirror during conversation.

Symptoms revolve around low back pain and limited spinal flexion, plus ankylosis and kyphosis advancing in a caudad to cephalad direction. With increasing ankylosis toward the point of "chin-on-chest" sign, dysphagia may follow, causing lack of oral hygiene, formation of mouth ulcerations, malnutrition, weight loss, anemia, fatigue, declining general hygiene, and eventually social estrangement.

Medical treatment is aimed at decreasing inflammation by use of immunosuppressant, DMARD, TNF-α antagonist, and NSAID therapy.

Surgery to stabilize the cervical spine is a challenging scenario for anesthesia providers, particularly when reaching the "chin-on-chest" stage (Fig. 12.2). Preoperative assessment of severe cervical kyphosis, difficult airway, or SCI often makes awake-FOI the safest airway management plan, especially when even the site for a tracheotomy is obliterated by the mandible juxtaposition. Often, the inhibited mouth opening will require preparations for a nasotracheal route. During nasal local anesthesia application, epistaxis must be avoided in an already compromised situation and contraindicates utilization of blind nasal intubation (BNI) methods. Cardiac, respiratory, renal, and malnutritional disorders present an interesting challenge, necessitating preoperative optimization and plans for extensive intraoperative monitoring.

c. **Osteomyelitis.** Osteomyelitis of the vertebrae and/or IVDs occurs in ≤2.4% of the population, particularly in older patients. The most typical site of infection is the lumbar spine and then the thoracic. Single-proton–emission computed tomography (PET scan) is the most sensitive early radiologic indicator of osteomyelitis.

Symptoms include back pain and spasm that can be treated with analgesics and a 4- to 6-week intravenous course of intravenous antibiotics, followed by oral therapy as outpatients.

Older patients are more susceptible to rare epidural abscess formation, primarily in multiple thoracolumbar and posterior column segments. Formation tends to develop from contiguous spread of infective osteomyelitic organisms, boney erosion, vertebral collapse, bacteremic seeding, and/or direct postsurgical inoculation or invasive needling. Pathologic expansion causes severe back pain, fever, radiculopathy, and myelopathy. Immediate antibiotic therapy plus debridement, drainage, and/or decompressive laminotomy are indicated for abscesses. In patients who pose high surgical risks, especially those with a fixed SCI (beyond 72 hours), antibiotics and possibly CT needle aspiration is a therapeutic alternative.

Anesthesia provider concerns for osteomyelitis or epidural abscess surgeries are similar to that for decompressive SCI in addition to addressing infection, its systemic effects, and intense pain, even during CT needle aspiration.

3. **Demyelinating diseases and upper neuron disorders of mixed origins.** Genetic, autoimmune, infectious, chemical, or idiopathic factors may result in myelin sheaths destruction or neuronal damage. Some demyelinating (e.g., multiple sclerosis) or upper motor neuron (e.g., amyotrophic lateral sclerosis) disorders originate within the CNS, while others begin more peripherally and spread centrally, perhaps gaining access through the blood–brain barrier. Symptomatology depends on regions affected and the degree of neurologic involvement. Most patients who develop SCI are treated with medical therapy and/or physical therapy and/or with surgery, as indications arise.

Anesthesia providers often choose monitored anesthesia care for these exceedingly debilitated patients with a view to minimize psychotropic, respiratory depressant, and cardiovascular depressant agents.

B. **Traumatic spinal cord disorders.** Traumatic SCI is defined exactly as stated, with symptoms ranging from mild pain to life-threatening myelopathy. Both traumatic cervical SCI and thoracic/lumbar/sacral SCI have singular characteristics. These patients must be placed in a system to treat existing damage and prevent secondary neurologic injury (SNI). SNI is CNS damage due to tissue ischemia, excessive spine movement, or spinal compression. Vale et al. [22] followed 77 patients who were hospitalized with SCI for whom immediate immobilization and resuscitative measures including intravenous fluids, blood products, and/or vasopressors were instituted to sustain a MAP of ≥85 mm Hg, in order to avoid secondary injury. Selected patients meeting criteria for decompression and/or stabilization and fusion had those surgeries performed. The authors found that neurologic outcomes improved on the average of one ASIA grade in most patients. Even those with complete injuries, had a 10% to 30% chance of walking, while 10% to 20% had a chance of returned bladder function within 12 months of injury.

The incidence of concomitant spinal cord injury (SCI) involved with any major blunt "head-trauma" patient is in the range of 5% to 8%, while for those suffering multiple, blunt bodily injuries it is almost 8%. Older patients have a 10-fold greater chance of simultaneous cervical SCI in comparison to children. Conversely, of patients admitted with known cervical SCI, approximately 33% have head injury. Approximately 20% of patients with SCI have multiple spinal levels of damage.

1. **Traumatic cervical spine injury.** In the setting of generalized trauma patients, the National Emergency X-radiography Utilization Study (NEXUS) group's prospective research with radiologic confirmation of damage, noted that cervical SCI was discovered in 2% of cases [16]. Over 50% of the cervical SCI patients who developed neuropathy or complete/incomplete tetraplegia suffered injury at C6 or C7, while approximately 33% had C2 damage.

Whiplash is the most frequent cervical spine injury and is most often caused by acceleration/deceleration forces. With frontal collisions, the upper vertebral areas are directed anteriorly while the lower ones appear to shift posteriorly. This may damage cervical muscles, IVDs, the alar ligament complex, and/or facet joints, causing dislocations and fractures. Rarely, IVDs suffer annular tears or herniation and ligaments can rupture, risking nervous system impingement.

Some human and simulation studies indicate that frontal impact is most likely to result in abnormal motion involving lower (C6–T1) and middle (C2–C5) cervical areas. Other simulation studies indicate that rear-end collision is most associated with a predominantly hyperextension effect and if violent, is more prone to injure the lower cervical (C5–T1) spine.

Symptomatology from sprained muscles, tissue damage, and/or SCI is dependent upon the pathologic insult. Patients with underlying spondylosis or other compromising disorders are subject to develop cervical myeloradiculopathy.

The development of the Emergency Medical Services (EMS) in 1971 and initiation of spinal immobilization decreased by 10-fold the occurrence of SNI in cervical spine risk patients. Subsequently, as a direct result, the historical estimate of ≥25% chance of suffering an SNI dropped to 1% to 3%.

For simple cervical injuries, such as neck strain or a mildly herniated disk, medical treatment, physical therapy, and/or soft collar immobilization is sufficient [23]. For more significant SCI, rigid immobilization devices and further therapy are recommended. Early surgical correction including decompression, diskectomy, and/or fusion for severe cervical spine trauma is advised.

Anesthesia providers must be diligent in preventing SNI by precise airway management and maintenance of appropriate monitoring and operative care. Concomitant bodily injuries, particularly to the head, should not be overlooked.

2. **Traumatic thoracic/lumbar/sacral spine injury.** Classically, spinal trauma tends to be inflicted on more mobile spinal locations. Thus, 75% of SCI insults involve C3–C7, while the next most commonly injured area is at L1, affecting 16% of SCI patients. Holmes et al.'s review found that thoracolumbar injuries were detected in 6.3% of patients suffering from general trauma [16].

At higher thoracolumbar levels of SCI, complete or incomplete paraplegia may result, whereas neuropathy is possible at any level. Frequently, there may be injuries to other organs since spinal trauma in the thoracic/lumbar/sacral regions requires more force to cause SCI. Cardiac, pulmonary, and chest wall injury are more likely to accompany thoracic spine trauma whereas fractures at the L1 transverse process may be associated with ipsilateral renal trauma. Lumbar spine trauma is often accompanied by intra-abdominal and diaphragmatic damage.

Most thoracic and many lumbar fractures tend to be more stable, reliably treated with immobilization and conservative therapy. In patients with thoracolumbar compression or burst fractures with no signs of neurologic injury, no loss of vertebral body height less than 50%, and no narrowing of the spinal column of less than 30%, random treatment protocols with braces, casts, physical therapy, and/or postural instructions for 6 to 12 weeks showed no difference in outcome. Sacral spine injuries, which are 20 times less frequent than lumbar injuries, are very amenable to conservative therapy.

For anesthesia providers, attendance to immobilization, invasive monitoring for hemodynamic control, and blood product acquisition will depend on the injury and type of surgery.

IV. **Special considerations with complete spinal cord injury.** Many bodily systems may be affected by complete SCI (paraplegias, tetraplegias, and so forth) prompting patients to undergo repeated surgeries and anesthetics. Some coexisting factors and complications related to SCI may have significant impact on patient care.

If patients require airway control, the presence of semirigid collars, halos, and cervical fusions all tend to spur anesthesia providers into implementing protocols for management of a difficult airway with minimal cervical motion.

SCI patients may incur a wide spectrum of respiratory aberrancies. Abnormal pulmonary functions include up to 32% drops in vital capacity during changes from seated to supine positions. In the supine position, decreases of up to 70% mean vital capacity and 45% forced expiratory volume in 1 second can occur. Complete injury at C3–C5 results in ventilator dependency. Some patients may be assisted and have fewer infections following special surgeries such as diaphragmatic pacing. Respiratory infection may result from hypoventilation following diaphragmatic, thoracic, and abdominal muscle paralysis with impaired coughing ability to clear secretions and increased aspiration risk. Pulmonary embolism is a complication associated with venous stasis and DVT. Also finally, hypotension due to neurogenic shock may provoke excessive fluid administration, resulting in pulmonary edema.

In these situations, providers have a heightened awareness of intolerance to hypoxemia and likelihood of respiratory deterioration, particularly during acute airway management. Supplementary oxygen, ventilatory techniques, and suctioning are worthwhile.

Patients with complete SCI are more susceptible to cardiovascular abnormalities such as early hypotension from neurogenic shock and/or concomitant organ injury. Treatment goals include limiting crystalloids to 2,000 mL to prevent pulmonary edema and acute respiratory distress syndrome, using fluid plus vasoactive therapy to achieve systolic BP levels ≥90 to 100 mm Hg and heart rates 40 to 100 beats per minute, maintaining oxygenation, and keeping urine output at ≥0.5 mL/kg/h. Days to months later, hypotension may develop from sympathectomy, infection, hypoproteinemia, anemia, and/or insufficient fluid intake.

SCI patients with complete levels at T6–T7 or higher have a greater possibility of autonomic dysreflexia. When planning for anesthetic management during surgery (more commonly nonspinal types), dysreflexia risks can be completely avoided if anesthesia providers choose neuraxial blocks. Continuation of epidural block postoperatively provides the same benefit, particularly in those with a history of frequent events.

Hypothermia is a significant problem in tetraplegics or paraplegics, both in the acute phase of spinal shock and in chronic cases, where patients have a relatively greater surface area due to weight loss. Active fluid warming, use of warming blankets, and increasing ambient temperature stave off excessive hypothermia and consequences such as infection, postoperative shivering, and adverse coagulation effects.

Patients with lack of sensation, contractures, and pressure sores may require special padding and diligence to prevent additional injury. Catheterizations, urine retention, and ureteral reflux expose SCI patients to repeated infections and kidney failure problems that anesthesia providers must consider. In addition to effects of sepsis in these situations, the safety of regional anesthesia must be evaluated.

Periodically, effects of SCI may actually alter anesthetic choices [24]. Spasticity may preclude the use of monitored anesthesia care if spastic movements have a chance of causing field motion or impeding surgical technique. Large-scale paralysis causing upregulation of acetylcholine receptors 12 to 24 hours beyond the onset of SCI is a contraindication to succinylcholine administration for fear of precipitating severe hyperkalemia. Prior to 12–24 hours, there is insufficient time for significant upregulation and administration is safe, theoretically. The duration of contraindication may span one or more years or even forever, especially in the face of fluctuating neurologic deficit.

Finally, after major spine surgery, pain control is most problematic in patients receiving chronic, high-dose analgesic regimens.

V. Management approaches for spinal cord injury. The main objective of therapy is to improve recovery from the effects of SCI, halt worsening of the condition from whatever caused the injury, and prevent secondary neurologic damage. Acute SCI is a more "immediate, therapy-intensive" situation and even subacute or chronic SCI cases may fall into an urgent status category. This discussion will provide an overview of the two major modes of treatment for acute SCI: Conservative medical and/or physical therapy or surgical therapy with anesthetic management.

A. Medical/physical therapy

1. External immobilization. Initial treatment phases of most trauma/suspicion for acute SCI frequently include immobilization in the prehospital setting. Immobilization consists of a hard collar (superior restriction to soft ones) for cervical injuries or a backboard plus strapping/taping, or orthopedic brace for cervical/thoracic/lumbar injuries. Interestingly, for penetrating trauma patients, immobilization is not recommended unless SCI is highly suspected, and may have been harmful to a small percentage of those immobilized, by causing twice the mortality rate, perhaps due to delayed definitive therapy. For thoracolumbar risk, there does not seem to be a consensus on the value of immobilization, unless criteria for surgery exist. Studies on thoracolumbar spinal fracture patients with no specific surgical criteria, who randomly underwent surgery versus conservative therapy and similarly treated lower cervical spine patients showed that surgically treated patients had greater speeds of recovery, less pain, and returned to work faster than conservatively treated ones. However, the middle long-term effects of the two therapeutic courses were comparable for residual pain, quality of life, and residual employment-limiting disability.

In cervical spine patients, immobilization may involve use of a halo. Halos are the most restrictive but do not totally prevent movement. Complications of halo fixators include scars, pressure sores, infection, pins getting loose, periorbital edema, burns at pin sites during MRI, osteomyelitis, penetration of the cranium and subdural abscess, VAE, nerve palsy, and failure to prevent motion.

Chan et al.'s [25] review revealed that of 21 healthy subjects immobilized for 30 minutes on a backboard, 100% developed head, sacral, lumbar, and mandibular pain. Indeed, half considered the degree of pain to be moderate to severe and 29% developed more symptoms within 48 hours. Considering these results, and the fact that backboards allow greater degrees of cervical motion compared to vacuum mattresses, perhaps this information should result in a recommendation that EMS services eliminate backboards in lieu of purchasing mattresses.

2. **Temporizing therapy (analgesics and anti-inflammatory drugs).** For conservative therapy, opioid analgesics, tramadol, oxycontin, gabapentin, pregabalin, or fentanyl patches alone or in combination may be administered to make pain tolerable. Judicious dosing avoids the loss of patient cooperation, prevents inability to perceive neurologic changes, and stays away from adverse hypoventilation. Attentiveness to ventilation must be greatest in the presence of coexisting respiratory embarrassment from SCI, other traumatic respiratory disorders, or concomitant cerebral injury with increased ICP.

   Beneficial nonsteroidal anti-inflammatory drugs (NSAIDs) such as ibuprofen, acetylsalicylic acid, naproxen, indomethacin, mefenamic acid, or piroxicam which all reduce prostaglandin synthesis, should be avoided in the face of "high risk-of-bleeding" acute SCI or contraindications. Acute pain from less-damaging SCI, such as a herniated disk, might be treated with a week-long course of potent anti-inflammatory steroids (prednisone) to inhibit lipid peroxidation and calcium influx. Epidural, interlaminal, or transforaminal steroid injections under fluoroscopy are useful, but best avoided if concerns for SCI are present, except in cases unlikely to be candidate for other therapy.

3. **Cervical traction or lumbar traction.** Cervical traction with cerebral tongs and a 20- to 40-lb weighted pulley system can be used for cervical radiculopathy, disk herniation, or neural foraminal stenosis. Lumbar traction with a hip padding system and pillows under the feet for acute SCI (<6 weeks from onset) has had considerable success. Vertebral separation can decrease spinal cord pressure, lessen disk herniation, or modify pressure on disk bodies. Length of immobilization time, possibility of pressure sores, and hygiene factors are disadvantages.

4. **Spinal cord protection**
   a. **Implementation of moderate hypothermia.** Hypothermia has been studied considerably as a protective strategy for cerebral ischemia. Because of the many parallels between the spinal cord and the brain regarding effects of metabolism, autoregulation, and ischemic injury, some clinicians think that hypothermia may be a "cord-protective" proposition. Hypothermia decreases metabolism fourfold per 10°C, maintains adenosine triphosphate (ATP), and reduces glutamate release, excitotoxicity, inflammatory changes, vasogenic edema, neutrophil response, calpain activation, and apoptosis. A prospective, definitive study is still needed to determine the relationship between SCI and hypothermia.

   b. **Recent/future therapeutic alternatives.** An assortment of therapies has been investigated in animal studies and human subjects with varying success while searching out the best treatment for SCI. These include angiogenic protein, Schwann cell transplantation, gangliosides, calcineurin inhibitors such as cyclosporin A and tacrolimus, omega-3 fatty acids, adult stem cell transplantation, riluzole, and transplantation of many cell types, such as bone marrow cells onto damaged spinal tissue.

   c. **The high-dose steroid therapy controversy.** In 1990, a prospective acute SCI outcome study by the Second National Acute Spinal Cord Injury Study (NASCIS II) used high-dose methylprednisolone (HDMP) with the object of ameliorating the effects of SCI and preventing secondary damage [26]. The study assessed only unilateral neurologic testing and found no benefit overall (according to ASIA, motor, or sensory scores) in the HDMP group, compared to naloxone or placebo groups. In the NASCIS III study, 24 to 48-hour infusions of HDMP compared to tirilazad showed no overall benefit between groups [27]. A trend toward sepsis, pneumonia, gastrointestinal bleeding (1.5-fold), wound infection (2-fold), pulmonary embolism (3-fold), and death was detected in the HDMP group.

On post hoc analysis, both studies found a subgroup that had improved neurologic changes, but the magnitudes were not objectified. In spite of this, the authors recommended that patients with acute SCI should be treated with HDMP for 23 hours, initially 8 hours postinjury, and after their next study, at 3 to 8 hours postinjury. Perceived pressure to administer anything that might be beneficial for SCI, made use of HDMP very popular.

Some researchers questioned this therapy's validity, particularly considering risky adverse side effects. Recently, meta-analysis of the literature found that significance of the subgroup data was unknown. Multiple independent reviewers had trepidation regarding randomization, clinical endpoints [28], statistical analysis, plus the lack of having levels I, II, or even the majority of level III evidence clearly demonstrated that HDMP definitely was *not* warranted to be considered as a standard of care *or* indeed, even as a recommendation for SCI patients. They warned of adverse complications with HDMP far outweighing the "limited suggested benefits." Presently, the Canadian Association of Emergency Physicians (CAEP) has renounced the use of HDMP and the Congress of Neurosurgeons has stated that its use is more likely to be associated with adverse side effects rather than clinical benefit.

B. Surgical management

1. **Indications for spinal cord injury surgery.** Halo immobilization may be insufficient to prevent cervical spine motion from deteriorating into acute SCI, progression of existing SCI, or development of SNI. Radiographic evidence of fracture site motion in the upright position may occur in 77% of patients with halos. Studies have additionally demonstrated that surgery can be more beneficial than immobilization techniques.

   Criteria for surgical treatment of SCI include: (1) Spinal instability, (2) intractable pain unresponsive to conservative therapy for ≥6 weeks, (3) progressive neurologic deficits, and/or (4) progressive spinal cord or nerve/nerve root compression with pain or neurologic deficit. Other indications may involve the following: (1) Adequate medical status and stability following numerous organ injuries, (2) radiographic evidence of intrinsic damage to the spinal cord, (3) significantly extensive bone, disk, fracture/dislocation, or hematoma compression, and (4) inability to immobilize or prevent spinal instability through closed reduction, rigid external immobilizers, or natural healing.

   Acute SCI is frequently considered an urgent problem if the need for decompression is apparent. The idea of urgency in timing was advocated because of numerous experimental projects suggesting greater chances of irreversibility or SNI beyond certain lengths of time. For acute spine or SCI what is the optimal timing for surgical correction and/or stabilization? Review articles researched this question and found no class I evidence to support improved neurologic outcome after "early" institution of surgery (8 to 72 hours). Studies were retrospective, poorly randomized, and had contradictory outcomes with levels II to IV evidence [29]. Regardless, some authors felt that newer evidence tended to be inclined toward the safety of early surgical therapy and that outcomes are associated with faster and potentially better recoveries following surgery within 24 hours of traumatic SCI onset.

2. **Types of surgical procedures and anesthetic caveats.** Once a patient meets surgical criteria, a number of techniques are available. Many are very beneficial, but even these are fraught with the possibilities of persistent or worsening symptomatology, adjacent degenerative changes due to motion abnormalities and complications.

   Newer surgical techniques are beginning to be explored. Among these are artificial disk replacement and artificial facet replacement techniques designed to permit more natural movement of the spine in contrast to fusion surgery. Although they boast shorter recovery periods, outcomes have not been encouraging. There was insufficient support in the literature to recommend these procedures and further intimated possibilities of hazardous revision after pre-existing artificial disk surgery. Disk replacement surgery in 93 patients with no control group revealed results indicating that adjacent spine degeneration was lessened by 10% [30]. However, many patients fared worse clinically than they were beforehand, with more limited motion and progression to facet joint degeneration. This finding was highly informative since facet joint disease and spondylosis are listed among contraindications to this surgery. Facet joint implant is yet another unproven technique, performed since 2007 in Europe. Studies there had no controlled outcome and the method is only now being researched in the United States.

a. **Anterior cervical diskectomy.** Anterior cervical diskectomy (ACD) is an approved technique employed for patients diagnosed with herniated cervical disks. Through anterior neck approaches, plans are executed for repairing a disk, removing fragments, or performing complete diskectomy, frequently with removal of nearby osteophytes.

These patients tend to have few risk factors regarding cervical motion. However, if present, then airway management techniques should be chosen according to the method with which anesthesia providers feel most expert [23]. If general anesthesia (GA) and ETT are planned, laryngotracheal anesthesia (LTA; 4% lidocaine) spray to the trachea minimizes surgical stimulation and lowers anesthetic requirements. Muscle relaxants help prevent movement, but may have to be abandoned if MEPs are monitored.

This surgery is less complex than diskectomy with fusion. IOM selection depends on the degree of SCI and risk of surgery. Invasive hemodynamic monitoring, additional intravenous access, or blood products are unlikely.

Anesthetic agents should be chosen with the object of early postoperative neurologic testing. Stomach decompression eliminates gastric distension and at least two good antiemetics assist in achieving a "quiet" emergence from anesthesia to avoid gagging, coughing, hypertension, and hematoma formation. Intravenous lidocaine, judicious lowering of inhalation agent, continuous small-dose remifentanil infusion or other narcotics, and "near the end of surgery" use of nitrous oxide/oxygen can make for a very smooth wake-up. Postoperative pain is minimal, especially after local anesthesia in the incision.

b. **Anterior cervical diskectomy or corpectomy with fusion.** For patients with unstable cervical spines or excessive spine motion, ACD and fusion (ACDF) is often chosen. Anterior corpectomy (removal of the vertebra) with fusion may be considered if the vertebral body is excessively eroded. A patient's hip site for a donor bone graft is usually is the greatest source of postoperative pain. This autograft or alternatively, an allograft from cadaver donation can be used as a solid stabilizing plug or groundup and packed into the fusion site between vertebrae and/or around instrumentation. Fusion will eventually result at vertebral levels above and below the disk site after the bone graft is inserted or if the entire disk endplate is excised.

Awake- or asleep-FOI, or other intubation method with manual in-line stabilization (MILS) is advised for at-risk cases. Anesthesia providers must avoid complications of ETT-surgical retractor-related RLN palsy associated with this surgery [31].

If IOM indicates little or no SCI, BP can be kept in the low normal range to lessen bleeding. An arterial line is recommended if tight BP control is required for adequate perfusion in the face of SCI or if greater blood loss is anticipated from ≥2 levels of fusion. Tumor pathology or corpectomy plans increase blood losses and needs for appropriate lines and blood products. IOM will mandate keeping inhalation agents at ≤0.5 MAC. Supplementary propofol or dexmedetomidine can assist with hypnosis. TIVA may be required if the initial EPs are so poor that inhalation agents are contraindicated.

Occasionally, a surgeon may request aid by asking for cervical traction to create sufficient space for boney grafts or "plugs." While carefully keeping fingers out of the surgical field, anesthesia providers exert a constant, slow cephalad pull on the angles of the mandible until the surgeon indicates when to maintain position. The provider can slowly let go after being informed that the graft is in place. An alternative is to pull on the cord of a cervicocranial traction device, if present. Subsequently, plates are added for further stability.

Similar to ACD, wake-up should be gentle and quite early. Postoperative pain is mild to moderate.

c. **Posterior diskectomy, hemilaminectomy, or laminectomy/fusion.** Posterior diskectomy surgery is targeted for patients with posteriorly protruding disks. Hemilaminectomy is a posterior body surface approach designed to eliminate encroaching bone, impinging ligaments, and/or herniated disks by cutting lamina to free up the spinal cord and nerve roots. With pre-existing spinal stenosis and myelopathy, the entire lamina at one or more levels needs to be excised (laminectomy). If boney removal is sufficient, an otherwise impinging disk may be left untouched because it is now "free." Vertebral movement is unlimited after this surgery. Motion-limiting fusions are undertaken to provide stability by performing a laminectomy and/or diskectomy followed by insertion of interbody stabilization instrumentation and ground-up bone for structural support.

Although these are lower-risk procedures, anesthetic concerns for venous access, blood availability, and invasive monitoring depend on the extent of surgery, patient comorbidities, and diagnosis. For cervical surgeries, care is required to avoid excessive neck flexion, particularly with pre-existing SCI. Soft, prone headframes or pins are employed for facial protection. Prone positioning is a concern for the usual reasons including ensuring sufficient room for abdominal and chest expansion to prevent restrictive ventilatory effects.

d. **PLIF, TLIF, ALIF, and XLIF.** These acronyms are attributed to approaches for fusion of at least two vertebrae for patients with diagnoses of scoliosis, spondylolisthesis, spinal fractures, or multiple severely deteriorated disks. Surgeries may be minimally invasive or may be quite extensive.

A posterior lumbar interbody fusion (PLIF) is approached through a posterior midline incision. After laminectomies and diskectomies, vertebral surfaces are prepared and ground-up bone and instrumentation is placed.

A transforaminal lumbar interbody fusion (TLIF) approaches from a posterior midline incision but aims more posterolaterally through less muscle with less risk of nerve disruption. Otherwise the salient objectives are similar to the PLIF.

Anterior lumbar interbody fusion (ALIF) is akin to PLIF but is approached anteriorly or laterally.

The extreme lateral interbody fusion (XLIF) is an analogous technique completed through a number of small incisions in the flank for a maximum of perhaps two vertebral levels.

These extensive surgeries frequently involve time spent on major boney stressing anesthesia considerations for airway management, respiratory status, invasive lines, IOM and anesthetic interactions, positioning, monitoring and treatment of major blood loss/coagulation abnormalities, temperature control, wake-up tests, ischemic optic neuropathy (ION), extubation, and postoperative concerns.

Providers are keenly aware of when pedicle screw testing is needed with regard to effects of neuromuscular blockade (NMB). The sought-for response is similar to watching for nervous system irritation on free-run EMG, except that the surgeons specifically use a probe to test on the screw. Needle electrodes record from appropriate nearby muscles that correlate with nerve root innervation. The purpose is to detect screws that have penetrated the spinal canal or breeched the pedicle wall, resulting in direct contact with nerve roots. Muscle responses to lower currents (<6–10 mA) indicate excessive proximity and suggest surgical adjustment. Chronically compressed nerves may have higher thresholds of concern.

Individual nerve root identification and threshold testing are performed in a similar fashion during surgeries where spinal tumor excision, boney work, or freeing up of a tethered spinal cord is planned. In these cases, a probe in the operative site emits low levels of electrical stimulation so that responses and thresholds are measured in corresponding muscles. Dermatomal EP responses are highly sensitive to volatile agents.

With the likelihood of chronically injured nerve roots, many anesthesia providers recommend against muscle relaxants. See Chapter 26: Electrophysiologic Monitoring for further details.

Transthoracic approaches for anterior and lateral pathology often necessitate one-lung ventilation by a double-lumen ETT or bronchial blocker, or hypoventilatory jet ventilation techniques. A double-lumen ETT in a patient in a prone head holder can be problematic if the ETT has shifted and is unable to isolate the lung. It may be very difficult to adjust through the small frame opening after softening body heat causes it to become excessively flexible.

  e. **Minimally invasive spinal surgery, microdiskectomy.** Endoscopic or minimally invasive spinal surgeries utilize small incisions. These posterior, posterolateral, anterior cervical spine, or extreme lateral endoscopic approaches have the advantage of using dilation technology to traverse soft tissues.

  Indications include spinal or foraminal stenosis, facet joint cysts, cauda equina syndrome, or radiculopathy accompanying smaller-sized disk herniation with motor dysfunction. Spinal instability and central canal impingement are contraindications.

  General ETT anesthesia is preferred, although monitored anesthesia care is possible in highly motivated patients unlikely to move body parts. Preparation must always be considered for conversion to GA.

  f. **Vertebroplasty and kyphoplasty.** During vertebroplasty under x-ray guidance, a hollow bore needle is inserted within a collapsed vertebral body for cement injection to strengthen its structure. The kyphoplasty method inserts a dilating balloon through the needle to expand the vertebral body. After the balloon is deflated and withdrawn, cement is injected into the "cavity."

  Both surgeries are easily amenable to monitored anesthesia care. Anesthetic providers should remember the distinctive problems that arose in Layton et al.'s series of patients, including a 1% incidence of rib fracture or rib pain secondary to prone positioning and an episode of cement-induced pulmonary embolism [20].

VI. **Anesthetic management for surgical spinal cord injury procedures.** The bulk of this description of anesthesia for SCI will be directed toward anesthetic strategies for patients with acute cervical SCI and/or surgery with the possibility of major blood loss. Preoperatively, patients should already have had maximal evaluation of history, physical examination, MRI and/or necessary testing. There are many unique aspects in anesthetic care. When indicated, five important areas include explanations for awake-FOI or other airway management, wake-up testing, use of invasive monitors, postoperative intubation, and postoperative pain management. The degree to which laboratory data can be obtained, preanesthetic discussions completed, and anesthetic plans developed, depends on the speed and urgency for surgery.

  A. **Optimization of patient status, psychological preparation, premedication.** The patient should be on optimal therapeutic regimens for surgery if possible, with regard to volume status, laboratory data, and major organ systems function. When anticipated, major spine surgery should prompt blood bank requests for availability of packed red blood cells (PRBC), platelets, cryoprecipitate, arginine vasopressin, coagulation factors, and/or FFP. Keeping eight units of PRBC or a major trauma protocol in nearby refrigerators is most efficient.

  Complete airway assessment and knowledge of neurologic examination data are extremely important. A thorough, reassuring, and explanatory preanesthetic visit is an extremely worthwhile psychological preparation of the sequence of events from induction to the postoperative phase. Discussing the importance of awake-FOI while giving reassurances and comparisons of local airway anesthesia to otolaryngology throat examinations with sedation makes it very tolerable.

  A case could be made for explaining the "wake-up test" to all patients undergoing SCI surgeries where risk to the motor system may occur. Fear is allayed by descriptions of being asleep throughout the surgery and having a wake-up test similar to waking up with heavy narcotics once the surgery is finished. Patients should be informed of not being able to open taped eyes to prevent injury, and not being able to speak temporarily because of a "breathing tube" that probably will not bother them. The provider should explain requests to squeeze their hands, move their feet, and most importantly, not move the rest of their bodies. Going back to sleep after a few moments of testing is also conveyed. Remarking that most patients typically do not remember anything bad about the wake-up test is very much appreciated.

An explanation of arterial, central, and peripheral intravenous lines should be given with reasons for placement, sensations felt after awakening, and possible risk.

Patients with difficult airways, complex cervical surgery (especially simultaneous anterior–posterior), lengthy surgery in the prone position, or high volume resuscitation are prime candidates for postoperative intubation. Explaining the benefits, concomitant sedation, sensations, and expectations for extubation is important.

One method of discussing postoperative pain relief expectations with patients might relate pain judged on a scale of 0 to 10, where 10 is the worst pain imaginable. Meeting expectations is more likely with descriptions for pain scores objectives ≤3 or 4 being better than zero, where concern may arise about too much narcotic and respiratory arrest. Preempting worry about awakening at a zero score can be achieved by describing extra vigilance at that level.

Premedication for patients with acute SCI depends on surgical urgency, overall medical status, aspiration risk, airway difficulty, hemodynamic circumstances, degree of cooperation required, anxiety, presence of pain, drug therapy, allergies, age, height, and weight. Anxiolytic agents and/or narcotics should be titrated carefully in patients with significant risk and at extreme ages.

Excepting contraindications, glycopyrrolate is recommended for awake oral approaches to airway management, to improve intraoral local anesthetic absorption and airway viewing by lessening secretions.

Drugs for significant comorbidities such as anticonvulsants, antihypertensives, immunologic suppressants, and so forth may be administered if benefits exceed disadvantages. It is advantageous to administer antibiotics prior to incision unless cultures of the wound are planned at which time antibiotics should be administered after the cultures are acquired.

B. Anesthetic management

   1. General anesthesia. GA is the most frequently chosen technique with benefits of controlled ventilation, freedom to deal with the complexity of anesthetic patient care, and a nonmoving field in the face of intricate spinal surgery. Complexities may involve airway management, monitoring, anesthetic choices, invasive techniques, and positioning.

   a. Airway management. Striking spinal deformities, SCI, respiratory restriction, and effects of patient positioning often lead to the selection of specialized airway devices and techniques. For intubated patients, if airway pressures rise significantly, but simple causes and solutions are not found, early institution of fiberoptic examination of the ETT and airway can be invaluable, particularly when prone, and may prevent hypoxemia, lung trauma, and/or accidental extubation from ETT manipulation.

   (1) Airway devices, cervical spine motion, maneuvers. Unique considerations for airway devices for spinal surgery include the use of reinforced anode ETTs, particularly in thoracic scoliosis patients to prevent boney deformity compromises of the ETT lumen. Some might consider this type of ETT to be beneficial during cervical spine surgery when the external pressure of surgical instrumentation might cause narrowing or occlusion of the ETT lumen. Two points argue against this. Firstly, external pressure might harm the RLN. If airway pressures rise during instrumentation, the surgeons should be informed so that they can make adjustments. Secondly, the wire spiraling may interfere with intraoperative radiologic studies.

   Classically, the use of a rigid laryngoscope for intubation with midline stabolization (MILS) is considered a relatively rapid and reliable technique that might be preferred particularly in urgent situations. Nevertheless, considerable difficulty with this method can arise. Difficult intubation occurs in 1% to 13% of patients and impossible intubation in 0.05% to 0.35%. Complications from difficult intubation can be devastating and cervical SCI with poor mobility may result in difficult intubation.

No retrospective or prospective studies have shown adverse SNI subsequent to airway management, but isolated case reports have raised concerns about cervical motion. Of the case reports none had preoperative scans. Most but not all had unknown preoperative pathologic states with no attempt made to limit cervical motion and of the postairway management deficits, most were transient.

Both location and cause of cervical spine instability (bony vs. ligament abnormality) are significant to airway management if at-risk areas are more susceptible to movement following the use of intubation equipment. Routinely during rigid laryngoscopy (RL) usage, 40 N of force (750 mm Hg) is applied. With the dramatically lowered incidence of SNI following the EMS recommendations for spinal immobilization (one-tenth of that previously found), Crosby's editorial noted another finding [23]. In terms of airway management, the popularity of immobilization broadened into an extrapolation of two suppositions: (1) That RL intubation causes cervical spine movement and (2) that awake intubation, when a patient could "theoretically protect the cervical spine due to intrinsic muscle tone and vocalization of symptoms" may be better than asleep intubation.

MILS is a maneuver that was developed to limit neck motion during airway management. To perform MILS, an assistant severely braces both hands and forearms on either side of the patient's neck, between the clavicles and occipital/ear/mandibular/maxillary regions, while at the patient's side facing cephalad or by the head facing caudally. Radiologic studies reveal that MILS decreases RL-provoked movements by 25% to 100% [32].

Problematically, employing MILS can result in 50% to 100% incidence of Cormack–Lehane grade 3 or 4 views with a doubling of RL force in an attempt to intubate the trachea, and an intubation failure rate of 10% to 33%. A doubling of motion may be encountered while using MILS while using RL in cadavers having complete C4–C5 ligamentous laxity versus RL use alone, due to the difficult view [33].

In contrast to RL usage, flexible FOI has a 98% to 99% success rate in the operating room and causes virtually no cervical motion (<5% to 10% of that with RL) in both live subjects and cadavers [34]. Note that patients can self-position after awake intubation. In anticipation of awake-FOI, antisialagogue administration (glycopyrrolate) is advantageous when given 15 to 20 minutes beforehand, particularly if local airway anesthesia is intended. Sedation must be judicious to prevent respiratory arrest and many anesthesia providers advocate supplemental oxygen. Airway conditions should be perfect by instituting glossopharyngeal, superior laryngeal, and transtracheal anesthesia. These can be accomplished by a number of approaches. For patients with significant aspiration risks, to keep airway protection intact, the latter two blocks should be carried out moments before ETT insertion by using a "spray as you go" technique down the fiberscope at the vocal cords and intratracheally. This is followed by immediate fiberscope insertion, ETT insertion, and ETT cuff inflation. FOI may also be successful after induction of GA. Coughing with local anesthetic application has not caused SNI.

ETTs with centrally bending tips improve rates of successful passage over the fiberscope and through the glottis. However, use of regular polyvinyl chloride ETT can also be successful if the most distal tip is rotated 90° or 180° from its customary direction so that the Murphy eye is parallel to the patient's frontal or coronal plane.

Many other intubating devices can be utilized in both awake and asleep states. The introduction of the videolaryngoscope (VL) has given rise to many similar devices with ≤60 degree-angled MacIntosh-like blades including some with ETT-loading channels. Decreased spinal motion with VL devices has been attributed to their superior capability for laryngoscopic visualization and intubation. Crossover studies of normal patients with MILS found a 50% motion reduction in C2–C5 segments with the VL (Glidescope) in comparison to RL, with little difference at Oc-C1, C1-C2 or C5-T1. There is no question, however that the glottic views during MILS were better with the VL and that successful intubations had a higher likelihood. Patients placed in semi-rigid collars with their heads taped to trolleys while intubated with the RL resulted in modified Cormack–Lehane views of three and four almost 100% of the time. In contrast, the VL views were Grade 1 or 2 over 90% of the time [35]. The viewing difficulties were partially related to the collar's anterior portion effectively reducing the mean interdental distance to 2 cm. Rigid halo fixators are even more likely to produce a difficult airway.

Decreased spinal motion has been observed with other VLs and optical laryngoscopes including the Pentax Airway Scope and the Airtraq, which are associated with 40% and 66% less cervical spine motion, respectively at Oc–C1, C2–C5, and C5–T1. Differences were negligible at C1–C2 [36].

Lightwands are battery-powered, malleable stylet-like devices with distal bulbs that can be inserted in an L-shape within an ETT for blind placement through observation of transillumination in the neck, while room lights are darkened. Jaw manipulation transmitted to the spine from lightwand usage incurred 41% to 72% less motion than RL at multiple segments involving Oc–T1 while employing MILS in normal spine patients. Successful lightwand intubation has been observed at over a 95% rate with a single attempt in elective surgery patients.

The Fastrach is an intubating LMA that employs a fixed metallic body within a much more angulated LMA covering. It is frequently used for blind intubation with its specialized silicone ETT having a very soft, centrally directed tip. Blind intubation in cadavers with no spinal instability elicited 25% to 50% of extension at C1–C3 in comparison to RL extension. In cadavers with unstable spine and axial traction, the Fastrach produced up to 50% of the movement caused by RL. Similar motion findings have been noted in living subjects. What is the success rate? In patients with cervical immobilization and position adjustments, blind intubation was successful in up to 90% by the third intubation attempt, whereas with concomitant use of a flexible fiberoptic bronchoscope through the device, successful intubation approaches 100% [37].

The Bonfils intubation fiberscope is a malleable optical stylet. In comparison studies during fluoroscopy in living subjects, it causes less extension at C1–C2 and C3–C4 than a MacIntosh RL, but atlanto-occipital distance was slightly more reduced with the MacIntosh RL [38]. When compared to Fastrach, the success rate for Bonfils intubation was 100% by the second attempt.

Cricoid pressure is another airway management technique that tends to worsen laryngeal views. It also may cause more cervical spine motion.

(2) **SCI airway management outcomes and recommendations.** What is expert opinion on the best intubation approach for SCI patients? Two techniques cause virtually no motion: (1) FOI, which requires patient cooperation in awake subjects or may be an expensive asleep alternative and (2) BNI, which has a smaller intubation success rate and is risky for epistaxis or other injury. Interestingly, for SCI patients, neither technique has been shown to be safer than any other intubation method. Practice surveys have yielded figures showing that a majority of anesthesiologists favor awake-FOI in 65% to 78% of cooperative patients with unstable cervical spines [39]. For the patients chosen for GA, RL use has trended downward from 66% to 8% due to greater preferences for techniques such as FOI (75%), VL (8%), and Lightwand (8%).

There are no outcome data that would support a recommendation for a best intubation technique in cervical spine at-risk patients. Experts support the idea that whichever technique is most practiced by the airway management provider is thought to be the best plan, with the caveat to include MILS. This is accepted with the recommendation for MILS by the American College of Surgeons as outlined in the Student Course Manual (7th ed., 2004) of the Advanced Trauma Life Support Program for Doctors, the Eastern Association for the Surgery of Trauma, and by experts in anesthesiology, trauma, and neurosurgery.

For supine and perhaps lateral position surgeries, supraglottic airways (SGA) could be chosen. Rarely, but more commonly in Western Europe, SGA is used in the prone position with the patient's bed nearby. These choices would be more likely in simple, shorter duration surgery with normal low airway-risk patients. SGA do have an advantage for "smoother wake-up."

> **CLINICAL PEARL** There is no known "best intubation technique" in cervical spine at-risk patients to prevent SNI. Experts recommend whichever technique is most practiced by the provider with the caveat to include MILS. Techniques associated with less spinal motion while improving glottic views by 1 to 2 grades, such as FOI or videolaryngoscopic intubation, are preferred to direct laryngoscopic (DL) intubation.

    b. Extubation following SCI surgery. Smooth emergence and extubation after cervical spine surgeries eliminate "bucking," sympathetic excitation, hematoma formation, and stressing any recent fusion components. Multiple techniques have been tried to achieve this end with varying success. Choices range from ultrashort-acting narcotics such as remifentanil (average maintenance ranges are 0.03 to 0.05 μg/kg/min) until extubation to longer-acting drugs such as hydromorphone. Small, incremental doses of propofol, dexmedetomidine, and ketamine toward the end of surgery have been utilized. Turning off volatile agents and continuous anesthetic infusions while instituting high concentrations of nitrous oxide (60% if no IOM is ongoing) in the last 10 minutes of surgery is often helpful. Lidocaine has been used in a variety of routes: Intravenously 2 to 10 minutes before extubation (1.5 mg/kg), intratracheal as 4% LTA prior to intubation for surgeries ≤2 hours or placed within an ETT cuff (40 mg combined with 2 mL 8.4% sodium bicarbonate).

    "Deep extubation" when surgery finishes can be used to achieve a "smooth emergence/extubation" in a nonaspiration risk and nondifficult airway patient. Drawbacks include extra waiting time for a patient to awaken or miscalculation of the depth of anesthesia resulting in coughing, laryngospasm, and/or airway loss.

    To achieve the same goal in a similar type of patient, the Bailey maneuver is an alternative technique performed approximately 30 minutes before surgery ends [40]. Increased anesthetic and/or relaxant is administered to prevent reaction to ETT movement. A lubricated SGA is seated behind the ETT until at the appropriate depth. While bracing the SGA, the ETT is removed. Before ETT removal, if desired, a fiberscope can be inserted down the SGA to observe the ETT entrance into the glottis and assure correct SGA placement. Subsequently, the SGA is inflated and used to ventilate the patient until surgery ends for a smoother emergence.

> **CLINICAL PEARL** Multiple techniques aid in prevention of "bucking," sympathetic excitation, hematoma formation, and stress to recent fusion components. Choices range from the use of ultrashort-acting narcotics such as remifentanil (continued at 0.03 to 0.05 μg/kg/min until just after extubation) to anesthesia with longer-acting narcotics. Similar aids include small, incremental doses of propofol, dexmedetomidine, ketamine, lidocaine (1.5 mg/kg within 5 minutes of extubation), and high concentrations of nitrous oxide (if no IOM is ongoing), while tapering inhalational agents toward the end of surgery. "Deep extubation" and the Bailey maneuver are alternatives.

Administering β-blockers and/or antihypertensives to combat sympathetic effects can also be used as needed.

Another concern with emergence that is currently gaining increased attention is the problem of difficult extubation resulting in respiratory complications where risk was second only to aspiration during intubation. A threefold higher incidence of adverse events during extubation is likely versus those following difficult intubation.

Some spinal surgeries present this challenging question: "Can we successfully extubate this patient?" Predictors supporting continued postoperative intubation include fiberoptic evidence of tracheal edema, ACF surgery involving C2, greater than 4 cervical spine level ACF, operating time more than 10 hours, ≥4 units of blood transfusion, ACF reoperations, same sitting anterior–posterior cervical surgery, difficult airway, obesity >100 kg, and significant respiratory comorbidities [41].

In instances when there is a concern for airway edema secondary to fluid resuscitation, studies have shown that the cuff leak test can help determine the likelihood of successful extubation. In a spontaneously breathing patient with no muscle relaxant effect, the ETT is detached from the circuit, the cuff is deflated, and the connector is occluded. If good respirations are not observed around the ETT, this is a warning of upper airway obstruction risk. Cuff leak can also be measured by observing the difference between inspired and expired volumes of a spontaneously ventilating patient with a deflated cuff. If the difference is ≥110 mL, the test is passed. Likewise some providers measure this difference as a percentage where ≥10% is a pass. Ultrasound can also be employed to delineate the diameter of the air column within the larynx around the ETT to assist in predictions.

> **CLINICAL PEARL** Predictors supporting postoperative intubation include fiberoptic bronchoscope (FB) evidence of tracheal edema, a failed cuff leak test, ACF surgery involving C2, greater than four cervical spine level ACF, ACF reoperations, same sitting anterior–posterior cervical surgery, difficult airway, operating time >10 hours, transfusion ≥4 units PRBC, obesity >100 kg, and significant respiratory comorbidities.

If extubation success is considered quite likely but perhaps not 100%, the patient can be extubated over a "conduit" as a guide for reintubation. Any conduit must be at least 70 cm long. A conduit for expedited reintubation must be inserted so that its distal end remains just above the carina. It can be left in the patient for up to 24 hours (Fig. 12.3). The Cook airway exchange catheter, a Teflon guide catheter, and Aintree catheter are conduits whose advantage over a retrograde intubation guide wire is the capability of jet ventilation if ETT reinsertion becomes difficult. In addition, their greater degree of rigidity makes them better conduits. The wire has an advantage in that it can be threaded up a fiberscope via the working channel toward the control area. For reintubation the fiberscope can follow the wire toward the larynx. All conduits can suffer unrecognized dislodgement within the patient.

2. **Neuraxial anesthesia.** Spinal and epidural neuraxial blocks have had successful roles during elective non-injured lumbar spine surgery. Advantages of spinal anesthesia versus GA include patient self-positioning, reduced surgical time, less blood loss, minimal hypertension, and decreased postoperative pain and nausea. Both techniques have had similar success in American Society of Anesthesiologists (ASA) 1 to 4 patients having microdiskectomies, multilevel fusions, nerve root decompression, or hardware removal. Patients would be either lightly sedated and cooperative, or more heavily sedated with target-controlled infusions of propofol. Less than 4% required phenylephrine to maintain BP and 100% were successful with significantly more hemodynamic stability in sicker patients [42]. Other studies have elicited similar results with a lower incidence of DVT. Neuraxial anesthesia may be particularly advantageous in preventing autonomic dysreflexia reactions.

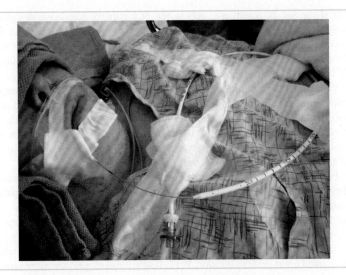

FIGURE 12.3 Cook retrograde teflon guide catheter placed through a pre-existing ETT during GA, followed by retrograde wire passage with subsequent withdrawal of the catheter and fixation of the wire.

When considering this anesthetic technique, surgeons must have sufficient surgical expertise to use this technique. Patients must be motivated with no contraindications, have adequate respiratory freedom, and be padded for comfort. Major concerns with this method include possibilities of increased risk for respiratory depression or airway obstruction, VAE because of spontaneous ventilation, delayed postoperative neurologic assessment, and medicolegal issues if neurologic damage is found postoperatively.

3. **Monitored anesthesia care and local anesthesia.** Monitored anesthesia care provides advantages of self-positioning and ongoing communication for clinical neurologic monitoring. Patient selection is similar to that for neuraxial blocks and risks are fewer and causes for new SCI injury are unlikely to be anesthetically related. Propofol (50 to 75 μg/kg/min) and small amounts of ketamine (0.67 to 1 mg/kg/h) cause minimal respiratory depression in most patients. Dexmedetomidine (1 μg/kg bolus over 10 minutes, followed by ~0.2 to 0.7 μg/kg/h) is even more advantageous because of analgesia, amnesia, sedation, and fewer effects on respiration. Titration of these regimens and judicious titration of supplementary narcotics is more efficacious while monitoring respiratory rate ($\geq$10 breaths/min), $PetCO_2 \leq 55$ torr, $SpO_2 \geq 92\%$ to 94%, and cerebral hypnotic measurement (bispectral index ~70). A Ramsay sedation scale (RSS) score of 2 or 3 should be maximal to prevent respiratory compromise.

4. **Monitoring, vascular access, drugs, and anesthetic choices.** Numerous monitors may crowd the operating room during SCI surgery: BP, electrocardiogram (EKG), pulse oximetry, neuromuscular stimulator, inspired and expired gas analysis, core temperature, urine output, arterial lines, central venous pressure (CVP) lines, IOM, precordial Doppler, and/or a cerebral hypnotic monitor (particularly useful to avoid awareness for TIVA or intravenous anesthesia plus low concentrations of inhalation anesthesia). Having two large-bore intravenous catheters is preferable if anticipating more than 1,000 mL blood loss. Central lines and excellent intravenous access are required for excessive losses.

Antibiotic prophylaxis is frequently administered within 1 hour of surgery or according to recommendations by institutional pharmacology/surgery protocols. This should be repeated intraoperatively for prolonged surgeries at appropriate intervals.

Anesthetic choices are driven by the desire for anesthesia, amnesia, analgesia, hemodynamic control, minimizing influences on IOM, and rapid postoperative awakening.

No single set of anesthetic agents for SCI surgery has been designated as the best possible choice. But some choices are better than others. One of them includes avoiding succinylcholine in patients with significant SCI beyond 12 to 24 hours of acute injury onset. This contraindication may last over 1 to 2 years or indefinitely, particularly with ongoing SCI pathology such as multiple sclerosis.

Pain control is tailored to a patient's age, weight, consciousness, preoperative analgesic requirements, and comorbidities. When significant pain is anticipated, drugs with longer half-lives such as fentanyl, hydromorphone, methadone, or morphine may be administered carefully. In anxious patients, particularly ones in considerable pain and who are on multiple analgesics preoperatively, low-dose ketamine and tranquilizers may prove to be of assistance, but must be used cautiously.

Prophylaxis and/or therapeutic measures against postoperative nausea and vomiting include antiemetic agents such as dexamethasone, ondansetron, compazine, transdermal scopolamine patch, and droperidol.

a. **Hemodynamics, fluid administration, and chemistries.** With pre-existing SCI, the operative team usually wants perfusion pressure ≥ high normal preoperative range, and if compromised enough, perhaps 10% to 20% higher. Acceptable BP should be agreed upon prior to incision. Periodically, patients who are more sensitive to anesthetics may need phenylephrine infusions as a complimentary background agent to offset vasodilatory effects. After a stable BP range has been achieved as a result of a constant rate of infusion for approximately an hour under conditions of varying surgical stimuli, reactions to subsequent increases or decreases in BP should not include changing the phenylephrine infusion rate. This will avoid masking circumstances where another factor is causing the hemodynamic change. In this case, the factor should be found and treated while other pharmacotherapies such as temporizing boluses of phenylephrine are delivered as short-term bridging measures. Of course, for extreme BP changes, this "background" agent infusion might need to be altered.

> **CLINICAL PEARL** An arterial line is recommended for BP, blood gas, and/or chemistry monitoring if there is a likelihood for new SCI, greater than two levels of open fusion, 1,000 mL blood loss, VAE, or the patient has significant comorbidities. More complex surgery such as greater than four levels of surgery, reoperation, or comorbidities may necessitate CVP monitoring and/or large bore intravenous access.

An arterial line is recommended for BP, blood gas, and/or chemistry monitoring if there is a likelihood for new SCI, greater than two levels of open fusion, 1,000 mL blood loss, VAE, or the patient has significant comorbidities. If more complex surgery is anticipated, such as more than four levels of surgery or reoperation, or if comorbidities warrant it, a CVP line is recommended. Assuming minor interim fluid administration and a decline to prepositioning BP has occurred following a supine to prone body change, a successful technique for situating the CVP transducer in prone patients is to place it at a level where the numerical value is identical to what it was while supine. In sitting positions, the arterial transducer should be kept at Circle of Willis level (external auditory meatus), while any intracardiac monitoring transducer is kept at right atrial level. Pulmonary arterial monitoring is indicated depending on pre-existing comorbidities such as congestive heart failure.

Minimizing undesirable hypotensive and vasoconstrictive effects on spinal circulation is more likely if patients are not hyperventilated.

Recommendations for fluid administration and chemistries for moderate to severe blood loss surgeries lasting more than several hours include nondextrose-containing crystalloid solutions to avoid deleterious neurologic associated effects of hyperglycemia. Large quantities of crystalloid (>2,000 to 3,000 mL) may be detrimental because of excessive extravascular accumulation.

Colloids and blood transfusions are administered as required to maintain acceptable blood volume, hemoglobin values, and avoid fluid overload. The ASA guidelines for high-risk spine surgery (HRSS) recommend a minimum hemoglobin range of 7 to 10 g% depending on comorbidities and rapidity of blood loss.

Among the colloids, high-molecular weight hetastarches (Hextend, Hespan) are often used for minor blood loss surgeries, but because they cause platelet dysfunction, dysfunction of clotting factors, and platelet surface coating, a consideration should be made to avoid using them when potential blood losses and/or development of coagulopathy are high (multiple level spine fusion, revision, or tumor surgery). Recently, some low- and medium-molecular weight hetastarches (Pentastarch, Voluven) have been shown to have lesser coagulopathic tendencies.

Pruritus is another adverse reaction caused by widespread deposition of hetastarch within macrophages, but relatively ignored by many caregivers. Bork et al. [43] reviewed reports of a 10% incidence of pruritus, frequently characterized as starting weeks after infusion, having a 44% refractory rate to treatment, and lasting 1 to 2 years. Pruritus tends to severely decrease patient's quality of life, cause sleep disturbances, and induce stress.

> **CLINICAL PEARL** High-risk spine surgery (HRSS) should prompt blood bank requests for availability of PRBC, platelets, cryoprecipitate, arginine vasopressin, coagulation factors, and/or FFP. Large quantities of crystalloid (>2,000 to 3,000 mL) may cause excessive extravascular accumulation. The ASA guidelines for HRSS recommend a hemoglobin 7 to 10 g% depending on comorbidities and rapidity of blood loss. Albumin is associated with less bleeding than high-molecular weight hetastarches and has less adverse effects.

While having similar half-lives and effects on oncotic pressure, the incidence of anaphylactoid reactions with hetastarches are 4.5 times that of albumin. Albumin has the advantage of a longer intravascular half-life than crystalloids with less tissue edema, better maintenance of BP (increased oncotic pressure), and at least equal safety to saline or hetastarch [44]. Albumin is associated with less bleeding than high-molecular weight hetastarches. Hetastarch had a 4.5% incidence of adverse events while the rate of 5% albumin's total adverse events was 6.1 to 6.8 per 10^5 infusions and for serious adverse events was 1.29 per 10^6 infusions.

Dealing with excessive blood loss can be effected by other methods. Cell-saver use is a consideration for major surgeries, particularly for anticipated losses over 2,000 mL. The technique cannot be used in infected cases, tumor surgery, or where red cell stasis and lack of oxygenation is a problem, such as sickle cell anemia. This method can be used occasionally along with hemodilution to decrease red blood cell loss in cases when nonautologous transfusion blood is unavailable because of matching problems, patients have a high risk of transfusion-related acute lung injury (TRALI); some Jehovah's Witness patients will accept its application. Hemodilution through infusion of 1,000 to 2,000 mL fluid is contraindicated in patients in whom volume overload might be detrimental.

An alternative technique, acute normovolemic hemodilution, involves the removal and storage at ambient temperature of a patient's own blood immediately before surgery, while maintaining euvolemia with crystalloids or colloids. Target hematocrits are usually 25% to 30%. Acute normovolemic hemodilution is contraindicated in the presence of severe anemia, infection, uncontrolled hypertension, or cardiopulmonary, renal, or hepatic disease. This time-consuming method requires intensive monitoring and may have only modest benefits in limiting blood loss or avoidance of allogeneic transfusions.

   b. Neurophysiologic monitoring and wake-up testing. IOM is an area of acute interest to anesthesia providers to (1) prevent injury from IOM, (2) understand IOM effects on anesthetic monitors and the patient's body, (3) limit impeding functions of IOM, (4) avoid mimicking or masking intraoperative neurologic injury, and (5) respond with therapeutic measures that might reverse deteriorating neurologic function [18]. Prior to patient anesthetization, collaboration with the surgical and IOM teams is useful to determine what types of IOM are planned so that the anesthetic agents and levels of perfusion pressure can be optimized for patient safety.

(1) **Prevention of injury from neurophysiologic monitoring.** Bite blocks prevent dental trauma during transcranial MEP stimulation.

(2) **IOM effects on patients and anesthetic monitors.** Transcranial electrical stimuli or application to peripheral nerves can also cause body movement which may interfere with surgery and cause concern that the patient is moving spontaneously. Awareness of this possibility will circumvent needless administration of anesthetic agents. IOM activity may additionally cause motion artifact and even interference with EKG, BP, or SpO_2 waveforms and number changes. In many IOM situations, saturations can plummet, BP can disappear, and the EKG can look like ventricular tachycardia. Lack of correct interpretation can lead to mistaken diagnoses. Checking BP cuff readings, feeling a pulse, and/or asking for a temporary cessation of IOM stimulation can differentiate IOM artifact from reality.

(3) **Anesthetic techniques to limit interference of IOM.** To prevent interfering with IOM anesthetic equipment and dressings for arterial lines should not inhibit placement of IOM electrodes.

During SSEP monitoring, IOM teammates may make requests to use muscle relaxants and/or increase anesthetic depth to prevent fine muscle movements, eliminate EP artifact, and improve "clean" waveform analysis. Conversely, volatile anesthetics cause dose-dependent drops in EP amplitudes and prolong latencies, confounding their interpretation [45]. For this reason, inhalation agents are kept at ≤0.5 MAC. For more sensitive potentials such as single/double impulse myogenic MEPs, even minute amounts of muscle relaxants cause inhibition, prompting avoidance of their usage.

(4) **Anesthetic drugs and interpretation of neurologic injury.** Since anesthetic-induced decreases in amplitudes and/or prolongations of SSEP and MEP latencies mimic neurologic damage, providers purposely maintain unchanging anesthetic levels to eliminate intermittent "worsening" or "improvement" in EP signals, which might confuse IOM interpreters. Although nitrous oxide has a negligible influence on latency, it is the most potent depressor of amplitude, and therefore, often excluded.

Muscle relaxants have similar dose-dependent effects but only on MEPs. The muscle relaxant effects on MEP thresholds show that NMB below 80% (<2/4) on the train of four is adequate for testing and was comparable to no blockade being present (assuming no pre-existing motor deficits). Many clinicians find that <45% to 65% NMB was acceptable and assists with prevention of movement during transcranial stimulation [46]. Of importance is that thresholds often are raised in nerve roots with a pre-existing state of chronic compression. In this situation, some chronically injured nerve roots might have added risk in the presence of muscle relaxants even though blockade was <80%. Because of this many providers avoid NMB.

Most intravenous agents have minimal depressant effects on SSEP, although barbiturates decrease MEP amplitudes considerably. Propofol infusions are frequent accompaniments to half-MAC inhalation usage. Assuming a compatible anesthetic regimen, EP decreases of ≥50% in amplitude and/or increases of ≥10% in latency are considered markers for new SCI through ischemia by direct pressure or indirect lack of oxygen supply (Fig. 12.4). Indirect factors might include surgical causes such as instrumentation interfering with blood supply, hypotension, or

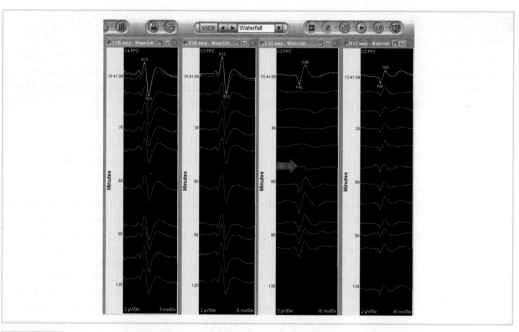

FIGURE 12.4 Waterfall SSEP during anterior–posterior fusion: The baseline EP waveforms are at at the top. The left two tracings show the left and right upper extremity responses and the right two tracings shown the left and right lower extremity responses. *Red arrow* points to the loss of left lower SEP resulting from iliac artery compression. (Photograph courtesy Mr. Carlos Munoz, Neurophysiology technician, Northwestern Memorial Hospital, Chicago.)

numerous other causes of poor oxygenation. Sensitivity can vary among different neural structures. For example, damage to a single dermatomal nerve root may not be noticed in SSEP or MEP tracings because multiple nerve roots are involved in the response. However, it could be very evident in the corresponding dermatomal EP waveform.

In the operating room prior to surgery, pre-existing SCI may result in initially impaired EP waveforms, necessitating TIVA to prevent volatile anesthetic effects. In some instances even after conversion to TIVA with no vestiges of inhalation agent, the initial EP signals may be almost nonexistent and monitoring might have to be abandoned. For these cases, etomidate or ketamine infusions may increase waveform amplitude 100% to 300% or more. In some circumstances this may make waveforms discernible and permit IOM. TIVA administration should not be scaled back by the addition of etomidate. A simple method includes administering two divided boluses of etomidate (0.15 mg/kg) 1 to 2 minutes apart, while observing for BP changes and treating them as needed. A constant infusion of 0.3 mg/kg/h is then begun. Administration can be stopped in the last 15 minutes or more of surgery. If EP amplitudes do not improve after the first 15 minutes of infusion, however, there is no need to continue. Many providers prefer to cover any cortisol depression with hydrocortisone (100 to 200 mg), although there is no evidence that this overcomes the drug effects [47].

In spite of having an augmenting effect on EP amplitude, ketamine is less likely to be used because of prolonged sedation. Does etomidate or ketamine use alter the interpretation of EPs? In other words, if surgery proceeds with interpretable EPs after institution of such an infusion and much later the markers for judgment of new SCI are reached, will the EPs' changes reflect SCI in exactly the same fashion as usual? No study has looked at these points.

CLINICAL PEARL The presence of presurgical impaired EPs may necessitate TIVA to prevent volatile anesthetic effects. In some instances, almost nonexistent initial EP signals might be improved 100% to 300% by etomidate or ketamine infusion to permit use of IOM throughout the surgery. If EP amplitudes do not improve after the first 15 minutes of infusion, however, there is no need to continue. To prevent masking injury these drugs should not be started for this purpose if EP responses spontaneously worsen during a case.

An important contraindication to infusion of these agents is that neither should be administered after intraoperative worsening of EP waveforms because these changes indicate that IOM unfavorable factors must be investigated to rule out new SCI.

(5) **Responses to deteriorating evoked potential signals.** Onset of abnormal EP changes should trigger a scan of the patient for causative factors. IOM interpreters should be checking equipment for malfunctions and testing to ensure that peripheral nerve injury is not the cause. Impaired perfusion or nerve compression in an extremity may worsen EPs, whether due to abnormal position, edema, or extrinsic pressure such as continuously inflated BP cuffs. Anesthetic factors mimicking neurologic injury include higher volatile anesthetic levels, muscle relaxants (if MEP used), hypotension, anemia, hypoxemia, hyperventilation, hypothermia, and extremity disorders. Surgical factors include instrumentation causing neurologic impingement, excessive distraction, massive bleeding, or vascular injury precipitating impaired extremity perfusion (Fig. 12.5). Adjustments by all personnel are made according to any discovered causative factors.

If no factor is present, consideration should be given to the possibility of local edema from tissue trauma at the surgical site, compromising nervous system perfusion. The anesthesia provider can institute deliberate hypertension by increasing BP ≥ 20% to 40% above previous levels to improve perfusion through this area. A case presentation at the 1996 Illinois Anesthesia Study Commission Meeting described a normotensive patient with a month-long history of 3/5 motor strength (no sensory loss) tetraparesis. Toward the end of a multilevel, decompressive cervical surgery, he developed worsening SSEPs with no obvious causative factor except for the possibility of surgical edema [48]. Almost complete resolution of changes occurred within 10 minutes of phenylephrine-induced deliberate hypertension by raising the MAP 30%. Strength testing after extubation was unaltered (3/5). The plan was to continue controlled hypertension in the postoperative anesthesia care unit (PACU) and ICU but twice, in the PACU, he deteriorated to 0/5 (complete motor and sensory loss tetraplegia) when the vasopressor was stopped for extraneous reasons. His MAP had drifted downward to within his normal preoperative range. Both times he recovered completely within minutes of restarting the infusion to keep the MAP 30% and then 40% above normal. High MAPs were kept for 48 hours in the ICU after which they were gradually and successfully tapered to normal levels. He was discharged with neurologic function identical to his preoperative status.

During placement of spinal hardware, if MEPs deteriorate intraoperatively or if only SSEPs are being monitored and they decline, without correctable causes, many surgeons will request the performance of a "wake-up test." This is a check for the presence of motor dysfunction and can be acted upon by surgical adjustments of instrumentation. Some surgeons routinely want testing after all major hardware insertions. Before performing the "wake-up test," the arms are immobilized to preclude injury. Anesthetic agents are eliminated as if awakening a patient toward the end of surgery, including full reversal of any muscle relaxants. At the appropriate moment, while holding the patient's head to prevent excessive motion or ETT dislodgement, the patient is reassured of the circumstances including inability to

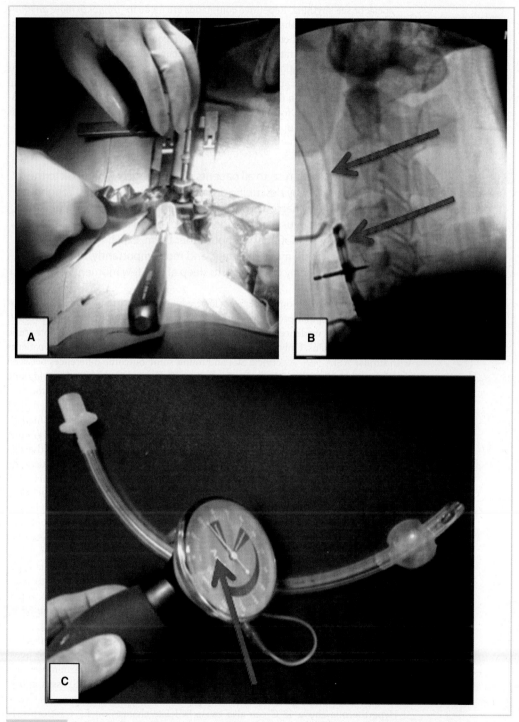

FIGURE 12.5 **A:** Anterior cervical fusion surgery with retractor pressure on airway; **B:** Radiographic evidence of close proximity of ETT and instrumentation (red arrows) anterior to cervical spine; **C:** Ambu manometer for cuff pressure assessment (blue arrow).

speak or see anything. Repetitive commands are made to "*try not to move anything unless told to do so.*" The patient is instructed to move an area thought to be neurologically intact, whether upper extremity (thoracolumbar surgery) or jaw (cervical surgery), to demonstrate presence of comprehension and response to command. Then, under observation by a teammate, movement of each at-risk extremity is requested. Once the appropriate response or lack of response is confirmed, half an intravenous induction dose is administered with return of prior continuous anesthetic agents (except for muscle relaxants). If readjustment of instrumentation is made, another wake-up test may be undertaken if EPs show no improvement.

CLINICAL PEARL   Explain the "wake-up test" to all patients preoperatively where risk to the motor system is possible. Allay anxiety by describing a similarity to being asleep throughout the surgery and waking up with heavy narcotics once the surgery is finished. Inform patients of having their eyes taped to prevent injury, and temporarily not being able to speak because of the "breathing tube" and that these probably will not bother them. Explain anticipated testing requests to squeeze their hands, move their feet, and most importantly, not move the rest of their bodies. Describe immediately going back to sleep after a few moments of testing.

c. **Temperature control.** Some caregivers have advocated the use of modest hypothermia (34.5°C) as a "spinal-protective" technique, similar to that for the brain. At present, no level I, II, or III evidence studies prove that outcomes are better with hypothermic techniques in humans. Only one retrospective analysis looked at two groups of patients with similar ASIA [49]. A cervical SCI and found some outcome differences between the groups: but 12 of the 14 hypothermic patients had spinal surgery within 24 hours, while only 7 of 14 normothermic controls were surgically treated within the same time period. Unlike any patients in the hypothermia group, the control group included three patients who were lost to follow-up and some patients who were treated with a methylprednisolone protocol. No statistical difference between groups for final ASIA grading was discovered but there seemed to be a trend toward better scores in the hypothermia group. Because of the group differences, it is difficult to evaluate the only statistically proven findings in the hypothermia group: An increased incidence of anemia (≥2.5 times that of the control) and pleural effusion (≥10 times the control) where $p = 0.01$ and 0.02, respectively. More study is needed in this area.

As discussed, significant difficulties can arise secondary to hypothermia. Core temperature drops can mimic neurologic injury by creating global EP amplitude decreases and latency increases.

Core temperature monitoring is important for prevention of hypothermia especially when large body surface exposure is present. Drops of 2°C are unlikely to cause significant bleeding diathesis but are associated with a higher propensity for wound infection. Regarding the coagulation system, the production of thromboxane B2 by platelets is decreased at temperatures <33°C, resulting in reversible platelet dysfunction. Greater degrees of hypothermia are also associated with prolongation effects of nondepolarizing muscle relaxants, interference with propofol and inhalation anesthetic kinetics, and postoperative shivering. Intravenous and body warming systems plus warmer room temperatures (69° to 70°F or 20° to 21°C for HRSS) assist in preventing excessive cooling.

Hyperthermia above 42°C can also cause SCI-like changes on EP waveforms. In addition, hyperthermia may have detrimental effects similar to those during cerebral hypoxia, at least on behavioral outcomes in the rat. Here, also, there are no definitive studies on effects related to human SCI patients.

d. **Monitoring/treatment of coagulation abnormalities.** HRSSs can be defined as those involving >6 spinal levels, >6 hours of surgery, complexity with a propensity for increased surgical risk, or patients with comorbidities that might impact on surgical outcome. Large blood losses are often accompanied by threatening decreases in coagulation factors usually at the 6-hour mark. Halpin et al.'s [50] review described a high-risk spine protocol to combat poor outcomes. In this HRSS protocol, arterial blood gases, sodium, potassium, calcium, glucose, lactic acid, hemoglobin, platelets, prothrombin time, partial thromboplastin time, and INR are measured every 2 hours until the 6-hour mark, and every hour, thereafter.

Cryoprecipitate is thawed at fibrinogen levels <200 mg/dL and administered at <150 mg/dL. Platelets are ordered when counts are <150,000/μL, and given at <100,000/μL. Desmopressin (0.3 μg/kg) is administered for oozing in spite of a platelet count >100,000/μL and normal fibrinogen. Recombinant factor VIIa (30 μg/kg) is given after desmopressin therapy if the INR is >2 and oozing is present. The protocol's main focus involves anesthesiologists, neurosurgeons, orthopedic spine surgeons, critical care physicians, and hospitalists in a multidisciplinary, methodized approach to assessing blood product losses and HRSS management. Most likely, protocols and recent advances such as continuous noninvasive hemoglobin monitoring devices can keep team members abreast of ongoing changes in the operating room in order to give appropriate therapy in a timely manner.

e. **Venous air embolism monitoring.** VAE during SCI surgery has the highest frequency in sitting cases. Since the spine is above heart level, low incidences during prone position surgery in the literature are most likely due to lack of monitoring and under-reporting, but the possibility of occurrence should not be discounted. Precordial Dopplers are underused because of effort needed to situate them with sufficient padding to prevent pressure injuries. Wills et al. [51] reviewed 53 reported, prone position VAE cases between 1995 and 2007, finding a 55% mortality rate. In addition to precordial Doppler and PetCO$_2$ monitoring for VAE, multiorificed CVP catheters (as opposed to multilumen) are recommended for sitting positions [52]. MicroDoppler catheters may be better for detecting emboli but need more investigation (see Chapters 21 and 22).

In contrast, VAE is rare in minimally invasive spine surgery while sitting, due to the small incision, making a CVP unnecessary. Studies find that a 0% incidence rate of VAE is most probable with ≤2 cm incisions in sitting microdiskectomy patients even while using nitrous oxide. Concern for VAE does not mean that nitrous oxide is a contraindication; rather, it should be eliminated if VAE transpires.

CLINICAL PEARL ACF surgeries are associated with RLN palsy due to dangers of nerve entrapment between the retractors and the ETT cuff. Test ETT cuff pressure during any retractor positioning to deflate them to just-seal pressures of 15 mm Hg or have the ETT recentered in the trachea with cuff adjustment. This can decrease the incidence of RLN palsy to <1/4 the 3.3% occurrence rate found in patients with "no-cuff adjustment."

---

f. **Prevention of recurrent laryngeal nerve palsy.** ACF or ACDF surgery is associated with RLN palsy due to dangers of nerve entrapment between the hardware and the ETT cuff (Fig. 12.5). Apfelbaum et al. studied 900 consecutive patients who underwent ACF surgery with plating. After the first 250 patients were intubated and cuffs inflated in "the normal fashion," ensuing patients had ETT cuffs kept at pressures of 15 mm Hg with pressure monitoring throughout the procedure. Cuff pressures rose to 40 to 52 mm Hg with surgical retractor placement. Consequently, they were deflated to just-seal pressures of 15 mm Hg or the ETT was recentered in the trachea with cuff adjustment. The incidence of RLN palsy was 3.3% in the "no-cuff adjustment" group, who had 5 times the chance of developing RLN paralysis. Permanent paralysis occurred in 3 of the 27 injuries. RLN complications were more likely with a history of previous anterior surgery, surgery near T1, or if multiple instrumentation levels were required [31].

TABLE 12.3 ASA advisory regarding ION and spine surgery

Preoperative advisories:
- Prone patients ≥6.5 h and/or blood loss ≥44.7% of estimated blood volume are at risk for vision loss.
- Inform HRSS patients of vision loss possibilities.
- Deliberate hypotension has not been associated with vision loss.

Intraoperative advisories:
- Colloids should be used with crystalloids to maintain volume in HRSS.
- No apparent transfusion threshold is recommended to eliminate vision loss.
- Maintain the head/neck neutral in a position at or higher than heart level when possible.
- Consideration should be given to staged spine procedures in HRSS.
- MAP should be maintained on average within 24% (range, 0%–40%) of estimated baseline MAP or with a minimum systolic BP of 84 mm Hg (range, 50–120 mm Hg).
- Central venous pressure monitoring should be used in high-risk patients.
- Hemoglobin should be maintained at a minimum average of 9.4 g/dL (range, 6–13 g/dL) or hematocrit 28% (range, 18%–37%).

g. **Ischemic optic neuropathy associations and advisories.** Spine, cardiac, dental, sinus, shoulder, and general surgeries have each been coupled with devastating, ophthalmologic complications. The occurrence of ION after spinal surgery is 0.2% [53], compared to a rate of ≥1% after cardiac surgery. In cases with visual loss, posterior ION, anterior ION, unspecified ION, and central retinal artery occlusion were causative factors in 60%, 20%, 9%, and 11% of the patients, respectively. Only 42% of all cases had at least partial recovery to "light/dark perception to hand motion" while bilateral loss was present in 30%. Age 50 years ±14 and male gender (72%) are among the demographic risk factors, while comorbidities include morbid obesity (53%), tobacco intake (46%), hypertension (41%), diabetes mellitus (16%), hyperlipidemia (13%), coronary artery disease (10%), or cerebrovascular disease (4%). In addition to the first four comorbidities, the 2006 ASA Practice Advisory for Perioperative Visual Loss Associated with Spine Surgery notes other influential factors: Preoperative anemia, glaucoma, and carotid artery disease. They also enumerated procedure-related risk factors: Surgical duration >6 hours (94%), blood loss >1,000 mL (82%), and prone positioning (72%) [54].

Theories for this complication include venous engorgement, increased intraocular pressure, and optic nerve compartment syndrome. What preventive measures can be taken? Conceivably, it may help to keep the patient as head-up as possible, increase perfusion pressure, prevent severe anemia, and perhaps have a preference for colloid fluids over crystalloids, to decrease extravascular edema. A number of salient points from the published advisory of the American Association of Anesthesiologists are summarized (see Table 12.3) [54].

Suspicions for this complication should prompt consultation with an ophthalmologist to assess vision. If loss is detected an MRI is necessary to rule out intracranial causes.

h. **Macroglossia.** Massive swelling of the tongue is another rare but impressive complication. Very likely, it develops from oropharyngeal pressure obstructing venous drainage, lymphatic drainage, and/or arterial perfusion. Lam et al.'s case report review from 1974 to 1999, in the sitting, park bench, prone, and supine positions, noted macroglossia incidences of 43%, 31%, 19%, and 6%, respectively [55]. Of these, 62% had more than one intraoral device. Keeping minimal number of objects in the mouth and preventing ETT impingement on the tongue is advised. Instead of "usual" bite blocks, very short, horizontally placed gauze blocks between the front teeth may be advantageous and can be taped in place to avoid falling out in the prone position.

i. **Knee chest position.** Some surgeons prefer "knee chest positions" for lower spine surgery by utilizing an Andrews table or Relton-Hall frame (Fig. 12.6). Achieving this position always seems to be a labor-intensive effort. Advantages include avoidance of epidural vein engorgement and better operative exposure with less injury risk to nearby

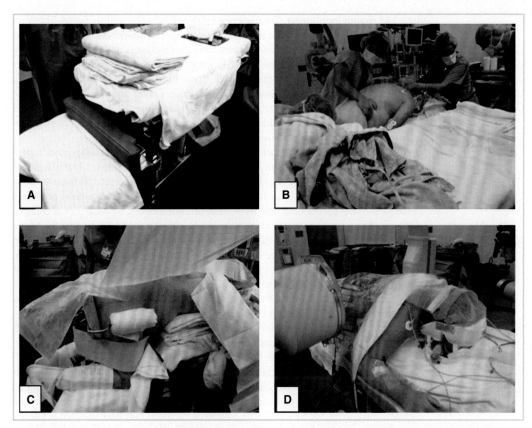

FIGURE 12.6 **A:** Andrews table; **B:** Moving the patient; **C:** Side view of strap supports; **D:** Upper body secured.

structures. Ventilation is relatively good but the CI can drop 20%. Compartment syndrome of the gluteal muscle region and the leg has been reported in some patients. Possibly, the cause is excessive hip and/or knee flexion precipitating a tourniquet-like effect.

j. **Lateral position.** Although less common during thoracic or lumbar surgery, this position may be chosen for expected lateral approaches or for patients who are too obese in other positions to allow adequate ventilation. It does restrict ventilation and drop CI. A 7.5% incidence of upper extremity SSEP abnormalities is twice that in the sitting position. An "axillary roll" should be placed under the chest wall near the axilla to avoid brachial plexus and long thoracic nerve palsy. Injury can occur to unpadded knees and to the peroneal nerve, particularly from bed straps.

5. **Positioning.** Positioning equipment requires: (1) A frame and/or bed, (2) supportive devices for the head and limbs, (3) adequate suspension in the air or padding (foam, donuts, heel cups) to guard against damage to pressure-liable points, and (4) safety straps, belts, tape, or beanbags. Elements that predispose to positioning complications include a large body mass index (BMI), older age, poor skin condition, range of motion limiters, implants, many comorbidities, and more complex surgery with "rougher" handling. Some clinicians feel that having an SCI or at-risk patient self-position is likely to suffer less nerve or pressure complications although there is no evidence of this in the literature. All common concerns for nonsupine positions are important in SCI patients.

a. **Prone position.** The prone position can be used for cervical, thoracic, and lumbar surgeries. Distribution of pressure points is important to prevent excesses in any single area; for the face this can be assisted by headframes, such as the ProneView Helmet System. After induction, this three-part frame is situated so that pressures are equally distributed to the forehead, cheeks, and chin, with the mirror's long axis perpendicular to the frame's long axis. This sideways rotation allows a wider view for intermittent eye, nose, and mouth monitoring. The neck must stay neutral or be slightly flexed. This "one size fits all" headframe does not fit everyone even with a towel between the forehead sponge and frame. Excessive chin pressure can cause ischemia and necrosis especially in heavier patients and prolonged surgeries where pinning is preferable.

This alternative is to use a Mayfield skull clamp for head support. Propofol (0.7 mg/kg), remifentanil (0.7 μg/kg), and esmolol (0.7 mg/kg) or similar regimens can blunt pinning stimulation in most hypertensive patients. Dosages are tailored to age, BMI, and health status. Keeping ≥3 cm chin to sternum or clavicle distance prevents excessive neck flexion and the patient's nose should be free.

Arms require padding, whether tucked by the sides or placed in a supported "superman" formation, with <90° flexion at the shoulders and elbows to prevent brachial plexus damage which has an incidence of 7%. Cylindrical axillary or chest roll foam in 6- to 8-inch lengths, placed vertically between the bed and the clavicle/acromial processes prevents shoulders from hunching over. IOM can often detect brachial plexus changes if the extremity position is not ideal, allowing modifications, which frequently return EPs to normal. An upright ETT elbow inhibits secretions from clogging the gas analyzer connection. Precautions must be taken for skin, joints, breasts, genitals, and so forth. Complications include injuries to other nerves such as the peroneal, the occurrence of meralgia paresthetica, and even tetraplegia from excessive neck flexion or extension.

Compression due to prone positioning increases intrathoracic pressure and decreases venous return, with declines in cardiac index (CI) approaching 24%. As stroke volume drops, systemic and pulmonary vascular resistances tend to rise. Patients with pre-existing pulmonary hypertension or cardiovascular compromise may develop life-threatening hemodynamic consequences.

What are the anesthetic effects? Interestingly, research work comparing TIVA with propofol versus isoflurane anesthesia discovered greater CI decreases on turning to the prone position in the propofol group (25.9% vs. 12.9%, respectively), with more hypotension and higher SVR [56]. The positional variation may have resulted in altered propofol pharmacokinetics.

Prone positioning can cause ETT migration toward the carina or endobronchially, with ensuing irritation, bronchospasm, shunting, and/or deoxygenation. External encroachment on the ETT lumen is particularly possible in scoliosis patients where the sternum and thoracic vertebrae may be in close proximity. Residual volumes are lower and airway pressures are higher with abdominal compression and restricted ventilation.

Prone compression of intra-abdominal contents tends to force intestines and the aorta toward the vertebra, increasing risks of surgical laceration. Higher intra-abdominal pressure increases pressure in venous conduits such as the inferior vena cava. This translates into more extradural venous plexus blood, a suboptimal surgical field, and greater blood loss. Restricted ventilation and hypercarbia can worsen vascular engorgement, which oddly, may be beneficial for avoiding VAE.

Increased lordotic curves close intralaminar spaces, causing worse surgical site viewing. A Wilson upwardly curved chest frame ameliorates this effect by supporting between the shoulders and hips while allowing the abdomen to protrude downward.

b. **Sitting position.** Advantages of sitting cervical surgery includes correct patient orientation, less blood in the field, better ventilation, less risk to eyes, and easier availability of the airway, chest, and limbs (see Chapter 21).

Hypotension is the most common adverse event when assuming the sitting position. Keeping lighter anesthetic levels, prior administration of 500 mL colloid to the average patient, constant arterial monitoring at the level of the Circle of Willis (external auditory meatus), and slow changes will tend to promote hemodynamic stability. Other possible difficulties and associated preventive actions include sciatic nerve injury (flex the hips and knees), cervical plexus injury (support under the forearms so they are not hanging), foot drop (employ a plantar support), VAE (use monitoring and avoid hypovolemia), macroglossia (avoid oropharyngeal pressure), and rarely, ventilatory restriction or compartment syndrome (examine high BMI patients to prevent abdominal pressure against flexed knees).

Further SCI and tetraplegia is one of the most feared, but rare complications of this position. Although reported in other positions, perhaps sitting seems so natural that it lends itself to excessive head and neck movement. Mechanisms responsible may involve impaired cervical spine perfusion from cervical spine stretching plus hypotension or thromboembolism. Pre-existing cervical spine pathology such as spondylitis has an increased association, requiring diligence to neck neutrality.

Sitting is contraindicated for patients with hypovolemia, low cardiac output states, pulmonary arteriovenous shunts, intracardiac shunts, and platypnea-orthodeoxia.

VII. **Immediate postoperative considerations.** Rapid awakening is desirable for assessing neurologic function. Most patients at risk for neurologic or medical compromise are sent to the intensive care unit (ICU).

During or after emergence from cervical spine surgery, signs of respiratory difficulty raise concerns for airway compromise from cervical edema and/or hematoma formation. However, the differential diagnosis of dyspnea must be considered to avoid missing other causes.

After any spinal surgery, the likelihood of successful extubation must be measured. Whether due to muscle weakness, edema, medical comorbidities, cervical manipulation, metabolic/respiratory disorder, or hematoma, patients who do not meet extubation criteria are often left intubated.

Reverse Trendelenburg can improve respiratory mechanics and lessen edema. However, after lumbar procedures, if CSF leak is possible, reverse Trendelenburg is discouraged to prevent increased CSF pressures tending toward further leakage and patency of a dural rent. For cervical rents this position is beneficial.

Intubated patients going to ICU are often sedated with short-acting infusions (propofol 50 μg/kg/min or dexmedetomidine 0.4 μg/kg/h) and/or narcotics so that neurologic testing can occur.

HRSS cases frequently require repeated laboratory studies if abnormalities are likely. Other testing depends on specific circumstances such as chest x-ray postcentral line insertion.

Pain control can be extremely difficult in patients who are already analgesic-dependent. Postoperative multidisciplinary pain control team interaction is highly advisable. Whenever possible, local anesthesia surgical site injections are useful for small-incision microdiskectomy or ACD surgery. A preoperatively designed oral multimodal analgesia regimen, utilizing a variety of nonnarcotics (acetaminophen, extended-release oxycodone, pregabalin, and gabapentin) may be assisted by narcotic bridging plans before a subsequent reinstitution of the regimen. Narcotic combinations with intravenous clonidine (3 to 6 μg/kg) and low-dose ketamine (83 μg/kg/h) have been efficacious in decreasing pain and narcotic requirements.

Patient-controlled epidural analgesia with 14 mL/h sufentanil (1 μg/mL) in ropivacaine 0.125% resulted in much better pain scores in comparison to intravenous patient-controlled analgesia with morphine 2 mg/mL when both were treated with appropriate boluses [57]. Benefits of epidural also include less nausea, vomiting, hypotension, and better gastrointestinal recovery. Fewer than 20% of the patients with spinal anesthesia had sensorimotor blocks of a short, transient nature. However, concern for hematoma, infection, and instrumentation impingement often make clinicians shy away from this technique. But some clinicians do place intrathecal narcotics either by direct injection intraoperatively or by intraoperatively placed catheters.

VIII. **Postoperative complications.** In the recovery room complications may arise that require immediate airway management. Uncommon but significant respiratory problems frequently involve entities such as postcervical surgery upper airway obstruction. More often, edema rather than hematoma is involved. Patients must be assessed for impending total obstruction and more than the simplest types of airway devices should be available including videolaryngoscopes, intubating supraglottic airways (Fastrach), flexible fiberscopes, and invasive airway equipment. Hoarseness of voice is often a heralding sign of airway compromise. Patients can be a particular challenge if lack of neck motion is important or if comorbidities might be adversely affected by hypoxemia and/or sympathetic discharge. It is important to follow the ASA difficult airway algorithm for approaches to difficult airways. A differential diagnosis of other respiratory problems encountered soon after surgery includes narcotic depression, secretions and laryngospasm, atelectasis, pulmonary edema, pulmonary embolism, pneumothorax, pneumonia, cardiac problems, allergic reactions, or TRALI.

CLINICAL PEARL   Postoperatively, respiratory obstruction is usually secondary to edema, not hematoma. Management includes assessment for impending total obstruction (hoarseness is a herald) and availability of a variety of airway devices: VL, intubating SGA, fiberscope, and invasive airway equipment. It is important to follow the ASA difficult airway algorithm. Remember a differential diagnosis of other respiratory problems.

Postoperative hemodynamic changes can develop such as hypertension due to pain. This is more of a problem for cervical surgery where hematoma and airway compromise is feared, in contrast to thoracolumbar surgeries. Treatment in this circumstance must be rapid to prevent the possibility of respiratory compromise. On the other hand, some patients may become hypotensive, particularly after HRSS cases. Differentiating blood loss and/or coagulopathy from drug or transfusion reactions and so forth may be challenging.

Compartment syndromes can also develop in the early postsurgical time frame and require rapid diagnosis and surgical correction.

IX. Summary. A thorough knowledge of anatomy and preoperative patient status, all phases of planned surgery including the impact of the entire anesthetic process, and postoperative diagnosis and treatment of adverse effects is the key to successful SCI surgical anesthesia. Diverse areas involving medications, airway management, hemodynamic monitoring, IOM, positioning, and postanesthetic care provide fascinating challenges. Key elements including team communication, planning, and specific protocols can facilitate approaches to problems as they arise. An array of tools and alternatives for each possible scenario is obligatory and enables anesthesia providers to stretch beyond simple single method techniques and escape narrow focusing on approaches to solutions.

REFERENCES

1. Standring S, ed. Section Editor: Newell RL. *Gray's Anatomy. The Anatomical Basis of Clinical Practice.* 40th Ed 2011. Elsevier.
2. Hata T, Todd MM. Cervical spine considerations when anesthetizing patients with Down syndrome. *Anesthesiology.* 2005;102(3):680–685.
3. Shields RW Jr. Functional anatomy of the autonomic nervous system. *J Clin Neurophysiol.* 1993;10(1):2–13.
4. Kudo K, Terae S, Asano T, et al. Anterior spinal artery and artery of Adamkiewicz detected by using multi-detector row CT. *AJNR Am J Neuroradiol.* 2003;24:13–17.
5. Nathan PW, Smith MC, Deacon P. The corticospinal tracts in man. Course and location of fibres at different segmental levels. *Brain.* 1990;113:303–324.
6. Hickey R, Albin MS, Bunegin L, et al. Autoregulation of spinal cord blood flow: is the cord a microcosm of the brain? *Stroke.* 1986;17(6):1183–1189.
7. American Spinal Injury Association. *International Standards for Neurological Classifications of Spinal Cord Injury,* revised ed. Chicago, IL: American Spinal Injury Association; 2000:1–23.
8. Dumont RJ, Okonkwo DO, Verma S, et al. Acute spinal cord injury, part I: pathophysiologic mechanisms. *Clin Neuropharmacol.* 2001;24(5):254–264.
9. Ditunno JF, Little JW, Tessler A, et al. Spinal shock revisited: a four-phase model. *Spinal Cord.* 2004;42:383–395.
10. Bilello JF, Davis JW, Cunningham MA, et al. Cervical spinal cord injury and the need for cardiovascular intervention. *Arch Surg.* 2003;138(10):1127–1129.
11. Krassioukov A, Warburton DE, Teasell R, et al. A systematic review of the management of autonomic dysreflexia after spinal cord injury. *Arch Phys Med Rehabil.* 2009;90(4):682–695.
12. Tator CH, Benzel EC., eds. Contemporary management of spinal cord injury: From impact to rehabilitation. *Thieme. 2nd ed.* Jan 1, 2000:27–28.
13. Schneider RC, Cherry G, Pantek H. The syndrome of acute central cervical spinal cord injury; with special reference to the mechanisms involved in hyperextension injuries of cervical spine. *J Neurosurg.* 1954;11(6):546–577.
14. Brown R, DiMarco AF, Hoit JD, et al. Respiratory dysfunction and management in spinal cord injury. *Respir Care.* 2006;51(8):853–870.
15. Baker RI, Coughlin PB, Gallus AS, et al. Warfarin reversal: consensus guidelines, on behalf of the Australasian Society of Thrombosis and Haemostasis. *Med J Aust.* 2004;181(9):492–497.
16. Holmes JF, Akkinepalli R. Computed tomography versus plain radiography to screen for cervical spine injury: a meta-analysis. *J Trauma.* 2005;58(5):902–905.
17. Stiell IG, Clement CM, McKnight RD, et al. The Canadian C-spine rule versus the NEXUS low-risk criteria in patients with trauma. *N Engl J Med.* 2003;349(26):2510–2518.
18. Sloan TB, Heyer EJ. Anesthesia for intraoperative neurophysiologic monitoring of the spinal cord. *J Clin Neurophysiol.* 2002;19(5):430–443.
19. Meyerding HW. Spondylolisthesis. *Surg Gynecol Obstet.* 1932;54:371–377.
20. Layton KF, Thielen KR, Koch CA, et al. Vertebroplasty, first 1000 levels of a single center: evaluation of the outcomes and complications. *AJNR Am J Neuroradiol.* 2007;28:683–689.

21. McDonnell MF, Glassman SD, Dimar JR 2nd, et al. Perioperative complications of anterior procedures on the spine. *J Bone Joint Surg Am.* 1996;78(6):839–847.

22. Vale FL, Burns J, Jackson AB, et al. Combined medical and surgical treatment after acute spinal cord injury: results of a pro-spective pilot study to assess the merits of aggressive medical resuscitation and blood pressure measurement. *J Neurosurg.* 1997;87:239–246.

23. Crosby T. Airway management in adults after cervical spine trauma. *Anesthesiology.* 2006;104:1293–1318.

24. Martyn JA, Richtsfeld M. Succinylcholine-induced hyperkalemia in acquired pathologic states: etiologic factors and molecular mechanisms. *Anesthesiology.* 2006;104(1):158–169.

25. Chan D, Goldberg R, Tascone A, et al. The effect of spinal immobilization on healthy volunteers. *Ann Emerg Med.* 1994;23(1):48–51.

26. Bracken MB, Shepard MJ, Collins WF. et al. Methylprednisolone or naloxone treatment after acute spinal cord injury: 1 year follow-up data. *J Neurosurg.* 1992;76:23–31.

27. Bracken MB, Shepard MJ, Holford TR, et al. Administration of Methylprednisolone for 24 or 48 Hours or Tirilazad Mesylate for 48 Hours in the Treatment of Acute Spinal Cord Injury. *JAMA.* 1997;277(20):1597–1604.

28. Short DJ, El Masry WS, Jones PW. High dose methylprednisolone in the management of acute spinal cord injury - a systematic review from a clinical perspective. *Spinal Cord.* 2000;38(5):273–286.

29. Vaccaro AR, Daugherty RJ, Sheehan TP, et al. Neurologic outcome of early versus late surgery for cervical spinal cord injury. *Spine.* 1997;22:2609–2613.

30. Siepe CJ, Zelenkov P, Sauri-Barraza JC, et al. The Fate of Facet Joint and Adjacent Level Disc Degeneration Following Total Lumbar Disc Replacement: A Prospective Clinical, X-Ray, and Magnetic Resonance Imaging Investigation. *Spine.* 2010;35(22):1991–2003.

31. Apfelbaum RI, Kriskovich MD, Haller JR. On the incidence, cause, and prevention of recurrent laryngeal nerve palsies during anterior cervical spine surgery. *Spine (Phila Pa 1976).* 2000;25(22):2906–2912.

32. Turner CR, Block J, Shanks A, et al. Motion of a cadaver model of cervical injury during endotracheal intubation with a bullard laryngoscope or a MacIntosh blade with and without in-line stabilization. *J Trauma.* 2009;67(1):61–66.

33. Thiboutot F, Nicole PC, Trépanier CA, et al. Effect of Manual in-line stabilization of the cervical spine in adults on the rate of difficult orotracheal intubation by direct laryngoscopy: A randomized controlled trial. *Can J Anesthe.* 2009;56(6):412–418.

34. Wong DM, Prabhu A, Chakraborty AS, et al. Cervical spine motion during flexible bronchoscopy compared with the Lo-Pro GlideScope®. *Br J Anaesth.* 2009;102:424–430.

35. Robitaille A, Williams S, Tremblay M, et al. Cervical spine motion during tracheal intubation with manual in-line stabilization: Direct laryngoscopy versus GlideScope® videolaryngoscopy. *Anesth Analg.* 2008;106:935–941.

36. Maruyama K, Yamada T, Kawakami R, et al. Upper cervical spine movement during intubation: Fluoroscopic comparison of the AirWay Scope, McCoy Laryngoscope, and Macintosh laryngoscopy. *Br J Anaesth.* 2008;100(1):120–124.

37. Bilgin H, Bozkurt, M. Tracheal intubation using the ILMA, C-TrachTM or McCoy laryngoscope in patients with simulated cervical spine injury. *Anaesth.* 2006;61:685–691.

38. Rudolph C, Schneider JP, Wallenborn J, et al. Movement of the upper cervical spine during laryngoscopy: a comparison of the Bonfils intubation fibrescope and the Macintosh laryngoscope. *Anaesth.* 2005;60:668–672.

39. Manninen PH, Jose GB, Lukitto K, et al. Management of the airway in patients undergoing cervical spine surgery. *J Neurosurg Anesthesiol.* 2007;19:190–194.

40. Nair I, Bailey PM. Review of uses of the laryngeal mask in ENT anaesthesia. *Anaesth.* 1995;50:898–900.

41. Epstein NE, Hollingsworth R, Nardi D, et al. Can airway complications following multilevel anterior cervical surgery be avoided? *J Neurosurg.* 2001;94(2 suppl):185–188.

42. Goddard M, Smith P, Howard C. Spinal anaesthesia for spinal surgery. *Anaesth.* 2006;61(7):723–724.

43. Bork K. Pruritus precipitated by hydroxyethyl starch: a review. *Br J Dermatol.* 2005;152(1):3–12.

44. Finfer S, Bellomo R, The SAFE Study Investigators, et al. A comparison of albumin and saline for fluid resuscitation in the intensive care unit. *N Engl J Med.* 2004;350:2247–2256.

45. Banoub M, Tetzlaff JE, Schubert A. Pharmacologic and physiologic influences affecting sensory evoked potentials. *Anesthesiology.* 2003;99:716–737.

46. van Dongen EP, ter Beek HT, Schepens MA, et al. Within-patient variability of myogenic motor-evoked potentials to multipulse tran-scranial electrical stimulation during two levels of partial neuromuscular blockade in aortic surgery. *Anesth Analg.* 1999;88:22–27.

47. Payen JF, Dupuis C, Trouve-Buisson T, et al. Corticosteroid after etomidate in critically-ill patients; a randomized controlled trial. *Crit Care Med.* 2012;20(1):29–35.

48. Gil KS. Case Presentation: Intraoperative reversal of SSEP changes and postoperative reversal of two episodes of new-onset quadriplegia occurring in the recovery room. Illinois Anesthesia Study Commission Meeting. 1996.

49. Levi AD, Casella G, Green BA, et al. Clinical outcomes using modest intravascular hypothermia after acute cervical spinal cord injury. *Neurosurgery.* 2010;66(4):670–677.

50. Halpin RJ, Sugrue PA, Gould RW, et al. Standardizing care for high-risk patients in spine surgery: the Northwestern high-risk spine protocol. *Spine (Phila Pa 1976).* 2010;35(25):2232–2238.

51. Wills J, Albin MS. Outcomes after Venous Air Embolism in the Prone Position during Spine Surgery – a Cause for Alarm. *ASA Abstracts.* 2008; A240.

52. Bunegin L, Albin MS, Helsel PE, et al. Positioning the right atrial catheter: a model for reappraisal. *Anesthesiology.* 1981;55:343–348.

53. Stevens WR, Glazer PA, Kelley SD, et al. Ophthalmic complications after spinal surgery. *Spine.* 1997;22:1319–1324.

54. Practice Advisory for Perioperative Visual Loss Associated with Spine Surgery. A Report by the American Society of Anesthesiologists Task Force on Perioperative Blindness. *Anesthesiology.* 2006;104:1319–1328.

55. Lam AM, Vavialala MS. Macroglossia: Compartment syndrome of the tongue. *Anesthesiology.* 2002;92(6):1832–1835.

56. Sudheer PS, Logan SW, Ateleanu B, et al. Haemodynamic effects of the prone position: a comparison of propofol total intrave-nous and inhalation anaesthesia. *Anaesthesia.* 2006; 61: 138–141.

57. Schenk M, Putzier M, Kugler B, et al. Postoperative analgesia after major spine surgery: Patient-controlled epidural analgesia versus patient-controlled intravenous analgesia. *Anesth Analg.* 2006;103(5):1311–1317.

13 Anesthesia for Intramedullary Spinal Cord Tumors

Stacie Deiner

KEY POINTS

1. Spinal cord tumors may be primary tumors of the spinal cord or secondary to metastases.
2. The type of tumor and surgical procedure will influence the choice of neuromonitoring, appropriate venous access, and need for invasive monitoring.
3. Intraoperative neuromonitoring can provide important information and the anesthesiologist can facilitate acquisition of signals by creating a supportive anesthetic plan.

I. Introduction

A. Spinal cord tumors: An unusual cause of back pain. The majority of spinal surgery is precipitated by a painful condition or neurologic deficit. Although spinal cord tumors are an unlikely cause of back pain, anesthesia for patients with a spinal cord tumor for surgical resection has important anesthetic considerations and merits discussion. Spinal cord tumors may be primary tumors of the spinal cord or secondary to metastases.

B. Spinal cord tumor chapter organization. We will begin with a description of the different types of spinal cord tumors and their treatment and prognosis. The remainder of the chapter will focus on intramedullary spinal cord tumors. We will discuss in depth the preoperative evaluation and intraoperative management of the patient presenting with a spinal cord tumor for surgical resection.

II. Evaluation of spinal cord tumors

A. Tumor types. Spinal cord tumors are classified according to their location: Extradural, intradural-extramedullary, and intramedullary-intradural (Fig. 13.1).

1. **Extradural tumors.** Extradural tumors are the most common type of spinal cord tumors, the most common of which are secondary metastatic lesions arising from the vertebral bodies. In contrast, primary extradural tumors are less common; an example is a chordoma.

2. **Intradural-extramedullary.** These tumors are located within the dura but outside the spinal cord. Examples of these are meningiomas and nerve sheath tumors. Meningiomas arise from arachnoid cells and are sometimes found in association with neurofibromas.

3. **Intramedullary-intradural tumors.** The majority of intramedullary tumors are subtypes of gliomas which bear histologic resemblance to normal glial cells. These include ependymomas, astrocytomas, and oligodendrogliomas.

B. Clinical presentation. Spinal cord tumors often cause symptoms secondary to disruption of neural pathways through extrinsic or intrinsic compression of normal neural tissue. Symptoms may be localized to the site of the tumor, or have distant effects. In the case of

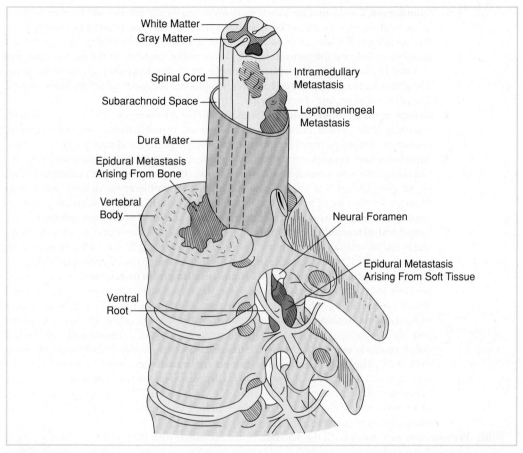

White Matter
Gray Matter
Spinal Cord
Subarachnoid Space
Dura Mater
Epidural Metastasis
Arising From Bone
Vertebral
Body
Ventral
Root
Intramedullary
Metastasis
Leptomeningeal
Metastasis
Neural Foramen
Epidural Metastasis
Arising From Soft Tissue

FIGURE 13.1 Original from Stubblefield and O'Dell's "Principles and Practice of Cancer Rehabilitation," Demos Medical Publishing.

the benign tumors, the disease process may be indolent and patients may have localized pain for months or years prior to diagnosis. Classically the pain is described as gnawing and unremitting and may result in nocturnal awakening [1]. Neurologic deficits may occur due to interruption of the spinal cord pathways and may be either sensory or motor. Often the symptoms are unilateral and then may progress to bilateral disease. In severe cases, cauda equina syndrome can occur.

C. **Treatment of spinal cord tumors.** The treatment for almost every spinal cord tumor involves surgical resection; the type of tumor determines whether adjunctive therapy with chemotherapeutic agents or radiation is indicated. If the patient has received chemotherapeutic agent, the anesthesiologists should familiarize themselves with the potential side effects. For example, cisplatin is associated with nephrotoxicity and electrolyte disturbance, and sirolimus is associated with thrombocytopenia. In all cases, complete resection is rarely a guarantee of cure. In many of the primary tumors, 5-year survival is >70%, but recurrence is likely.

CLINICAL PEARL   If the patient has received chemotherapeutic agent, the anesthesiologists should familiarize themselves with the potential side effects.

1. **Chordomas.** Chordomas are rare tumors which are locally invasive and frequently recur. Wide local excision is attempted, although complete resection is often not possible [2]. Postoperative radiation therapy is frequently employed [3]. Chemotherapeutic agents with activities include the following: Imatinib plus or minus cisplatin, sirolimus, sunitinib, and erlotinib [4]. Sarcomas and lymphomas may be primary or secondary disease in the spine. These tumors are generally treated with a multimodal approach, which includes surgical resection, radiation, and chemotherapy.

2. **Benign primary bone lesions.** These may occur in the spine and are treated with resection alone. These include osteoid osteomas, osteoblastomas, osteochondromas, chondroblastomas, giant cell tumors, vertebral hemangiomas, and aneurysmal bone cysts.

3. **Intramedullary tumors.** Intramedullary gliomas are preferentially treated surgically [5]. The initial step is an attempt at curative resection. There have not been randomized trials of radiation therapy. The roles of radiotherapy and chemotherapy have been as adjuvants to surgery in the case of noncurative resections or recurrence. The most recent guidelines suggest that patients who have had curative resections should not receive radiation.

4. **Intradural-extramedullary tumors.** These tumors include meningiomas, schwannomas, and ependymomas and are preferentially treated with surgery. Radiation has been used for recurrence which is not amenable to resection; chemotherapy is not indicated [6,7].

5. **Treatment options for spinal cord tumors resulting from metastases.** Several cancers are likely to result in metastases to the spine; 90% of patients dying of prostate cancer and 75% of patients dying of breast cancer have metastases to the spine [8]. Metastatic cancer of the spine may require surgical treatment when it results in a pathologic fracture causing pain and instability or epidural spinal cord compression (ESCC) resulting in a neurologic deficit or cauda equina syndrome. Vertebral metastases are significantly more common than ESCC. The three most common tumors are prostate cancer, breast cancer, and lung cancer. Use of radiation or chemotherapy is dependent on the type of tumor.

   Because of their potential for invasion of local tissues and generous blood supply, the resection of metastatic lesions of the spine can have significant potential for intraoperative blood loss (especially metastatic renal cell carcinoma).

III. Preoperative assessment. All the standard issues associated with the preparation of any patient for anesthesia apply to patients with spinal tumors, including an underlying understanding of their physical status, their medication regimens, any potential allergies, and their surgical history. In addition, preparation for anesthetic care of patients with spinal tumors starts with an understanding of the chief complaint that brought the patient to surgery.

A. Pain. Pain is the most common symptom present among patients with spinal cord tumors and may be associated with varying levels of neurologic deficit. Use and schedule of pain medications should be noted, including current medications and medications used previously. This history will help the anesthesia team instruct the patients how to manage their medication regimen prior to surgery, will influence the intraoperative approach, particularly for opioid usage, and will assist in managing acute postoperative pain.

> **CLINICAL PEARL** Pain is the most common symptom present among patients with spinal cord tumors and may be associated with varying levels of neurologic deficit.

1. **Opioids.** Use of transdermal systems, for example, fentanyl patch should also be continued, although not necessarily initiated. If an opioid-tolerant patient is unable or does not take his pain medication on the morning of surgery, then the patient's daily opioid consumption should be calculated and converted into the equivalent intravenous morphine dosage. This calculation will provide the anesthesiologist with an approximate idea of the patient's daily opioid intake, some of which will have to be given intravenously during the surgery. The details of converting the patient's oral opioids to an intravenous dose is somewhat controversial, however the underlying principle is correct; namely that surgical patients who are opioid tolerant will require opioid dosing based on their previous consumption [9].

Some patients with spinal cord tumors have been taking extremely high doses of opioid medication for an extended period of time. The perioperative period is not an appropriate time to attempt to wean these medications. For patients with drug-seeking behavior, attempting to minimize analgesic consumption in the perioperative period is ill-advised.

2. **Adjuncts.** Continuation of adjunctive medications like gabapentin is recommended; however, use of nonsteroidal anti-inflammatory drugs (NSAIDs) should be discussed with the surgeon because of the potential for postoperative bleeding. Implementing gabapentin therapy immediately prior to surgery is controversial. While gabapentin has been shown to decrease postoperative morphine requirements, effective dosages can be associated with significant side effects, most notably dizziness [10]. A recent study found that beginning a preoperative multimodal regimen of medications, including gabapentin, acetaminophen, and an oral opioid, continued into the perioperative period was associated with better pain control and fewer side effects than intravenous morphine PCA [11].

B. **Neurologic deficits.** The presence of weakness, paresthesias, and bowel or bladder function should be documented in the preoperative record. The neurologic history will determine how the patient is moved and positioned as well as the quality of the neuromonitoring signals which can be expected.

C. **Location and etiology.** Some types of tumors may be located at the skull base or cervical cord and/or be associated with a syrinx. In these cases, particular attention should be paid to the stability of the cervical spine and any concerns related to manipulating the cervical spine during endotracheal intubation. The anesthesia team should be aware of the primary cancer when metastatic disease is suspected, including an appreciation for the therapies that have been received to date, including surgeries, chemotherapy, and/or radiation. The presence of metastatic disease in other areas of the body may raise important considerations. Breast and lung cancers may also have concomitant metastases to the brain, potentially resulting in space-occupying lesions. Patients who have undergone breast cancer surgery with axillary node dissection may not be able to have intravenous access or noninvasive blood pressure monitoring on that side.

CLINICAL PEARL   Some types of tumors may be located at the skull base or cervical cord and/or be associated with a syrinx. In these cases, particular attention should be paid to the stability of the cervical spine and any concerns related to manipulating the cervical spine during endotracheal intubation.

D. **Multidisciplinary preoperative care.** The ideal preoperative preparation would optimize patient outcomes with a multidisciplinary approach. One study reported improved outcomes with active efforts of presurgical rehabilitation. The study protocol included an intensive exercise and nutrition program, and optimization of the analgesic treatment. The early postoperative rehabilitation included balanced pain therapy with self-administered epidural analgesia, doubled intensified mobilization, and protein supplements [12]. In this small study, patients in the intervention group reached the recovery milestones faster than the control group (1 to 6 days vs. 3 to 13 days), and left hospital earlier (5 [3–9] vs. 7 [5–15] days).

IV. **Intraoperative management**

A. **Induction and maintenance.** The plan for induction and maintenance of anesthesia should be established with respect to the patient's medical comorbidities and in concert with the neuromonitoring plan.

1. **Neuromonitoring.** While standard of care for neuromonitoring during spinal cord tumor surgery has not been established, multimodality monitoring with motor evoked potential (MEP), somatosensory evoked potential (SSEP), and electromyography (EMG) is useful and common (see Chapter 26). The use of intraoperative SSEPs, MEPs, and EMG allows for continual intraoperative assessment of the dorsal columns, anterior spinal cord, and nerve roots. In deformity surgery and tumor surgery, several studies have demonstrated that no single modality monitors the entire spinal cord [13,14]. When used in combination with SSEP, MEPs are associated with a higher sensitivity and specificity of motor tract

injury than single modality monitoring [15]. Utility of monitoring for spinal tumor surgery in specific includes dorsal column mapping during intramedullary surgery and evaluation of temporary clipping of spinal nerve roots in thoracic tumor resection [16].

The anesthesiologist must be aware of which monitoring modalities will be utilized during the surgery, since each has anesthetic implications.

> **CLINICAL PEARL**   While standard of care for neuromonitoring during spinal cord tumor surgery has not been established, multimodality monitoring with MEP, SSEP, and EMG is useful and common (see Chapter 26).

> **CLINICAL PEARL**   SSEPs and MEPs are sensitive to all anesthetic agents (inhalational >> intravenous), while MEPs and EMGs are sensitive to paralytic drugs. Although initial studies suggested that <0.5 MAC of inhalational agent still allow for adequate monitoring of signals, a recent study suggests that this may not be the case for older patients with diabetes and/or hypertension [17].

2. **Anesthetics and neuromonitoring.** Management of TIVA during spine surgery and neuromonitoring for the patient with a spinal cord tumor has several goals, which may be challenging to achieve simultaneously. Often the patient needs to be immobile without the use of paralytic medication, have steady state anesthesia compatible with neuromonitoring, and maintain adequate blood pressure to avoid blindness, loss of neuromonitoring signals, and perfusion pressure to the vital organs. In addition, rapid awakening after surgery is desirable to facilitate a neurologic examination. The anesthesiologist should be aware of the context-sensitive half-time of the agents they are using, and whether their patient has any renal or hepatic insufficiency, which may further complicate the recovery from intravenous anesthetic infusions.

   a. **Timing.** An anesthetic technique compatible with consistent IOM needs to be established well in advance to obtain monitoring signals. This is important because the transition from the relatively rapid dissipation of inhalational agents to the relatively slower onset of steady state blood levels of drug infusion may take significantly longer than several minutes when not temporally associated with an induction dose.

   b. **Specific anesthetic agents.** The anesthesiologist should select a combination of agents with a favorable effect profile and start their maintenance infusion around the time of induction (Table 13.1). Examples include the addition of ketamine to a propofol infusion and the use of dexmedetomidine to decrease propofol and opioid requirements. If it is necessary to use inhalational agents (e.g., propofol shortage, patient history of adverse reaction, expense of TIVA), then there must be clear communication with the monitoring team. A single gas, either halogenated agent or nitrous oxide should be used. In any

TABLE 13.1   Anesthetics and evoked potentials

	Latency	Amplitude
Halogenated agents	increase	decrease
Nitrous oxide	increase	decrease
Narcotics	mild increase	mild decrease
Benzodiazepines	minimal effect	mild decrease
Barbiturates	increase	decrease
Propofol	increase	decrease
Dexmedetomidine[a]	minimal effect	mild decrease
Ketamine	decrease	increase
Etomidate	decrease	Increase

[a]At clinically relevant concentrations.

case, whichever technique used during the acquisition of baseline signals must be continued throughout the case to avoid loss of signals at the critical portions of the procedure.

(1) **Intravenous anesthetics.** The effect of intravenous agents on evoked potentials is related to their affinity for neurotransmitter receptors (e.g., GABA, NMDA, glutamate, etc.). The effect varies with the specific receptor and pathways affected. Propofol, benzodiazepines, and barbiturates cause significant depression of the amplitude waveforms. Benzodiazepine and barbiturate infusions are out of favor as maintenance anesthetics for spine surgery, for various reasons including their extremely long context-sensitive half-time, potential for hyperalgesia (barbiturates), and prolonged depression after a bolus induction dose. While bolus induction doses of propofol can cause depression of SSEPs, its context-sensitive half-time is significantly more favorable and easier to titrate. Hence propofol has become an important component of maintenance anesthesia during a monitored spine surgery. Some intravenous anesthetics, which do not depress SSEP waveform amplitude include etomidate and ketamine. These drugs increase signal amplitude, potentially by attenuating inhibition [18]. In addition to its beneficial effects on neuromonitoring signals, ketamine is powerfully analgesic and may be especially helpful in opioid-tolerant patients.

(2) Opioids affect SSEP signals less than inhalational agents, making them an important component of evoked potential monitoring. Bolus doses of opioids can be associated with mild depression of amplitude and an increase of latency in responses recorded from the cortex. Infusion doses are generally conducive to monitoring and many neuroanesthesiologists have taken advantage of extremely short-acting opioids such as remifentanil to supplement intravenous maintenance anesthetic.

(3) Dexmedetomidine: Recent studies have examined the effect of dexmedetomidine on the acquisition of neuromonitoring signals. Several studies have found that the use of dexmedetomidine is compatible with the acquisition of SSEPs [19]. The effect of inhalational and intravenous agents on SSEP monitoring, with suggested dosage range is summarized in Table 13.1.

(4) Neuromuscular blocking agents have their effect at the neuromuscular junction and therefore do not negatively affect the acquisition of SSEP signals. If anything, this class of drugs improves the acquisition of SSEP signals by decreasing movement artifact. However, if EMG or MEP signals are planned, then neuromuscular blockade should be avoided, or at least attempted with caution and the use of a twitch monitor with an accelerometer.

3. **Physiology and neuromonitoring**

   a. **Maintenance of intraoperative blood pressure.** The ventral portion of the spinal cord is particularly vulnerable to injury because of its relatively tenuous blood supply; a single anterior spinal artery supplies 75% of the entire cord which includes the motor tracts. Therefore the anterior portion of the cord is more susceptible to hypoperfusion injury due to anemia, hypotension, and blood vessel compression. MEPs monitor the anterior spinal cord directly and can be exquisitely sensitive to changes in blood pressure, especially in susceptible patients, that is, those with myelopathy or certain medical comorbidities such as diabetes or hypertension [17]. Anesthesiologists should strive to maintain normotension throughout the surgery, and if the motor evoked signals decline, the patient's blood pressure should be additionally augmented to ensure adequate blood flow to areas of the cord which have been chronically compressed.

CLINICAL PEARL MEPs monitor the anterior spinal cord directly and can be exquisitely sensitive to changes in blood pressure, especially in susceptible patients.

   b. **Other physiologic factors.** Neuromonitoring signals can be sensitive to temperature, anemia, electrolyte disturbance, and arterial blood gas perturbations but only at extremes [18].

4. **Access.** Prior to the surgical procedure, a discussion regarding the surgical plan and tumor type will give the anesthesiologist an understanding of the need for large bore venous access and invasive monitoring. Patients with metastatic disease may have indwelling venous access for administration of chemotherapy. In general, this access can be used for administration of drugs, provided there is venous return; the appropriate volume is aspirated if the access has been flushed with heparin, and that the external access will not cause soft tissue injury if the patient is prone. Of note, these lines are rarely adequate for volume resuscitation, which if anticipated requires placement of a large bore peripheral cannula or central access. Discussion of the surgical plan also allows appropriate ordering of blood and blood products. Resection of primary tumors of the spinal cord (intramedullary tumors, and extradural–intramedullary tumors) rarely involves large volume blood loss.

5. **Intraoperative choice of opioids.** Appropriate management of chronic pain during spinal cord tumor surgery involves "big picture" planning for postoperative pain control. As mentioned above, continuation of the patient's chronic medications, preoperative administration of oral adjunctive medication, and calculation of daily opioid requirements help assist in finding the appropriate dosage.

   a. **Remifentanil.** Use of short-acting opioids like remifentanil should be used with care in this population. While still controversial, the use of high dose remifentanil has been associated with the development of acute tolerance, higher morphine requirements in the recovery room, and hyperalgesia [20,21]. One study suggested that use of propofol infusion for maintenance as opposed to sevoflurane prevents the development of hyperalgesia [22]. Another suggested that ketamine infusion may be effective in preventing remifentanil-induced hyperalgesia [23]. With these studies in mind, the use of remifentanil for spine surgery should be carefully considered especially in patients who are tolerant to opioids prior to surgery. These patients should receive an anesthetic, which includes enough longer-acting opioids to avoid withdrawal and facilitate pain control.

   b. **Methadone.** Administration of 0.2 mg/kg of methadone given as an intravenous bolus at the beginning of complex spine is associated with lower opioid requirements, lower VAS scores, and without a higher incidence of opioid-associated side effects [24].

   c. **Ketamine.** In chronic pain patients, the intraoperative use of ketamine (0.5 mg/kg as a loading dose, and then an infusion of 10 μg/kg/min) has been associated with lower 48-hour postoperative morphine requirements, also facilitates signal acquisition, and was not associated with an increase in side effects [25].

B. **Emergence.** If the patient is to awaken in a timely fashion at the end of the procedure, it is extremely important that the anesthesiologist is aware of the context-sensitive half-time of the drugs they are using to maintain amnesia.

1. Context-sensitive half-time is the time for the plasma concentration to decrease by 50% from an infusion that maintains a constant concentration; context refers to the duration of the infusion. Time to 50% decrease in plasma concentration was chosen because a 50% reduction in drug concentration appears to be necessary for recovery after the administration of the most intravenous hypnotics (Fig. 13.2). During a long spine surgery this knowledge must be used to aggressively taper the intravenous anesthetic at the appropriate time, often more than 40 minutes prior to surgical finish. Fortunately, often during closure of the incision, the neuromonitoring team will conclude monitoring and inhalational gas can be added if necessary.

2. **Processed EEG monitoring.** The utility of processed EEG to detect awareness under anesthesia is controversial [26]. Processed EEG may be somewhat helpful to determine when infusions can be tapered, although it is not an index of immobility. Studies have shown that sevoflurane and propofol effect movement to noxious stimuli differently. At an equivalent depression of BIS, sevoflurane suppresses the blink reflex more than propofol, indicating different pharmacodynamic properties of these anesthetics at brainstem level [27]. The differential level of immobility at similar levels of hypnosis makes titration of TIVA during spine surgery, without the use of paralytic drugs, somewhat complex.

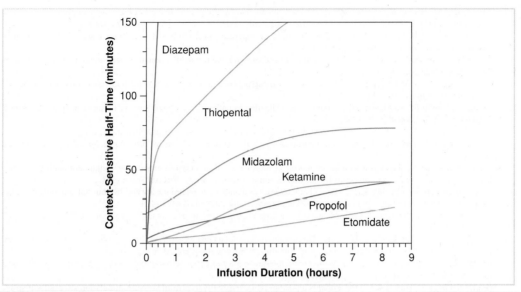

FIGURE 13.2 Plot of the context sensitive half-time versus duration of infusions of several anesthesia medications. (Redrawn from Hughes MA, et. al. Context-sensitive half-time in multicompartment: Pharmacokinetic models for intravenous anesthetic drugs. *Anesthesiology.* 1992;76:334–341, with permission).

    3. **Importance of smooth emergence.** Care should be taken to avoid prolonged coughing and bucking on the endotracheal tube since this will stress the dural repair. Strategies to facilitate a smooth emergence include the following: Allowing the patient to return to spontaneous ventilation prior to emergence, titration of intravenous opioids at the end of the procedure, and use of drugs like dexmedetomidine during emergence which may blunt the discomfort associated with intubation.

V. Conclusion. Providing anesthesia for the patient undergoing resection of a spinal tumor requires an understanding of the tumor type and location. The anesthesiologist needs to discuss the planned procedure with the surgeon, including the need for intraoperative monitoring. Since many patients with spinal cord tumors have chronic back pain related to their tumor, it is also important to understand the patient's pain history. This information will guide the preoperative evaluation, choice of intraoperative technique, need for venous access and invasive monitors, and challenges for postoperative management.

REFERENCES

1. Welch WC, Jacobs GB. Surgery for metastatic spinal disease. *J Neurooncol.* 1995;23(2):163–170.
2. Stacchiotti S, Casali PG, Lo Vullo S, et al. Chordoma of the mobile spine and sacrum: A retrospective analysis of a series of patients surgically treated at two referral centers. *Ann Surg Oncol.* 2010;17(1):211–219.
3. Park L, Delaney TF, Liebsch NJ, et al. Sacral chordomas: Impact of high-dose proton/photon-beam radiation therapy combined with or without surgery for primary versus recurrent tumor. *Int J Radiat Oncol Biol Phys.* 2006;65(5):1514–1521.
4. Stacchiotti S, Marrari A, Tamborini E, et al. Response to imatinib plus sirolimus in advanced chordoma. *Ann Oncol.* 2009;20(11):1886–1894.
5. Abdel-Wahab M, Etuk B, Palermo J, et al. Spinal cord gliomas: A multi-institutional retrospective analysis. *Int J Radiat Oncol Biol Phys.* 2006;64(4):1060–1071.
6. Pica A, Miller R, Villa S, et al. The results of surgery, with or without radiotherapy, for primary spinal myxopapillary ependymoma: A retrospective study from the rare cancer network. *Int J Radiat Oncol Biol Phys.* 2009;74(4):1114–1120.
7. Bagley CA, Wilson S, Kothbauer KF, et al. Long term outcomes following surgical resection of myxopapillary ependymomas. *Neurosurg Rev.* 2009;32(3):321–334; discussion 334.
8. Quraishi NA, Gokaslan ZL, Boriani S. The surgical management of metastatic epidural compression of the spinal cord. *J Bone Joint Surg Br.* 2010;92(8):1054–1060.
9. Anderson R, Saiers JH, Abram S, et al. Accuracy in equianalgesic dosing. conversion dilemmas. *J Pain Symptom Manage.* 2001;21(5):397–406.

10. Van Elstraete AC, Tirault M, Lebrun T, et al. The median effective dose of preemptive gabapentin on postoperative morphine consumption after posterior lumbar spinal fusion. *Anesth Analg.* 2008;106(1):305–308, table of contents.

11. Rajpal S, Gordon DB, Pellino TA, et al. Comparison of perioperative oral multimodal analgesia versus IV PCA for spine surgery. *J Spinal Disord Tech.* 2010;23(2):139–145.

12. Nielsen PR, Jorgensen LD, Dahl B, et al. Prehabilitation and early rehabilitation after spinal surgery: Randomized clinical trial. *Clin Rehabil.* 2010;24(2):137–148.

13. Sala F, Bricolo A, Faccioli F, et al. Surgery for intramedullary spinal cord tumors: the role of intraoperative (neurophysiological) monitoring. *Eur Spine J.* 2007;16(2):S130–S139.

14. Tsirikos AI, Howitt SP, McMaster MJ. Segmental vessel ligation in patients undergoing surgery for anterior spinal deformity. *J Bone Joint Surg Br.* 2008;90(4):474–479.

15. Hyun SJ, Rhim SC, Kang JK, et al. Combined motor- and somatosensory-evoked potential monitoring for spine and spinal cord surgery: Correlation of clinical and neurophysiological data in 85 consecutive procedures. *Spinal Cord.* 2009;47(8):616–622.

16. Eleraky MA, Setzer M, Papanastassiou ID, et al. Role of motor-evoked potential monitoring in conjunction with temporary clipping of spinal nerve roots in posterior thoracic spine tumor surgery. *Spine J.* 2010;10(5):396–403.

17. Deiner SG, Kwatra SG, Lin HM, et al. Patient characteristics and anesthetic technique are additive but not synergistic predictors of successful motor evoked potential monitoring. *Anesth Analg.* 2010;111(2):421–425.

18. Sloan TB, Heyer EJ. Anesthesia for intraoperative neurophysiologic monitoring of the spinal cord. *J Clin Neurophysiol.* 2002;19(5):430–443.

19. Anschel DJ, Aherne A, Soto RG, et al. Successful intraoperative spinal cord monitoring during scoliosis surgery using a total intravenous anesthetic regimen including dexmedetomidine. *J Clin Neurophysiol.* 2008;25(1):56–61.

20. Guignard B, Bossard AE, Coste C, et al. Acute opioid tolerance: Intraoperative remifentanil increases postoperative pain and morphine requirement. *Anesthesiology.* 2000;93(2):409–417.

21. Schmidt S, Bethge C, Forster MH, et al. Enhanced postoperative sensitivity to painful pressure stimulation after intraoperative high dose remifentanil in patients without significant surgical site pain. *Clin J Pain.* 2007;23(7):605–611.

22. Shin SW, Cho AR, Lee HJ, et al. Maintenance anaesthetics during remifentanil-based anaesthesia might affect postoperative pain control after breast cancer surgery. *Br J Anaesth.* 2010;105(5):661–667.

23. Joly V, Richebe P, Guignard B, et al. Remifentanil-induced postoperative hyperalgesia and its prevention with small-dose ketamine. *Anesthesiology.* 2005;103(1):147–155.

24. Gottschalk A, Durieux ME, Nemergut EC. Intraoperative methadone improves postoperative pain control in patients undergoing complex spine surgery. *Anesth Analg.* 2011;112(1):218–223.

25. Loftus RW, Yeager MP, Clark JA, et al. Intraoperative ketamine reduces perioperative opiate consumption in opiate-dependent patients with chronic back pain undergoing back surgery. *Anesthesiology.* 2010;113(3):639–646.

26. Avidan MS, Jacobsohn E, Glick D, et al.; BAG-RECALL Research Group. Prevention of intraoperative awareness in a high-risk surgical population. *N Engl J Med.* 2011;365(7):591–600.

27. Sadean MR, Glass PS. Pharmacokinetic-pharmacodynamic modeling in anesthesia, intensive care and pain medicine. *Curr Opin Anaesthesiol.* 2009;22(4):463–468.

28. Hughes MA, Glass PSA, Jacobs JR. Context-sensitive half-time in multicompartment pharmacokinetic models for intravenous anesthetic drugs. *Anesthesiology.* 1992;76:334–341.

14

Functional Neurosurgery

Hélène G. Pellerin and Rosemary Ann Craen

KEY POINTS

1. Deep brain stimulation is the surgical treatment of choice for movement disorders, especially Parkinson's disease.
2. Continuous monitoring of the patient during transfer from MRI to OR is of utmost importance.
3. If the procedure is done under sedation, management of the airway will be more difficult because of the stereotactic frame and strategies to manage the airway should be planned prior to surgery.
4. Confusion, airway obstruction, venous air embolism, intracranial hemorrhage, high blood pressure, and seizure are some of the intraoperative complications that can occur and require prompt diagnosis and treatment.
5. Use of surgical electrocautery and MRI in a patient with implanted DBS should be done with extreme caution to prevent burns and dysfunction of the generator.

I. **Introduction.** Functional neurosurgery is concerned with the treatment of conditions where central nervous system function is abnormal although the structure or anatomy may be normal. Examples of conditions include movement disorders such as Parkinson's disease and essential tremor, chronic pain, and some psychiatric conditions. This chapter will mainly focus on deep brain stimulation (DBS). The underlying principle behind DBS is based on neutralizing or disrupting neuronal dysfunction to improve or restore brain function or on driving the circuitry in underperforming circuits to enhance activity and improve brain function. A better understanding of the brain circuitry, improved brain imaging and brain mapping, improved neurosurgical techniques, and improved stimulating devices have led to the increased growth of functional neurosurgery.

A. **History.** Prior to the 1990s, surgical options that could be offered to patients with movement disorders were destructive lesionectomy, including thalamotomy and pallidotomy. Unfortunately, these procedures were irreversible, and caused several permanent side effects. They were thus used as a last option when medical treatment failed. Interest in surgery was renewed by the first description of DBS surgery in 1987 as an alternative to ablative procedures to reduce the symptoms of Parkinson's disease [1]. DBS, unlike lesionectomy, is reversible and allows tailoring to reduce cognitive and motor side effects. Current instrumentation provides multiple programmable options, which allow for adaptation to the electrophysiologic changes that develop in the neuronal circuitry of patients which in turn allows long-term symptom control. DBS has become the primary treatment for patients with Parkinson's disease who are debilitated with symptoms which remain refractory to medical therapy. Indications for DBS are slowly expanding outside the circle of movement disorders. There is however, an ongoing

201

TABLE 14.1	Indications for deep brain stimulation
Movement disorders (Parkinson's disease, dystonia, essential tremor)	
Psychiatric conditions (depression, obsessive–compulsive disorder)	
Epilepsy	
Chronic pain (trigeminal neuralgia, sympathetic dystrophies, hemifacial spasm)	

debate about the exact mechanism of action of DBS and it may differ depending on the site of stimulation [2–4].

II. Indications

A. **Movement disorders.** Movement disorders are conditions that produce inadequate or excessive movement and medical therapy is directed at reducing symptoms. The majority of movement disorders result from alteration in function of the basal ganglia, a group of interconnected subcortical nuclei comprising the substantia nigra, putamen, caudate, globus pallidus, thalamus, and subthalamic nucleus (STN) (Fig. 14.1). DBS is an expanding field for the treatment of movement disorders and is considered a treatment of choice for adult movement disorders that are refractory to medical therapy. The aim of DBS is to improve the quality of life of the patient.

1. **Parkinson's disease.** Parkinson's disease is a neurodegenerative condition due to loss of dopaminergic cells in the substantia nigra. Dopamine inhibits the rate of firing of the neurons that control the extrapyramidal motor system. Depletion of dopamine results in diminished inhibition of these neurons and unopposed stimulation by acetylcholine. Diagnosis is clinical and based on cardinal symptoms of resting tremor, bradykinesia, rigidity, and gait disturbance. Treatment is designed to increase the concentration of dopamine in the basal ganglia or to decrease the neuronal effects of acetylcholine. Replacement therapy with the dopamine precursor levodopa is the standard medical treatment but is associated with numerous side effects including dyskinesia. Bilateral DBS of the STN is the most commonly performed procedure for surgical treatment of advanced Parkinson's disease, and when successful, it results in reduced motor disability, reduced motor fluctuations, and a reduction in levodopa-induced dyskinesia. Medication dosages can be lowered postsurgically, with a resultant reduction in medication-induced adverse effects. DBS can add value to the best medical treatment and it is a cost-effective intervention, although it is not curative of Parkinson's disease and it does not alter the progression of disease [5]. Optimal outcome primarily depends on patient selection and accuracy of lead placement in the proximity of the target nucleus. Patient selection is

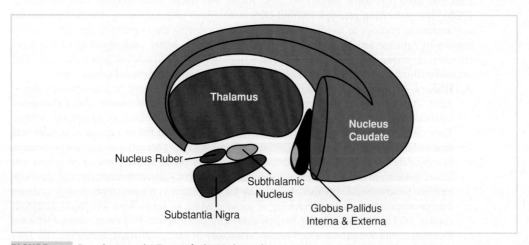

FIGURE 14.1 Deep brain nuclei: Targets for brain electrodes.

done by a multidisciplinary team. Patients are selected on the basis that they respond to dopaminergic medications, exhibit medically refractory motor fluctuations or dyskinesia, and they do not have significant cognitive decline or depression.

2. **Dystonia.** Dystonia is a clinical syndrome characterized by muscle contractions causing abnormal repetitive and twisting movements resulting in painful and debilitating postures. There is no medical cure, and medical therapy is aimed at symptom relief. Stimulation of the globus pallidus internus (GPi) has been shown to reduce symptoms and significantly improve the quality of life of these patients [6].

3. **Essential tremor.** Essential tremor is the most common form of pathologic tremor. It affects mainly the hands, head, voice, and tongue but lower extremities can also be involved. Essential tremors can be treated with DBS of the ventral intermediate thalamus [4,7].

B. Other indications. Indications of DBS have now expanded and include many other neurologic and psychiatric conditions. For each specific disease, such as Tourette's syndrome, cluster headaches, chronic pain and Alzheimer's disease, a specific target is developed [4,8,9]. Severe depression and obsessive–compulsive disorder have been treated with stimulation of the subcallosal cingulate gyrus, the anterior limb of the internal capsule, or the nucleus accumbens [10]. Some studies have shown positive effects of anterior thalamus stimulation for refractory epilepsy (Table 14.1) [11,12].

III. The procedure. Through a burr hole, a stimulating electrode is placed within the vicinity of a deep brain nucleus using brain mapping and fluoroscopy. Following confirmation of placement, this electrode is connected to a generator inserted in the subclavian space using a subcutaneous lead (Fig. 14.2). The pulse generator produces high-frequency electrical stimulation. Electrical stimulation of the target nucleus is programmed to obtain the best symptom relief and to allow for flexibility and potential long-term symptom control. In Parkinson's disease, bilateral electrodes are usually inserted and controlled separately with one single pulse generator. Target nuclei are localized using a combination of methods. First, magnetic resonance imaging (MRI) is used to

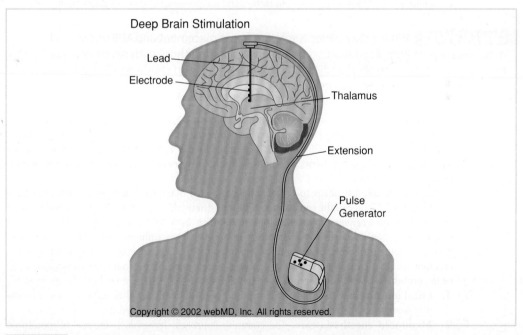

Deep Brain Stimulation

Lead
Electrode
Thalamus
Extension
Pulse Generator

FIGURE 14.2 An electrode is placed in the vicinity of a deep brain nucleus and via a subcutaneous lead is connected to a pulse generator which has been inserted in the subclavian space. Two electrodes can be inserted into one generator and still operate independently. (Reproduced with permission)

locate the nucleus and identify stereotactic coordinates. STN and GPi are visualized on MRI, however, the thalamic nucleus is usually not visible on standard MRI and target localization is instead performed based on proportional system coordinates or stereotactic superimposition of standardized brain atlases. Intraoperatively, target location is confirmed by electrophysiologic monitoring. Each nucleus has a characteristic neural firing profile allowing its identification. An electrode is inserted 10 to 15 mm above the target nucleus and then it is advanced in steps of 0.5 to 1 mm while spontaneous neuronal discharges are recorded (microelectrode recordings [MER]) until the electrode is in close proximity to the target. A stimulation trial (macrostimulation) allows for assessment of clinical improvement and side effects such as dysarthria, dyskinesia, sensory deficits, eye movement, and muscle cramps. This last step requires an awake, cooperative patient. Anesthetic agents may reduce the quality of MER although some studies have reported good quality of MER of the STN under general anesthesia [5,13]. Macrostimulation may be difficult to interpret if the patient is fatigued.

A. **Description of surgery.** On the day of surgery, a rigid frame is fixed on the patient's head following a scalp block or local anesthetic infiltration at the pin insertion sites. Local anesthetics most commonly used include bupivacaine 0.5%, ropivacaine 1% alone or in combination with lidocaine 1%. A blend of mepivacaine 1% and tetracaine 0.2% is used in one of the authors' institutions. Tetracaine, is a long-acting ester-type local anesthetic. In addition, small sedative doses of propofol can be given at the time of head fixation with the stereotactic frame. With the frame in place, MRI is performed to define the target nucleus. Images are used to map and localize the area of interest and to plan the path for the introduction of the electrode. The patient is then transferred to the operating room and placed in a semi-sitting position for burr hole and electrode placement. After the position of the electrode is confirmed, a final quadripolar electrode is inserted and sutured in place. If bilateral electrodes are required, all the steps are then repeated on the contralateral side. At the end of the procedure or on a subsequent day depending on local practices, electrodes are internalized, the leads are tunneled and the pulse generator is inserted in a subcutaneous pocket below the clavicle. This second stage of the procedure is almost always done under general anesthesia. The implanted electrode remains inactive during this second stage so choice of anesthetic technique will be influenced by patient factors and the presence of comorbidities [8,14].

CLINICAL PEARL While many patients tolerate frame placement and MRI under local anesthesia with minimal sedation, some patients including those with severe cervical dystonia or with uncontrolled body and limb movements, and children will require moderate sedation or general anesthesia.

B. **Anesthesia.** The anesthesiologist faces many challenges during a DBS procedure. The anesthetic goals are to provide maximum patient comfort with minimal interference with intraoperative MER and macrostimulation. The procedure is relatively long in duration, usually several hours, and most patients who present for surgery are disabled as a consequence of their neurologic condition.

The anesthesiologist needs to be prepared to rapidly diagnose and treat any intraoperative complications. Choice of the most appropriate anesthetic modalities has been widely discussed in the literature because of the possible interference with MER, by altering neuronal firing frequency. It is not known to what extent anesthetic drugs influence the MER as the effect depends on the individual agent and the intended target. Controversy is compounded by the fact that anesthetic management differs among centers and ranges from local anesthesia alone, or in combination with supplemental sedation, to the use of general anesthesia for every case.

1. **Local anesthesia.** The traditional method is to use only local anesthetic for burr hole placement and keep the patient unsedated throughout the procedure.

2. **Monitored anesthesia care.** The common approach; however, is the use of monitored anesthesia care with sedation when patient cooperation is not needed. Propofol sedation should be stopped approximately 15 to 20 minutes before neurophysiologic mapping to allow dissipation of drug effects. Propofol infusion, 25 to 75 μg/kg/min alone, or in

combination with remifentanil infusion 0.02 to 0.05 μg/kg/min is commonly used [2,3]. The pharmacokinetic behavior of propofol in patients with Parkinson's disease may differ from the general population and its sedative effect may be more profound [8]. Close monitoring with frequent adjustment of infusion rates may be necessary. Dexmedetomidine, an α-2 receptor agonist, administered at a dose of 0.3 to 0.6 μg/kg/h, may be the drug of choice, as it provides sedation with minimal respiratory depression, and has little or no effect on electrophysiologic mapping and functional testing. Dexmedetomidine also decreases the intraoperative use of antihypertensive medications. Hypotension and bradycardia, however may occur with dexmedetomidine [15]. Oversedation can still lead to upper airway obstruction due to relaxed muscle tone. Some patients, especially the older, are more sensitive to the effects of dexmedetomidine and the risks of oversedation and longer recovery times need to be carefully addressed. It might be necessary to reduce the infusion rate of dexmedetomidine after a couple of hours in order to maintain the same level of sedation [15]. Benzodiazepines are not used because they can abolish MER, increase the threshold of stimulation and may induce dyskinesia [3]. It can be difficult to predict a patient's response to sedation during brain surgery as every patient responds differently. The key is careful and gentle titration of sedative(s). And in some cases, no sedation may be the safest option.

> **CLINICAL PEARL** Anesthesia agents may interfere with microelectrode recordings and therefore sedation should be discontinued or decreased to a minimum during recordings and stimulation.

3. **General anesthesia.** General anesthesia may be the only option for patients with severe diseases and uncontrolled movements or for pediatric patients. The advantages of using general anesthesia include reduced anxiety, reduced neck and back pain, and reduced painful dystonia in patients. It has been reported that general anesthesia can produce surgical outcomes similar to that found using local anesthesia alone [5,13,16]. However, a recent report showed comparable long-term motor outcome between general anesthesia and local anesthesia but significant cognitive decline and higher stimulation side effects in the general anesthesia group [17]. In these studies, adequate MER were obtained with all agents: propofol, dexmedetomidine, remifentanil, and volatile agents. It should be noted that DBS surgery can be done without MER. MRI-guided only DBS surgery under general anesthesia or local anesthesia may be a viable option [16]. The use of depth of anesthesia monitors such as bispectral index (BIS) has been studied to help titrate sedation, or anesthesia depth during recordings. However, the reliability of BIS has not yet been proven and conflicting results have emerged [18,19].

4. **Specific anesthetic considerations (Table 14.2)**
   a. **Preoperative evaluation.** Preoperative evaluation includes an assessment for the presence of comorbidities, especially of the cardiovascular and respiratory systems, and a detailed review of the patient's medications. For the patient with Parkinson's disease, side effects of levodopa treatment such as orthostatic hypotension should be evaluated (Table 14.3). Withdrawal of parkinsonian medication that is necessary before DBS implantation can increase patients' symptoms and should be anticipated. The patient's

TABLE 14.2 Anesthetic considerations for deep brain stimulation

Cooperative patient (if general anesthesia is not planned)
Long procedure, need to maximize comfort
Semi-sitting position—risk for venous air embolism
Standard monitors +/− arterial line
Have a plan for airway management
Minimize interference during functional testing and microelectrode recording
Ensure safety during transfer from MRI to OR

TABLE 14.3   Anesthetic considerations for Parkinson's disease

Cardiovascular:
- Autonomic neuropathy—orthostatic hypotension, increased perioperative hemodynamic instability, and altered responses to vasopressors, such as norepinephrine
- Intravascular volume depletion and inadequate response to hypotension due to depletion of noradrenaline stores secondary to levodopa therapy and resultant fluctuations in heart rate and blood pressure
- Muscle tremors mimicking ventricular fibrillation on the ECG

Airway and respiratory:
- Cervical and facial muscle rigidity—reduces mouth opening and neck movement
- Muscle rigidity can impair airway manipulation and ventilation
- Intermittent upper airway obstruction due to involuntary movements of glottis and supraglottic structures
- Laryngospasm and diaphragmatic spasm
- Respiratory dysfunction
- Restrictive lung disease secondary to chest wall rigidity

Gastrointestinal/urinary:
- Dysphagia, gastroparesis which may be asymptomatic, leading to increased risk of pulmonary aspiration
- Urinary retention

Central nervous system:
- Violent tremors
- Increased risk of postoperative confusion, agitation, and hallucinations after general anesthesia
- Neuroleptic malignant syndrome
- Dementia

Potential drug interactions/side effects:
- Propofol can cause dyskinesia and ablation of resting tremor
- Opioids may cause muscle rigidity
- Phenothiazines, haloperidol, and metoclopramide may precipitate or exacerbate Parkinson's symptoms
- Levodopa causes dyskinesia
- Muscle relaxants: Depolarizing and nondepolarizing muscle relaxants can be used but there was a case report of succinylcholine-induced hyperkalemia
- Ondansetron, a serotonin antagonist, is safe to use for emesis.

ability to cooperate during surgery done under local anesthesia with or without sedation should be confirmed by the anesthesiologist in consultation with the neurosurgeon.

b. **Monitoring.** Intraoperative monitoring includes electrocardiography, pulse oximetry, noninvasive blood pressure monitoring, and end-tidal CO_2. End-tidal CO_2 and respiratory rate can be monitored reliably using nasal prongs equipped with a monitoring channel. Invasive blood pressure monitoring with an arterial line may be indicated depending on comorbidities and to better manage hypertension. An arterial line also eliminates the discomfort of regular cuff inflation during a long procedure. It should also be considered in patients with severe tremor in whom noninvasive blood pressure monitoring might be nonreliable. Some centers routinely use invasive arterial monitoring. Urinary catheterization can be omitted in awake patients if omitting it improves comfort. However, the combination of a lengthy procedure together with the potential difficulty in using a urinal or bed pan while the head is fixed in place, leads some centers to insert indwelling urinary catheters in all cases. Temperature control needs to be checked regularly and adjusted according to patient comfort. It is not unusual for patients to feel cold at the beginning of the procedure and warm during stimulation. Temperature should be monitored routinely if the patient is under general anesthesia [3,20]. The anesthesiologist should ensure that equipment is adequate to closely monitor the patient in all locations: MRI suite, operating room, and during transfers [3,14].

CLINICAL PEARL   All lines (IVs, arterial line) and monitors should preferentially be on the side ipsilateral to the procedure to allow for intraoperative testing of stimulation effects on the contralateral side. If bilateral procedure is planned, line placement should be on the side being operated first.

c. **Positioning.** There are operating tables designed for DBS. If the procedure is done under local anesthesia and sedation, meticulous attention should be paid to adequate positioning of the patient, especially neck and head posture. The degree of flexion of the neck should be minimized as much as possible. The patient's speech, swallowing and ease of breathing when in final position should be assessed by the team. In the semi-sitting position, there is a tendency for the patient to slip down on the surgical table and this can be prevented by providing a firm support under the knee and flexing the legs. The degree of sitting position should be as little as possible to decrease the risk of venous air embolism. Frequent interactions with the patient, reassurance, regular adjustment of arms and legs, moistening of lips and mouth are all essential to ensure patient comfort [3,14].

CLINICAL PEARL In a semi-sitting position, there is a tendency for the patient to slip down on the surgical table. A firm support under the knees and flexing the legs is necessary.

d. **Intraoperative management.** Good communication between all team members is essential to allow coordination of the action of each team member. Deepening or lightening the sedation or the anesthesia at specific surgical times necessitates good collaboration between the neurosurgeon and the anesthesiologist.

(1) **Airway management during conscious sedation.** Oxygen supplementation through nasal prongs is recommended throughout the procedure. As endotracheal intubation will be more difficult with the stereotactic frame in place, strategies to manage the airway in an emergency should be discussed prior to surgery. Equipment such as oral and nasal airway adjuncts, different sizes of endotracheal tubes, laryngoscope with a variety of blades, and a fiberoptic bronchoscope should be readily available. The laryngeal mask airway can be a lifesaving tool to facilitate ventilation of the patient during an emergency. A tool to remove the fixed frame in case of an emergency should be readily available. Vigilance at all stages of the procedure is the central element of success to detect any changes in respiratory pattern as early as possible.

(2) **Hemodynamic management.** Tight control of systolic blood pressure throughout the procedure is important to prevent intracranial hemorrhage. Labetalol, esmolol, hydralazine, nitroglycerin, and sodium nitroprusside can be used to treat intraoperative arterial hypertension. Dexmedetomidine can reduce hypertension. Although the optimal level of blood pressure is still the subject of debate, maintaining systolic blood pressure below 160 mm Hg and within 20% of preoperative value has been suggested [15,21]. High blood pressure can create pulse artifacts during MER so treating hypertension may improve quality of recordings. However, metoprolol reduces tremor, and can modify the spiking activity of the STN and interfere with MER [22]. While it would be prudent to avoid β blockers altogether during MER, direct vasodilators have the disadvantage of causing reflex tachycardia. To date, labetalol has not been associated with alterations in STN and is the preferred choice if a β blocker is needed to treat hypertension.

e. **Postoperative management.** In order to detect complications in a timely manner, patients should be monitored in a specialized unit for at least the first night following surgery. Routine checks of neurologic signs and monitoring of patient's vital signs will allow the early detection of most complications. DBS insertion is a procedure causing minimal postoperative pain therefore pain management should not be a problem. Medication causing minimal alteration in the level of consciousness and minimal respiratory depression should be prescribed.

C. **Complications**

1. **Perioperative complications.** Information regarding perioperative complications is limited and comes mainly from retrospective studies (Table 14.4). The incidence of adverse

4

TABLE 14.4 Complications of deep brain stimulation
Uncooperative patient, agitation
Excessive sedation
Respiratory: Hypoventilation, hypoxia, airway obstruction
Cardiovascular: Hypertension, bradycardia
Venous air embolism
Intracranial hemorrhage
Seizures
Infection
Hardware, e.g., broken or misplaced lead

events has been reported between 7% and 16% [8,14,23]. Respiratory complications including airway obstruction, respiratory arrest, dyspnea, aspiration, and pulmonary edema have a reported incidence between 1% and 2%. Oversedation can lead to decreased respiratory rate, airway obstruction, and respiratory arrest. Prompt management of these complications is required. Intracranial hemorrhage is the most frequent neurologic complication and can be devastating. Its incidence has been estimated between 2.5% and 5% and it mainly presents as a focal neurologic deficit or a change in mental status such as agitation or confusion. Suspicion of intracranial hemorrhage might require an urgent computerized tomography. Chronic arterial hypertension and acute intraoperative hypertension have been associated with increased risk of intracranial hemorrhage. Seizures have also been reported during or after DBS procedure but are often self-limited and rarely necessitate treatment. Small doses of midazolam and/or propofol should be used as the first-line treatments to stop seizures.

Venous air embolism has been reported to occur in 1% to 9% of DBS procedures, especially if the procedure is done in the sitting position with the surgical site above the level of the heart, creating a negative pressure gradient between the operative site and the right atrium. A retrospective review of 467 cases reported an incidence of venous air embolism of only 1.3% but the retrospective nature of the study may have underestimated the incidence [24]. If the patient is awake, coughing, oxygen desaturation, and hypotension are possible symptoms and signs suggestive of venous air embolism. A decrease in end-tidal CO_2 may also be observed. Management includes identification of the source of air entry, irrigation of the surgical field, application of bone wax, lowering the head of the bed, oxygen supplementation, and hemodynamic support. Some authors have recommended screening patients for the presence of a patent foramen oval prior to neurosurgery planned in the sitting position to decrease the risk of paradoxical air embolism.

CLINICAL PEARL The incidence of intracranial bleeding is about 3%. Blood pressure should be maintained less than 160 mm Hg systolic (or locally agreed upon limits). There is an increased risk of venous air embolism with the patient in the semi-sitting position. In the awake patient, coughing may be the first sign of venous air embolism.

2. **Long-term complications.** Long-term complications are mainly related to the hardware and include infection, lead migration, lead fracture, generator malfunction, and skin erosion. Superficial infections of the wound can be treated with intravenous or oral antibiotics but deep infections involving hardware often require device removal [25]. Mood changes such as depression, decreased working memory performance and impulsivity have also been attributed to DBS implantation [8,14]. A case of akinetic-rigid state was reported postoperatively after stimulator replacement when the neurostimulator was not

activated [26]. Parkinsonism hyperpyrexia, a rare and potentially fatal syndrome, can occur in patients with Parkinson's disease following reduction or cessation of dopaminergic medication [27]. This syndrome is clinically similar to neuroleptic malignant syndrome and presents with rigidity, hyperpyrexia, a decreased level of consciousness, autonomic instability, and increased serum creatine kinase. Dopaminergic drug replacement and supportive measures are the only treatments. A case of parkinsonism hyperpyrexia syndrome was reported in a patient with bilateral DBS of STN in whom there was a rapid reduction in antiparkinsonian drugs [28].

IV. Anesthesia for patients with deep brain stimulator in situ

A. Nonrelated surgery. There is little published information on the anesthetic management of patients with DBS devices. Most of the knowledge has been extrapolated from literature resulting from other implantable devices such as the cardiac pacemaker and implantable defibrillators. Extreme care must be taken with patients with DBS device undergoing an MRI. MRI can induce heating of the leads and potentially produce a thermal lesion in the brain. The magnetic field may also produce movement of the neurostimulator, alter its function, and modify its programming. MRI examinations should be done only if absolutely necessary and communication with the manufacturer should identify specific recommendations. To decrease the risk of distortion in images, it has been suggested that the neurostimulator be turned off temporarily for the duration of the MRI examination. Surgical electrocautery might also interfere with DBS. Surgical electrocautery can damage DBS leads, cause potential thermal injury, and temporarily suppress or interfere with the programming of the neurostimulator. Whenever possible, bipolar diathermy should be used. If use of unipolar electrocautery is essential, the lowest possible level of energy should be programmed, and the ground plate should be placed as far from the neurostimulator as possible and it should be used in short irregular bursts. The best approach is to turn the neurostimulator off just before the induction of general anesthesia and reactivate after surgery. Use of an external defibrillator may also modify the function of the neurostimulator. Paddles should be placed as far as possible from the stimulator and perpendicular to the lead system. The DBS system should be interrogated after defibrillation. The DBS generator can also cause distortion in electrocardiography and turning the device off will reduce artifact in cardiac monitoring [2,14].

B. Battery replacement. The battery life of the generator is around 2 to 5 years so battery replacement will need to be planned regularly. The procedure lasts less than an hour and is most often done under general anesthesia with the patient in the supine position and the shoulder elevated to better expose the subclavicular area. The airway can be managed either with a laryngeal mask airway or an endotracheal tube. In order to avoid underlying symptom recurrence, DBS generator should be turned off after the induction of general anesthesia and activated immediately after replacement.

V. Future. DBS has changed the face of stereotactic and functional neurosurgery by allowing exploration of discrete subcortical gray and white matter targets that had previously been thought too dangerous to manipulate. New surgical techniques are being developed and studied such as frameless stereotaxy and MRI-guided only DBS surgery which could potentially increase the tolerance to surgery by eliminating the need for a cooperative patient. Indications for DBS are expanding and optimal targets for specific diseases are being actively searched for. We will see an increase in the rate of DBS surgery, and in the number of patients presenting to the operating room with implanted devices.

VI. Summary. DBS surgery is a complex procedure that necessitates excellent collaboration among all members of the surgical and anesthesia teams, especially if the patient is minimally sedated. Interactions between anesthetic agents and MER have not yet been fully determined so the choice of anesthesia is mainly based on local practice. As well, the best tool to precisely localize each target nucleus is still under investigation. It is important to maintain constant vigilance throughout the procedure to promptly detect, diagnose, and treat complications. As the number of DBS cases grows, clinicians will need to become familiar with the anesthetic implications of implanted devices.

REFERENCES

1. Benabid AL, Pollak P, Louveau A, et al. Combined (thalamotomy and stimulation) stereotactic surgery of the VIM thalamic nucleus for bilateral Parkinson disease. *Appl Neurophysiol.* 1987;50(1–6):344–346.
2. Dobbs P, Hoyle J, Rowe J. Anaesthesia and deep brain stimulation. *Contin Educ Anaesth Crit Care Pain.* 2009;9(5): 157–161.
3. Venkatraghavan L, Luciano M, Manninen P. Anesthetic management of patients undergoing deep brain stimulator insertion. *Anesth Analg.* 2010;110:1138–1145.
4. Lyons MK. Deep brain stimulation: current and future clinical applications. *Mayo Clin Proc.* 2011;86(7):662–672.
5. Sutcliffe AJ, Mitchell RD, Gan YC, et al. General anaesthesia for deep brain stimulator electrode insertion in Parkinson's disease. *Acta Neurochir.* 2011;153:621–627.
6. Sebeo J, Deiner SG, Alterman RL, et al. Anesthesia for pediatric deep brain stimulation. *Anesthesiol Res Pract.* 2010;: 401–419.
7. Mandat T, Koziara H, Rola R, et al. Thalamic deep brain stimulation in the treatment of essential tremor. *Neurol Neurochir Pol.* 2011;45(1):37–41.
8. Venkatraghavan L, Manninen P. Anesthesia for deep brain stimulation. *Curr Opin Anaesthesiol.* 2011;24(5):495–499.
9. Laxton AW, Tang-Wai DF, McAndrews MP, et al. A phase I trial of deep brain stimulation of memory circuits in Alzheimer's disease. *Ann Neurol.* 2010;68:521–534.
10. Holtzheimer PE, Mayberg HS. Deep brain stimulation for psychiatric disorders. *Annu Rev Neurosci.* 2011;34:289–307.
11. Fisher R, Salanova V, Witt T, et al. Electrical stimulation of the anterior nucleus of thalamus for treatment of refractory epilepsy. *Epilepsia.* 2010;51(5):899–908.
12. Cukiert A, Cukiert CM, Argentoni-Baldochi M, et al. Intraoperative neurophysiological responses in epileptic patients submitted to hippocampal and thalamic deep brain stimulation. *Seizure.* 2011;20(10):748–753.
13. Harries AM, Kausar J, Roberts SA, et al. Deep brain stimulation of the subthalamic nucleus for advanced Parkinson disease using general anesthesia: long-term results. *J Neurosurg.* 2012;116(1):107–113.
14. Poon CC, Irwin MG. Anaesthesia for deep brain stimulation and in patients with implanted neurostimulator devices. *Br J Anaesth.* 2009;103(2):152–165.
15. Rozet I, Muangman S, Vavilala MS, et al. Clinical experience with dexmedetomidine for implantation of deep brain stimulators in Parkinson's disease. *Anesth Analg.* 2006;103:1224–1228.
16. Nakajima T, Zrinzo L, Foltynie T, et al. MRI-guided subthalamic nucleus deep brain stimulation without microelectrode recording: can we dispense with surgery under local anaesthesia? *Stereotact Funct Neurosurg.* 2011;89(5):318–325.
17. Chen SY, Tsai ST, Lin SH, et al. Subthalamic deep brain stimulation in Parkinson's disease under different anesthetic modalities: a comparative cohort study. *Stereotact Funct Neurosurg.* 2011;89(6):372–380.
18. Schulz U, Keh D, Barner C, et al. Bispectral index monitboring does not improve anesthesia performance in patients with movement disorders undergoing deep brain stimulating electrode implantation. *Anesth Analg.* 2007;104:1481–1487.
19. Lefaucheur JP, Gurruchaga JM, Pollin B, et al. Outcome of bilateral subthalamic nucleus stimulation in the treatment of Parkinson's disease: correlation with intra-operative multi-unit recordings but not with the type of anaesthesia. *Eur Neurol.* 2008;60:186–199.
20. Kalenka A, Schwarz A. Anaesthesia and Parkinson's disease: how to manage with new therapies? *Curr Opin Anaesthesiol.* 2009;22(3):419–424.
21. Gorgulho A, De Salles AA, Frighetto L, et al. Incidence of hemorrhage associated with electrophysiological studies performed using macroelectrodes and microelectrodes in functional neurosurgery. *J Neurosurg.* 2005;102:888–896.
22. Coenen VA, Gielen FLH, Castro-Prado F, et al. Noradrenergic modulation of subthalamic nucleus activity in human: metoprolol reduces spiking activity in microelectrode recordings during deep brain stimulation surgery for Parkinson's disease. *Acta Neurochir (Wien).* 2008;150:757–762.
23. Khatib R, Ebrahim Z, Rezai A, et al. Perioperative events during deep brain stimulation: the experience at cleveland clinic. *J Neurosurg Anesthesiol.* 2008;20(1):36–40.
24. Chang EF, Cheng JS, Richardson RM, et al. Incidence and management of venous air embolisms during awake deep brain stimulation surgery in a large clinical series. *Stereotact Funct Neurosurg.* 2011;89:76–82.
25. Deiner S, Hagen J. Parkinson's disease and deep brain stimulator placement. *Anesthesiol Clin.* 2009;27(3):391–415.
26. Dagtekin O, Berlet T, Gerbershagen HJ, et al. Anesthesia and deep brain stimulation: postoperative akinetic state after replacement of impulse generators. *Anesth Analg.* 2006;103(3):784.
27. Newman EJ, Grosset DG, Kennedy PG. The Parkinsonism-hyperpyrexia syndrome. *Neurocrit Care.* 2009;10:136–140.
28. Factor SA. Fatal Parkinsonism-hyperpyrexia syndrome in a Parkinson's disease patient while actively treated with deep brain stimulation. *Mov Disord.* 2007;22(1):148–149.

15 The Approach to the Pediatric Neurosurgical Patient

Karen A. Dean and Rita Agarwal

KEY POINTS

1. Children differ slightly from adults in spinal cord and cranial anatomy. They also have altered myelination, cellular development, cerebral blood flow, and pain processing. These changes may affect monitoring and maintenance during anesthesia.
2. Differences in body composition, hepatic function, and renal function account for altered drug distribution, metabolism, and elimination in young children. The selection and dosing of neuro-anesthetic drugs may need to be modified as a result.
3. Thorough preoperative evaluation is essential to a successful pediatric neuroanesthetic, and should include documentation of the extent of neurologic compromise, as well as investigation into potential comorbidities.
4. The fundamental goals of pediatric neuroanesthesia are to avoid worsening of neurologic injury, to provide excellent operating conditions for the surgeon, and to enable prompt emergence and neurologic assessment at the end of surgery. Multiple induction and maintenance techniques will serve to this end.
5. Maintaining normal ventilation, body temperature, fluid and electrolyte balance, and glucose level is the key to a successful neuroanesthetic. Disruption of homeostasis in these areas can lead to secondary neurologic injury.

I. **Basic neurophysiology.** The central nervous system (CNS) of the newborn is immature, and CNS development continues after birth. The practice of pediatric neuroanesthesia includes understanding the implications of this incomplete neural development. It also requires knowing how children and adults differ in the physiology of other organ systems; these differences will affect the selection and dosing of drugs in neuroanesthesia.
   A. **Neural development**
      1. **Anatomic differences**
         a. **Spinal cord.** At birth, the conus medullaris extends to the L3 or L4 level, and it reaches the adult level of L1 by 1 year of age.
         b. **Dura.** The dural sac extends to S3 or S4 at birth, and rises to S2 by 1 year of age. This elevates the risk of inadvertent dural puncture during caudal anesthesia in very young infants.
         c. **Incomplete bony development.** At birth, vertebrae are largely cartilaginous and sacral vertebrae are not yet fused. The skull sutures are open to accommodate growth. The posterior fontanelle generally closes by 3 months of age, and the anterior fontanelle usually closes between 9 and 18 months of age. Increases in intracranial pressure (ICP) can cause bulging fontanelles and suture separation in the neonate.

> **CLINICAL PEARL** Unlike older children with rigid calvaria, very young children may be able to partially compensate for rises in ICP with skull expansion at the suture lines. This is particularly true if intracranial hypertension occurs gradually and will result in increased head circumference.

2. **Physiologic differences**
   a. **Delayed myelination.** Central and peripheral myelination may not be complete before adolescence. This shortens onset time for local anesthetics, and affects morphology and latencies of normal waveforms during neurophysiologic monitoring.
   b. **Neural cellular development.** The cerebral cortex is immature at birth, and cellular elements continue to develop during early life. There is a growing body of evidence, mostly in animals, that exposure to general anesthesia during infancy may induce neuronal apoptosis and lead to long-term cognitive-behavioral impairment [1,2]. More research is required in this area to clarify the potential for damage in humans, the cellular mechanisms of such damage, and the anesthetic agents responsible. Future anesthetic techniques may be altered based on this research.
   c. **Cerebral blood flow.** Cerebral blood flow (CBF) is estimated to be 50 mL/100 g/min in adults. CBF is slightly lower in neonates (40 mL/100 g/min), and much higher in older children (100 mL/100 g/min). As in adults, autoregulatory mechanisms should maintain constant CBF in children over a wide range of blood pressures. However, these autoregulatory mechanisms are markedly impaired in premature neonates.

> **CLINICAL PEARL** With impaired autoregulation of CBF in premature neonates, increased blood pressure is transmitted to the fragile cerebral vessels and can easily result in vessel rupture and intracerebral hemorrhage. Conversely, low blood pressure can compromise cerebral perfusion and lead to ischemia. It is important to avoid extremes of blood pressure in this population.

   d. **Nociceptive pathways.** Pain pathways are operational at birth, but continue to undergo structural and functional changes in early life [3]. Descending inhibition of pain pathways develops late in gestation and is still immature at birth. Premature infants have lower pain thresholds and impaired inhibitory control mechanisms. Persistent stimulation of peripheral nociceptors in neonates may lead to sensitization, with permanent modulation of pain processing at the spinal and supraspinal levels; adequate perioperative analgesia is imperative. Dose requirements for analgesics will vary with development, based on changes in body composition, drug–protein binding, and drug elimination systems. This necessitates frequent titration of analgesics in young children based on clinical response.

B. **Developmental pharmacology**
   1. **Body Composition.** A term infant has a higher total body water content, lower muscle mass, and lower fat content than an adult (Fig. 15.1). These alterations in body composition are even more extreme in the premature infant.
      a. Total body water is approximately 85% in the preterm infant, 75% in the term infant, and approaches the adult level of 60% by about 6 months of age [4].

> **CLINICAL PEARL** In neonates, high total body water content means that water-soluble drugs will have a larger volume of distribution, and will require a larger initial dose to reach the desired blood level and produce clinical effect.

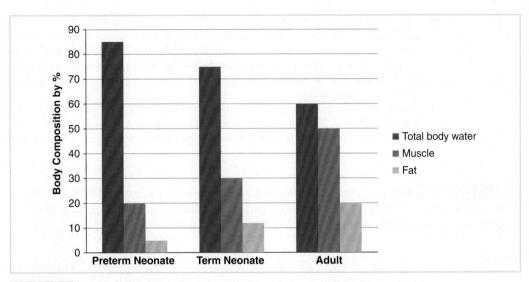

FIGURE 15.1 Variation in body composition with age. Neonates have elevated total body water content relative to adults, but reduced fat and muscle stores.

A larger volume of distribution explains why the infant dose of succinylcholine (2 mg/kg) is double the adult dose. With a larger initial dose requirement and a larger volume of distribution, the excretion of many water-soluble drugs will also be prolonged.

    b. Muscle mass is less than 20% in the preterm infant, about 30% in the term infant, and over 50% in an adult. Drugs that redistribute to muscle tissue will have less uptake in infants, and thus a swifter washout.

    c. Fat content is <5% in a preterm infant, 10% in a term infant, and peaks at 20% to 30% in the first year of life before reaching normal adult levels of 15% to 20%. Since the neonate has less fat, a drug like thiopental that depends on initial redistribution into fat for termination of effect may have a higher plasma concentration and prolonged clinical effect.

  2. **Hepatic function.** In infancy, a smaller proportion of cardiac output reaches the liver than in older children and adults. Hepatocellular enzymatic function is also immature. These factors combine to slow the hepatic metabolism of many drugs in neonates. Older children, on the other hand, usually have rapid drug elimination because of increased hepatic blood flow and robust enzymatic activity.

CLINICAL PEARL   Lower hepatic perfusion in neonates limits the delivery of drugs to the liver, prolonging the elimination half-life of all medications metabolized by the liver. Those drugs that do successfully reach the liver are metabolized slowly because of limited hepatocellular enzyme function. This means that drugs administered to these patients may have prolonged clinical effect or require reduced dosing.

    a. Many drugs require biotransformation by the liver to more water-soluble forms before they can be eliminated. Phase I reactions transform drugs through oxidation, reduction, or hydrolysis. The cytochrome P450 system is a key contributor to phase I metabolism, and its various enzymes are involved in the transformation of many anesthetic drugs. Components of the cytochrome P450 system are at significantly reduced capacity in neonates relative to adults.

  b. Phase II reactions transform drugs through conjugation. Impaired ability to complete phase II reactions can lead to prolonged elimination times for drugs that rely on hepatic conjugation before renal excretion. Slow phase II conjugation of morphine to morphine 3- and 6-glucuronide is partially responsible for the prolonged clinical activity of morphine in the neonate. Conjugation pathways do not reach full maturity until several months of age.

  c. Plasma levels of albumin and α-1-acid glycoprotein are lower in neonates than in older infants and adults. The limited capacity for protein binding in neonates (and especially preterm neonates) results in a greater free portion of acidic drugs (e.g., thiopental) and basic drugs (e.g., local anesthetics).

> **CLINICAL PEARL** Reduced protein binding in neonates results in increased free fractions of drugs, swifter clinical onset, and increased danger for toxicity. Certain drugs, including barbiturates and local anesthetics, may require dose reduction.

  3. Renal function. Glomerular and tubular functions are immature at birth, and perfusion pressure to the kidneys is lower in infants than in adults because of increased renal vascular resistance. Together, these physiologic differences mean that glomerular filtration in the term infant is less than one-third of adult levels when indexed to size, and is almost nonexistent in the extremely premature infant. Glomerular filtration rates develop rapidly, and approach adult levels by 1 year of age, with full maturation of renal function by the age of 2 years.

> **CLINICAL PEARL** Reduced renal perfusion and immature glomerular function mean that very young children cannot readily excrete excess fluid and solutes through glomerular filtration. Immature tubular function impairs urine concentrating and diluting abilities. Limited modification of the glomerular filtrate can lead to obligate sodium losses, which cause hyponatremia if not balanced by appropriate intake.

  a. The half-life of medications excreted by the kidneys will be prolonged. Morphine 6-glucuronide, an active metabolite of morphine, is dependent on renal elimination and thus its accumulation will lead to prolonged opiate effect in infants with immature renal function.

> **CLINICAL PEARL** Morphine has prolonged clinical effect in neonates for two reasons: (i) Decreased hepatic perfusion and reduced conjugation enzymes result in slow metabolism of the native drug, and (ii) renal excretion of the active metabolite morphine 6-glucuronide is impaired. Fentanyl is usually a better choice in the neonatal population.

  4. Minimum alveolar concentration. The minimum alveolar concentration (MAC) for most volatile agents increases from birth through early infancy, peaks at 3 to 6 months of age, and then gradually decreases throughout life (Fig. 15.2). The exception is sevoflurane, which actually has a slightly higher MAC in neonates than in infants 3 to 6 months old. The MAC for all agents is lower in preterm neonates than in term neonates.

   Physiologic explanations for the lower anesthetic requirement of desflurane and isoflurane in neonates relative to older infants include: CNS immaturity, higher levels of endorphins, and the persistence of maternal progesterone. It is unknown why the MAC pattern of sevoflurane differs from that of the other agents.

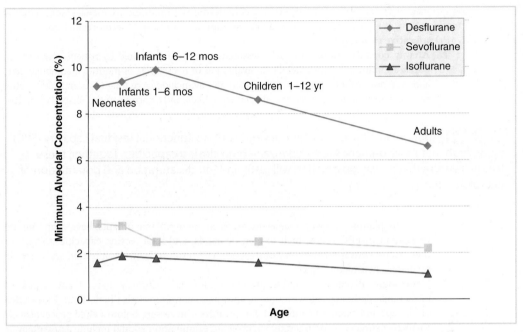

FIGURE 15.2 Minimum alveolar concentration (MAC) of common volatile anesthetic agents throughout childhood. For desflurane and isoflurane, MAC peaks at approximately 6 months of age. Sevoflurane differs from the pattern and has an elevated MAC in neonates. (Data from references 5–7.)

CLINICAL PEARL   Children have elevated MAC requirements relative to adults, especially around 6 months of age. When choosing a maintenance dose, higher anesthetic requirements in children must be balanced against the deleterious effects of volatile anesthetics in neurosurgery, particularly increased CBF.

     5. **Anesthetic uptake.** Inhalation induction is much faster in infants than in adults for several reasons (Table 15.1). The rapidity of anesthetic induction is determined by the rate of rise of the alveolar concentration of volatile agent relative to inspired concentration. Alveolar concentration is determined by the balance between anesthetic delivery and uptake.

        a. As in adults, volatile anesthetics cause a dose-dependent increase in CBF in children, and with swift anesthetic uptake it is easy to create rapid increases in CBF during inhalation induction.

  II. **Anesthetic management.** A carefully planned anesthetic for pediatric neurosurgery starts with a thorough preoperative evaluation. Special attention should be paid to anything that might

TABLE 15.1   Causes of faster inhalation induction in children compared to adults

Factors that speed up equilibration of alveolar and inhaled concentrations

Increased anesthetic delivery to the lungs

1. Increased ratio of alveolar ventilation to functional residual capacity

Decreased anesthetic uptake from the lungs

1. Greater proportion of cardiac output directed to the vessel-rich group (including brain), with rapid equilibration and decrease in the alveolar–venous partial pressure gradient

2. Lower tissue/blood solubility

3. Lower blood/gas solubility

compromise airway access and to pre-existing comorbidities. Intraoperative management requires attention to maintenance agents, fluid and glucose administration, and thermoregulation.

A. Preoperative evaluation

1. **Airway considerations.** Airway assessment in a child is limited by patient cooperation, but at a minimum should include an evaluation of neck range of motion, mandibular size, and dentition. Unique features of the infant airway include large tongue-to-oral cavity ratio, cephalad positioning of the larynx, slanted vocal folds, and a narrow omega-shaped epiglottis.

CLINICAL PEARL   Infants have high minute ventilation-to-functional residual capacity (FRC) ratios, high metabolic demands for oxygen, and high closing capacities. Together, these features ensure that airway obstruction will result in swift desaturation and potentiation of neurologic injury.

When planning airway management, keep in mind that infants have high minute ventilation-to-FRC ratios, high oxygen demands, and high closing capacities. Together these factors ensure that airway obstruction will result in swift desaturation and possible secondary neurologic injury.

2. **Neurologic disease.** Children presenting for neurosurgery have many types of intracranial pathology, all with unique anesthetic considerations (Table 15.2). Knowledge of the type and extent of neurologic compromise is necessary before a child proceeds with corrective surgery. A preoperative neurologic examination should include assessment of level of consciousness, motor and sensory function, reflexes, and cranial nerve function. If symptoms of increased ICP are present, extra caution must be exercised during induction to avoid worsening the situation.

   a. In neonates and infants, intracranial hypertension may present with irritability, lethargy, refusal to feed, or bulging fontanelles.

   b. In older children, signs of elevated ICP include headache, nausea or vomiting, confused speech, and depressed consciousness.

3. **Other comorbidities.** A thorough history and physical examination to uncover relevant comorbidities is essential. This is especially true in very young children, whose high risk of perioperative arrest may be partially related to failed recognition of coexisting congenital heart defects or airway syndromes [8].

4. **Fasting status.** Appropriate fasting intervals should be observed for elective surgery (Table 15.3). The guidelines published by the ASA are based on healthy patients undergoing elective surgery [9], so fasting intervals may need to be extended if there is reason to suspect delayed gastric emptying.

CLINICAL PEARL   Gastrointestinal motility disorders, metabolic disorders (e.g., diabetes), fever, infection, trauma, pain, narcotic use, and anxiety can all delay gastric emptying. Children with nausea, vomiting, and intracranial hypertension may also require extended fasting intervals or a rapid sequence induction (RSI).

B. Premedication

1. Children with normal ICP may benefit from a sedative to reduce anxiety during the induction of anesthesia. The most popular choice is oral midazolam, although other medications and routes can be considered (Table 15.4).

CLINICAL PEARL   Sedatives are best avoided in children with symptoms of intracranial hypertension, as they can lead to respiratory depression, hypercarbia, hypoxia, and further elevation of ICP.

TABLE 15.2 Key elements of preoperative assessment for common neurosurgical diseases and their anesthetic considerations

Type of cranial pathology	Further information needed	Anesthetic considerations
Seizures	Types of seizures and their clinical presentation	If patient taking phenytoin, consider increasing doses of fentanyl and muscle relaxants
	Recent control of seizure frequency	Avoid ketamine, methohexital, meperidine, and other epileptogenic agents
	Medications used for control, and any toxicities	Consider lab tests for hematologic and hepatic function
Hydrocephalus	Evidence of increased ICP (nausea, vomiting, lethargy, irritability, confused speech, poor feeding)	Consider rapid sequence induction, avoid increasing ICP
	If vomiting, check fluid and electrolyte status	Prophylactic antibiotics to prevent shunt infection
Traumatic brain injury	Presence of other injuries, especially to cervical spine	Spinal cord precautions
	Extent of neurologic injury	Avoid increases in ICP
	Assessment of airway protective reflexes	Avoid hypoxia, hypercarbia, hyperglycemia, and other causes of secondary neurologic injury
Intracranial mass	If vomiting, check fluid and electrolyte status	Prepare for massive blood loss
	Evaluate for signs of increased ICP	Intraoperative stress-dose steroids
	Chemotherapy agents, and any toxicities	For posterior fossa surgery, consider use of an armored or nasotracheal ET tube
		Alert surgeon immediately to sudden swings in BP or heart rate during surgery
Meningocele/ encephalocele	Look for concurrent hydrocephalus or Chiari malformation	Latex allergy precautions
	Determine if neonate has comorbidities or prematurity	Avoid muscle relaxants if nerve stimulator to be used by surgeon
	Assess renal function	Careful positioning of defect
	Look for stridor, apnea, swallowing difficulty, loss of gag reflex	Reduce narcotics if defect is below sensory level
	Assess sensory/motor level	
Craniosynostosis	Look for craniofacial syndrome (Crouzon disease, Apert syndrome), maxillary hypoplasia	If syndrome present, anticipate difficult mask fit and possibly difficult intubation
	Assess for increased ICP	Avoid further increases in ICP
	If syndrome present, evaluate for sleep apnea and difficult airway	Anticipate rapid blood loss and possible venous air embolism
Arnold–Chiari malformation	Assess for swallowing difficulty, stridor, apnea, and loss of airway reflexes	Consider postoperative ventilation if respiratory drive or airway reflexes are compromised
Aneurysm/AVM	Document preoperative deficits	Controlled hypotension
	Evaluate for signs of high-output heart failure in neonates	Avoid light anesthesia and hypertension before lesion secured

TABLE 15.3 Appropriate fasting intervals for children having elective surgery

Type of food	Fasting interval[a]	Examples
Clear liquids	2 h	Apple juice, water, pediatric electrolyte solutions
Breast milk	4 h	—
Other liquids, Light meal	6 h	Infant formula, cow's milk, orange juice, dry toast
Solids	8 h or more	Fatty foods

[a]Appropriate fasting interval does not guarantee gastric emptying.

TABLE 15.4 Choice of agents for premedication, with doses and routes of administration

Drug name	Route of administration				
	Intravenous	**Oral**	**Rectal**	**Nasal**	**Intramuscular**
Midazolam (mg/kg)	0.05–0.1	0.2–0.5	0.75–1.0	0.1–0.2	0.1–0.2
Dexmedetomidine (μg/kg)	—	2.5–4	—	1–2	—
Ketamine (mg/kg)	0.5–1	3–5	6–10	2–4	2–10
Thiopental (mg/kg)	—	—	20–40	—	—
Clonidine (μg/kg)	—	4	—	—	—

2. If the benefits of sedation are thought to outweigh the risks of further neurologic compromise, dexmedetomidine is an excellent choice because it has minimal effects on respiratory drive. There are studies to support the use of dexmedetomidine as an oral or nasal premedication [10,11].

3. In situations where pharmacologic anxiolysis is contraindicated, behavioral interventions may be helpful. Child life specialists can meet with the child preoperatively to explain the process of induction through visual aids, thereby building rapport and reducing anxiety. Clowns, video games, or low-stimulation environments during induction have also been shown to be helpful. Currently available evidence does not support the routine use of parental presence to reduce a child's anxiety [12], but may be considered at the discretion of the anesthesiologist.

4. In children having epilepsy surgery with intraoperative seizure monitoring, midazolam is contraindicated because of its tendency to suppress seizure foci and interfere with electroencephalography. Dexmedetomidine is an acceptable alternative.

CLINICAL PEARL In many situations in pediatric neurosurgery, premedication is avoided either because of the risk of respiratory depression and elevated ICP, or because of potential interference with neurologic examination and EEG monitoring. Anxious children with unsecured aneurysms are an important exception to this general principle. Sedatives should be given as needed in this population to prevent agitation, hypertension, and aneurysm rupture with anesthetic induction.

C. **Induction techniques**
1. In children with increased ICP, it is critical to prevent episodes of hypoventilation, hypoxemia, hypotension, coughing, or straining during induction of anesthesia.
2. **IV techniques.** Many children with intracranial lesions already have an IV in place, and proceeding with an IV induction can be a safe and simple option. A variety of induction agents can be used, including propofol, thiopental, and etomidate. Induction can be supplemented with a muscle relaxant, fentanyl (2 to 5 μg/kg), remifentanil (1 to 5 μg/kg), and/or lidocaine (1 to 1.5 mg/kg) to provide optimal intubating conditions.
   a. With the exception of ketamine, all IV induction agents will cause a decrease in CBF and cerebral metabolic rate for oxygen ($CMRO_2$).

CLINICAL PEARL Ketamine should be avoided in children with intracranial hypertension because of its tendency to raise CBF and ICP.

   b. Keep in mind that dosage requirements of commonly used anesthetic agents will vary with age. For example, the effective dose of propofol is 2 to 3 mg/kg in older children and adults, but increases to 3 to 5 mg/kg in infants.

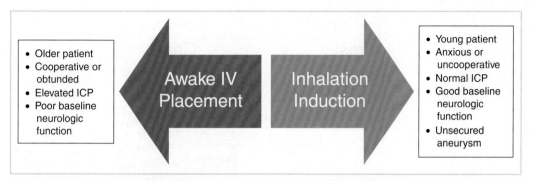

FIGURE 15.3 Methods of anesthetic induction in a child who presents for neurosurgery without an intravenous line.

   c. An RSI is necessary for patients with a full stomach to reduce the risk of aspiration. Gastric emptying may be delayed in patients with elevated ICP despite adherence to fasting guidelines, so these patients should also get an RSI or a modified RSI. In children, a modified RSI with low-pressure manual ventilation may be just as effective as a strict RSI at preventing aspiration [13].

  3. **Inhalation techniques.** Some children present for neurosurgery without an IV, so options include inhalation induction or preoperative (awake) placement of an IV. There are several factors to consider, including patient age, cooperativeness, and the type and severity of neurologic compromise (Fig. 15.3). All potent inhalation agents will cause a dose-dependent increase in CBF and decrease in $CMRO_2$, which leads to a net increase in ICP. The increase in CBF may be offset by mild hyperventilation to an arterial carbon dioxide tension ($PaCO_2$) of 30 to 35 mm Hg.

   a. For the young or uncooperative child with a vascular lesion, all possible precautions must be taken to avoid agitation and lesion rupture, so inhalation induction may be the best choice.

   b. For the child with symptoms of increased ICP or impending herniation, it is best to avoid high doses of volatile agent required for inhalation induction, and IV placement is advised. The children with the worst neurologic impairment are usually the most tolerant of awake IV placement.

D. **Maintenance of anesthesia**

  1. A variety of maintenance agents have been used successfully in pediatric neurosurgery, including low-dose potent volatile agents, nitrous oxide, propofol, dexmedetomidine, and narcotics. In most situations, a balanced technique is preferred. Inhalation agents may be reduced or avoided in patients with intracranial hypertension, in favor of IV agents that will reduce CBF, ICP, and $CMRO_2$ while maintaining cerebral perfusion pressure (CPP). Inhalation agents may also be reduced or avoided in cases requiring monitoring of somatosensory evoked potentials (SSEPs) or motor evoked potentials (MEPs) (Chapter 26).

   a. In children with intracranial hypertension, desflurane may have a more exaggerated effect on ICP than other potent inhalational agents. In this situation, isoflurane or sevoflurane are preferred over desflurane.

  2. Controversy persists over whether the routine use of nitrous oxide has a place in pediatric neurosurgery (Fig. 15.4). Relative contraindications to its use include the presence of pneumocephalus, or the need for MEP monitoring. Many would also argue against the use of nitrous oxide in cases where there is high risk for venous air embolism (VAE). If nitrous oxide is used for maintenance, it must be discontinued at the first sign of VAE.

E. **Monitoring**

  1. **Routine monitors.** Standard ASA monitors should be used for all cases.

  2. **Invasive blood pressure monitoring.** Placement of an arterial line is advisable whenever there is the potential for rapid fluid shifts or blood loss. It is also important when blood

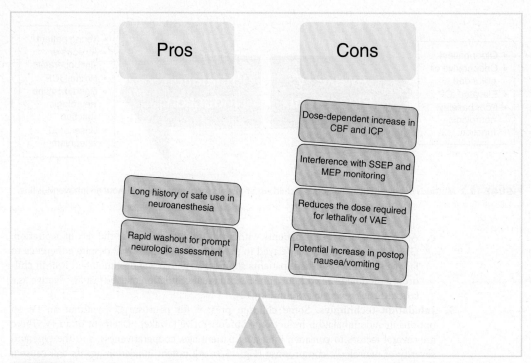

FIGURE 15.4 Evaluation of the use of nitrous oxide for maintenance during neurosurgical procedures.

pressure must be tightly controlled at all times, such as to provide adequate mean arterial pressure (MAP) and CPP in the patient with elevated ICP, or to avoid hypertension in a patient with an unsecured aneurysm. An arterial line is also useful for frequent blood gas sampling, or for measuring systolic pressure variation and predicting fluid responsiveness.

CLINICAL PEARL   Continuous blood pressure monitoring is critical in posterior fossa surgery, where traction on the brainstem and cranial nuclei can lead to rapid swings in blood pressure and heart rate. If hemodynamic changes occur, the most important intervention is immediate notification of the surgeon.

3. **Urine output monitoring.** Placement of a Foley catheter should be considered for all large intracranial cases. If the surgical dissection is near the hypophysial fossa, compromise of the posterior pituitary gland can result in central diabetes insipidus and copious urine output. This diagnosis can be confirmed by comparing urine and serum osmolality.

4. **Central venous pressure (CVP) monitoring.** There are many indications for central line use during neurosurgery (Table 15.5). Placement of a central line can be useful for cases in which large fluid shifts are anticipated, to assist with monitoring volume status. Keep in mind, however, that prone positioning may compromise the accuracy of the values obtained. A central venous line may be considered in cases with high risk for VAE, as a means of aspirating air; placement at the atriocaval junction should be confirmed by radiography or electrocardiography. However, the small diameter of pediatric central venous catheters means they will have high resistance to flow that may limit their ability to rapidly aspirate air. In a patient with increased ICP, one may want to use a smaller catheter in a jugular vein or pick another site entirely, so as not to impede cerebral venous drainage.

TABLE 15.5   Indications for central line placement during neurosurgery

Indication

1. To guide fluid management in a case with anticipated large fluid shifts or blood loss
2. Administration of vasoactive agents, treatment of hemodynamic instability
3. Insufficient peripheral venous access
4. Aspiration of air from the atriocaval junction in cases with high risk for VAE
5. Frequent lab sampling
6. Administration of hypertonic saline to treat ICP

5. **VAE monitors.** Monitoring for VAE can be accomplished by Doppler ultrasonography, echocardiography, end-tidal nitrogen monitoring, or a combination of techniques. The risk of VAE is particularly high in the sitting position, but is increased above normal anytime the patient's head is above their heart. Clinically significant VAE will present with hemodynamic and ventilatory abnormalities (Table 15.6) (see chapter 22).

  a. The Doppler probe should be placed in the fourth intercostal interspace to the right of the sternum. In neonates, it is also possible to position the probe on the posterior chest. Proper positioning should be checked by rapidly administering a few milliliters of agitated saline and listening for the characteristic churning sound. Doppler ultrasonography is one of the most sensitive monitoring methods, detecting as little as 1 mL of air. Its reliance on sound for detection means that the anesthesiologist can monitor the Doppler continually while attending to other tasks.

  b. Echocardiography is an even more sensitive technique, detecting air volumes as small as 0.3 to 0.5 mL. However, maximum sensitivity requires that a skilled individual be continuously watching the screen. Currently available TEE probes are recommended for use in children as small as 3 kg.

  c. End-tidal nitrogen monitoring has limited sensitivity and is not standard equipment on anesthesia machines.

  d. Pulmonary artery catheters and end-tidal CO_2 monitors can provide supportive evidence in the diagnosis of VAE, but are not sensitive or specific by themselves.

CLINICAL PEARL   The high incidence of atrial-level shunt in the pediatric population means that the risk of paradoxical embolism and stroke is high. Patients who survive the hemodynamic collapse associated with a larger air embolism may have permanent stroke deficits.

TABLE 15.6   Signs and symptoms of clinically significant venous air embolism

Clinical signs of venous air embolism

1. Cough
2. Tachycardia
3. Hypotension
4. Jugular venous distention, increased central venous pressure
5. Nonspecific ST-segment and T-wave changes on EKG
6. S wave in lead I, Q wave and inverted T wave in lead III
7. Pulmonary hypertension
8. Tachypnea
9. Wheezing
10. Hypoxia, cyanosis
11. Decreased end-tidal carbon dioxide
12. Increased arterial carbon dioxide (increased alveolar–arterial gradient)
13. Increased airway pressures
14. Millwheel murmur

6. **Neurophysiologic monitors.** Neurophysiologic monitoring is recommended for complex surgeries involving central or peripheral nervous structures. For example, the activity of adjacent structures may be monitored during tumor resection to help maximize the area that can be safely resected without loss of function in neighboring areas. Available monitoring modalities include SSEPs, brainstem auditory evoked potentials (BAEPs), visual evoked potentials, transcranial electric motor stimulation, electromyography (EMG), and electroencephalography (Table 15.7). In order to ensure accurate monitoring, it is necessary to minimize fluctuations in anesthetic depth, ventilation, oxygenation, and body temperature (see Chapter 26).

   a. SSEPs measure the integrity of ascending sensory pathways of proprioception and vibration, from peripheral nerves to dorsal spinal columns to the sensory cortex. SSEPs are usually obtained by stimulation of the posterior tibial nerve, and recording of signal from cortical or subcortical electrodes. In general, a significant change is defined as a 50% decrease in amplitude or a 10% increase in latency from baseline values. Anesthetic medications can interfere with the latency and amplitude of recordings [14].

   CLINICAL PEARL Successful SSEP monitoring requires constant anesthetic depth and avoidance of physiologic disturbances like anemia, hypoperfusion, hypo/hyperthermia, and hypoxia. Inhaled agents are best avoided in favor of IV anesthetic infusions. The effects of anesthetic agents on signal amplitudes may be even greater in children under the age of 3 years because of the immaturity of neural pathways.

   b. MEPs measure the integrity of descending motor pathways, from motor cortex to anterior corticospinal tracts to motor end plates. MEPs are most often obtained by transcranial electrical stimulation of the motor cortex, and recording of muscle action potentials in the limbs. Scalp electrode placement for transcranial stimulation is contraindicated in infants with an open anterior fontanelle (up to the age of 18 months). MEP monitoring is sensitive to anesthetic technique, blood loss, changes in blood pressure, and neuromuscular blockade.

   CLINICAL PEARL MEPs are even more sensitive to the presence of volatile anesthetics than are SSEPs, and if possible, halogenated agents and nitrous oxide should be avoided entirely. Young children have higher thresholds for elicitation of MEPs than adult patients.

   c. EMG monitors for electromyographic potentials in areas of potential nerve injury. Recording of bursts or discharges from the area of interest indicates nerve root irritability, and the need to limit surgical manipulation. EMG is commonly used during tethered cord release or myelomeningocele repair, with EMG recordings taken from the muscles innervated by lower lumbar and sacral nerve roots. EMG also has application in selective dorsal rhizotomy surgery for spasticity.

   d. BAEPs (also know as ABR: auditory brainstem response) use surface scalp electrodes to monitor for activation of the eighth cranial nerve and brainstem auditory pathways in response to click stimulus in the ear. They are used to monitor cranial nerve function during resection of tumors in the cerebellopontine angle. BAEPs are more resistant to changes in anesthetic technique or dose than SSEPs or MEPs. Incomplete myelination in the cochlear nucleus and other brainstem structures means that latencies are extended in children under the age of 3 years.

   CLINICAL PEARL BAEP latencies are prolonged in preterm neonates. The normalization of BAEP recordings generally coincides with maturation of other brainstem structures, notably the respiratory control center.

TABLE 15.7   Characteristics of neurophysiologic monitors commonly used in neurosurgery

Type of monitor	Description	Potential uses	Anesthetic considerations
Somatosensory evoked potentials (SSEPs)	Measure activity of ascending sensory pathways from peripheral nerves to cortex (via dorsal columns)	Monitor integrity of posterior and lateral spinal cord in spine surgery Predict postop neurologic deficit in surgery for anterior circulation aneurysms	Recordings sensitive to changes in anesthetic depth, ventilation, or temperature. Avoid anemia and hypotension Reduce or eliminate potent volatile agents (<0.5 MAC) and nitrous oxide for best recordings Ketamine and etomidate can augment signal amplitude
Motor evoked potentials (MEPs)	Measure activity of descending motor pathways from cortex to motor end plates (via anterior corticospinal tracts)	Monitor integrity of anterior spinal cord in spine surgery	Recordings sensitive to changes in anesthetic depth, ventilation, or temperature. Avoid anemia and hypotension Eliminate potent volatile agents and nitrous oxide for best recordings, avoid benzodiazepines and paralytics Contraindicated in patients with recent seizures, intracranial metal, or skull defects – including children <18 months
Electromyography (EMG)	Measure muscle action potentials as an indicator of nerve function and irritability	Monitor cranial or peripheral nerve irritability to warn against potential surgical injury—e.g., facial nerve monitoring for resection of vestibular schwannoma Assess level of nerve function—e.g., myelomeningocele Differentiate nerve from nonnervous structures— e.g., tethered cord release	Avoid muscle relaxants
Brainstem auditory evoked potentials (BAEPs, ABRs)	Measure activation of eighth cranial nerve and brainstem auditory pathways in response to audible click stimulus	Resection of vestibular nerve schwannoma	More resistant than SSEPs and MEPs to type of anesthetic used Avoid sudden changes in anesthetic depth
Electroencephalography, electrocorticography (EEG/ECoG)	Measure electrical activity of the brain via scalp electrodes (EEG) or subdural electrodes (ECoG)	Confirm adequate blood flow to the cortex (e.g., moyamoya surgery, aneurysm clipping) Induce barbiturate coma Identify and resect seizure focus Help gauge depth of anesthesia Map eloquent areas of brain during awake craniotomy	Maintain constant ventilation, temperature, and anesthetic depth Avoid benzodiazepines Reduce or avoid propofol and potent volatile agents in favor of opiates, dexmedetomidine, or nitrous oxide May need to help provoke a seizure with hyperventilation or methohexital

e. Electroencephalogram (EEG) monitors the brain's electrical signals using scalp electrode recordings. It is useful in monitoring for cerebral ischemia (e.g., controlled hypotension), trending anesthetic depth, or for identifying a seizure focus for resection.

f. Electrocorticography (ECoG) uses a subdural grid of electrodes to monitor the EEG directly from the exposed cortical surface. It is used in epilepsy surgery to identify the origin of epileptiform discharges, with better localization than scalp EEG recordings. In most cases, intracranial grid placement is followed by days of seizure monitoring/recording, and then resection is completed under a second anesthetic. In future, grid placement, monitoring, and resection may be completed under one anesthetic. ECoG can also be used to map critical areas of motor or language function using direct cortical electrical stimulation (DCES) in awake (older) children.

   (1) For ECoG procedures, avoid benzodiazepines for premedication, as they will suppress seizure activity; intranasal dexmedetomidine is an acceptable alternative.

   (2) Also avoid maintenance with propofol or volatile agents, as these may affect the ECoG recording. Our group uses dexmedetomidine (bolus 1 μg/kg over 10 minutes, maintenance infusion 0.1 to 2 μg/kg/h) and remifentanil (0.05 to 1.3 μg/kg/min) for maintenance, with or without 50% to 70% nitrous oxide.

F. **Thermoregulation**

1. Small children are especially prone to hypothermia because of key physiologic differences. First, they have a large body surface area to weight ratio, providing more surface area for heat loss. They also have thin skin and limited fat stores. In addition, infants <3 months of age have minimal ability to produce heat by shivering, so they rely on nonshivering cellular thermogenesis by the metabolism of brown fat.

2. Hypothermia is undesirable because it leads to impaired coagulation, decreased metabolism of anesthetic drugs, delayed emergence, arrhythmias, and increased postoperative oxygen consumption.

3. While hypothermia has traditionally been used during neurosurgery for cerebral protection, current evidence does not support this practice. A Cochrane Review of cooling for cerebral protection did not reveal any evidence that hypothermia is more effective than normothermia for neuroprotection in patients undergoing brain surgery [15]. Multiple studies have suggested possible adverse effects of cooling, including increased blood loss, increased rate of wound infection, delayed emergence, and increased perioperative cardiac complications.

   a. The pediatric data for hypothermia is largely limited to the treatment of traumatic brain injury in the ICU setting. A randomized controlled trial published in 2008 compared normothermia versus 24 hours of prophylactic hypothermia (to 32.5°C) in children with traumatic brain injury [16]. No mortality or neurodevelopmental benefits were seen with hypothermia, and there was more hemodynamic instability and a trend to higher mortality.

CLINICAL PEARL Given the current state of the evidence, maintaining normothermia or very mild hypothermia is a reasonable target during neurosurgery. Hyperthermia is to be strictly avoided.

4. Heat loss occurs in the operating room by four primary mechanisms: radiation, convection, evaporation, and conduction.

   a. Radiant heat loss is the primary mechanism of operative heat loss, and involves the transfer of heat from a warm body to the environment by infrared emission. It can be prevented by reducing the gradient for radiant heat transfer by warming the OR environment to at least 80°F, by keeping the patient covered, or by applying radiant heat in the form of warming lights.

   b. Convection is also a critical mode of heat loss in the OR, and occurs when cool air travels over the warm patient. It can be prevented by the use of a forced-air warming blanket.

TABLE 15.8 Assessment of preoperative fluid deficit in children based on history and physical examination findings

Severity of dehydration	Decrease in weight (%)	Symptoms	Estimated deficit in mL/kg
Mild	5	Dry mouth, poor skin turgor	50
Moderate	10	Tachycardia, sunken fontanelles, decreased urine	100
Severe	15	Hypotension, anuria, absent tears	150

    c. Evaporation is the heat loss that occurs when the patient's moisture transfers into gaseous phase, most notably with perspiration or the vaporization of moisture in the lungs. Evaporative losses can be reduced by prewarming the sterile preparative solution. Insensible heat losses due to breathing can be reduced by using humidified respiratory gases.

    d. Conduction is the transfer of heat from the patient to a cold object, usually the operating table. It contributes only a small amount to operative heat loss. Conduction can be prevented by using a warm mattress pad.

  5. Hyperthermia is also to be avoided, with strong evidence that hyperthermia leads to increased secondary neurologic injury in at-risk brain. Forced-air warmers and cooled IV or irrigation fluids can be used to help maintain normothermia.

    a. The differential diagnosis for intraoperative hyperthermia includes iatrogenic overwarming, infection/sepsis, blood transfusion reaction, thyroid storm, hypothalamic injury, and malignant hyperthermia.

G. Fluid management

  1. Fluid balance may be perturbed preoperatively in neurosurgical patients because of poor oral intake, vomiting, fluid restriction, or the use of osmotic diuretics. Findings in the history and physical examination can help determine the extent of a child's preoperative fluid deficit (Table 15.8).

CLINICAL PEARL   Note that hypotension is a very late finding of dehydration in children. Blood pressure should not be relied upon to indicate mild or moderate levels of dehydration.

---

  2. In addition to large preoperative fluid deficits, neurosurgical patients have the potential for significant intraoperative fluid losses. These losses are usually due to bleeding, or to the use of osmotic diuretics.

  3. Fluid deficits and ongoing losses should be replaced to maintain euvolemia. Administration of isotonic crystalloid solutions should not exacerbate cerebral edema, so there is no benefit to aggressive intraoperative fluid restriction. Rather, fluid restriction and hypovolemia may lead to decreased MAP and CPP, and should be carefully avoided.

  4. Maintenance fluid requirements in children are calculated based on a formula developed by Holliday and Segar in 1957 [17], as described in Table 15.9. This formula accounts

TABLE 15.9 Calculation of maintenance fluid requirements in children

Body weight in kg	Fluid requirements
0–10	4 mL/kg/h × (weight under 10 kg)
10–20	4 mL/kg/h × (10 kg) + 2 mL/kg/h × (weight above 10 kg)
>20	4 mL/kg/h × (10 kg) + 2 mL/kg/h × (10 kg) + 1 mL/kg/h × (weight above 20 kg)

for maintenance needs only, and does not include pre-existing fluid deficit, blood loss replacement, or third space losses.

CLINICAL PEARL The best replacement and maintenance fluids for neurosurgery are isoosmolar or slightly hyperosmolar, including normal saline and Plasma-Lyte. Hypoosmolar fluids like Lactated Ringers are best avoided because they can worsen brain edema.

5. Glucose levels can be disrupted perioperatively because of prolonged fasting, vomiting, steroid administration, or the stress response to illness. Both hypoglycemia and hyperglycemia can lead to exacerbation of secondary neurologic injury in patients with acute cerebral damage. Typical pediatric intravenous maintenance fluids include 5% dextrose. However, there is no evidence that glucose-containing fluids should be continued during surgery, except in the case of premature neonates or patients on total parenteral nutrition. There is a particularly large body of evidence linking hyperglycemia to poor outcome in adult ICU populations with traumatic brain injury or subarachnoid hemorrhage. Hyperglycemia causes osmotically induced cerebral swelling, and contributes to fluid and electrolyte loss through glucosuria-induced diuresis.

a. Current trends in adult neurosurgical ICU management favor conventional glucose control (target <140 to 180 mg/dL) rather than more intensive insulin therapy (target 80 to 110 mg/dL) because of the increased risk of iatrogenic hypoglycemia and mortality with the latter as demonstrated by the NICE-SUGAR trial [18].

b. Randomized controlled trials examining glycemic control in critically ill children are few at the time of publication. The 2009 study by Vlasselaers et al. [19] compared intensive insulin therapy with age-adjusted goals (50 to 79 mg/dL for infants; 70 to 99 mg/dL for children of 1 to 16 years) to conventional insulin therapy (goal 180 to 215 mg/dL), and found that the intensive insulin group had shorter ICU stays and lower inflammatory markers. However, they also had a much higher risk of hypoglycemic episodes.

c. Given the available evidence, the authors' recommendation is to monitor glucose frequently in the perioperative neurosurgical setting in an attempt to avoid both hypoglycemia and hyperglycemia. Particular caution is required with patients receiving hyperalimentation, steroids, or transfusion.

CLINICAL PEARL Except in the case of established parenteral nutrition, glucose should be eliminated from routine maintenance fluids and only administered as needed to treat hypoglycemia.

H. Positioning

1. Neurosurgical procedures are often lengthy and limit the anesthesiologist's access to the head and airway. For these reasons, proper patient positioning requires that all pressure points are padded, and that the airway is well secured. Additional considerations apply depending on the type of position (Table 15.10).

2. Supine positioning is the simplest, but the anesthesiologist should know whether the head is to be secured on a horseshoe headrest or in pins. Use of pins by the surgeon may require a deeper anesthetic or the use of muscle relaxation to prevent patient movement and self-injury. Another consideration with supine positioning is the degree of head rotation required by the surgeon. Turning the head severely can impede venous return, increase bleeding from the surgical field, or increase ICP. Brachial plexus injuries have also been reported.

3. Prone positioning is frequently used for access to the posterior fossa in children, and typically involves significant cervical flexion to aid exposure. Excessive neck flexion can

TABLE 15.10 Anesthetic considerations related to type of patient positioning for neurosurgery

Position	Factor	Anesthetic considerations
Supine	Type of headrest	Use of pins may require deeper anesthesia or paralytic use
	Head rotation	Over-rotation can prevent venous drainage, increase ICP, increase bleeding, and lead to stretch injury of the brachial plexus
	Head elevation	Risk of VAE exists whenever the surgical site is above the level of the heart, which can occur even while supine in infants with large occiputs
Prone	Type of headrest	Use of pins may require deeper anesthesia or paralytic use
	Neck flexion	Potential for massive tongue swelling requiring postop ventilation
		Risk of ET tube kinking, consider armored or nasal tube
		Rarely reported cervical cord ischemia and quadriplegia
		Risk of inadvertent mainstem intubation
	Abdominal pressure	Increased abdominal and thoracic pressure can prevent cerebral venous drainage and increase bleeding
Sitting	Head elevation	High risk for venous air embolism

exert pressure on the tongue and prevent venous drainage, resulting in massive tongue swelling and inability to extubate following the procedure. Another potential complication of extreme neck flexion is kinking of the endotracheal tube, and placement of an armored endotracheal tube (with a bite block) or a nasotracheal tube is a good option. In rare cases, extreme neck flexion has led to cervical spinal cord ischemia and quadriplegia. Finally, head flexion will advance the ET tube down the trachea, which could result in mainstem intubation.

CLINICAL PEARL Before a child is placed prone, it is recommended to auscultate for breath sounds in flexed and neutral neck positions, and retract the endotracheal tube if necessary.

4. VAE can occur whenever an open vein is above the level of the patient's heart. In an infant, this can occur even in a supine position because the large occiput elevates the head above the rest of the body. Significant VAE is most common, however, with seated positioning. A plan for a sitting craniotomy should prompt special VAE precautions, including a mode of detection and placement of a central line.

I. **Postoperative care**

1. In general, a smooth and swift emergence is desirable for neurosurgery. Coughing, straining, agitation, and hypertension should be minimized, because these can lead to transient increases in ICP and risk of intracranial bleeding.

   a. A controlled awake extubation may require the use of narcotics or lidocaine to reduce stimulation from the endotracheal tube. Any hypertension on emergence should be aggressively treated with short-acting antihypertensives like esmolol or nitroprusside.

   b. Another option is to remove the endotracheal tube when the child is still deeply anesthetized. This is only possible in children with intact airway reflexes and good overall neurologic function. Any child with airway swelling, preoperative obtundation, or poor secretion management is not a good candidate.

2. Failure to emerge from anesthesia in a timely fashion should prompt an immediate review of likely physiologic or pharmacologic causes including hypoglycemia, hypothermia, hyponatremia, excess sedation, and persistent neuromuscular blockade. If no cause is immediately apparent, the child should have an emergent CT scan to look for new ischemia, mass effect, or hemorrhage. Perioperative seizure is also a possibility.

3. Postoperative mechanical ventilation should be considered if the patient has demonstrable facial swelling and suspected airway edema, or if the surgery is likely to have compromised airway reflexes or respiratory drive. This may be true in posterior fossa craniotomies

where the surgical dissection is in close proximity to cranial nuclei and respiratory control centers.

4. Immediate postoperative management should include frequent assessment of neurologic status to monitor for signs of stroke, seizure, or intracranial hemorrhage.

5. Electrolytes and urine output should also be monitored postoperatively, as neurosurgical patients may develop central diabetes insipidus or syndrome of inappropriate ADH secretion (SIADH).

REFERENCES

1. Stratmann G. Neurotoxicity of anesthetic drugs in the developing brain. *Anesth Analg.* 2011;113(5):1170–1179.
2. McCann ME, Soriano SG. Is anesthesia bad for the newborn brain? *Anesthesiol Clin.* 2009;27(2):269–284.
3. Walker SM. Pain in children: recent advances and ongoing challenges. *Br J Anaesth.* 2008;101:101–110.
4. Friis-Hansen B. Body composition during growth. In vivo measurements and biochemical data correlated to differential anatomical growth. *Pediatrics.* 1971;47(1):S264–S274.
5. Lerman J, Sikich N, Kleinman S, et al. The pharmacology of sevoflurane in infants and children. *Anesthesiology.* 1994;80(4):814–824.
6. Taylor RH, Lerman J. Minimum alveolar concentration of desflurane and hemodynamic responses in neonates, infants, and children. *Anesthesiology.* 1991;75:975–979.
7. Cameron CB, Robinson S, Gregory GA. The minimum anesthetic concentration of isoflurane in children. *Anesth Analg.* 1984;63:418–420.
8. Bhananker SM, Ramamoorthy C, Geiduschek JM, et al. Anesthesia-related cardiac arrest in children: update from the Pediatric Perioperative Cardiac Arrest registry. *Anesth Analg.* 2007;105(2):344–350.
9. Apfelbaum JL, Caplan RA, Connis RT, et al. Practice guidelines for preoperative fasting and the use of pharmacological agents to reduce the risk of pulmonary aspiration: application to healthy patients undergoing elective procedures: an updated report by the American Society of Anesthesiologists Committee on Standards and Practice Parameters. *Anesthesiology.* 2011;114(3):495–511.
10. Zub D, Berkenbosch JW, Tobias JD. Preliminary experience with oral dexmedetomidine for procedural and anesthetic premedication. *Paediatr Anaesth.* 2005;15(11):932–938.
11. Yuen VM, Hui TW, Irwin MG, et al. A comparison of intranasal dexmedetomidine and oral midazolam for premedication in pediatric anesthesia: a double-blinded randomized controlled trial. *Anesth Analg.* 2008;106(6):1715–1721.
12. Yip P, Middleton P, Cyna AM, et al. Non-pharmacological interventions for assisting the induction of anaesthesia in children. *Cochrane Database Syst Rev.* 2009;3:CD006447.
13. Cook-Sather SD, Tulloch HV, Cnaan A, et al. A comparison of awake versus paralyzed tracheal intubation for infants with pyloric stenosis. *Anesth Analg.* 1998;86:945–951.
14. Pajewski TN, Arlet V, Phillips LH. Current approach on spinal cord monitoring: the point of view of the neurologist, the anesthesiologist and the spine surgeon. *Eur Spine J.* 2007;16(S2):S115–S129.
15. Milani WR, Antibas PL, Prado GF. Cooling for cerebral protection during brain surgery. *Cochrane Database Syst Rev.* 2011;10:CD006638.
16. Hutchison JS, Ward RE, Lacroix J, et al. Hypothermia therapy after traumatic brain injury in children. *N Engl J Med.* 2008;358(23):2447–2456.
17. Holliday MA, Segar WE. The maintenance need for water in parenteral fluid therapy. *Pediatrics.* 1957;19:823–832.
18. NICE-SUGAR investigators. Intensive versus conventional glucose control in critically ill patients. *N Engl J Med.* 2009;360(13):1283–1297.
19. Vlasselaers D, Milants I, Desmet L, et al. Intensive insulin therapy for patients in paediatric intensive care: a prospective, randomized controlled study. *Lancet.* 2009;373(9663):547–556.

16

Pediatric Congenital Lesions

Michael Chen and Cynthia Tung

KEY POINTS

1. Latex precautions are essential in patients with neural tube defects to avoid early sensitization.
2. The size of the defect affects the volume of insensible fluid losses during surgery.
3. Patient positioning and laryngoscopy may be challenging depending on the location and size of the defect.
4. Spinal dysraphisms can produce clinical signs and symptoms via structural abnormalities, mass effect from the lesion, or tethering of the spinal cord.
5. Surgical repair of spinal dysraphisms usually requires intraoperative motor and sensory nerve root mapping, therefore muscle paralysis should be spared to facilitate neuromonitoring.
6. Risk of bleeding and venous air embolization is greater in patients with larger cranial defects.
7. Thermoregulation is important in patients with spinal and cranial dysraphisms because of potential fluid losses and possible dysfunctional autonomic control.

I. **Spinal dysraphisms.** Spinal dysraphisms are lesions where the dorsal midline structures fail to fuse during embryogenesis. Spinal dysraphisms are categorized into two types: Spina bifida aperta (open) or spina bifida occulta (occult). Spina bifida aperta is easily identifiable by the sac-like lesion containing meninges (meningocele) or neural tissue and meninges (myelomeningocele). As the name implies, spina bifida occulta are more difficult to recognize because they often do not have cutaneous manifestations. Rachischisis consists of exposed neural tube with no covering.

II. **Spina bifida aperta**
   A. **Background and anatomy**
      1. Neural tube defects occur secondary to failure of the posterior neural tube to close. Closure of the neural tube begins at gestational age 22 to 23 days, with complete closure around days 26 to 27 [1]. Closure starts near the cervical spine region and extends cephalad and caudad. Therefore, most commonly defects occur along the thoracic or lumbosacral region, but can occur along the cervical region as well.
         a. A **meningocele** consists of a herniation of meninges through the defect.
         b. A **myelomeningocele** consists of a herniation of meninges and spinal cord elements through the defect.
      2. The incidence of neural tube defects is approximately 2 to 5/1,000 live births [2].
      3. These lesions are associated with Arnold–Chiari malformations, hydrocephalus, and neurologic deficits. Cervical cord or brainstem compression is possible in patients with concomitant Arnold–Chiari malformations.

    4. There is no association with congenital cardiac anomalies.

    5. Patients may have poor autonomic control below level of the defect.

B. Surgery

    1. After birth, defects are usually covered with sterile, saline-soaked gauze [3]. The patient is typically positioned prone to avoid pressure on the defect.

    2. Timely surgical closure is important to reduce risk of infection [4].

    3. Occasionally, rotational or myocutaneous flaps are required for closure [4].

C. Anesthetic considerations

    1. Preanesthetic evaluation

       a. The antenatal history, birth history, prematurity, other comorbidities and congenital anomalies should be thoroughly reviewed prior to surgery.

       b. One should document any preoperative neurologic deficits.

       c. Latex precautions/avoidance is essential to prevent early sensitization in this vulnerable patient population.

    2. Monitoring and intraoperative management

       a. Standard ASA monitors include ECG, noninvasive BP, pulse oximeter, and core temperature. An arterial line may be appropriate based on other comorbidities.

       b. Ensure adequate peripheral or umbilical IV access for fluid replacement or blood transfusion. The size of the defect affects volume of insensible fluid losses during surgery; thus, the larger the defect, the larger the volume of fluid loss expected. Typically, blood loss during the procedure is not significant enough to necessitate blood transfusions.

       c. May consider inhalation or IV induction with muscle relaxant for intubation. A presumed difficult airway may warrant an awake intubation, in which case preoxygenation and atropine premedication prior to laryngoscopy may be useful.

       d. Positioning patient for laryngoscopy may be challenging given the size of defect. Lateral decubitus position of patient may be necessary to accommodate both the defect and the laryngoscopy. If patient is supine, padding is necessary to avoid pressure or compression on the defect.

       e. Prone positioning for the surgery requires careful padding to prevent increased abdominal pressure, and to protect eyes and pressure points.

       f. Thermoregulation is important in this neonate population and can be achieved with forced-air warming blankets, warming lights, hot water warming mattresses, increased ambient temperature, and/or humidified inhalational agents.

    3. Postoperative management

       a. Common complications after closure include cerebral spinal fluid (CSF) leak, infection, poor wound healing, hydrocephalus, and tethered cord syndrome (TCS).

       b. Some patients return for VP shunt secondary to hydrocephalus.

       c. TCS occurs in 15% to 20% of patients during their lifetime [3] and such patients return for surgical untethering.

III. Spina bifida occulta

A. Background

    1. Spina bifida occulta is a bit of a misnomer since some of these lesions have intact vertebral bodies. A better way to describe this constellation of disorders is occult spinal dysraphisms (OSD). There are over a dozen disorders that are classified as OSDs.

       a. Examples of OSDs include thickened filum terminale, lipomyelomeningocele, split cord malformations (SCMs), dermoid sinus, inclusion cyst, and terminal syringohydromyelia.

       b. Since all OSDs share a common embryologic origin, patients with one form of OSD can also express other forms of OSD as well [5].

    2. Advances in magnetic resonance imaging (MRI) have allowed for a better understanding of OSD; there have been three important observations made:

       a. Most neurologic symptoms come from tension caused by traction on the spinal cord, TCS, which will be discussed later.

   b. There is a steady progression of neurologic compromise with time.

   c. Once a neurologic deficit occurs, it is usually irreversible [6].

B. **Anatomy/pathophysiology**

   1. Patients with OSD often have skin covering over their underlying pathology. These patients can also present with neurologic, orthopedic, urologic, and cutaneous lesions.

   2. There are a number of cutaneous lesions that are associated with OSD. Most cutaneous lesions are found at the midline in the lumbosacral region corresponding to the level of the OSD. Common cutaneous manifestations are hypertrichosis (tuft of hair), capillary hemangioma (nevus), dermal sinus, subcutaneous lipoma, and pseudotail.

   a. A popular misconception is that cutaneous lesions are a predictor for OSD. This clinical correlation is only found in 3% of the patients with cutaneous lesions. However, having two cutaneous lesions raise the predictive value to 70% [7].

   b. In infants, cutaneous manifestations are often the only sign of OSD. However, as the child gets older, other manifestations will appear. These include scoliosis, vertebral abnormalities, foot deformities, lower extremity asymmetry, neurogenic bladder, abnormal reflexes, pain, and delayed motor skills.

   3. There are three mechanisms by which OSDs produce clinical signs and symptoms:

   a. The lesion itself can be an abnormal neural structure.

   b. The lesion may cause a mass effect.

   c. The lesion may tether the spinal cord. Tethering of the spinal cord is the primary reason that most OSDs cause neurologic deficits. The cord can be tethered cranially, caudally, ventrally, or dorsally [5].

   4. The most common OSDs that occur include filum terminale, lipomyelomeningoceles, intramedullary lipomas, SCMs, and congenital dermoid sinus.

   a. The **filum terminale** is normally a thread-like structure that connects the lower end of the spinal cord to the bony spinal column. A thickened filum terminale results in tethering of the spinal cord and is associated with a low conus. Surgical resection is usually required.

   b. **Lipomyelomeningoceles** are fibrolipomatous masses that can extend from the intramedullary canal to the skin. They are associated with unfused vertebral bodies.

   c. **Intramedullary lipomas** are closely related to lipomyelomeningoceles. These lipomas originate in the conus and do not extend beyond the dura. Both lipomyelomeningoceles and intramedullary lipomas grow and can create a mass effect as well as a tethered effect on the spine.

   d. **SCMs** are a condition in which the spinal cord is split at the end. These two entities that were classically referred to as diastematomyelia and diplomyelia have now been renamed SCM I and SCM II, respectively, based on unified theory of embryogenesis. SCMs usually result in TCS [8].

   e. **Congenital dermoid sinuses** result from the abnormal adhesion between the ectoderm (destined to form the neural tube) and the dermis. When cells from the dermis are trapped beneath the skin, it creates an epithelial lined track which may extend anywhere from the skin to the spinal cord.

   (1) The primary concern is risk for infection.

   (2) **Dermoid cysts** are formed by the same mechanism and can cause TCS or create a mass effect on the spinal cord.

   (3) **Dermoid sinus tracts** are found in the lumbosacral region or higher. Dimples in the lower sacrum are not associated with dermoid sinuses. Probing the sinus tract or injecting radiopaque contrast is not recommended. Instead, MRI is the study of choice.

   5. Diagnosis of OSD and determining the extent of the disease is highly dependent on MRIs. Prenatal ultrasonography, amniocentesis, and amniotic alpha-fetoprotein have all proven to be poor diagnostic tools for the disease. Very often, the diagnosis of OSD is missed at birth because of the lack of clinical findings. As a result, the incidence of OSD is not known [5]. However, with improved neonatal screening and better radiologic imaging, the diagnosis of OSD is being made more frequently. Females are twice as often likely as males to have OSD. There are no known environmental causes of OSD; however, there appears to a higher incident between siblings than when compared to the general public.

C. Anesthetic considerations

1. **Preanesthetic evaluation**

   a. The most important issue is to determine, preoperatively, whether the OSD is causing traction on the spinal cord. A reliable history and physical examination can help make the diagnosis, otherwise a recent MRI may be required.

   b. It is also important to determine if the patient has any evidence of scoliosis, neurogenic bladder, incontinence, positional limitations, spasticity, back pain, or leg pain. Sometimes the excision of the OSD can aggravate the aforementioned conditions.

2. **Monitoring and intraoperative management**

   a. For simple OSD repairs, it is appropriate to use any standard anesthetic technique. If patients are placed in a prone position, pressure points should be appropriately padded. Placing bolsters so the patient's abdomen hangs freely will improve ventilation and decreases venous engorgement of the spine.

   b. Complex OSD repairs will often require intraoperative monitoring of electromyography (EMG), somatosensory (SSEPs), and motor evoked potentials (MEPs).

      (1) If neuromuscular relaxants are used for induction, they should not be redosed if EMGs and MEPs are being measured. Volatile anesthetics should be limited to 0.5 mean alveolar concentration (MAC). Opioids have a minimal effect on action potentials; therefore, fentanyl or remifentanil infusions are popular techniques.

      (2) Bite blocks should be placed if MEPs are being used.

      (3) Intraoperatively, some surgeons may give high-dose steroids because of supporting data from spinal cord trauma [9].

      (4) Placement of a foley catheter may be necessary for patients with neurogenic bladders.

   c. Patients with OSDs who are having a procedure unrelated to their OSD should not undergo a lumbar neuraxial block for uncomplicated pain management. The low position of the conus may put the patient at risk for spinal cord injury. In addition, many of these patients do not have a normal epidural space, which may increase the risk of wet spinal taps.

   d. Some anesthesiologists feel it is acceptable to place caudal epidural blocks with ultrasound guidance in patients with sacral dimpling [10]. However, it should be remembered that patients with OSDs can have abnormal sacral anatomy and that there is evidence to show that patients with tethered cord can develop cord ischemia when the spine is flexed [11]. Therefore, it may be best to conclusively rule out both of these conditions before proceeding with caudal epidural blocks.

3. **Postoperative management**

   a. Patients should lay flat to decrease the orthostatic pressure of CSF on the dural closure. While the adult population may require large doses of opioids postoperatively, this is generally not the case in the pediatric population after OSD surgery [5].

CLINICAL PEARLS • For complex OSD repairs, intraoperative monitoring of EMGs, SSEPs, and MEPs are often required. Therefore neuromuscular blockade should be avoided.
• Patients with OSDs who are having a procedure unrelated to their OSD should not undergo a lumbar neuraxial block for uncomplicated pain management.
• In the pediatric population, there is generally not as great of an opioid requirement after an OSD repair compared to the adult population.

IV. Tethered cord

A. Background

1. **TCS results from abnormal tension on the spinal cord.** Clinical presentation of TCS varies widely and may include motor weakness, sensory deficit, gait disturbances, scoliosis, pain, orthopedic deformities, and urologic dysfunction [1,12].

2. Neonates and infants with midline cutaneous stigmata such as nevi or hairy tufts along the sacrum, sacral dimpling, lipomas, or anorectal malformations should be highly suspected for spinal cord tethering [1].

3. Older children and adults may have a history of orthopedic surgeries, urologic surgeries, or trauma before a diagnosis of TCS is recognized [1].

B. **Anatomy and pathophysiology**
   1. Source of tethering varies widely depending on the type of spinal dysraphism.
      a. Prior meningocele or myelomeningocele surgery can result in TCS.
      b. For defects such as dermoid sinus tracts, abnormally thick filum terminale, and lipomas, TCS can occur from the resultant low-lying conus medullaris or mass effect from the abnormal fatty tissue [1].
   2. The pathophysiology of TCS has been attributed to impaired blood flow and oxidative metabolism from traction or stretching of the spinal cord [13].

C. **Surgery**
   1. The goal is to untether the spinal cord, and release tension without causing further nerve damage. Surgical technique will vary depending on the cause of tethering. For example, a tethered cord after prior myelomeningocele repair may require release of the cord from scar tissue, whereas lipomas may require surgical debulking of the mass.

D. **Anesthetic considerations**
   1. **Preanesthetic evaluation**
      a. Obtain a thorough history including antenatal and birth history, other comorbidities, and congenital anomalies.
      b. Obtain a thorough neurologic examination to document preoperative motor and sensory deficits. Urodynamic studies are typically performed to measure and follow neurologic function pre- and postoperatively.
      c. Obtain an MRI to evaluate and localize level of tethered cord
   2. **Monitoring and intraoperative management**
      a. Anesthetic induction may include inhalation or IV. A muscle relaxant can be used to facilitate intubation, followed by an anesthetic maintenance plan with no further muscle paralysis in order to facilitate neuromonitoring by the surgeon.
      b. Motor and sensory nerve root mapping with a hand-held nerve stimulator and EMG are used to discern between fibrous tissue and nerve roots [14]. Motor evoked and somatosensory evoked potentials are also used as a way to continuously monitor the entire circuit.
      c. Standard latex precautions are taken to avoid early sensitization.
   3. **Postoperative management**
      a. Common complications include CSF leak, new neurologic or urologic dysfunction, VP shunt malfunction secondary to a low-pressure hydrocephalus.
      b. Prone positioning postoperatively is generally preferred.

CLINICAL PEARLS • Neonate and infants may present with midline, cutaneous stigmata that suggests TCS.
• Older children and adults may have a history of orthopedic surgeries, urologic surgeries, or trauma before a diagnosis of TCS is recognized.
• Surgical repair usually requires motor and sensory nerve root mapping, so muscle paralysis should be spared to facilitate neuromonitoring.

V. Encephaloceles
A. **Background**
   1. Cranial dysraphism are neuro tube defects that are characterized by a calvarial defect.
      a. When the defect is associated with an extracranial herniation of leptomeninges in a form of a sac, it is known as a cranial meningocele or simply as a meningocele.

   b. When the herniation involves neuro tissue and leptomeninges, it is known as an encephalocele or meningoencephalocele.

   c. Cranium bifidum occultum is a calvarial defect in which there is no prolapse of intracranial matter.

   d. The incidence of all encephaloceles is approximately 1 to 3/10,000 live births [16].

2. Encephaloceles can appear on any part of the skull and are best classified by location [15].

   a. In Western countries, 85% of the encephaloceles are located on the back of the head (occipital encephaloceles) [16].

   b. In Asian countries, most encephaloceles are located anteriorly including those involving the nose (sincipital encephaloceles). Occipital and sincipital encephalocele each have special anesthetic considerations, which are discussed below.

B. Anatomy/pathophysiology

1. On physical examination, encephalocele appear as a sac-like protrusion and are usually covered by an intact layer of skin.

   a. Encephaloceles are often pulsatile and can sometimes become very large, sometimes greater than 20 cm in diameter [17].

   b. Infants with small encephalocele may present acting otherwise normally, whereas those with large ones usually have associated neurologic defects such as cranial nerve abnormalities, developmental delay, growth delay, poor feeding, blindness, and seizures.

   c. Occasionally, smaller encephaloceles can escape notice until adulthood. Patients with certain encephalocele (such as sincipital encephalocele) are likely to have near-normal intelligence. Patients with occipital encephalocele are more likely (83%) to have significant mental or physical impairments [18].

2. Primary (congenital) encephalocele are often diagnosed in utero by fetal ultrasonography. Infants with large encephaloceles should be delivered via cesarean sections.

3. Secondary (acquired) encephalocele are relatively uncommon and result from trauma or postsurgical cranial defects.

4. The exact cause of encephaloceles is not known and there does not appear to be a hereditary component for isolated encephaloceles [19]. However, encephaloceles are commonly associated with several syndromes [20], including Meckel's syndrome and amniotic band syndrome. They are also associated with other craniofacial abnormalities and brain abnormalities such as anencephaly, microcephaly, ataxia, and quadriplegia. The incidence of hydrocephalus may be as high as 65% [21].

C. Surgery

1. Recent innovations in surgical techniques, including image guidance and multidisciplinary reconstruction techniques, have improved the outcome for patients.

2. Without treatment, encephaloceles will continue to grow in size. The only effective treatment is surgical repair. These surgeries are usually elective as long as the overlying skin is intact.

   a. Sincipital encephaloceles usually contain fibrous gliotic neuro tissue. This nonfunctional tissue can be safely transected at the level of the skull, and the defect closed primarily. When the surgical approach is intranasally, the closure can be difficult. The postop course is complicated by CSF leaks and sometimes meningitis. Consulting an ENT surgeon and using image guidance surgery is highly recommended in these cases.

   b. Occipital encephaloceles can often have functional neuro tissue in the sac. All efforts should be made to preserve any functional tissue. Often the defect is large and an "expansion cranioplasty" maybe required to accommodate the larger herniated neural tissue. Consulting a plastic surgeon to create split thickness calvarial grafts can be useful. When primary closure is not possible, then a staged secondary repair is often necessary. The surgical outcome is highly dependent on the condition of the patient prior to the surgery which correlates with the location and severity of the lesion. The long-term survival of occipital encephaloceles is only about 50% [18].

D. **Anesthetic considerations**

1. **Preanesthetic evaluation.** Encephaloceles are not a homogenous population. Their management varies based on the severity as well as the location of the lesion. This section will focus on the anesthetic consideration for the two groups: Sincipital and occipital encephalocele.

   a. Sincipital encephaloceles should be differentiated from other midline nasal masses including nasal polyps, dermoid sinus cyst, and tumors. Cases of mistaken biopsies of nasal encephaloceles have resulted in disastrous consequences. The diagnosis should be done with computed tomography (CT) or magnetic resonance (MR) scan. Depending on the surgical approach, image guidance based on 3D image reconstructions and radionuclide ventriculography may also be useful. Sincipital encephaloceles can have involvement of the pituitary and hypothalamic centers. An endocrinology consult should be considered to rule out hypothyroidism, adrenal insufficiency, and diabetes insipidus. Complete blood count (CBC) and blood should be crossmatched for complex lesions.

   b. In severe cases, patients with an occipital encephalocele may have inadequate respiratory effort if the pontomedullary respiratory control center is affected by the lesion. Aspiration risk may also be increased because of decreased pharyngeal coordination and an absent gag reflex. Depending on the size of the lesion, significant blood loss may be expected in the intraoperative and postoperative period.

2. **Monitoring and intraoperative management**

   a. Some sincipital encephalocele preclude the possibility of effective mask ventilation because of the location of the lesion. In these patients, preservation of spontaneous ventilation during induction should be considered. Manipulation of these lesions should be limited because of the risk of meningitis. In a large series ($n = 102$) of sincipital encephaloceles, only one patient was found to be a difficult intubation. One other patient in this series required reintubation because of postop airway edema [22].

   b. Intraoperatively, significant hypotension can be an indication of hypothyroidism, adrenocortical deficiency, or diabetes insipidus. This can manifest as a reduction of plasma volume, anemia, hypoglycemia, hyponatremia, or impaired hepatic drug metabolism. Patients who develop diabetes insipidus should be treated with a vasopressin infusion and urinary output replaced with crystalloid. Foley catheter and arterial lines should be considered for any complex lesions. If risk for postop CSF leak is significant, then surgeons may place a ventricular drain.

   c. Positioning the patient supine may be a challenge with occipital encephaloceles. Foam or gel donuts are used to support the patient's head without putting pressure on the encephalocele. Patients with extremely large encephaloceles may need to be induced and intubated laterally. Mask ventilation may be difficult in this position so an assistant can support the head as the anesthesiologist applies a mask seal. Intubation may also be more difficult in the lateral position and may require the use of a flexible fiberoptic bronchoscope or video laryngoscope.

   d. The surgical repair is performed in a prone position so the patient's face should be well supported by a padded horseshoe. In this position, precaution should be taken so that the endotracheal tube (ETT) is well secured and there is no pressure on the eyes.

   e. The risk of bleeding and venous air embolization is greater in patients with larger cranial defects.

   f. Temperature control can potentially be an issue because of possible dysfunctional autonomic control.

   g. Latex precautions are advisable in patients with neuro tube defects to avoid early sensitization [23].

3. **Postoperative management**

   a. Patients with sincipital encephaloceles should go to an intensive care unit postoperatively to be closely monitored for adrenal cortical deficiency, diabetes insipidus, and airway obstruction.

b. Steps should be taken to minimize the need for positive pressure mask ventilation because of the possibility of pneumoencephaly and resultant meningitis. These patients should also be instructed not to blow their noses.

c. Mild sedation may be required for some pediatric patients.

d. Chronic CSF leaks are not an uncommon complication. It can be confused with normal sinus drainage. Some patients may need additional surgical repair or have a ventriculostomy drain placed if the leak does not stop.

e. For complex occipital encephalocele repairs, some surgeons may not want patients to be supine, to avoid pressure on the incision. The patient will often continue to lose blood into the subgaleal space so serum hemoglobin should be monitored carefully.

CLINICAL PEARLS • Intraoperatively, significant hypotension can be an indication of hypothyroidism, adrenocortical deficiency, or diabetes insipidus.

• It may be difficult to position a patient with occipital encephalocele supine for induction. Foam or gel donuts are used to support the patient's head without putting pressure on the encephalocele.

• Steps should be taken to minimize the need for positive pressure mask ventilation because of the possibility of pneumoencephaly and resultant meningitis.

• The perioperative management of encephaloceles is often complex, requiring input from neurosurgeons, otolaryngologists, plastic surgeons, radiologists, intensivists, endocrinologists, and anesthesiologists to give optimum care.

REFERENCES

1. Lew SM, Kothbauer KF. Tethered cord syndrome: an updated review. *Pediatr Neurosurg.* 2007;43:236–248.
2. Motoyama EK, Davis PJ. *Smith's Anesthesia for Infants and Children.* 7th ed. Philadelphia, PA: Mosby; 2006.
3. Gaskill SJ. Primary closure of open myelomeningocele. *Neurosurg Focus.* 2004;16(2):E3.
4. McClain CD, Soriano SG. The central nervous system: pediatric neuroanesthesia. In: Holzman RS, Mancuso TJ, Polaner DM, eds. *A Practical Approach to Pediatric Anesthesia.* Philadelphia, PA: Lippincott Williams & Wilkins; 2008:177–214.
5. Albright L, Pollack I, Adelson D, eds. *Principals and Practice of Pediatric Neurosurgery.* New York, NY: Thieme; 1999:321–351.
6. Wu H, Kogan B, Baskin L, et al. Long-term benefits of early neurosurgery for lipomyelomeningocele. *J Urol.* 1998;160:511–514.
7. Bruce DA, Schut L. Spinal lipomas in infancy and childhood. *Childs Brain.* 1979;5:192–203.
8. Pang D, Dias MS, Ahab-Barmada M. Split cord malformation. *Neurosurgery.* 1992;31:451–480.
9. Walton M, Bass J, Soucy P. Tethered cord with anorectal malformation, sacral anomalies and presacral masses: an under-recognized association. *Eur J Pediatr Surg.* 1995;5:59–62.
10. Schwartz D, Al-Najjar H, Connelly NR. Caudal block in a child with a sacral dimple utilizing ultrasonography. *Pediatr Anesth.* 2011;21:1073–1074.
11. Yamada S, Iacono RP, Andrade T, et al. Pathophysiology of tethered cord syndrome. *Neurosurg Clin North Am.* 1995;6:311–323.
12. Hudgins, RJ, Gilreath, CL. Tethered spinal cord following the repair of myelomeningocele. *Neurosurg Focus.* 2004;16(2):E7.
13. Yamada, S, Won, DJ, Yamada SM. Pathophysiology of tethered cord syndrome: correlation with symptomatology. *Neurosurg Focus.* 2004;16(2):E6.
14. Kothbauer, KF, Novak, K. Intraoperative monitoring for tethered cord surgery: an update. *Neurosurg Focus.* 2004;16(2):E8.
15. Suwanwela C, Suwanwela N. A morphological classification of sincipital encephalomeningoceles. *Neurosurgery.* 1972;36:201–211.
16. Mealey J Jr, Dzenitis AJ. The prognosis of encephaloceles. *J Neurosurg.* 1970;15:89–112.
17. Shokunbi T, Adeloye A, Olumid A. Occipital encephaloceles in 57 Nigerian children: a retrospective analysis. *Child's Nerv Syst.* 1990;6:99–102.
18. French BH. Midline fusion defects and defects of formation. In: Youman JR, ed. *Neurological Surgery.* Philadelphia, PA: WB Sunders; 1990:1164–1169.
19. Drolet BA, Clowry L, McTigue MK, et al. The hair collar sign: marker for cranial dysraphism. *Pediatrics.* 1995;96(2):309–313.
20. Naidich TP, Altman NR, Braffman BH, et al. Cephaloceles and related malformations. *AJNR.* 1992;13:655–690.
21. Lorber J, Schonfield JK. The prognosis of occipital encephaloceles. *Z Kinderchir.* 1979;28:347–351.
22. Leelanukrom R, Wacharasint P, Kaewanuchit A. Perioperative management for surgical correction of frontoethmoidal encephalomeningocele in children: a review of 102 cases. *Pediatr Anesth.* 2007;7:856–862.
23. Hamid RKA, Newfield P. Pediatric neuroanesthesia: neural tube defects. *Anesthesiol Clin North Am.* 2001;10:219–228.

17

Chiari Malformation

Penny P. Liu, Krystal Tomei, and J. Brad Bellotte

KEY POINTS

1. The Chiari malformations should be viewed as a spectrum of defects involving the brainstem, cerebellum, cervical spine, spinal cord, clivus, and subocciput.
2. Chiari I malformations are more common and the least severe of the forms. It most often presents in young adulthood.
3. Chiari II malformations are less common and more severe in this spectrum of defects. It is frequently associated with myelomeningocele, hydrocephalus, and other associated spinal cord malformations such as syrinx and tethered spinal cord.
4. Important anesthetic considerations include positioning, establishing adequate intravenous access, venous air embolism, invasive blood pressure monitoring, and neurophysiologic monitoring.
5. The type of anesthetic technique and drugs used in maintaining general anesthesia is not nearly as important as the appreciation that the ultimate anesthetic goal is a rapid, though carefully planned emergence. It should be the goal of both the anesthesiologist and surgeon to optimize postoperative neurologic assessment.

1 **THE CHIARI MALFORMATIONS (CM)** represent four types of hindbrain anomalies. It can be said that they are a spectrum of defects involving the craniocervical junction including the brainstem, cerebellum, cervical spine, spinal cord clivus, and subocciput.

I. Historical considerations

A. In 1883, Cleland [1] described nine cases of infants found at autopsy to have hindbrain malformations.
B. In 1891, Chiari described what was later classified as the Chiari II (CM-II) malformation [2].
C. In 1894, Arnold reported on a collection of individuals with congenital defects in the hindbrain and hydrocephalous (consistent with the later named Chiari I malformation CM-I).
D. The term Arnold–Chiari malformation was used interchangeably throughout the 1950s and 1970s to refer to CM-I and CM-II malformations. However, there are differences in the etiology of the conditions and this grouping should be avoided.

II. Chiari malformation I

A. Anatomy

2
1. Cerebellar tonsils descend through the foramen magnum due to overcrowding of the hindbrain.
2. The cerebrospinal fluid (CSF) is displaced by the abnormal anatomy. This causes alterations in the flow of the CSF. It is believed that this altered CSF flow can lead to the development of a cervical spine syrinx (fluid-filled segment within the spinal cord) in a number of instances.

3. The cerebellar tonsils can cause direct compression of the brainstem leading to neurologic signs and symptoms.

B. Signs and symptoms
1. Valsalva-induced suboccipital headache are common.
2. Visual complaint such as blurred vision, flashing lights, diplopia, and sensitivity are associated with Chiari I malformation.
3. Otologic complaints can include tinnitus, feelings of pressure, vertigo, or decreased hearing.
4. Dysphagia, apnea, nausea, and ataxia are other complaints that can arise from the brainstem compression by the cerebellar tonsils.
5. A syrinx in the cervical spine will cause motor and sensory deficits of the extremities.
6. Many patients with Chiari I malformation may have various other complaints that are not as easily attributable by the local anatomy.

C. Diagnosis
1. MRI scan of the brain is regarded as the definitive test in the diagnosis of Chiari I malformation. It will show descent of the tonsils through the foramen magnum. This causes crowding of the brainstem at the foramen and even at the C1 and C2 vertebrae at times.
2. MRI scan of the cervical spine is useful in the diagnosis of a syrinx associated with the Chiari I malformation. Sometimes the disorder is first detected on a cervical MRI ordered to work up cervical complaints. Usually the tonsils and foramen magnum are imaged on the sagittal images. A close inspection of the area around the brainstem can identify patients with Chiari I malformation.
3. It is important to appreciate that there is not just a sole criterion used to make the diagnosis of Chiari I malformation. There is increasing evidence that careful interpretation of imaging studies, clinical picture, and even the quantitative analysis of CSF dynamics aids in the accurate diagnosis of this condition [3–6].

D. Treatment
1. **Surgical considerations**
   a. The goal of surgical treatment is to provide more room at the base of the brain and posterior cervical spine. This involves a suboccipital craniectomy in which a window of occipital bone down to the foramen magnum is removed. If necessary, a C1 and C2 laminectomy can provide additional room. There are several accepted techniques to provide additional room. This often involves opening the dura and resecting the herniated cerebellar tissue. An expansion duraplasty is commonly used as part of the closure.
2. **Risks**
   a. **General surgical risks**
      (1) These risks include, but are not limited to, bleeding, venous air embolism, infection, pulmonary, and cardiovascular risks.
   b. **Specific procedure**
      (1) The vertebral artery is vulnerable during the initial dissection as it courses over the arch of C1 laterally. Injury to the vertebral artery at this level will result in profuse bleeding. A stroke may develop depending on collateral flow.
      (2) The posterior inferior cerebellar artery (PICA) lies deep to the cerebellar tonsils. The PICA supplies blood to the lateral medulla, posterior cerebellum, and tonsils. An infarct due to an injury to PICA will result in Wallenberg syndrome. Signs and symptoms of Wallenberg syndrome include dysphagia, hoarseness, nausea/vomiting, vertigo, nystagmus, and gait and balance disturbances.
      (3) The nuclei of the sixth and seventh cranial nerves are vulnerable in the floor of the fourth ventricle. Injuries to these structures will result in occulomotor dysfunction and facial paresis, respectively.
      (4) The eleventh cranial nerve enters the foramen magnum on the lateral side of the spinal cord. Injury to this nerve is less common. However, it is very excitable and will result in muscle contraction with even very little manipulation.

E. Anesthetic considerations
   1. Positioning
      a. Typically, the corrective procedure is performed with the patient in prone position.
         (1) The patient is placed in three-point head fixation.
         (2) The neck is flexed to create an opening of the craniocervical junction.
            (a) Check the position of the endotracheal tube after neck flexion by auscultation to rule out a mainstem intubation.
            (b) The goal is to achieve a balance of neck flexion that facilitates optimal exposure and the reassurance of adequate venous outflow.

> **CLINICAL PEARL** Venous obstruction of the head and neck can lead to intracranial hypertension. Ideally, both surgeon and anesthesiologist should agree on the extent of neck flexion acceptable for surgical exposure, adequacy of ventilation, as well as venous outflow. Poor venous outflow of the head and neck region could potentially lead to macroglossia and intracranial hypertension.

            (c) A good starting point is at least two to three fingerbreadths between the anterior mandible and the sternal notch.
         (3) Next, the shoulders are retracted inferiorly with tape.
            (a) Excessive inferior retraction of the shoulders can lead to brachial plexus injury.
            (b) If somatosensory evoked potentials (SSEPs) are used for the case, monitor brachial plexus.
   2. General

> **CLINICAL PEARL** Ensure adequate IV access and consider the benefits in placement of a radial arterial line especially if the symptoms are severe or if the patient has comorbidities. Detection of venous air embolism can be accomplished by placement of a precordial Doppler.

      a. Whereas there is no one best anesthetic technique, one must keep in mind the ultimate goal of an expedited, though carefully planned, emergence. The postoperative neurologic assessment of the patient is of paramount importance.
   3. Neuromonitoring
      a. SSEP monitoring can provide useful information with respect to the dorsal sensory elements.
      b. Changes in SSEP can be indicative of problems with positioning or as a result of a surgical insult and ischemia.
      c. Prompt recognition of SSEP changes and a thorough assessment should lead to either of a combination of surgical correction or repair of the surgical injury if needed, blood pressure manipulation, addition of corticosteroids, or administration of rheologic agents.

III. Chiari malformation II
   A. Anatomy
      1. It is a constellation of intracranial findings isolated to the myelomeningocele population. It can be found in approximately 98% of patients with myelomeningocele [7].
         a. It is characterized by the presence of hindbrain herniation resulting in downward displacement of the cerebellar vermis, fourth ventricle, and medulla through the foramen magnum, tectal beaking, medullary kink [7].
         b. Patients with Chiari II malformation may have associated hydrocephalus. Between 80% and 90% of patients with myelomeningocele and Chiari type II will ultimately require ventricular shunting for symptomatic hydrocephalus or symptomatic Chiari Type II malformation [7]. Prenatal repair of myelomeningocele has been shown to decrease shunt dependence by approximately 50% [8].

    c. Other intracranial findings that are not a part of the Chiari type II malformation include polymicrogyria, agenesis of the corpus callosum, enlarged massa intermedia, or fused thalami [9].

  2. Patients with Chiari II malformations may have associated spinal cord malformations.

    a. There can be the presence of a syrinx in approximately 68% of patients [7].

    b. Every attempt is made during spinal cord reconstruction surgery to prevent the late tethering of the spinal cord. A placode is the thickening of the embryonic epithelial layer from which organs and structures (i.e., spinal cord) later develop. Thus, in myelomeningocele repair, surgical closure of the neural placode, although may not completely prevent retethering, may make the untethering of the spinal cord easier to perform later on.

B. Epidemiology

  1. Approximately 1,500 babies are born each year with spina bifida [10], overall prevalence of 2:10,000 [11], between 2.64 and 4.17 babies per 10,000 births in certain race subgroups [12].

  2. Over 90% survive the first year, 75% reach adulthood [13].

C. Signs and symptoms

  1. Chiari II malformation

    a. Headaches

    b. Apnea

    c. Bradycardia

    d. Impaired auditory evoked potentials

    e. Spasticity

    f. Torticollis

    g. Eye movement abnormalities such as saccadic dysmetria, impaired vestibulo-ocular reflex, impaired smooth pursuit, nystagmus, internuclear ophthalmoplegia.

  2. Hydrocephalus

    a. May exacerbate symptoms of Chiari II malformation

    b. Headache

    c. Nausea/vomiting

    d. Lethargy

    e. Upgaze palsy

  3. Tethered cord

    a. Worsening bowel and bladder function

    b. Progressive lower extremity motor or sensory deficit

    c. Worsening spasticity

    d. Increasing symptoms of Chiari II malformation and brainstem compression

D. Diagnosis

  1. Chiari II malformation

    a. The history of myelomeningocele must be present.

    b. MRI brain

      (1) There is hindbrain herniation through foramen magnum including cerebellar vermis, medulla, and fourth ventricle.

      (2) Medullary kink

      (3) Tectal beaking

      (4) May have associated hydrocephalus

      (5) Low-lying venous sinuses and torcula

      (6) Small posterior fossa

  2. Myelomeningocele

    a. This condition is often diagnosed prenatally via quad screen or ultrasound. The quad screen tests maternal blood for α-fetoprotein, hCG, estriol, and inhibin-A.

    b. There is the protrusion of meninges and neural elements through a bone and skin defect.

  3. Tethered spinal cord

    a. Almost all patients will show radiographic evidence of tethered cord after myelomeningocele repair [14].

  b. Between 10% and 30% will require surgical release to ameliorate symptoms, and almost 15% will require a secondary tethered cord release [14].

  c. The combination of MRI showing low-lying conus or tether and the below symptoms can be an indicator of tethered cord. Symptoms include:

  (1) Worsening of lower extremity motor function

  (2) Worsening of bowel/bladder dysfunction

  (3) Increasing symptoms of Chiari II malformation

  (4) Sensory deficit

  (5) Spasticity

E. Treatment

  1. Surgical considerations

  a. Chiari II malformation

  b. Surgical decompression of the posterior fossa for symptomatic Chiari II malformation is required in 8% to 17% of patients [15].

  c. Hydrocephalus

  (1) Between 80% and 90% of patients with myelomeningocele and Chiari II malformation will require shunting for symptomatic hydrocephalus.

  (2) Shunt may be performed simultaneously with the myelomeningocele repair or in a delayed fashion; however, there is conflicting evidence on increase in infection rate with simultaneous shunting [16].

  d. Tethered cord

  (1) Aim of surgical procedure is to release scar tissue or tethered filum terminale.

  (2) By doing so, it may improve the symptoms of lower lumbosacral nerve root dysfunction or Chiari II malformation.

  2. Surgical risks

  a. Chiari II decompression

  (1) The vertebral artery is at risk of injury during its course around C1 laminae through the foramen magnum.

  (2) The Posterior inferior cerebellar artery (PICA) is vulnerable due to its location deep within the cerebellar tonsils.

  (3) Cranial nerve injury is possible though rare given the deep location of the cranial nerves at risk during this exposure. The nuclei of cranial nerves six and seven are found in the floor of the fourth ventricle. Finally, cranial nerve eleven courses lateral to the spinal core and enters the foramen magnum.

  b. Ventriculoperitoneal shunting for hydrocephalus

  (1) Potential surgical risk includes intraparenchymal hemorrhage

  (2) Bowel injury

  c. Tethered cord release

  (1) Surgical risk in tethered cord release procedures involves potential injury to lower spinal cord and lumbosacral nerve roots.

F. Anesthetic considerations

  1. Positioning

  a. Prone

  (1) Typically, the prone position is used for surgical procedures involving suboccipital craniectomy and/or C1 laminectomy for Chiari decompression, and tethered cord release.

  b. Lateral/supine

  (1) Either lateral of the supine position can be used for procedure of shunt placement.

  2. General

  a. Ensure adequate IV access and consider the benefits in placement of an arterial line especially if the symptoms are severe. A precordial Doppler should be used to detect venous air emboli.

  b. There is no one best anesthetic technique. The main goal is a rapid emergence from anesthesia for the purpose of a postoperative neurologic assessment.

3. Neuromonitoring

CLINICAL PEARL Information from neurophysiologic monitoring can be useful in tethered cord release and EMG and bladder sphincter monitoring can be useful to guide the surgical dissection.

a. Depending on the patient's presentation, monitoring of the lower cranial nerves along with SSEP/MEP and/or EMG in Chiari decompression may be useful.

b. SSEP and MEP can detect vascular compression secondary to positioning, anesthetic effects of cardiovascular circulation, and other physiologic changes associated with anesthesia [17].

c. Anemia in the setting of blood loss has been shown to affect neuromonitoring, with restoration of signal following blood transfusion [18].

d. Apart from the known effects of inhaled anesthetics on intraoperative neuromonitoring and preference for TIVA, different intravenous anesthetics have been shown to minimally affect SSEP, such as remifentanil [19,20]. Monitoring in pediatric patients has been successful utilizing ketamine.

e. Tethered cord release monitoring

(1) Series of 44 adult patients with tethered cord in whom SSEP and EMG was utilized for detethering with a SSEP sensitivity of 50% and specificity of 100% and EMG sensitivity of 100% and specificity of 19% [21].

REFERENCES

1. Cleland J. Contribution to the study of spina bifida, encephalocele, and anencephalus. *J Anat Physiol.* 1883;17:257–291.
2. Carmel PW, Markesbery WR. Early descriptions of the Arnold–Chiari malformation. The contribution of John Cleland. *J Neurosurg.* 1972;37(5):543–547.
3. Sekula RF Jr, Jannetta PJ, Casey KF, et al. Dimensions of the posterior fossa in patients symptomatic for Chiari I malformation but without cerebellar tonsillar descent. *Cerebrospinal Fluid Res.* 2005;2:11.
4. Barkovich AJ, Wippold FJ, Sherman JL, et al. Significance of cerebellar tonsillar position on MR. *Am J Neuroradiol.* 1986;7(5):795–799.
5. Elster AD, Chen MY. Chiari I malformations: clinical and radiologic reappraisal. *Radiology.* 1992;183(2):347–353.
6. Loth F, Yardimci MA, Alperin N. Hydrodynamic modeling of cerebrospinal fluid motion within the spinal cavity. *J Biomech Eng.* 2001;123(1):71–79.
7. Talamonti G, D'Aliberti G, Collice M. Myelomeningocele: long-term neurosurgical treatment and follow-up in 202 patients. *J Neurosurg.* 2007;107:368–386.
8. Adzick NS, Thom EA, Spong CY, et al. A randomized trial of prenatal versus postnatal repair of myelomeningocele. *N Engl J Med.* 2011;364:993–1004.
9. Kawamura T, Morioka T, Nishio S, et al. Cerebral abnormalities in lumbosacral neural tube closure defect: MR imaging evaluation. *Childs Nerv Syst.* 2001;17:405–410.
10. Canfield MA, Honein MA, Yuskiv N, et al. National estimates and race/ethnic-specific variation of selected birth defects in the United States, 1999–2001. *Birth Defects Res A Clin Mol Teratol.* 2006;76:747–756.
11. Roberts HE, Moore CA, Cragan JD, et al. Impact of prenatal diagnosis on the birth prevalence of neural tube defects, Atlanta, 1990–1991. *Pediatrics.* 1995;96:880–883.
12. Boulet SL, Yang Q, Mai C, et al. Trends in the postfortification prevalence of spina bifida and anencephaly in the United States. *Birth Defects Res A Clin Mol Teratol.* 2008;82:527–532.
13. Bowman RM, McLone DG, Grant JA, et al. Spina bifida outcome: a 25-year prospective. *Pediatr Neurosurg.* 2001;34:114–120.
14. Mehta VA, Bettegowda C, Ahmadi SA, et al. Spinal cord tethering following myelomeningocele repair. *J Neurosurg Pediatr.* 2010;6:498–505.
15. Wagner W, Schwarz M, Perneczky A. Primary myelomeningocele closure and consequences. *Curr Opin Urol.* 2002;12:465–468.
16. Radmanesh F, Nejat F, El Khashab M, et al. Shunt complications in children with myelomeningocele: effect of timing of shunt placement. Clinical article. *J Neurosurg Pediatr.* 2009;3:516–520.
17. Seyal M, Mull B. Mechanisms of signal change during intraoperative somatosensory evoked potential monitoring of the spinal cord. *J Clin Neurophysiol.* 2002;19:409–415.
18. Lyon R, Lieberman JA, Grabovac MT, et al. Strategies for managing decrease motor evoked potential signals while distracting the spine during correction of scoliosis. *J Neurosurg Anesthesiol.* 2004;16:167–170.
19. Strahm C, Min K, Booos N, et al. Reliability of perioperative SSEP recordings in spine surgery. *Spinal Cord.* 2003;41:483–489.
20. Asouhidou I, Katsaridis V, Vaidis G, et al. Somatosensory evoked potentials suppression due to remifentanil during spinal operations; a prospective clinical study. *Scoliosis.* 2010;5:8.
21. Paradiso G, Lee GY, Sarjeant R, et al. Multimodality intraoperative neurophysiologic monitoring findings during surgery for adult tethered cord syndrome: analysis of a series of 44 patients with long-term follow-up. *Spine.* 2006;31:2095–2102.

18

Craniofacial Surgery—Pediatric Considerations

Petra M. Meier and Susan M. Goobie

KEY POINTS

1. Optimal care for pediatric craniofacial surgery patients is best accomplished by interdisciplinary teams of pediatric specialists which may include craniofacial surgery, neurosurgery, otolaryngology, ophthalmology, oro-maxillofacial surgery, and pediatric intensive care.
2. Infants who present for craniofacial surgery under one year of age, with a body weight less than 5 kg, and/or an associated syndrome have a significantly increased peri-operative morbidity and mortality.
3. Many infants and children with craniofacial abnormalities present with a compromised airway including a high incidence of sleep disorder and central/obstructive airway symptoms. If these are unrecognized/untreated and longstanding, there is the potential for associated pulmonary hypertension. Thorough preoperative airway evaluation/imaging is recommended.
4. In syndromic children, additional congenital malformations should be sought, especially congenital heart disease.
5. Anesthetic management is based on the type of surgical repair and the presence of associated anomalies. Craniofacial repair can be associated with significant ongoing blood loss, and episodes of sudden abrupt blood loss caused by venous sinus bleeding, increased intravenous and/or intracranial pressure, venous air embolism, paradoxical air emboli if cardiac right to left shunting is present, and other rare but life threatening situations like transfusion induced hyperkalemia.

I. Introduction. Craniofacial anomalies encompass a wide spectrum of defects of the cranial vault, and/or facial skeleton. The major objective of craniofacial surgery is to correct these skeletal anomalies with a combination of osteotomies, cranial bone remodeling, calvarial bone grafts and fixation. Pediatric craniofacial reconstruction surgery frequently involves a team approach involving pediatric anesthesia, neurosurgery, plastic surgery, and oromaxillofacial surgery. Multiple-staged procedures may be required for craniofacial reconstruction. Some children with craniofacial anomalies have associated syndromes that will significantly influence the anesthetic management. This review will build on the principles outlined in Chapter 15 and examine the specific anesthetic management issues associated with the diverse surgical approaches to these anomalies.

II. Cranial vault and craniofacial anomalies

    A. Craniosynostosis

        1. Classification

            a. Classic craniosynostosis has been traditionally regarded as an event that occurs early in fetal development, resulting in a characteristic skull shape at birth that is determined by the specific sutures involved (Fig. 18.1). This condition can be either an isolated single suture craniosynostosis, of which sagittal craniosynostosis is the most prevalent form, or a multiple-suture synostosis (complex craniosynostosis) that can be syndromic (Table 18.1) or nonsyndromic. The abnormal cranial suture development results in failure of growth perpendicular to the affected suture and overgrowth of skull parallel to the affected suture often visible and palpable as a bone ridge (Fig. 18.1). The etiology of most cases is sporadic, although there is a strong genetic component. Genetic mutations that may be responsible include mutations in the fibroblast growth factors (FGFR 1, FGFR2, FGFR3), *TWIST,* and *MSX2* genes.

b. **Progressive postnatal craniosynostosis** is characterized by a normal skull shape and normal radiologic study results at birth followed by midface hypoplasia and occasionally hypertelorism as the infant grows. Frequently, an association with the classic Crouzon syndrome phenotype occurs. These cases are significant because, although they have open sutures in infancy and do not initially display the physical manifestation of craniosynostosis, they develop multiple-suture craniosynostosis over time with slow development of symptoms of increased intracranial pressure (headaches, vomiting, irritability, papilledema, progressive optic atrophy, seizures, and/or bulging fontanels) that ultimately requires surgical interventions.

c. **Shunting craniosynostosis.** Shunting procedures in early infancy may result in overlapping of the calvarial bones and can induce secondary craniosynostosis.

d. **Positional plagiocephaly** also known as deformational plagiocephaly is a condition most commonly found in infants and is characterized by a flat spot on the back or one side of the head caused by remaining in one position for too long. These changes are not related to premature closure of cranial sutures and treated nonsurgically by orthotic treatment using a helmet if done early enough.

CLINICAL PEARL   In keeping with the general philosophy of the correction of congenital defects, there is consensus that surgical correction of craniosynostosis during early infancy is advantageous.

2. **Surgical management.** Craniofacial surgical treatments vary with age, location, and number of sutures involved. Many surgeons prefer to operate early in life to capitalize on the ameliorating effects of brain growth on skull shape. The following are some of the surgical management techniques:

a. **Endoscopic strip craniectomy (ESC)** is considered for infants (1 to 6 months) for all single suture and simple multiple suture craniosynostoses. ESCs are short surgical procedures (approximately 45 minutes) associated with small amount of blood loss, low incidence of blood transfusions, and ICU admissions. The average length of hospital stay is between 1 and 2 days with the majority of patients discharged on the first postoperative day [1].

Small skin incisions are performed perpendicular to the stenosed sutures. Cranial burr holes are made through the midline of each scalp incision. An endoscope is used to visualize the fused suture, identify emissary veins, dural attachments, and assure hemostasis. The closed suture is resected and removed through the burr hole.

CLINICAL PEARL   Less-invasive surgical techniques (e.g., ESC) are associated with a significant reduction in blood transfusions, intensive care unit (ICU) admissions, and costs. It remains to be determined whether the indications for less-invasive surgical techniques and open reconstruction procedures for single- and multiple-suture craniosynostosis can be better defined to further improve risk/benefit profile and costs.

b. **Spring-assisted cranioplasty** utilizes implanted cranial springs that allow gradual correction of the skull malformation over time and is used in infants older than 3 months of age. Optimal results are achieved in infants younger than 6 months of age while the skull still being relatively pliable. This technique involves an osteotomy and resection of the prematurely closed suture combined with the insertion of one to three

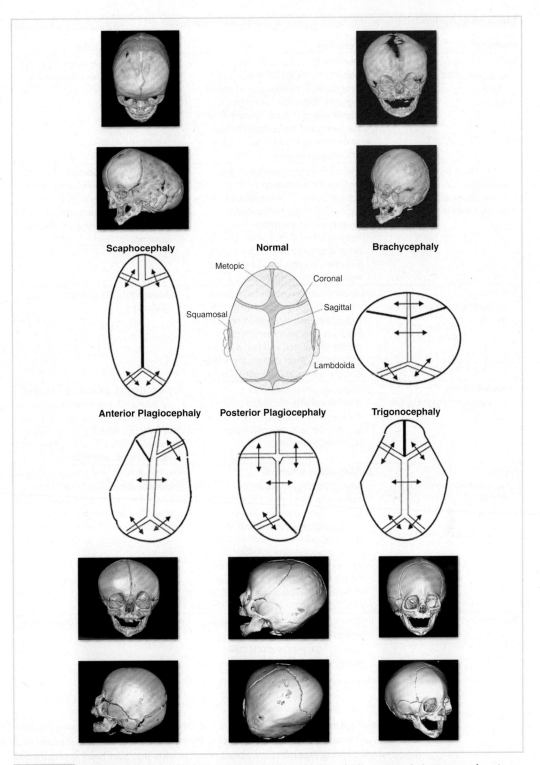

FIGURE 18.1 Morphologic types of craniosynostosis. Diagrammatic views of different morphologic types of craniosynostosis are shown in the center of the figure. The premature closed suture is marked as a bold line. The sutures involved determine the shape of the skull. The diagrammatic view of each synostosis type is matched with the corresponding radiologic findings. The fused suture is seen as a hypertrophic keel or ridge on the x-rays.

TABLE 18.1   Common craniofacial syndromes associated with craniosynostosis

Syndrome	Description	Anesthesia implication
Apert (acrocephalopolysyndactyly type I)	Most common coronal synostosis, possibly increased ICP, maxillary hypoplasia, exophthalmos, choanal stenosis, obstructive sleep apnea, cognitive impairment, syndactyly of the hands and feet, partial cervical spine fusion C5/6, renal anomalies, CHD may be present.	Evaluation for CHD, possible difficult intubation, possible increased ICP.
Crouzon, craniofacial dysostosis (acrocephalopolysyndactyly variant type II)	Multiple suture synostosis, possibly increased ICP, intracranial abnormalities (Chiari), maxillary hypoplasia, airway obstruction, exophthalmos, proptosis, hypertelorism, parrot peak nose, renal anomalies, high arched palate, 55% have hearing loss, C2–C3 spinal fusion, normal mental capacity.	Possible difficult intubation, nasal obstruction, possible increased ICP, elective tracheostomy might be indicated, eye protection, renal excretion of drugs might be impaired.
Carpenter (acrocephalopolysyndactyly type II)	Multiple suture synostosis (acrocephaly, cloverleaf skull) mental deficiency, hypoplastic mandible and/or maxilla, brachydactyly with absence of middle phalanges, additional or fused fingers/toes, short stature, short neck, obesity, cardiac abnormalities (50%).	Evaluation for CHD, possible difficult intubation.
Saethre–Chotzen (acrocephalopolysyndactyly type III)	Multiple suture synostosis (brachycephaly), possibly increased ICP, maxillary hypoplasia, syndactyly, possible cervical vertebral fusion, clavicular anomalies.	Possible difficult intubation, possible increased ICP, may have seizures and mental deterioration, possible difficult placement of a subclavian venous catheter, careful positioning secondary to contractures.
Pfeiffer (acrocephalopolysyndactyly type V)	Multiple suture synostosis (brachycephaly), maxillary hypoplasia, cervical vertebral fusion. Type 1: Classic, variable degree of syndactyly; Type 2: Hand and foot anomalies, cloverleaf skull, severe ocular proptosis and ankylosis of the elbows, diminished life expectancy; Type 3: Similar to Type 2, no cloverleaf skull, severe ocular proptosis, visceral malformations.	Possible difficult airway, evaluate lower airway patency (tracheobronchial anomalies), obstructive sleep apnea, possible seizures (interaction of anticonvulsants with anesthetic drugs), evaluation for CHD.
Muenke syndrome	Coronal craniosynostosis, macrocephaly, possible obstructive sleep apnea, hearing loss, short stature, mild abnormalities of hand/feet.	Possible mild obstructive sleep apnea.

CHD, Congenital heart disease; ICP, Increased intracranial pressure.

stainless steel springs across the newly created false suture to allow ongoing dynamic correction of the skull anomaly over the following months. The ends of the stainless steel omega-shaped spring expanders are placed under tension into burr holes approximately 1 to 2 cm apart with the body of the spring bent to conform to the curvature of the skull. The expansion of a spring is a slow process and is monitored both clinically and radiologically. The springs are surgically removed after adequate cranial expansion [2].

TABLE 18.2 Common craniofacial syndromes not associated with craniosynostosis

Syndrome	Description	Anesthesia implication
Oculo-auriculo-vertebral syndrome; Goldenhar syndrome or hemifacial microsomia	Features are variable, asymmetric and unilateral. Primary features are hypoplasia of the mandible, maxilla, and auricle. Facial dysmorphia including hypoplasia of the zygoma, facial muscles, eye, tongue, parotid gland, cardiac disease (TOF or VSD), renal maldevelopment. Called Goldenhar when it accompanies vertebral anomalies (commonly cervical; C2–C3 fusion, hemivertebrae, and spina bifida) and bulbar dermoid.	Difficult mask fit due to asymmetry; difficult intubation due to asymmetrical hypoplasia of mandible and maxilla and c-spine fusion.
Treacher–Collins syndrome (mandibulofacial dysostosis)	Symmetric hypoplasia of facial bones (zygomas, mandible, pterygoids, and temporomandibular joint); ocular manifestations (coloboma, vision loss), velopharyngeal insufficiency, hearing loss, cleft palate.	Obstructive sleep apnea due to retrognathia and malocclusion; difficult mask fit due to cleft; difficult intubation; eye protection to avoid corneal abrasion/orbital compression.
Pierre–Robin syndrome	Cleft palate, micrognathia, glossoptosis. CHD in some. Neonates: respiratory obstruction/apnea may occur and lead to cor pulmonale. Maintain airway by nursing prone. May require tongue suture, intubation, or tracheostomy	CHD; central and obstructive sleep apnea; intubation may be very difficult: consideration for awake technique. In skilled hands, fiberoptic intubation under general anesthesia may be used. Patient should be fully awake before extubation.

CHD, Congenital heart disease.

    c. Open reconstruction procedures represent a variety of surgical procedures that are usually performed in infants older than 6 to 12 months of age to limit operative morbidity and mortality. However, the deformities are more severe at this late stage. Open reconstruction procedures include simple strip craniectomy, π cranioplasties (paramedian strip craniectomies and a transverse craniectomy in the shape of the Greek letter pi for scaphocephaly secondary to sagittal synostosis), anterior calvarial remodeling procedures including bicoronal craniectomy with fronto-orbital advancement (FOA) and posterior cranial vault remodeling (CVR) with and without barrel stave osteotomies. These techniques are associated with significant blood loss, varying between 0.2 and 4 blood volumes, lengthy surgical times (3 to 8 hours) and hospital stays (4 to 7 days), and require often postoperative monitoring in an ICU.

B. Craniofacial syndromes

  1. Clinical issues

    a. Common craniofacial syndromes associated with craniosynostosis include Apert, Crouzon, Carpenter, Saethre–Chotzen, Pfeiffer, and Muenke (Table 18.1).

    b. Common craniofacial syndromes not associated with craniosynostosis are Goldenhar/hemifacial microsomia, Treacher-Collins, and Pierre-Robin sequence (Table 18.2). However, these syndromes are associated with difficult airway management issues.

  2. Surgical management

    a. Syndromes associated with craniosynostosis. Infants may present for craniosynostosis surgery between 3 and 6 months of age or older and require surgical correction of midface/maxillary hypoplasia usually between the ages of 5 and 8 years. In adolescence, the maxillary deficiency may be corrected. In more severe cases, hypertelorism may accompany midface flattening and may require further surgical intervention.

b. **Syndromes not associated with craniosynostosis.** In Goldenhar/hemifacial microsomia, skeletal reconstruction involves correction of mandibular hypoplasia and soft tissue reconstruction (ear cartilage and lobe anomalies). In Treacher-Collins (mandibulofacial dysostosis) and Pierre-Robin syndrome, airway management is the primary concern, and early distraction osteogenesis (DO) to treat mandibular hypoplasia or retrognathia may avert the need for tracheostomy in severely affected neonates. Additional surgery in Treacher-Collins to correct facial bone hypoplasia is most successfully accomplished in staged procedures that address the zygomas, maxilla, and mandible along with the colobomas, macrostomia, and microtia. These reconstructions are ideally preformed between 4 and 10 years of age.

> **CLINICAL PEARL** Craniofacial surgery includes reconstructive surgery for craniosynostosis, cranial base tumors, encephalocele, hypertelorism, facial clefts, midface/maxillary hypoplasia, and mandibular hypoplasia. Multiple-staged procedures may be required for craniofacial reconstruction.

C. **Anomalies of the face and jaw**
1. **Clinical issues**
    a. **Craniofacial cleft.** Craniofacial clefts are caused by failure of midline closure and lack of fusion of facial prominences. Defects involve the underlying cranial and/or facial skeletal and/or brain and/or soft tissue. Various combinations of eye, ear, and central nervous system deformities are associated with clefts. Thirty percent of patients with clefts have associated cardiac anomalies.

    The most severe clefts are the midline craniofacial clefts associated with cerebrofacial dysmorphogenesis. The most severe form, holoprosencephaly, derives from the failure of the anterior portion of the neural tube to form the cerebral hemispheres, resulting in a single (holo) forebrain (prosencephaly). Infants with lobar brain morphology are mentally deficient but have a good prognosis for life expectancy and are generally repaired.

    Treacher-Collins syndrome (mandibulofacial dysostosis) is characterized by eyelid coloboma, aplasia/hypoplastic zygomas and pterygoids, mandibular and midface hypoplasia, ear deformities, and poorly developed supra-orbital ridges. Intelligence is usually normal. Oculoauriculovertebral spectrum (hemifacial microsomia or Goldenhar syndrome) is the most common craniofacial malformation other than cleft lip and palate. Frontonasal dysplasia (median cleft face syndrome) is characterized as a combination of hypertelorism and median facial clefting of the nose, upper lip, premaxilla, and palate.

    b. **Hypertelorism.** Hypertelorism is a descriptive term for an increased intraorbital distance and can lead to strabismus and abnormal binocular vision. It is caused by craniofrontonasal dysplasia, facial clefting, encephalocele, trauma, craniofacial dysostosis, and others (fibrous dysplasia, tumors, Grieg's syndrome, and Optiz syndrome) and is often associated with one of the craniofacial dysmorphic malformations (Apert, Crouzon, Pfeiffer, and Carpenter syndromes).

    Children with severe hypertelorism may not be able to develop stereoscopic vision if treatment is delayed. However, early repair may affect normal growth of the cranial skeleton. Surgery is typically delayed until 6 to 8 years of age if vision impairment is not an issue and may be staged. An intracranial approach consisting of a bifrontal craniotomy frees the orbital frame from the surrounding bone through intra- and extraorbital osteotomies.

    c. **Midface/maxillary hypoplasia.** In Apert and Crouzon syndromes, midface hypoplasia may be treated by a Leforte III osteotomy, which involves dysjunction of the entire midface and advancement of the nose, maxilla and orbits via a bicoronal scalp incision, various osteotomies to free and advance the entire facial block with bone grafts and rigid internal fixation.

    d. **Mandibular hypoplasia.** Various manifestations of mandibular hypoplasia are characterized by the following syndromes: Hemifacial microsomia (Goldenhar syndrome), mandibulofacial dysostosis (Treacher-Collins syndrome), and Pierre-Robin sequence. The classic syndrome of mandibular hypoplasia is Pierre-Robin sequence and is associated with acute airway obstruction, failure to thrive, and chronic hypoxia, which may lead to cerebral impairment, pulmonary hypertension, cor pulmonale, and death. Treatment depends on the following factors: (1) Extent and severity of desaturation during sleep, (2) correction of desaturation with supplemental oxygen, (3) a persistently high end-tidal carbon dioxide level, (4) failure to thrive despite nutritional and oxygen therapy.

2. **Surgical management**
  a. **Midface/maxillary hypoplasia**
     (1) Leforte I osteotomy corrects malocclusion due to underdevelopment of the maxilla. It involves separating the maxilla and the palate from the skull above the roots of the upper teeth through an intraoral incision, which is made horizontally across the nasal floor, anterior maxilla, and through the pterygomaxilllary junction. The maxilla is mobilized downward, advanced and stabilized with titanium screws and plates using bone grafts to fill in the spaces to insure healing and union across the bone cuts. The bone graft is frequently harvested from the iliac crest but may be harvested from the chin or lower jaw if a mandibular sagittal split osteotomy is performed at the same time.
     (2) Leforte II osteotomy is used to advance the lower maxilla and entire nose forward. It is a much more involved operation than the Leforte I, as it takes longer and incurs more significant blood loss. It involves a bicoronal scalp incision combined with an intraoral incision. The osteotomy involves mobilization and advancement of the lower maxilla via osteotomies across the nasal bridge, bilaterally down the nasal bridge and through the inferior orbital rim, across the maxilla to the pterygomaxillary junction. Rigid internal fixation devices are used and defects are filled in with bone grafts.
     (3) Leforte III osteotomy is used for complete underdevelopment of the midface involving the upper jaw, nose and cheek bones (as seen in Apert and Crouzon syndromes). It involves dysjunction of the entire midface and advancement of the nose, maxilla, and orbits through a bicoronal scalp incision and various osteotomies to free and advance the entire facial block. Bone grafts are used to fill in the spaces and rigid internal fixation is utilized.

     Midface dysjunction, advancement, and reconstruction procedures with osteotomies can be performed simultaneously or in stages. Timing is usually not until the child is 4 or 5 years old or later but may be delayed until adolescence to allow for eruption of permanent dentation.
  b. **Mandibular hypoplasia.** Surgical interventions depend on the severity of patency of the patient's airway. Most infants are treated with conservative measures such as prone positioning, especially during feeding. Infants who have continued severe apnea often require surgical intervention, which traditionally consists of a tongue lip adhesion or tracheostomy. In most centers, these techniques have given way to early mandibular distraction osteogenesis.

     Distraction osteogenesis (DO) is also called *callotasis* (stretching of the callus, as in a fracture). An osteotomy is used to fracture the bone and thereby induce a callus at which point the proximal and distal bone ends are gradually distracted and moved apart to allow new bone growth. It has the benefit of simultaneously increasing bone length and the volume of the surrounding soft tissues and has been primarily applied to treat mandibular hypoplasia. However, its use is expanding to treat other facial bone defects including midface hypoplasia (maxilla and zygoma are hypoplastic in children with severe hypoplasia as in Crouzon's, Apert's and hemifacial microsomia), and calvaria. External and/or internal uniplanar or multiplanar fixation devices are inserted. The three clinical phases of DO are (1) latency phase, 5 to 7 days after corticotomy and/or osteotomy when the initial fracture healing bridges cut the bony surface; (2) distraction phase, the 3 to 5-week period of active stretching when the bone is moved in three dimensions by rotating screws to increase the distraction by millimeters on a daily basis; and (3) mineralization phase, the 7 to 9-week period after distraction when the primary mineralization and strengthening of the bone occurs.

CLINICAL PEARL   Pediatric patients with craniofacial abnormalities because of their complexity, associated syndromes and co-morbidities continue to provide the anesthesiologist with some of the most challenging cases that present to the operating room.

III. Anesthetic management. The approach to the patient undergoing craniofacial surgery should closely follow the principles of pediatric neuroanesthesia as outlined in Chapter 15. However, there are unique aspects of craniofacial anomalies that merit special attention. Anesthesia management is based on the type of surgical repair and the presence of associated abnormalities. Children under 1 year of age need special attention because long-term assessments reveal that these children have a significantly increased risk related to anesthesia and surgery compared to children over 1 year of age. Open craniosynostosis reconstruction procedures in infants in the age group of 1 month to 1 year are the most common noncardiac surgical procedures with the highest blood loss and blood transfusion per weight. If a less-invasive surgical technique can be chosen with less blood loss, which is the single greatest intraoperative challenge, morbidity and mortality in these patients will be reduced. There are multiple associated conditions that have immediate impact on the course of anesthesia, which should be addressed in the preoperative evaluation of the patient.

A. Preoperative

1. Syndromes. Craniofacial abnormalities can be associated with more than 130 different syndromes, the most common ones are detailed in Table 18.1. Patients with Apert, Crouzon, Pfeiffer, and Saethre–Chotzen syndromes have a high prevalence of elevated ICP (21% to 53%), obstructive sleep apnea (approximately 30%), as well as hearing and visual problems (>50%). Apert, Crouzon, Pierre-Robin, Treacher-Collins, Goldenhar, and craniosynostosis related to mucopolysaccharidosis are associated with specific difficult airway management issues.

2. Airway. Airway management in patients with craniofacial syndromes poses many challenges. Particular attention needs to be paid to the anatomy of the oral cavity, anterior mandibular space, maxilla, temporomandibular joint, and vertebral column. Upper airway obstruction occurs because craniofacial anomalies change and reduce the physical dimensions of the upper airway [3]. Obstructive sleep apnea both from peripheral anatomical anomalies and central neurologic dysfunction is common. Preoperative history of mouth breathing, snoring, noisy breathing, apnea, daytime irritability, or somnolence should alert the anesthesiologist to further investigate. If apnea is severe, continuous positive airway pressure (CPAP) or tracheostomy may be required prior or during the planned surgery. In addition, some patients may have such severe preoperative apnea, which may predispose them to pulmonary artery hypertension. Facial asymmetry, facial clefts, mandibular hypoplasia, an enlarged tongue, and nasal deformities may make mask/bag ventilation difficult especially in patients with craniofacial syndromes. In a child with mandibular hypoplasia and retrognathia, the tongue is displaced posteriorly and thereby the diameter of the oro-, naso-, and hypopharynx is reduced. Retrognathia and hypoplasia of the mandible in Pierre Robin sequence and Treacher-Collins, and abnormal mobility of the temporomandibular joint may decrease mouth opening. Scar tissue from repeated surgeries may also limit mouth opening. Midface hypoplasia (as seen in Apert, Crouzon, Pfeiffer, Treacher-Collins syndromes) along with choanal narrowing and septal deviation, diminish dimensions of the nasal airway making a nasal intubation potentially challenging. Airway evaluation based on physical appearance may be misguided and unreliable as a predictor of difficult intubation.

Cervical vertebral anomalies including fusion of the cervical vertebrae may limit C-spine movement and is a characteristic of common craniofacial syndromes such as Goldenhar/hemifacial microsomia, Crouzon, Apert, and Pfeiffer. Previous anesthetics should be reviewed for intraoperative or postoperative problems with airway management.

CLINICAL PEARL   Anesthesia considerations include those of a pediatric patient, a shared and difficult airway, associated anomalies including cardiac defects, a prolonged procedure, excessive blood loss, and an intracranial approach.

3. **Cardiac.** A history of fatigue or sweating with feedings, cyanosis, or syncope is suggestive of an underlying cardiac abnormality. Craniofacial syndromes that have associated cardiac anomalies include Apert, Crouzon, Goldenhar, Carpenter, and Pfeiffer. Physical examination should focus on heart rate rhythm and abnormal heart sounds, particularly murmurs. An ECG, chest x-ray, or cardiac echocardiograph may aid in the diagnosis. Furthermore, a preoperative cardiac consult may be warranted and subacute bacterial endocarditis (SBE) prophylaxis should be considered for patients with congenital heart disease.

4. **Pulmonary.** Associated pulmonary pathology may include reactive airway disease caused by chronic aspiration or cor pulmonale due to increased pulmonary artery pressure.

5. **CNS.** If the patient with a craniofacial syndrome has craniosynostosis, consideration needs to be given to the presence of increased intracranial pressure, which is manifested as optic atrophy, papilledema, nausea, and vomiting, headaches, or decreased/altered level of consciousness. Intracranial pressure, however, may be elevated due to a restricted cranium with no overt physical manifestation. Chronically raised intracranial pressure may be detected on preoperative skull x-ray or CT scan as a "beaten copper" appearance.

6. **Miscellaneous.** Hearing, vision, and speech impairment may be present especially in the syndromic patient. In patients with proptosis (Crouzon, Apert, Saethre–Chotzen), it may be difficult to close the eye and protect the cornea from drying and abrasion intraoperatively. In addition, prone positioning may increase the risk for orbital compression and perioperative blindness. Infants with syndactyly (Apert, Carpenter, Pfeiffer) may present with difficult intravenous and arterial line placement. Bleeding tendencies need to be identified and investigated preoperatively.

B. Intraoperative

1. **Airway.** The surgeons and the anesthesia team typically share the airway, hence close communication and planning is paramount to ensure safety, and an uncomplicated intraoperative course. Even with careful planning and consideration, unanticipated difficulties with airway management may be encountered. Therefore, having multiple backup plans for airway management is prudent. Adequate planning not only involves having all the necessary equipment available but also having personnel experienced in the use of this equipment (which may include having a pediatric otorhinolaryngologist immediately available). Difficult mask fit may be overcome using a clear mask with moldable cushions, high gas flows, using gauze to fill in gaps or placing an LMA awake (with topical anesthetic) prior to or soon after induction prior to endotracheal intubation. An intravenous induction may be preferred to secure the airway expeditiously and to avoid stage II excitations during an inhalation induction. In a patient with an anticipated difficult intubation, keeping the patient breathing spontaneously until the airway is secured may be the safest option. Upper airway obstruction may occur with inhalation induction and may require various techniques including the use of an oral or nasopharyngeal airway, using sniffing position and a jaw thrust. As direct visualization of the larynx may be challenging, a variety of alternative difficult intubation equipment should be available including oral or nasopharyngeal airway, masks of various sizes, laryngeal masks, fiberoptic scope, tracheal light or lightwand, video laryngoscope, and endotracheal tubes of various sizes (including oral and nasal RAE tubes). Preoperative elective tracheostomy may be considered if extensive multiple complicated facial osteotomies are planned in a small child or if inadvertent tracheal extubation is a possibility with reintubation being impossible or extremely challenging. Once placed, the endotracheal tube may be secured intraoperatively by wiring it to the mandible.

2. **Anesthetic drugs.** A balanced technique is usually the technique of choice, which includes muscle relaxants, narcotics, inhalational agents, and antiemetics. The depth of anesthesia is titrated to maintain hemodynamics to keep blood pressure and heart rate within normal limits (within 20% baseline). Narcotics are titrated as needed. Pain is more significant postoperatively if iliac crest or rib graft is harvested. Dexamethasone is used to

reduce airway swelling. The goal is an awake and comfortable patient postoperatively who maintains a natural airway and cooperates for appropriate neurologic assessment.

3. **Associated conditions.** Anesthetic techniques that avoid increases in intracranial pressure (i.e., avoiding of hypertension, tachycardia, or hypercapnia) are preferred for patients who might have decreased intracranial compliance. Coexisting cardiac and pulmonary anomalies ultimately will guide the anesthetic technique. Orbital manipulation during FOA, Leforte II and III procedures may cause bradycardia. There are several reports of endotracheal tube damage/surgical transection of the nasoendotracheal tube during orognathic surgery.

4. **Temperature control.** Utilization of an underbody warming blanket, forced hot air warmer, warming lights, and a warmed operating room will help to avoid unnecessary hypothermia. Intravenous and irrigation solutions should be warmed. Airway gases should be heated and humidified.

5. **Fluid and blood transfusion**

    a. **Intravenous and intra-arterial access.** The placement of two large bore intravenous lines is advantageous for most cases. An arterial line should be considered in major craniofacial surgery where ongoing blood loss is a concern or in an infant or smaller child in whom small volumes of blood loss may cause hemodynamic instability. An arterial line also affords the anesthesiologist a means to rapid drawing of blood for analysis of blood gas and coagulation parameters. The placement of a central line should be considered if massive blood loss is considered or vascular access is limited. A urinary catheter should be used to ensure a minimum urine output of 0.5 mL/kg/h during the case.

    b. **Fluid management.** The goal of fluid management should be to maintain normovolemia but avoid hypervolemia so as to avoid swelling and edema and allow for safe uneventful extubation if planned. Children undergoing major craniofacial surgery develop varying degrees of metabolic acidosis which may last for several hours. Ringer's lactate is the preferred crystalloid solution over normal saline as it is associated with less severe acidosis in pediatric craniofacial surgery. Crystalloid given as maintenance solution and colloids to replace blood loss initially is prudent. In an infant or child less than 10 kg, the administration of blood to replace blood loss 1:1 when the blood loss is greater than 20% of the estimated blood volume may be required to maintain hemodynamic stability. These surgeries may involve rapid and massive blood loss (the extent and duration of the surgical procedure determining the amount). The anesthesia team should be prepared with blood and blood products in the operating room, and a blood transfusion device warmed, primed, and ready to go. Packed red blood cells for a patient less than 1 year or less than 10 kg should be less than 7 days old to avoid hyperkalemia during rapid transfusion or washed by the blood bank prior to use.

    c. **Blood conservation techniques.** Blood conservation techniques include tissue infiltration of a dilute vasoconstrictor solution (epinephrine 1:200,000 or less concentrated) to decrease blood loss upon scalp incision, intraoperative cell salvage techniques, and antifibrinolytic drugs. Tranexamic acid has been shown to decrease blood loss and blood transfusion requirement in craniosynostosis surgery and for other major craniofacial surgery [4]. In the older patient, preoperative autologous blood donation may be an option to reduce blood loss. Recombinant human erythropoietin increases the hematocrit preoperatively and may be used as an adjuvant. Massive blood loss should prompt a coagulation screen and replacement therapy with platelets, fresh frozen plasma, or cryoprecipitate if indicated.

CLINICAL PEARL   A combination of blood conservation techniques and an appropriately chosen surgical technique may best reduce the transfusion rate for extensive open reconstruction procedures.

5

6. **Potential intraoperative complications** include endotracheal tube dislodgement, rapid blood loss causing hemodynamic compromise, electrolyte and metabolic disturbances, bradycardia from the occulocardiac reflex, and venous air embolism [5] (the preemptive placement of a precordial Doppler ultrasonic probe is a noninvasive method for the early intraoperative detection of a VAE).

C. **Postoperative.** Postoperative intubation and admission to the ICU or PACU/ward depends on the duration of surgery, hemodynamic stability, pre-existing comorbidities (obstructive sleep apnea, difficult intubation), and potential complications during surgery including hypothermia, massive fluid resuscitation, electrolyte disturbances, etc. Since most of the surgical intervention is localized to the cranium, the airway rarely becomes edematous except by mechanical irritation of the vocal cords caused by the tube secondary to frequent surgical head repositioning. In selected cases if facial morphology permits noninvasive ventilatory support, CPAP or BiPAP may be an alternative. The initial management centers upon airway monitoring, sedation, pain management, thermoregulation, and correction of any residual volume deficits, acidosis, or coagulopathy. Isotonic solutions are maintained until fluid shifts are complete. Close hemodynamic and neurologic monitoring is provided until bleeding risk has past. Coagulopathy may be consumptive or dilutional in nature and requires specific correction. Continued blood loss via drains needs to be monitored and replaced appropriately and vigilance maintained for additional concealed losses.

CLINICAL PEARLS • In keeping with the general philosophy of the correction of congenital defects, there is consensus that surgical correction of craniosynostosis during early infancy is advantageous.

- Less-invasive surgical techniques (e.g., ESC) are associated with a significant reduction in blood transfusions, ICU admissions, and costs. It remains to be determined whether the indications for less-invasive surgical techniques and open reconstruction procedures for single- and multiple-suture craniosynostosis can be better defined to further improve risk/benefit profile and costs.
- Craniofacial surgery includes reconstructive surgery for craniosynostosis, cranial base tumors, encephalocele, hypertelorism, facial clefts, midface/maxillary hypoplasia, and mandibular hypoplasia. Multiple-staged procedures may be required for craniofacial reconstruction.
- Pediatric patients with craniofacial abnormalities, because of their complexity, associated syndromes, and comorbidities continue to provide the anesthesiologist with some of the most challenging cases that present to the operating room.
- Anesthesia considerations include those of a pediatric patient, a shared and difficult airway, associated anomalies including cardiac defects, a prolonged procedure, excessive blood loss, and an intracranial approach.
- A combination of blood conservation techniques and an appropriately chosen surgical technique may best reduce the transfusion rate for extensive open reconstruction procedures.

REFERENCES

1. Meier PM, Goobie SM, DiNardo JA, et al. Endoscopic strip craniectomy in early infancy: the initial five years of anesthesia experience. *Anesth Analg.* 2011;112(2):407–414.
2. Lauritzen CG, Davis C, Ivarsson A, et al. The evolving role of springs in craniofacial surgery: the first 100 clinical cases. *Plast Reconstr Surg.* 2008;121(2):545–554.
3. Nargozian C. The airway in patients with craniofacial abnormalities. *Paediatr Anaesth.* 2004;14(1):53–59.
4. Goobie SM, Meier PM, Pereira LM, et al. Efficacy of tranexamic acid in pediatric craniosynostosis surgery: a double-blind, placebo-controlled trial. *Anesthesiology.* 2011;114(4):862–871.
5. Faberowski LW, Black S, Mickle JP. Incidence of venous air embolism during craniectomy for craniosynostosis repair. *Anesthesiology.* 2000;92(1):20–23.

19

Epilepsy Surgery

Hubert A. Benzon, Craig D. McClain, and Heidi M. Koenig

KEY POINTS

1. Advances in neuroimaging and neurophysiology are identifying resectable lesions and surgical technique to mitigate medically intractable seizure disorders.
2. Chronic anticonvulsant drug therapy has multiple side effects such as hematologic derangements and increased hepatic metabolism of drugs.
3. Intraoperative monitoring of central nervous function will significantly alter the choice of the anesthetic technique.

I. Background. Epilepsy is one of the most common neurologic disorders. There has been significant improvement in the medical management of epilepsy. Despite the development of new drugs and treatment regimens, the prevalence of pharmacologically intractable seizures is still high, leading to significant developmental delays. Intractable epilepsy is defined as failure of more than two antiepileptic drugs and having more than one seizure per month over a period of 18 months. Advances in neuroimaging techniques and electroencephalography (EEG) have provided epileptologists with surgically resectable anatomic targets that mediate some of these medically intractable seizure disorders [1]. Neurosurgeons have utilized these technologies to dramatically improve outcomes in these patients.

II. Physiologic considerations

A. There are several features of pediatric epilepsy that differ from adult epilepsy:

1. The developing brain has a lower seizure threshold, which results in a more frequent occurrence of catastrophic epilepsy in young children.
2. In adults, mesial temporal lobe epilepsy is the most common form whereas in children, lesional epilepsy is more common. The presence of auras or focal manifestations of the seizure are relatively uncommon in the pediatric population.
3. Cerebrovascular physiology is different. Compared to adults, a larger percentage of the cardiac output is directed toward the brain, resulting in a greater cerebral blood volume in infants. Coupled with the fact that children have a lower baseline mean arterial pressure than adults, infants are at greater risk of hemodynamic instability during neurosurgical procedures.
4. Hepatic function is decreased in neonates leading to delayed metabolism of drugs. Renal function is also decreased in neonates, limiting the ability to compensate for changes in fluid and solute loads. Combined, these may alter the clearance of medications given to these patients.

B. Other considerations

1. Side effects of medical treatments.

254

2. Possible cranial nerve dysfunction resulting in impaired protective airway reflexes.
3. Significant comorbidities such as degenerative diseases, cerebral palsy (CP), scoliosis, inborn errors of metabolism with respiratory, myocardial effects, and hypo- or hyperglycemia.

III. Imaging techniques. Various imaging techniques are utilized to assess structural or functional epileptogenic zones. Magnetic resonance imaging (MRI) is the modality of choice for structural imaging. If the MRI is nonlocalizing and functional neuroimaging is necessary, newer modalities such as positron emission tomography (PET), single photon emission computed tomography (SPECT), MR spectroscopy (MRS), functional MRI (fMRI), magnetoencephalography (MEG), and diffusion tensor imaging (DTI) can be utilized. None of these have emerged as the best modality.

Adults in general will be able to tolerate these imaging modalities without sedation. However, since infants and patients are uncooperative, anesthesiologists. Anesthesiologists may be asked to sedate or anesthetize these children for MRI studies which can last almost one hour and require the patient, to be kept still for optimal imaging. Typically IV sedation is given to these patients, but occasionally a general anesthetic is necessary in the MRI suite to obtain optimal imaging while protecting a patient's airway.

IV. Surgical treatment

A. Surgical treatment of seizures often involves resection of a lesion or area of cortex that has been shown to be related to seizure generation and propagation.
   1. The most common location of seizure foci is the temporal lobe.
   2. The temporal lobe is involved with complex partial seizures (50% of new epilepsy cases each year) that are often related to mesial temporal sclerosis or a structural lesion of the temporal lobe.
   3. Approximately one-third of patients with complex partial seizures are not adequately controlled with medication alone.
   4. Although many epileptogenic foci are located in the region of the temporal lobe, such foci may be located in any area of the cerebral cortex.
   5. The mechanisms by which such foci contribute to seizure generation include alteration of vascularization, alteration of regional CBF, and irritation of adjacent cortex by compression or mass effect.

V. Surgical resection of seizure foci. A major concern for resection of seizure foci is to avoid harming brain tissue that controls vital functions such as motion, sensation, speech, and memory, especially if a seizure focus is adjacent to these cortical areas.

Advances in neurophysiologic monitoring (EEG and electrocorticography [ECoG]) have increased the ability to safely perform resections in functional areas of the brain. Typically low levels of anesthetic are necessary for these types of monitoring. Sometimes, cortical stimulation of the motor cortex is performed to observe motor movement of the area of the homunculus. Here, muscle relaxants must be avoided to enable visualization of the stimulated area. Asleep craniotomy is appropriate for lesions that are not located in or deep to eloquent areas of the brain. Awake neurosurgical procedures are most important for those patients requiring interventions close to or partially overlapping eloquent brain.

Potentially cooperative patients (adolescents and adults) can assist in determination of the limits of safe cortical resection if speech and motor functions can be continually assessed intraoperatively while performing an awake craniotomy. This technique incorporates a variety of techniques with the common goal of allowing intraoperative neurologic assessment and feedback to determine if eloquent cortex is at risk during surgical resection. Eloquent cortex is defined as a cortical region that serves a critical neurologic function such as motor, language, memory, or special sensory function. Removal of this area and loss of that specific function would have a deleterious effect on neurologic outcome. There are no randomized controlled trials comparing the safety or efficacy of these various techniques. Overall, there is a 33% to 86% seizure reduction with follow-up times of 6 months up to 7.9 years.

A. **Awake craniotomy.** There are different anesthetic approaches for an awake craniotomy:
   1. All procedures including line placement, local anesthetic infiltration for surgical exposure, skull and dural opening, and surgical resection of the seizure focus can be done with the patient completely awake or with minimal sedation. If intraoperative electrocorticography is being utilized, benzodiazepines and barbiturates should be avoided, unless specifically

accepted by the monitoring team. Patient completely awake or with minimal sedation. This requires an extremely motivated and cooperative patient.

2. Alternatively, short-acting sedatives and analgesics, such as propofol, fentanyl, or dexmedetomidine, can be titrated to unconsciousness but maintaining spontaneous ventilation for the infiltration of local anesthetic, catheter insertion for monitoring, placement of head pins, and skull opening. Then patients are allowed to awaken or kept slightly sedated for the surgical resection of the seizure focus. After surgical resection has been completed, then sedatives and analgesics can be restarted or increased for patient comfort during surgical closure.

B. **Asleep–awake–asleep technique.** This technique allows the painful portions of the procedure such as line placement and placement of head pins to be performed under general anesthesia. The patient does not have to tolerate a potentially uncomfortable and claustrophobic position for a long duration as a totally awake craniotomy.

1. Induce general anesthesia and maintain airway control with a supraglottic device (i.e., laryngeal mask airway [LMA]). Maintain general anesthesia for line placement, placement of head pins, and skull and dural opening.

2. The patient is then awakened, the supraglottic airway carefully removed, and resection of the seizure foci may then proceed.

3. When surgical resection has been completed, general anesthesia is again induced and the supraglottic airway reinserted for closure of the dura, skull, and skin. Following skin closure, the patient may then be awakened from general anesthesia.

4. Disadvantages of the asleep–awake–asleep approach:

   a. Airway management while the patient is in head pins can be quite difficult.

   b. Cervical spine injuries or scalp lacerations can occur during intraoperative emergence and reinduction should the patient cough or buck while the head is immobilized in head pins.

   c. Brain swelling is a major concern. It may worsen during spontaneous ventilation from elevated carbon dioxide in conjunction with the cerebrovasodilatory effects of a volatile agent and possibly nitrous oxide. Mannitol and furosemide can be given, but the patient then becomes very uncomfortable with sensations of thirst and urinary urgency in the awake patient. Hyperventilation or Doxapram have been used, but the patients quickly tire of this effort. These maneuvers have not proven satisfactory. Slight elevation of the head of the bed, assuring the neck veins are not compromised by clothing and monitors or extreme rotation often quickly relieve the problem. If none of these maneuvers work, the patient may have to undergo general anesthesia and controlled ventilation.

   d. Regardless of which technique is chosen, it is crucial for the anesthesiologist to have a discussion with the patient with respect to intraoperative needs and expectations. The preoperative evaluation is the time to determine whether or not the patient is a potential candidate to undergo an "awake" craniotomy.

   e. In general, children who are younger than 10 years old or uncooperative patients of any age will not tolerate the awake craniotomy approach and will require general anesthesia throughout the procedure. In these scenarios, a variety of intraoperative electrophysiologic techniques such as somatosensory evoked potentials, EEG, ECoG, and motor stimulation may be used to help localize and determine the function of the site of the planned resection. If EEG studies are performed, a nitrous oxide/high-dose narcotic technique enables all potent volatile agents that depress cerebral electrical activity to be minimized by the time of study. If direct cortical motor stimulation is planned, muscle relaxants must wear off by the time of study as well. Occasionally, a seizure focus is difficult to identify intraoperatively. In these situations, hyperventilation or methohexital (in small doses, 0.25 to 0.5 mg/kg) may be helpful in lowering the seizure threshold and evoke EEG seizure activity (see chapter 26).

VI. **Subdural grids and strips electrodes**

A. In some patients, the seizures are so generalized that detecting the site of origin can be very difficult. When this occurs, further evaluation with perioperative intracranial EEG monitoring ("grids and strips") may be accomplished by direct ECoG.

1. During a craniotomy under general anesthesia, leads are placed on the surface of the cerebral cortex.

2. Intraoperative EEG monitoring during the initial placement ensures that all leads are functional. The actual monitoring for seizures and mapping of seizure foci takes place

over the next several days to see if a focus can be identified and eventually surgically resected.

3. The patient must be observed carefully during this postoperative period because several complications can develop with these electrodes in place. Infections can develop from a foreign body in the brain. Pneumocephalus can occur as air persists in the skull for up to 3 weeks after a craniotomy. These patients should not have nitrous oxide administered to them for subsequent procedures (i.e., seizure focus resection and/or removal of the ECoG leads) until their dura has been opened to avoid the development of tension pneumocephalus.

4. A peripheral intravenous central catheter (PICC line) can be placed during the initial surgery for placement of "grids and strips." This is helpful as patients will receive IV antibiotic therapy during the time the electrodes are in place and avoids the discomfort of multiple IV catheter insertions.

5. These patients typically return in 1 week for repeat craniotomy for the removal of the grids and strips and resection of the seizure foci.

VII. Nonfocal surgical resection

A. When a focal resection is not possible, a lobectomy or corpus callosotomy may be attempted. Patients undergoing the corpus callosotomy are often somnolent for the first few postoperative days, particularly if a "complete" callosotomy is performed. This also occurs in children who have undergone insertion of multiple subdural grids and strips. It is more common for surgeons nowadays to initially perform a partial callosotomy, and to then perform a complete callosotomy if necessary. Since the surgical approach is near the sagittal sinus, this procedure can be associated with hemorrhage and venous air embolism (VAE).

Occasionally, small children will undergo a hemispherectomy because their seizures are attributed to an abnormal hemisphere that is already severely dysfunctional, such as when a hemiparesis is already present [2]. Hemispherectomies are being performed more often in younger children because it is thought to improve developmental and functional outcome later on in life.

1. Anatomic hemispherectomy consists of the resection of an entire hemisphere.

2. Functional hemispherectomy consists of a partial temporal lobectomy and disconnection of interhemispheric neural networks. The functional hemispherectomy generally involves less blood loss.

3. This procedure is usually performed when patients are very young. The intent is to permit the contralateral hemisphere to assume function of both hemispheres.

4. These can be very challenging cases for the anesthesiologist because blood loss can be significant. Multiples of estimated blood volume can be lost, and therefore adequate IV access is necessary. This can be difficult in very young children. If necessary, large-bore catheters can be placed into central veins to facilitate rapid volume resuscitation and treatment with medications.

5. One might consider the use of tranexamic acid, which has a prothrombotic effect, and may help decrease the blood loss.

6. Invasive arterial pressure monitoring is routine for such cases. Some practitioners utilize central venous pressure monitoring as well.

VIII. Vagal nerve stimulator

A. The vagal nerve stimulator (VNS) is another advance in the surgical treatment of epilepsy. Although its exact mechanism of action is not understood, it appears to inhibit seizure activity at the brainstem or cortical levels. Its placement has shown benefit with minimal side effects in many patients who are disabled by intractable seizures. It is estimated that there is a 60% to 70% improvement in seizure control in children receiving VNS, with the best results in those who suffer from drop attacks.

1. The VNS is a programmable device similar to a cardiac pacemaker, and that is placed subcutaneously under the left anterior chest wall.

2. Bipolar platinum stimulating electrode coils, which are implanted around the left vagus nerve, are connected to the generator by subcutaneously tunneled wires.

3. The device automatically activates for up to 30 seconds every 5 minutes.

4. Stimulation of the vagal nerve in this manner may affect vocal cord function, and sudden bradycardia or transient asystole has been reported but without resultant morbidity.

5. When patients with VNSs return for subsequent surgeries, it may be appropriate to deactivate the stimulator while the patient is under general anesthesia to prevent vocal cord motion. A magnet placed over the generator will deactivate the stimulator.

IX.　**Anesthesia issues**

　　A.　**Preoperative evaluation**

　　　　1.　A thorough preoperative evaluation is necessary for any patient presenting to the operating suite. A history must be undertaken and a thorough physical examination must be carefully performed as many of these patients have significant comorbidities. One should pay careful attention to the respiratory and cardiac systems. Cardiac function should be optimized prior to surgery especially in older patients who may have coronary heart disease or hypertension, as there can be significant blood loss with fluid and blood administration, and swings in blood pressure that can affect myocardial contractility. A complete airway examination should be performed as some craniofacial anomalies may require special techniques to secure the airway. The evaluation should also attempt to detect underlying conditions that are leading to the seizures, as well as describing disabilities resulting from progressive neurologic dysfunction.

　　　　2.　Special consideration should be given to those patients with a history of tuberous sclerosis. The intracranial lesions can lead to medically intractable epilepsy. This hamartomatous disease presents with cutaneous and intracranial lesions, with lesions infiltrating the cardiac, renal, and pulmonary systems. Preoperative electrocardiograph (EKG) and echocardiogram should perform to assess for functional defects from the possible cardiac rhabdomyomas leading to obstruction of intracardiac blood flow, dysrhythmias, or abnormal conduction pathways. Renal lesions can lead to hypertension or decreased renal function.

　　　　3.　Preoperative laboratory testing should include a complete blood count to assess for a baseline hematocrit level and coagulation studies to look for any unknown coagulation disorders. This is necessary as significant blood loss can occur during the procedure and underlying coagulopathies should be corrected prior to surgery. Type and cross-matched blood should be available for these procedures.

　　　　4.　The anticonvulsant medications that most of these patients require may have side effects that affect the anesthetic:

　　　　　　a.　Abnormalities of hematologic function such as abnormal coagulation, depression of red or white blood cell production, or decreased platelet counts are especially concerning during intracranial surgery (in particular from valproic acid and carbamazepine). Steroidal NMBs are more affected by this than the benzoisoquinolones NMBs such as Atracurium and cisatracurium. Continuous quantitative NMB monitoring can facilitate safe degrees of NMB administration in anticonvulsant treated patients.

　　　　　　b.　Alterations in hepatic function, in particular the upregulation of the cytochrome P450 system, also occur. Serum anticonvulsant levels should be determined preoperatively to detect subtherapeutic or toxic concentrations. These anticonvulsants enhance the metabolism of nondepolarizing muscle relaxants and opioids. Therefore, an increased amount of these drugs may be necessary during the surgical procedure. Newer anticonvulsants seem to have less of an effect on the metabolism of anesthetic drugs.

　　　　5.　A ketogenic diet that is a high-fat, low-carbohydrate diet that promotes ketosis, has been used as an adjuvant for intractable epilepsy. This ketosis can promote a metabolic acidosis, which can be exacerbated with the use of carbohydrate-containing solutions. These patients should be given normal saline instead of lactated Ringer's solution. Intraoperatively, these patients should have their acid base status and plasma glucose levels measured frequently.

　　B.　**General anesthesia**

　　　　1.　**Positioning**

　　　　　　a.　The positioning of the patient will depend mostly on the location of the seizure focus.

　　　　　　b.　Typically the seizure focus is located over one of the temporal or parietal lobes. Therefore, the most common position for this type of surgery is supine with the head turned over one shoulder. Often, the neurosurgeons place a shoulder roll to aid with optimal positioning for surgery.

　　　　　　c.　The head of the patient is usually placed in a pinning system for the duration of the procedure. Care should be taken to assure that the endotracheal tube is properly positioned with the expectation of the head being turned laterally for the procedure. The supine position is also utilized for many other types of seizure surgery such as VNS placement, hemispherectomy, and corpus callosotomy.

   d. For the awake craniotomy, the face must always be accessible to the anesthesiologist in case airway manipulation is necessary due to oversedation or the generation of a seizure. This also facilitates communication and facial observation during the neuropsychological assessment. The patient must also be in a comfortable position.

   e. In many of these procedures, the site of operation is elevated (relative to the heart) to facilitate venous and CSF drainage from the surgical site. This leads to pressure decreases in the sagittal sinuses, leading to an increased chance of venous air emboli.

2. **Typical surgical time**

   a. Intraoperative mapping of seizure foci and/or intraoperative imaging can add significant time onto the procedure.

   b. The typical VNS placement takes approximately 1.5 to 2 hours.

   c. A hemispherectomy is a procedure that takes several hours and can potentially last all day.

3. **Induction and maintenance**

   a. Induction and maintenance of general anesthesia in patients who are undergoing seizure surgery is similar to that of other patients undergoing intracranial procedures. Care should be taken not to exacerbate any existing intracranial hypertension. Also, if intraoperative seizure mapping is planned, one may have to alter the anesthetic technique (see later sections for details). Discussion with the neurosurgical team is essential to generate the anesthetic plan preoperatively.

   b. As mentioned earlier, consideration of the effects of anticonvulsant drugs on the metabolism of other drugs, specifically muscle relaxants and narcotics, is important to consider. It seems that first-generation antiepileptic drugs (AEDs) (i.e., phenytoin, phenobarbital, valproate) tend to have a higher potential for interactions and adverse effects due to hepatic enzyme induction or inhibition, whereas the newer AEDs have a greater safety profile and fewer drug interactions, but still can have significant adverse side effects. In terms of affecting anesthetic drug dosing, the requirements for muscle relaxants and narcotics are increased to maintain the same depth of anesthesia and muscle relaxation. Phenytoin, which is commonly given intraoperatively, can lead to hypotension and arrhythmias when given rapidly and fatalities have been reported, so careful consideration must be taken when giving drugs not familiar to the anesthesiologist.

   c. The induction can be performed via either an inhalational agent or an intravenous agent, depending on the clinical circumstances. There is some concern that sevoflurane has epileptogenic potential, however it has a much faster uptake than isoflurane and less of an airway irritant, making it more ideal to perform an inhaled induction with a child. If there is concern for aspiration from vomiting due to increased intracranial pressure, a rapid sequence induction should be performed.

   d. The maintenance of anesthesia can be performed with several techniques as long as one is aware of the effects of the type of anesthetic chosen. Inhaled agents can depress the metabolic supply and demand of the brain tissue, but at the same time can lead to cerebrovascular dilation. They can decrease cerebral perfusion pressure mostly by decreasing the patient's mean arterial pressure. Inhaled agents also depress the EEG and ECoG. Intravenous agents decrease the cerebral metabolic demand but do not lead to cerebrovascular dilation. They also can depress the EEG. Opioids depress the EEG less and are good analgesics, but can lead to side effects of respiratory depression and sedation postoperatively.

   e. There is much controversy as to whether anesthetic agents can increase or lower the seizure threshold. In fact, some anesthetics can produce both proconvulsant and anticonvulsant properties at different doses or with different physiologic situations. It seems that lower anesthetic doses have a proconvulsant tendency while higher doses have anticonvulsant tendencies. A drug like sevoflurane, for example, may have lead to epileptiform activity, but usually does not convert to convulsions. Low doses of propofol have definite anticonvulsant effects.

   f. Adequate intravenous access is essential. These procedures are associated with significant amounts of blood loss and this tends to be the most significant intraoperative complication. Large-bore intravenous access is necessary for volume resuscitation. If those are difficult to obtain, then central venous access should be considered. Normal saline is typically used for neurosurgical procedures as it is mildly hyperosmolar and should minimize cerebral edema; however, one should realize that large quantities of normal saline are associated with hyperchloremic acidosis. Significant blood loss should be replaced with colloid such as 5% albumin or packed red blood cells. Blood loss and replacement therapy can tax the cardiovascular system. Therefore, vasopressor support with a dopamine infusion may provide some hemodynamic stability.

g. Approximately 16% of patients experience a seizure during craniotomy for seizure focus excision. Most often, this occurs as the neurosurgeon stimulates the area of interest. It may be typical of the patient's seizures before surgery or different, depending on the relationship of the surgical stimulation to the patient's intrinsic seizure focus. It is important to quickly communicate to the surgeon that you are observing a physical seizure. Often the seizure is localized to the face or an extremity initially but rapidly becomes generalized if not immediately interrupted. The neurosurgeon can irrigate the area with iced Ringer's lactate to rapidly and reliably interrupt the seizure. A small bolus of propofol (10–20 mg) intravenously will stop a seizure. Both of these interventions also interrupt the electrocorticography briefly, but both are quickly completely reversible. Administration of intravenous barbiturates or benzodiazepines as anticonvulsants will interrupt the ability to stimulate and monitor for seizures for a longer time. These longer acting medications also take longer to control the seizure and may cause significant delays until effective monitoring can resume. If the patient goes into a persistent seizure you must protect them from personal injury, protect the airway and administer medications such as thiopental, propofol or benzodiazepines.

C. Monitoring. Monitoring for these patients is similar to that for other patients undergoing intracranial procedures:

1. Invasive BP monitoring is almost always used for intracranial procedures to ensure adequate mean arterial pressure and therefore cerebral perfusion pressure throughout the case. An arterial line also allows for serial blood gas sampling and lab draws. VNS placement typically does not require invasive BP monitoring.

2. Often it is useful to use a precordial Doppler to monitor for VAE. The precordial Doppler in conjunction with end-tidal CO_2 monitoring should enable the practitioner to detect minute VAE early enough before any significant hemodynamic instability can develop. The probe is best placed on the anterior chest, usually over the right of the sternum at the fourth intercostal space (see chapter 22).

3. A variety of neuromonitoring techniques are often used during these procedures. These techniques may include evoked potential monitoring, EEG, ECOG, and motor stimulation. If an awake craniotomy is performed, the patient will act as her or his own monitor.

4. Blood glucose levels should be monitored intraoperatively as well. Neonates with underdeveloped gluconeogenesis may require glucose to maintain IV fluids; however, this should be done cautiously as hyperglycemia should always be avoided in neurosurgical procedures as it may exacerbate neurologic injury if ischemia should develop.

5. Continuous monitoring of NMB as the response to NMBs is quite unpredictable.

D. Neuromonitoring. Anesthetic goals for epilepsy surgery are similar to other similar neurosurgical procedures (i.e., craniotomies). Detail of the age specific differences in the ECoG are discussed in Chapter 26. During seizure surgery, however, various modes of intraoperative neuromonitoring are often used to aid in delineation of seizure foci. Such techniques may involve ECoG, cortical stimulation, or electromyography. It is important to discuss the requirements of intraoperative mapping and neuromonitoring with the neurosurgeon, neurologist, and neurophysiologist in order to tailor the anesthetic technique. For example, if it will be necessary to induce seizure activity, long-acting agents that elevate the seizure threshold may be avoided. In the case of concurrent ECoG monitoring, one may minimize the dosage of a benzodiazepine given preoperatively for the anxious child. Occasionally, it may be necessary to induce seizure activity (i.e., administration of methohexital) to help locate seizure foci.

E. Postoperative considerations

1. For patients who have undergone primary resection of a seizure focus, or temporal lobectomy, the postoperative considerations are similar to those other patients who have undergone craniotomy. Typically, these patients are sent to the intensive care unit (ICU) postoperatively for serial neurologic examinations and invasive hemodynamic monitoring. Low dose dexmedetomidine (alpha 2 agonist) decreases the narcotic requirements greatly and the patients are much more calm and more readily arousable than if only narcotic sedation is utilized.

2. Monitoring for seizure activity should continue and a plan for treatment should be agreed upon. When patients have subdural electrodes (grids/strips) placed, the goal is to have the patient seize postoperatively in a controlled and monitored setting in order to generate a map of the seizure focus. However, there should be a plan in place to address longer, uncontrolled seizure activity that does not cease on its own.

   a. These patients may be somewhat somnolent depending on the number of electrodes left in place with higher numbers seeming to increase somnolence.

   b. Pain may be more significant in these patients and analgesic technique should be adjusted correspondingly. Typically, intravenous opioids are titrated to treat pain. However, opioid-induced respiratory depression can lead to hypoxemia and hypercarbia. If the patient requires large amounts of opioids and is old enough to do so, patient-controlled analgesia (PCA) can be administered.

   c. In addition, these patients will need continued IV antibiotic coverage while the electrodes are in place (which may be up to 2 weeks). Our practice is to place a PICC line in these patients during the same anesthetic to ensure longer-term IV access. The PICC line can be left in place while the patient is in the hospital and all medications administered through it. When the patient returns to the OR for the definitive resection, the PICC line may be used for induction of anesthesia.

3. Patients who undergo hemispherectomy or corpus callosotomy are often extremely somnolent for the first several days postoperatively. Therefore, the patient is often kept intubated at the conclusion of the surgical procedure. These patients are commonly taken to the ICU intubated and will most often be ready for extubation within 1 to 2 days of surgery.

4. These intracranial procedures can be associated with the syndrome of inappropriate antidiuretic hormone secretion (SIADH) leading to hyponatremia, or diabetes insipidus or cerebral salt wasting syndrome leading to hypernatremia.

5. Patients undergoing VNS can be sent home the day of surgery as long as there are no anesthetic or surgical concerns after the procedure has been completed.

CLINICAL PEARLS **1.** These surgeries in general are associated with significant blood loss. One should always be prepared with adequate intravenous access and blood products for resuscitation of the patient.
2. Depending on the surgical conditions, different types of neuromonitoring may be implemented. It is important to know ahead of time if the surgeons plan on using EEG, ECOG, motor stimulation, or the neurologic examination from an awake patient. The type of anesthetic must be altered to optimize the conditions for adequate neuromonitoring.
3. Given the numerous AEDs and the differing effects on metabolism of other drugs, the anesthesiologist must be attentive to the effects they can have on anesthetic agents, particularly muscle relaxants and narcotics. Careful attention should be applied toward monitoring for muscle relaxation (when used) and depth of anesthesia as these can be altered when compared to other types of surgery.

REFERENCES

1. Depositario-Cabacar DT, Riviello JJ, Takeoka M. Present status of surgical intervention for children with intractable seizures. *Curr Neurol Neurosci Rep.* 2008;8(2):123–129.
2. Flack S, Ojemann J, Haberkern C. Cerebral hemispherectomy in infants and young children. *Paediatr Anaesth.* 2008;18(10):967–973.
3. Kofke WA. Anesthetic management of the patient with epilepsy or prior seizures. *Curr Opin Anaesthesiol.* 2010; 23(3):391–399.
4. Soriano SG, Bozza P. Anesthesia for epilepsy surgery in children. *Childs NErv Syst.* 2006;22(8):834–843.

20

Pediatric Neurovascular Lesions

Hubert A. Benzon, Edward R. Smith, and Craig D. McClain

KEY POINTS

1. Maintaining cerebral perfusion pressure is essential in these patients. While one may desire some hypotension (particularly for AVMs or aneurysms) to minimize bleeding and avoid potential rupture of these neurovascular lesions, it is just as important to avoid ischemia in the surrounding brain tissue. Therefore, maintaining adequate perfusion to the brain tissue is critical.

2. Adequate intravenous access is necessary as these patients can lose blood very quickly, should a rupture of the vessel occur intraoperatively.

3. Many of these cases are being performed in interventional radiology. Whether it be for coiling of the lesion or serial embolizations prior to a surgical intervention, the anesthetic plan may actually need to take into account the fact that multiple anesthetics will be performed on the same patient on consecutive days. This can affect the intravenous access placed or the hemodynamic monitors used. Also, given the fragility of the lesions prior to and after both the embolization and surgical procedure, the numerous inductions and emergences from anesthesia, and the sedated period in between procedures, the anesthesiologists involved in the care must be very careful to avoid any significant swings in hemodynamics, as the shearing forces could lead to rupture of any of the lesions mentioned above.

I. Background

A. Cerebrovascular disease (CVD) is rare in pediatric patients and typically presents as either hemorrhagic or ischemic stroke. The underlying vascular anomalies that can result in stroke can be categorized as the following:

1. Structural changes in pre-existing blood vessels, that is, aneurysms or arterial dissections.

2. Pathologic vascular structures including arteriovenous malformations (AVMs), vein of Galen malformations (VOGMs), arteriovenous fistulas, and cavernous malformations (CMs)/hemangiomas.

3. Progressive arteriopathies such as moyamoya syndrome or heritable arteriopathies.

II. Patient assessment

A. Afflicted patients will present with headaches, seizures, cognitive deficits, focal neurologic deficits (weakness, numbness, or visual field problems), previous transient ischemic attacks (TIAs), or cerebral vascular accidents (CVAs). However, most patients with neurovascular lesions have no symptoms or specific physical findings on examination. Associated systemic illnesses such as systemic lupus erythematosus (SLE), congenital cardiac disease, high-output cardiac failure, and illicit drug use such as cocaine are associated with neurovascular lesions.

B. A systolic bruit over the eye, head, or neck (which is present in 15% to 40% of patients with an AVM or carotid dissections) may be detectable. AV shunts may be associated with tachycardia, cardiomegaly, and cardiac failure, especially in infants with a VOGM.

1 **CLINICAL PEARL** In general, the perioperative management of pediatric patients undergoing imaging studies and endovascular or surgical correction of their vascular anomalies should focus on optimizing cerebral perfusion and oxygen delivery to the brain tissue. Anesthetic management is focused on maintaining hemodynamic stability to assure adequate cerebral perfusion. However, it may be complicated by intracranial hypertension. Since the surgical resection of these lesions can be associated with significant blood loss, these patients require adequate intravenous (IV) access and invasive hemodynamic monitoring. Maintaining intravascular volume is key for these goals. Therefore, blood products should be available to replenish sudden massive blood loss. Hypotension from hypovolemia can be temporized with vasopressor agents such as ephedrine, phenylephrine, or infusions of dopamine, norepinephrine, or epinephrine. Alternatively, hypertension needs to be avoided as well, as one would not want to rupture these delicate vessels prior to, during, or after surgical repair. If an endovascular procedure be performed in the interventional radiology (IR) suite, the anesthesia team should be prepared that there may need to be an emergent surgical intervention should any complications occur during any IR procedure.

III. Radiographic studies

A. Several different modalities are used to aid in the diagnosis of neurovascular lesions.

1. Intracranial ultrasonography: Can be used as an initial, nonurgent screening test in infants with an open fontanel and for detecting hemorrhage, hydrocephalus, large infarcts, or lesions such as an AVM or VOGM.

2. Duplex ultrasonography is useful in the diagnosis of an extracranial carotid dissection.

3. Computerized tomography (CT)/computerized tomography angiography (CTA): CT is typically the initial study for any patient with neurologic symptoms and diagnosing hemorrhage, delayed stroke, or large vascular lesions. CTA is excellent for the evaluation of an AVM, aneurysm, and moyamoya disease.

4. Magnetic resonance imaging (MRI)/magnetic resonance angiography (MRA) is useful for the evaluation of stroke with diffusion-weighted images (DWIs), CMs (susceptibility imaging), and most vascular lesions.

5. Digital subtraction angiography (DSA) is the gold standard for all vascular lesions except CMs.

B. Pediatric anesthesiologists frequently anesthetize these patients with neurovascular lesions for an imaging study to obtain a definitive diagnosis. Due to reasons such as the invasiveness of the CTA to obtain venous and arterial access and to obtain optimal images, and the length of time a patient needs to stay still for an MRI, anesthesiologists are needed to keep the patients still for optimal images while maintaining a patient's normal physiology during a general anesthetic.

C. For MRI, these anesthetics can typically be performed under a deep sedation. Should the patient have a full stomach or other complicating conditions, the anesthetic for MRI may be done under general anesthesia. A discussion between the primary service and radiology service can help determine the type of anesthetic necessary. If deep sedation is chosen, typically, agents such as propofol or dexmedetomidine can be used. General anesthetic requires that airway control be secured by either a laryngeal mask airway (LMA) or endotracheal tube (ETT). The usual concerns for performing an anesthetic in the MRI suite (different sets of monitors, equipment, distance from the patient, and lack of familiar resources available in the main operating room) must be considered for these imaging studies. Hemodynamic stability should be maintained in patients with neurovascular lesions, since hypo- and hypertension can precipitate ischemia and hemorrhage respectively. Typically, a deep sedation provides a smoother hemo-dynamic course.

D. CTA can also be performed under a deep sedation with local anesthesia. However, an unco-operative infant or child will require a general anesthetic. Furthermore, interventional radiolo-gists may need episodes of apnea or hypercarbia to optimize the images during angiography. Apnea or hypoventilation can be achieved under general anesthesia.

IV. Arteriovenous malformations

A. **AVMs** result from improper formation of the arteriolar-capillary network that provides a direct connection between arteries and veins in the brain without intervening capillaries. This produces low resistance and leads to a high-flow shunt. They can occur in the cerebral hemi-spheres, brainstem, and spinal cord. The embryonic origins of these malformations are unclear. Functional neural tissue does not reside within the lesion. Surrounding tissues are deprived of blood supply and nutrients.

1. Anatomically, these malformations consist of large arterial feeding vessels, dilated communicating vessels, and large draining veins carrying arterialized blood.

2. Cerebral damage can result from AVMs due to the steal phenomenon, ischemia, hemorrhagic infarct from thrombosis, cerebral atrophy, or alterations of flow during surgery.

3. Saccular dilation of the vein of Galen (see the following text) may present later in infancy or childhood with hydrocephalus secondary to obstruction of the aqueduct of Sylvius.

4. In the pediatric population, the most common presentation is an intracerebral bleed, a seizure and hydrocephalus, or congestive hearing failure (rarely) in the neonatal period.

   a. Malformations not large enough to produce congestive heart failure (CHF) usually remain clinically silent unless they cause seizures or stroke, or until the acute rupture of a communicating vessel results in subarachnoid or intracerebral hemorrhage. Initial presentation is typically hemorrhage (80% to 85%) with an associated mortality of 25%. They present as seizures, headache, or focal neurologic deficits (from either mass effect from bleeding or from cerebral ischemia due to diversion of blood to the AVM from the normal cerebral circulation, known as the "steal" phenomenon). Ninety percent of AVMs occur supratentorially, most commonly in the distribution of the middle cere-bral artery.

5. Mortality seems to be higher in younger patients as compared to adults.

6. If amenable, treatment is usually embolization or radiation of deep AVMs, surgical excision usually for more superficial AVMs that are located in noneloquent areas of cortex, or some combination of these modalities (with the intent of decreasing the size and blood flow through the AVM during embolization, leading to a solid brittle mass that can then be surgically resected later). The purpose is to eliminate the malformation from the cerebral circulation in order to prevent intracranial hemorrhage. If surgically it is too difficult to approach, then treatment is with gamma knife over several months.

7. Rebleeding can occur approximately 6% during the first 6 months and then 3% per year afterward.

8. Sometimes, emergency surgery is necessary for increasing intracerebral hematoma that can be a significant risk for brain herniation, so a ventricular drain may be placed to treat acute hydrocephalus.

B. Anesthetic considerations

1. Anesthetic management for embolic procedures in the IR suite usually involves a standard general anesthetic with neuromuscular blockade and secure IV access. The anesthesiologist should be knowledgeable about the types of embolic agents that will be used and their potential complications.

   a. Bleeding, especially from the femoral arterial puncture site (which cannot always be visualized), should always be a consideration. This is especially true as the patient will be heparinized during the time the sheaths and catheters are in place.

   b. Fluid overload can occur due to the large amount of contrast agents administered, espe-cially in a young infant who may already be in high-output CHF. Newborns with CHF may be receiving several inotropic agents. It is possible to get some idea of the degree of cardiac compromise in newborns by obtaining a detailed feeding history—frequency, length of time per feeding, amount, respiratory distress during feeding, and so on.

   c. One should always be prepared for an emergency craniotomy should a vessel rupture occur.

      (1) If rupture occurs, one may have to induce hypotension in order to minimize the blood loss. If an occlusion occurs during embolization, then blood pressure should be augmented (with or without thrombolysis) to increase perfusion distally. Blood products should be readily available and adequate IV access obtained prior to any embolization.

2. If the AVM is amenable to surgical resection, then a craniotomy is performed in the operating room. Similar to other craniotomies, the anesthetic goals center on optimizing cerebral perfusion pressure (CPP) and oxygen delivery, which includes maintaining adequate mean arterial pressure. Avoiding large swings in blood pressure is the key to avoid any rupture of the AVM [1,2].

   a. Again, being prepared for a sudden loss of blood is essential. Multiple IV lines and an arterial line are helpful.

   b. Techniques to reduce cerebral edema such as moderate hyperventilation or osmotic diuresis may aid in providing an optimal surgical field.

   c. Titrating the anesthetic to a wake-up that avoids significant hypertension and allows the neurosurgeon to perform a complete neurologic examination shortly after surgery is ideal.

3. Currently, the treatment for AVMs involves embolization in IR prior to a surgical excision. The intent is that embolization will lower the high-flow circulation through the AVM, making the surgical resection less bloody. This also allows the tissue around the AVM to adjust gradually to the change in perfusion in that region.

4. Inhalational agents and IV agents have been used safely for the anesthetic for these lesions. Both decrease the cerebral metabolic rate of oxygen consumption (with the exception of ketamine). Inhalational agents can cause vasodilation whereas IV agents cause vasoconstriction. Theoretically, vasodilators may produce the steal phenomenon while the vasoconstrictors can lead to inverse steal and potentially protect the brain or prevent damage. There is no evidence favoring one or the other in terms of outcome for these patients. Likely, the most important thing is to maintain normotension and avoid large swings in blood pressure.

5. Since seizures are a common presenting symptom in these patients, they are often on anticonvulsant therapy. Therefore, the anesthesiologist needs to take into account the considerations previously mentioned regarding these drugs, in particular the need for increased doses of narcotics and muscle relaxants to maintain an adequate depth of anesthesia and muscle relaxation. Furthermore, the anticonvulsants should be continued in the perioperative period.

C. **Perioperative complications**

1. Hydrocephalus can result from subarachnoid blood and is initially managed with an external drain to lower CSF volume and to monitor ICP. Approximately one-third of all SAH patients will ultimately require ventricular shunt.

2. Rehemorrhage or stroke can occur from a faulty clip placement or a residual AVM. Residual lesions should be investigated with postoperative vascular imaging if possible and treated with evacuation of a clot if necessary and/or repositioning of the vascular clip.

CLINICAL PEARL   Normal perfusion pressure breakthrough (NPPB) can occur in a small number of patients with high-flow AVMs and results in postoperative parenchymal hemorrhage and cerebral edema from markedly increased blood flow in cerebral vessels (that were previously hypoperfused) after embolization or surgical resection of the AVM. NPPB should be anticipated after treatment of a high-flow lesion and can sometimes be avoided via staged embolizations prior to surgical resection and maintenance of normal to slightly low blood pressure postoperatively.

V. Vein of Galen malformation

    A. **A VOGM** is the result of an anomalous connection between the arteries of the posterior cerebral circulation and an enlarged vein of Galen in the deep cerebral circulation. The result of this type of direct connection is markedly increased cerebral venous pressure leading to elevated intracranial pressure and potential hemorrhage or venous stroke. Hydrocephalus, intracranial bleeding, and high-output CHF (often with pulmonary hypertension) may be presenting signs; hydrocephalus is the typical presenting sign in an infant because of the obstruction of venous drainage, in particular the aqueduct of Sylvius.

> **CLINICAL PEARL** In some VOGMs, there are such rapid flow rates that children can develop high-output CHF. The mortality with associated CHF is 40%; operative mortality with CHF approaches 100%. If left untreated, mortality is very high as well. In general, prognosis is very poor. If patients present in high-output cardiac failure, they may be on digoxin, lasix, inotropic drugs for hemodynamic support, or mechanical ventilation for respiratory support.

        1. Treatment consists of occlusion of the inflow (arterial) feeders followed by embolization of the venous side; this may be accomplished by IR, vascular microsurgical techniques, or both, in staged procedures. Staging the procedure decreases the risk of postocclusion hypertension and cerebral hyperemia. Typically, access is obtained through the femoral vein. The endpoint of treatment is not complete occlusion of the fistula, but is related to improvement in cardiac function.

        2. The open surgical approach typically involves access through a subtemporal, midline, or lateral occipital craniotomy. A burr hole at the confluence of venous sinuses may be used to approach the venous side of the malformation in a retrograde manner.

        3. Multidisciplinary efforts are now directed at IR procedures as the initial intervention, control of high-output CHF, and subsequent open craniotomy if required.

        4. Operative concerns are airway control, prone positioning, precautions for massive blood loss, and typical concerns for surgery on a newborn.

        5. Newborns with cardiac failure may be receiving several inotropic agents. It is possible to get some idea of the degree of cardiac compromise in newborns by obtaining a detailed feeding history—frequency, length of time, and amount per feeding, respiratory distress during feeding, etc.

        6. Postocclusion hypertension and cerebral hyperemia should be treated aggressively with antihypertensives such as vasodilators.

    B. **Anesthetic considerations**

        1. IV or inhalation induction can both be used, again the goal being to maintain normal hemodynamics during induction.

        2. If the child is in CHF, induction with an agent such as ketamine (which is typically avoided in neurosurgical procedures) or etomidate may be less of a myocardial depressant.

            a. Occasionally for an AVM, a hypotensive technique is requested. However, in the case of the patient with heart failure, a hypotensive technique should be avoided as an elevated blood pressure is necessary to maintain perfusion to the myocardium.

            b. If necessary, a central venous catheter or transesophageal echocardiogram can be used to assess for adequate cardiac filling pressures.

        3. Blood products should be available as significant blood loss can occur with the repair of a VOGM.

VI. Aneurysms

    A. **Intracranial aneurysms** are most often due to a congenital malformation in an arterial wall, but can be due to trauma, infection, or predisposing genetic disorders. Patients with coarctation of the aorta or polycystic kidney disease have an increased incidence of aneurysms, which usually remain asymptomatic during childhood. However, some aneurysms do rupture during childhood, and most of these are fatal. Symptoms of subarachnoid or intracerebral hemorrhage usually appear suddenly in a previously healthy young adult.

1. When technically feasible, surgical clipping or ligation is the treatment of choice. Similar to the AVM, the purpose is to eliminate the structural lesion from the cerebral circulation in order to prevent intracranial hemorrhage.

2. A patient's blood pressure is typically controlled prior to the procedure. If necessary, they may be on antihypertensives such as labetalol, nicardipine, or even sodium nipride. The use of nimodipine (typical in the adult patient) is controversial in children. Sometimes these patients are also on antiepileptic medications as well. If intracranial pressure is a concern, these patients may have an external ventricular drain placed to prevent hydrocephalus.

B. **Anesthetic considerations.** Aneurysm resection (similar to the AVM) involves the typical anesthetic concerns for a craniotomy with other specific considerations:

1. Deep preoperative sedation may be preferable to avoid sudden hypertensive episodes that can lead to aneurysmal rupture.

2. Blood products should be available in the operating room and checked before the start of the procedure. Blood-warming devices should be ready.

3. Ensuring adequate depth of anesthesia before any invasive maneuver such as endotracheal intubation or placement of head pins is essential to prevent precipitous hypertension.

4. Adequate large-bore peripheral venous access to deal with sudden and massive blood loss is crucial, but can usually be established after the induction of anesthesia.

CLINICAL PEARL Controlled hypotension for brief periods of time may be valuable in some situations to reduce shearing forces in the abnormal blood vessels and improves the safety of surgical manipulation. If needed, controlled hypotension may be induced with potent inhalation agents combined with vasodilators (nitroprusside or nitroglycerin). Intermediate-acting adrenergic antagonists, such as labetalol and esmolol, are also effective. Controlled hypotension should not, however, be used in the presence of elevated intracranial pressure because of the risk of decreasing CPP with resultant ischemia in the face of an elevated ICP. It is not clear whether or not controlled hypotension is worth the risks, particularly in small children. Although the absolute limits of acceptable hypotension are unknown, a mean BP >40 mm Hg (for infants) and 50 mm Hg (for older children) generally appears safe.

At the conclusion of the procedure and before closing the dura, the operative site should be inspected after the BP has been permitted to return to normal to ensure adequate hemostasis.

5. Hemodynamic stability is important during emergence. Excessive hypertension should be avoided to prevent postoperative bleeding. However, in most cases of aneurysm clipping, a slightly elevated BP may be desirable postoperatively to minimize the risk of vasospasm. BP control is also essential in the intensive care unit.

6. Prompt awakening after aneurysm clipping is particularly important to assess neurologic status. Postoperatively, after resection of an aneurysm, there can be the situation with serious consequences due to cerebral edema with increased ICP or hemorrhage. Just as in AVMs, NPPB is believed to be caused by hyperemia of the areas surrounding the previous aneurysm site where vessels suffer from continued vasomotor paralysis and cannot vasoconstrict. Treatment (although controversial) generally involves therapy for increased ICP (including diuretics, moderate hyperventilation, head elevation) with moderate hypotension but maintaining CPP, and moderate hypothermia.

C. **Postoperative complications**

1. Hydrocephalus can result from a subarachnoid bleed. This can be treated initially with an external drain to lower CSF volume and monitor the ICP. Approximately one-third of all SAH patients will ultimately require a ventricular shunt.

2. Vasospasm is extremely rare in children, but has been reported. It typically occurs 4 to 14 days postoperatively. It can be identified with transcranial Doppler (TCD) and angiography. Treatments include the calcium-channel blocker nimodipine (controversial in children), "triple-H" therapy (hydration, hemodilution, and hypertension), and angioplasty or intra-arterial vasodilators. Due to the rarity of this event in children and the lack of pediatric literature, these treatment modalities are extrapolated from evidence in the adult literature (see chapter 9).

3. Hyponatremia can result from either cerebral salt wasting resulting in hypovolemic hyponatremia (treated with IV replacement of isotonic fluids), or the syndrome of inappropriate antidiuretic hormone (SIADH) resulting in hypervolemic hyponatremia (treated with water restriction). Laboratory evidence to differentiate between the two is important as the treatment is very different between the two (see chapter 3).

4. Rehemorrhage or stroke can occur from faulty clip placement (very rare). This is treated with evacuation of a clot if necessary and/or repositioning of a clip.

VII. Moyamoya disease

A. **Moyamoya disease** is an anomaly that results in progressive stenosis and possible occlusion of intracranial vessels, primarily the internal carotid arteries (ICAs) (proximal anterior cerebral arteries and middle cerebral arteries) near the circle of Willis, resulting in stroke. Moyamoya disease is the idiopathic form of moyamoya while moyamoya syndrome is the arteriopathy found in association with other conditions.

1. An abnormal vascular network of collaterals develops in the cerebral cortex giving rise to the "puff of smoke" appearance during cerebral angiography.

   a. In the congenital form, the dysplastic process may involve other systemic arteries, especially the renal arteries.

   b. The acquired variety may be associated with a number of pathologies including meningitis, craniopharyngiomas, pituitary tumors, neurofibromatosis, chronic inflammation, connective tissue diseases, certain hematologic disorders (particularly sickle cell disease), Down syndrome, or prior intracranial radiation. For reasons that are unknown, this disease appears to be more common in children of Japanese ancestry. Moyamoya disease appears to have a bimodal age distribution with one peak in the first decade of life and the other in the fourth decade of life.

2. Moyamoya disease usually presents as TIAs progressing to strokes and fixed neurologic deficits in children. The attacks may be precipitated by hyperventilation. There is a high morbidity and mortality rate if left untreated.

3. Medical management consists of antiplatelet therapy such as aspirin. Calcium-channel blockers are also used as prophylactic agents.

4. Surgical management is often recommended for children who have experienced repeated or progressive attacks. The goal of surgery is to improve cerebral perfusion distal to the lesion in order to prevent cerebral infarction.

5. Techniques to bypass the stenosis of the ICA and the middle cerebral artery (MCA) have been employed with some success in selected patients.

6. Other techniques have been developed to take advantage of the ischemic brain's tendency to attempt to augment blood flow through the development of collateral vessels. This occurs when the chronically ischemic cortex has a source to develop such collateral blood flow from. This type of procedure, synangiosis, may involve procedures such as placement of a vascularized temporalis muscle flap or the superficial temporal artery (STA) directly onto the cortical surface.

7. The most common surgical operation for correction in the pediatric population is pial synangiosis, which involves suturing a scalp artery (usually the STA) onto the pial surface of the brain to enhance revascularization.

B. **Anesthetic considerations [3]**

1. Preoperatively, these patients should be neurologically stable prior to surgery and at least 1 month should have transpired after the last significant ischemic stroke. Patients should be medically optimized prior to surgery. They should be admitted the night before surgery and given IV prehydration.

2. Preoperative imaging is critical to planning vessel selection (the parietal branch of the STA may be small or absent, necessitating utilization of a frontal or retroauricular branch for the bypass). Preservation of spontaneous collateral vessels (as identified by the preoperative angiogram) from the external carotid system should be maintained during the craniotomy.

> **CLINICAL PEARL**   The anesthetic technique must minimize wide hemodynamic and respiratory swings in this patient population because preservation of CBF is of paramount concern. Hypotension should be avoided at all times to ensure adequate perfusion to brain tissue and prevent the occurrence of an intraoperative stroke.

3. Patients with moyamoya disease have reduced hemispheric blood flow in both hemispheres. Hyperventilation and resultant hypocapnia may further reduce regional blood flow and cause significant EEG and neurologic changes by causing cerebral vasoconstriction. Therefore, it is critical that normocapnia be maintained throughout the procedure and careful and continuous monitoring of end-tidal CO_2 tension is essential. In effect, this is one of the conditions in pediatric neuroanesthesia in which mild hyperventilation is inappropriate. Hyperventilation should be avoided at all times.

4. Adequate hydration and maintenance of baseline BP are therefore extremely important with the goal of maintaining CBF and CPP. Most of these patients are admitted to the hospital the night before surgery to have an IV catheter placed and then started on 1.5 times maintenance fluids to avoid dehydration during the perioperative period (as mentioned earlier).

5. There may be a benefit in EEG monitoring during these procedures to detect and potentially treat ischemia (manifested as either focal or global slowing) that appears to be a result of cerebral vasoconstriction in response to the direct surgical manipulation of the brain itself. The EEG technicians should communicate any changes in the EEG to the operative team. Appropriate changes can be made to the patient's blood pressure, partial pressure of carbon dioxide, and anesthetic agents to ensure an optimal EEG study without interference (see chapter 26).

6. Normothermia is maintained, particularly at the end of the procedure, to avoid postoperative shivering and the subsequent stress response.

7. A smooth extubation that avoids hypertension or crying is desirable. It appears that most complications (in particular strokes) occur postoperatively and are associated with dehydration and crying episodes (that leads to hyperventilation and hence cerebral ischemia).

8. Postoperative pain control is also essential because inadequate analgesia can lead to crying, hyperventilation, and ultimately cerebral ischemia and possibly death.

9. IV fluids should be continued at 1.5 times maintenance for at least 48 to 72 hours or until the patient is taking oral liquids. Frequent neurologic examinations should be performed to identify any signs of ischemia early.

REFERENCES

1. Millar C, Bissonnette B, Humphreys RP. Cerebral arteriovenous malformations in children. *Can J Anaesth.* 1994;41(4):321–331.
2. Sinha PK, Neema PK, Rathod RC. Anesthesia and intracranial arteriovenous malformation. *Neurol India.* 2004;52(2):163–170.
3. Soriano SG, Sethna NF, Scott RM. Anesthetic management of children with moyamoya syndrome. *Anesth Analg.* 1993; 77(5):1066–1070.

21

Sitting Position during Surgery

Antoun Koht and James P. Chandler

KEY POINTS

1. Blood pressure values are influenced by the location of the site of measurement and therefore the transducer position should be adjusted to the head level for better assessment of blood pressure at the head while CVP transducer should be at the heart level.
2. CVP catheter, used for monitoring of air embolism, is usually placed with the tip near the junction of the superior vena cava and the right atrium to optimize the ability to withdraw air and this position can be confirmed by x-ray, pressure transducer, or EKG tracing.
3. Air embolism is usually monitored by examining the changes in precordial Doppler ultrasound, decrease in end-tidal exhaled CO_2, and a rise in CVP, other monitors can be used.
4. Air embolism is more common in sitting position than in supine position; however, the morbidity is not greater.
5. High percentage of patients in sitting position will have pneumocephalus, which can last for days, and may influence some of the neurophysiologic monitoring parameters.
6. Excessive neck flexion in the sitting position can cause massive tongue swelling, quadriparesis/quadriplegia and therefore at least two finger width should be maintained between the chin and sternum.
7. Positioning the patient in sitting position may be associated with nerve and body injuries during table movements and should be closely observed.

I. Historical background

A. With advances in medicine and anesthesia in particular, the nineteenth century saw significant advances in surgery of the posterior fossa. Early surgeons found access to the posterior fossa via a sitting position to be particularly advantageous on the basis of the following:
   1. Providing relatively comfortable direct access to superficial and deep structures (Fig. 21.1).
   2. Maximum brain relaxation due to gravitational forces and optimal cerebrospinal fluid (CSF) drainage (Fig. 21.2).
   3. Decreased blood loss as a consequence of reduced venous congestion.
   4. Schede utilized this technique in 1905, however, Gardner in a 1935 publication credited de Martel of using this position in 1911 [1].

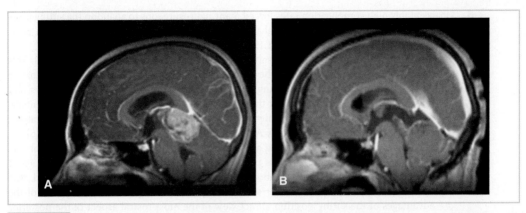

FIGURE 21.1 **A:** Sagittal MRI of the brain with gadolinium demonstrating large pineal region mass compressing the tectal plate and effacing the posterior third ventricle. **B:** Sagittal MRI following sitting position suboccipital craniotomy and tumor resection.

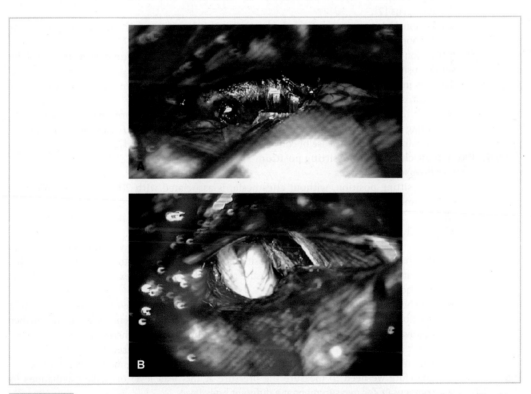

FIGURE 21.2 **A:** Intraoperative high magnification view of sitting position access to pineal region tumor. Note the relaxation of the cerebellar hemispheres and excellent access to the infratentorial and pineal region corridors. **B:** Postoperative view demonstrating complete tumor resection and exposure of the posterior third ventricle and dorsal brainstem.

B. Unacceptably high complication rates forced many neurosurgeons to abandon the sitting position approach, and gave birth to several alternative routes of access including the lateral position, first described by Lester Mount in 1945 [2], and the prone position [3].

    1. The lateral sitting position was described by Garcia-Bengochea in Cuba in 1956 [4]. This position utilized a modification of the sitting position. The patient is positioned such that he or she sits on the side of the operating room table, legs to the side supported by pillows, and one side of the body leaned against the OR table [4]. The lateral sitting position potentially allows the team to reposition the patient to the lateral position if unanticipated complications arise. This position was criticized by Albin for unfavorable cardiovascular alterations [5].

    2. A compromise between the sitting and the prone position is the concorde position [6]. In this arrangement, the patient is positioned prone with head of the bed up to about 45 degrees, the knees flexed to about 30 degrees and the neck maximally flexed. The operating surgeon stands to either side of the patient. This position offers some of the advantages of the sitting position, direct view of the most rostral aspect of the posterior fossa, significant brain relaxation, and reduced venous congestion relative to the prone position. The most significant disadvantage is the potentially long reach and angled access for the operating surgeon.

C. Utilization of the sitting position has been on the decline, both in Europe and USA [7,8].

    1. The decline is due to the complications associated with this position, such as venous air embolism (VAE), paradoxical air embolism, hypotension, and medical legal concerns [7].

    2. Personal observation suggests a slow return of the sitting position. This impression is supported by a recent publication from Helsinki by Lindroos [9].

D. In addition to neurosurgery, surgical advances in shoulder surgery have increased the use of the sitting position.

    1. This increase is due to frequent complications and injuries of the brachial plexus during arthroscopic shoulder surgery done in the lateral position.

    2. For this reason, many orthopedic surgeons have started to perform this operation in the sitting position, which provides less strain on the brachial plexus, excellent intra-articular visualization, and the ease of converting to open procedure [10,11,12].

II. Physiologic changes in the sitting position

A. Cardiovascular changes

    1. The sitting position, without anesthesia, is associated with 20% reduction in stroke volume and cardiac output; this may be compensated by rising vascular resistance from 50% to 80%. However, this compensatory mechanism may be blocked under anesthesia [13].

    2. Buhre et al. [14] found a 14% decrease in intrathoracic blood volume associated with the change from supine to sitting positions without changes in total blood volume. This indicates that the drop in blood pressure and stroke volume index is due to a decrease in preload.

    3. Cerebral perfusion pressure decreases by 15% in nonanesthetized patients in the sitting position. This decrease will be higher in an anesthetized patient, and can be further aggravated by jugular venous obstruction caused by unfavorable head and neck position.

    4. In the sitting position, blood pressure at the head level is decreased by gravity. For every 1 in. of height above the heart there is approximately 2 mm Hg drop in blood pressure. Therefore we need to measure the pressure at the head level or make calculations to compensate for measurement at a different body level.

    5. The reason for the relationship between height and blood pressure is the higher density of mercury, which is 13.54562 g/cm^3 at 20°C compared to that of water.

    6. If only noninvasive cuff pressure is used, then calculations to compensate for height differences should be used to avoid cerebral ischemia.

    7. The lack of such compensation may mask cerebral hypotension, leading to cerebral ischemia and postoperative neurologic deficits [13].

8. Improper position may lead to hypotension caused by blood pooling which is magnified during the use of potent anesthetic agents that promote vasodilation.

9. Hypotension in patients having surgery under general anesthesia in the sitting position requires treatment with vasopressors to maintain cerebral blood flow which can be maintained as long as mean blood pressure is kept above 70 mm Hg [15].

B. Respiratory changes

1. Spontaneous ventilation and changes in ventilatory patterns have been used to monitor brainstem function during surgery in the posterior fossa until it was replaced by cardiovascular parameters. However, recently there has been a report of using spontaneous ventilation to monitor surgery done in the sitting position [16].

2. Hyperventilation and low CO_2 are not recommended during surgery in the sitting position due to the relatively lower intracranial pressure (ICP) in the sitting position and possible cerebral ischemia caused by severe vasoconstriction.

C. Intracranial pressure

1. The sitting position is ideal for patients with increased ICP since it facilitates blood return to the heart and shifts CSF to the spinal canal.

2. Such decrease in ICP is enhanced by proper neck and head position which enhances venous drainage [13].

III. Placing the patient in sitting position

A. Preparation

1. Sitting position starts with the patient supine. After all lines are inserted and monitors applied, the patient will be moved to the sitting position.

2. Lines inserted include arterial line, multiorifice central line, intravenous lines, and urinary catheter.

3. The central line is inserted either via the central vessels or in the antecubital veins. The tip location of the multiorifice catheter is confirmed by x-ray, pressure transducer (obtain ventricular pressure tracings and pull back to the junction of the superior vena cava to the atrium), or by utilizing the EKG and connecting lead five to the special adaptor at the end of the catheter to locate the biphasic P-wave (Fig. 21.3).

4. Recording of the EKG from the central venous pressure (CVP) is facilitated by removing any air bubbles in the line and by filling the catheter with 7.5% sodium bicarbonate solution.

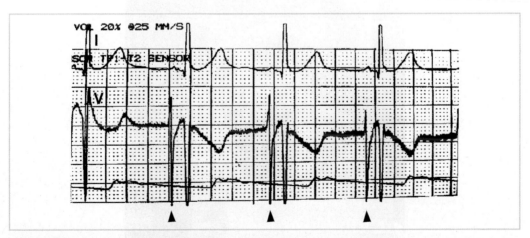

FIGURE 21.3 EKG, upper tracing is from lead I while lower tracing is from lead V which shows the biphasic P-wave. The biphasic P-wave is recorded from the metal adaptor located at the distal CVP line and reflecting signals at the tip of the multiorifice, saline-filled CVP line.

B. Positioning

1. The Mayfield head holder will be placed, the table sections will be adjusted by flexing the table in the middle toward 90 degrees and lowering the legs section at the knees by 30 degrees. The table head section is brought upward. During the previous movements, the table may be brought into Trendelenburg position to further help achieving the sitting position by allowing the head section more room to move. In this position, the knees will be at the level of the heart to minimize the drop in blood pressure.

2. Once the table is in position, the arch bar located toward the feet, which have the holding part, will be extended to connect securely with the Mayfield frame (Fig. 21.4). The arch bar can be placed on the same back section of the table where the patient's back is resting. This will eliminate accidental movement of the table which can put strain on the head. However, applying the normal-size arch bar at this location may be difficult and can generate pressure on the patient body trunk. The second location to place this bar is toward the end of the second section of the table where the patient is sitting.

3. Once the patient is in the sitting position, special attention is paid to the table movements. It is important to move the table as a unit and not to move sections of the table which can severely damage the cervical spine. Special attention is directed to the head–neck position to secure good blood drainage, assure free airway, and unkinked endotracheal tube. Attention, also, should be directed to the cross table bar, which holds the Mayfield frame, and to the straps to prevent pressure injuries which can be minimized by proper padding of the patient's body pressure points.

CLINICAL PEARL Once the patient is in the sitting position, special attention should be directed to table movements to prevent accidental neck movements.

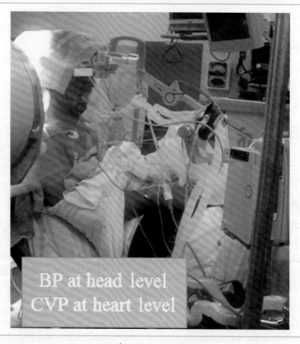

BP at head level
CVP at heart level

FIGURE 21.4 Patient in sitting position with BP transducer at head level, CVP transducer at heart level, arm comfortably on the abdomen.

CLINICAL PEARL   Position with two or more fingers' width from chin to sternum.

4. At the foot of the table, an upright padded foot section should be placed, to support the feet and prevent the patient from sliding down.
5. The arms can be placed across the abdomen, protected and secured before a Doppler ultrasound probe is placed on the chest and tested by injecting 5 mL of agitated saline into the central line.
6. The arterial-line transducer should be placed at the head level to measure the blood pressure at the head.

CLINICAL PEARL   Measure blood pressure at head level by A-line or adjust for the different heights.

7. The central-line transducer can be placed at heart level for accurate measurement of the CVP. The central line should be tested for blood aspiration, and a 20-mL syringe is placed in an easily accessed location to facilitate blood aspiration; if sizable air embolism is detected.

CLINICAL PEARL   Measure CVP at heart level.

8. During shoulder surgery, the head pins are not used and instead, the head is secured by straps and soft head holder.

IV. Clinical utility of the sitting position
  A. Utilization
  1. The sitting position is used for surgery in the posterior fossa, posterior cervical spine, and more recently, shoulder joint surgery [7,9,11]. Also, the sitting position may be used for neurosurgical operations during the later stage of pregnancy [17].
  2. Neurosurgeons who prefer to use this approach for pineal region tumors and other tumors and vascular pathology of the posterior fossa, cite the better exposure, the drop of the structure by gravity, the dry field, and the low ICP.
  3. Neurosurgeons find the position particularly useful for posterior cervical decompressions and discectomies and suboccipital and foramen magnum decompressive procedures.
  4. In addition, orthopedic surgeons are using the sitting position for shoulder surgeries.
  5. In more recent years, the sitting position has also been used for selective peripheral denervation for spasmodic torticollis [18].

  B. Contraindications. The contraindications for sitting position include patients with right to left cardiac shunt, severe spinal canal stenosis, severe hypotension or hypertension, and severe atherosclerotic vascular diseases.

  C. Advantages
  1. In most instances, the sitting position provides reasonable access to the apex of the posterior fossa, facilitates blood and CSF drainage, decreases intracranial pressure [7], and decreases blood loss.
  2. These features enable the sitting position to have the following advantages over traditional approaches: 1) Fewer blood transfusions, faster surgery [19]; 2) unhindered diaphragm movements and better ventilation which is used to monitor the brainstem; 3) more direct surgical access; 4) no position-related ocular pressure and blindness; 5) more optimal anatomical orientation particularly when accessing the midline lesions; 6) a more physiologic neck torsion which potentially facilitates access to the cerebellopontine angle region; and 7) significant reduction of cerebellar retraction during the surgical approach to the pineal region [7,9,19].

3. Advantages to the anesthesiologists include easy access to the airway, better ventilation, less problems with obstruction of the urinary catheter, easy access to the arms, and easy cardiovascular resuscitation in case of emergency [8].

4. The sitting position enables the visualization of the patient's face to monitor movements related to cranial nerve manipulation [5]. (Albeit, now this can be better tested with neurophysiologic monitoring utilizing free and triggered EMG.)

5. In a retrospective study, in children, complications in the sitting position were not more in the prone position and the postoperative course appears to have fewer complications [20]. These findings and other advantages of the sitting position have prompted some centers to utilize the sitting position more frequently [8].

D. **Disadvantages**

1. Cardiovascular alteration, air embolism, cervical cord ischemia, quadriplegia, macroglossia, pneumocephalus, and peripheral nerve compressions are among the many complications associated with the sitting position.

2. The lack of experience among young neurosurgeons and anesthesiologists has inhibited the use of this position.

3. Hypotension can occur in sitting position, but may be ameliorated by fluid infusion, proper position of the legs, and treated with vasopressor medications.

4. In sitting position, the drop in blood pressure and disturbed autoregulation may lead to cerebral and spinal cord ischemia and increased incidence of thromboembolic events [13].

5. Under anesthetic agents, that disturb autoregulation, blood pressure should be supported, and other measures such as good sitting position and sequential compression devices can be used to maintain blood pressure and enhance cerebral oxygenation as measured by the NIRS [21].

6. In addition to length of surgery and comorbidities, sitting position is still among the top three causes of complications during surgery [22].

V. **Complications in the sitting position**

A. **Air embolism** (for in-depth information please refer Chapter 22)

1. Air embolism occurs when the surgical site is above the heart level. It can be monitored and detected by transesophageal echocardiography (TEE) (threshold of detection approximately 0.02 mL/kg), Precordial Doppler (0.05 mL/kg when given as a bolus injection) [23], pulmonary artery pressure (PAP), end-expiratory carbon dioxide ($EECO_2$) (0.25 mL/kg), end-expiratory nitrogen (EEN_2) (0.5 mL/kg), esophageal stethoscope (1.5 mL/kg), and EKG (1.25 mL/kg) [24,25].

2. Few studies found that nitrous oxide (N_2O) will not enhance Doppler or TEE detection of VAE, but it does enhance the detection by $EECO_2$ and pulmonary pressures.

3. The lethal dose of air embolism is decreased by a factor of 3.4 in the presence of N_2O, and thus it is recommended not to use N_2O if air embolism is a possibility [26]. The air bubble size will increase due to the difference in blood solubility (34-fold) between nitrous oxide and nitrogen. This phenomenon is the reason for increase in CSF pressure associated with intrathecal air injection and during middle ear surgery.

4. Air embolism is more common in the sitting position than in the supine position, however the morbidity is not greater [27].

5. The most sensitive method for detecting air embolism, although not commonly used, is intracardiac echocardiography. This technique is more sensitive than both TEE and precordial Doppler, and can help guide repositioning of the multiorifice catheter to facilitate the aspiration of midsize to large amount of VAE [28].

CLINICAL PEARL   The most sensitive method for detecting air embolism is TEE, but the most clinically used method is the precordial Doppler.

6. The most clinically used monitor is precordial Doppler. The $EECO_2$, CVP, PAP, and airway pressure are all good monitors that detect larger amount of air which can be clinically significant.

CLINICAL PEARL Alert the surgeon to small air embolism to avoid the larger ones.

7. Early reports cited high percentage of air aspiration; however, more recently, some centers have discontinued the routine use of a central line on the basis of low yield with attempted air aspiration [9]. Although we do place central lines for monitoring, teaching, and possible aspiration, successful aspiration has rarely been productive. This may be due to early detection by Doppler and surgical interventions which may have prevented a larger amount of air aspiration.

8. Recently, there was a report of the association of air embolism encountered during posterior fossa surgery with platelet dysfunction. This suggests platelet function testing may be appropriate if a significant air embolism is encountered [29].

9. In a human study, Pandia et al. [30] found that VAE detected with TEE, and not with EECO$_2$, was not associated with changes in either tachycardia or hypotension. However, changes in both monitors were associated with 20% tachycardia and 30% hypotension.

10. The incidence of air embolism and hypotension are equal in children and adults [31].

B. **Pneumocephalus.** This is a common complication found, but not limited to patients who undergo surgery in the sitting position; the incidence of minor nonsymptomatic pneumocephalus is as high as 100%, while symptomatic cases are much less common and tension pneumocephalus can occur.

1. In a recent study and review, Sloan [32] found pneumocephalus to occur at 42.1%. The size as recorded on CT scan, ranged from 6 to 260 cc when measured within 4 hours of surgery. They used somatosensory evoked potential (SSEP) as an identifier of the onset of pneumocephalus.

2. Clinically, significant pneumocephalus may create mass effect and can be associated with headache, lethargy, confusion, hemiparesis, and seizures.

3. Changes of SSEPs, as a consequence of pneumocephalus, were reported by Watanabe et al. [33] in 1989 and are due to air accumulation between the brain and the recording sites which decrease the SSEP amplitude.

4. The use of N$_2$O in subsequent craniotomies is not clear. The calculation by Sloan [32] for the possible dissipation of the 280-mL air to less than 0.5 cc would have been 13 days.

C. **Macroglossia.** This complication was reported in adults and may be related to extreme neck flexion and the use of a hard large airway during prolonged operations. Such position, which interferes with blood flow and venous drainage of the tongue, may be minimized by the use of soft bite block, observing tongue, and proper head and neck position [34]. Macroglossia may lead to airway compromise after tracheal extubation at the end of surgery.

D. **Airway obstruction.** This may be related to excessive neck flexion, kinking of the endotracheal tube, oral edema, macroglossia, and by foreign bodies such as TEE and large airway devices [35].

E. **Quadriplegia.** Such complication is a serious, but rare, complication that can occur in the sitting position. The reason for this complication is thought to be blood flow disturbance to the spinal cord due to stretching of the spinal cord during flexion of the head [36].

F. **Peripheral nerve injury.** The sitting position may be associated with multiple nerve injuries, all of which can be avoided with extra padding and attention to the pressure points. Nerves susceptible to injury include sciatic, peroneal, and brachial plexus.

VI. **Anesthetic management.** Anesthetic management in the sitting position requires the basic knowledge of the physiologic changes due to anesthesia drugs (see Chapter 1) and due to the sitting position.

A. The anesthetic management should include preparations to deal with all potential complications [37], while optimizing anesthesia to accommodate the sitting position and the use of neurophysiologic monitoring.

B. Neurophysiologic monitoring may include SSEPs, transcranial motor evoked potentials (MEPs), and auditory brainstem evoked responses (ABRs), in addition to cranial nerve EMG monitoring (see Chapter 26).

    C. ABR can be conducted with almost all anesthetic regimens while SSEP can tolerate muscle relaxants, but have a dose-dependent depression from inhalation agents. MEP is affected by both inhalation agents (more than 0.5 MAC) and muscle relaxants, while cranial nerve monitors are affected only by muscle relaxants [38].

VII. **Conclusion.** Safe anesthesia in the sitting position is possible and requires the anesthesiologist to understand this position, the physiologic changes associated with it, in addition to the different monitoring modalities needed during surgery. Such knowledge is important for the safe anesthesia and this is especially important with the renewed interest in this position [39]. Anesthesiologists and surgeons both should get familiar with the mechanics of the sitting position and the associated physiologic changes, so that they may gain all the benefits of sitting position with minimal complications.

REFERENCES

1. Gardner WJ. Intracranial operations in the sitting position. *Ann Surg.* 1935;101(1):138–145.
2. Mount LA. The lateral position for operations in the cerebellopontine angle. *J Neurosurg.* 1945;2(5):460–461.
3. Anderton JM. The prone position for the surgical patient: a historical review of the principles and hazards. *Br J Anaesth.* 1991;67(4):452–463.
4. Bengochea FG, Fernandez JC. The lateral sitting position for operations in the posterior fossa and in the cervical and upper thoracic regions of the spine. *J Neurosurg.* 1956;13(5):520–522.
5. Albins MS, Chang J, Tung AS, et al. Anesthesia for the sitting position. *Anesth Analg.* 1977;56(2):325–326.
6. Kobayashi S, Sugita K, Tanaka Y, et al. Infratentorial approach to the pineal region in the prone position: Concorde position. Technical note. *J Neurosurg.* 1983;58(1):141–143.
7. Porter JM, Pidgeon C, Cunningham AJ. The sitting position in neurosurgery: a critical appraisal. *Br J Anaesth.* 1999;82(1):117–128.
8. Gale T, Leslie K. Anaesthesia for neurosurgery in the sitting position. *J Clin Neurosci.* 2004;11(7):693–696.
9. Lindroos AC, Niiya T, Randell T, et al. Sitting position for removal of pineal region lesions: the Helsinki experience. *World Neurosurg.* 2010;74(4–5):505–513.
10. Papadonikolakis A, Wiesler ER, Olympio MA, et al. Avoiding catastrophic complications of stroke and death related to shoulder surgery in the sitting position. *Arthroscopy.* 2008;24(4):481–482.
11. Peruto CM, Ciccotti MG, Cohen SB. Shoulder arthroscopy positioning: lateral decubitus versus beach chair. *Arthroscopy.* 2009;25(8):891–896.
12. Dippmann C, Winge S, Nielsen HB. Severe cerebral desaturation during shoulder arthroscopy in the beach-chair position. *Arthroscopy.* 2010;26(9 suppl):S148–S150.
13. Pohl A, Cullen DJ. Cerebral ischemia during shoulder surgery in the upright position: a case series. *J Clin Anesth.* 2005;17(6):463–469.
14. Buhre W, Weyland A, Buhre K, et al. Effects of the sitting position on the distribution of blood volume in patients undergoing neurosurgical procedures. *Br J Anaesth.* 2000;84(3):354–357.
15. Soeding PF, Wang J, Hoy G, et al. The effect of the sitting upright or 'beachchair' position on cerebral blood flow during anaesthesia for shoulder surgery. *Anaesth Intensive Care.* 2011;39(3):440–448.
16. Pandia MP, Bithal PK, Sharma MS, et al. Use of spontaneous ventilation to monitor the effects of posterior fossa surgery in the sitting position. *J Clin Neurosci.* 2009;16(7):968–969.
17. Giannini A, Bricchi M. Posterior fossa surgery in the sitting position in a pregnant patient with cerebellopontine angle meningioma. *Br J Anaesth.* 1999;82(6):941–944.
18. Girard F, Ruel M, McKenty S, et al. Incidences of venous air embolism and patent foramen ovale among patients undergoing selective peripheral denervation in the sitting position. *Neurosurgery.* 2003;53(2):316–319; discussion 319–320.
19. Black S, Ockert DB, Oliver WC Jr, et al. Outcome following posterior fossa craniectomy in patients in the sitting or horizontal positions. *Anesthesiology.* 1988;69(1):49–56.
20. Orliaguet GA, Hanafi M, Meyer PG, et al. Is the sitting or the prone position best for surgery for posterior fossa tumours in children? *Paediatr Anaesth.* 2001;11(5):541–547.
21. Kwak HJ, Lee D, Lee YW, et al. The intermittent sequential compression device on the lower extremities attenuates the decrease in regional cerebral oxygen saturation during sitting position under sevoflurane anesthesia. *J Neurosurg Anesthesiol.* 2011;23(1):1–5.
22. Aleksic V, Radulovic D, Milakovic B, et al. A retrospective analysis of anesthesiologic complications in pediatric neurosurgery. *Paediatr Anaesth.* 2009;19(9):879–886.
23. Furuya H, Suzuki T, Okumura F, et al. Detection of air embolism by transesophageal echocardiography. *Anesthesiology.* 1983;58(2):124–129.
24. Mirski MA, Lele AV, Fitzsimmons L, et al. Diagnosis and treatment of vascular air embolism. *Anesthesiology.* 2007;106(1):164–177.
25. Chang JL, Albin MS, Bunegin L, et al. Analysis and comparison of venous air embolism detection methods. *Neurosurgery.* 1980;7(2):135–141.
26. Losasso TJ, Black S, Muzzi DA, et al. Detection and hemodynamic consequences of venous air embolism. Does nitrous oxide make a difference? *Anesthesiology.* 1992;77(1):148–152.

27. Duke DA, Lynch JJ, Harner SG, et al. Venous air embolism in sitting and supine patients undergoing vestibular schwannoma resection. *Neurosurgery.* 1998;42(6):1282–1286; discussion 1286–1287.

28. Schafer ST, Lindemann J, Brendt P, et al. Intracardiac transvenous echocardiography is superior to both precordial Doppler and transesophageal echocardiography techniques for detecting venous air embolism and catheter-guided air aspiration. *Anesth Analg.* 2008;106(1):45–54, table of contents.

29. Schafer ST, Sandalcioglu IE, Stegen B, et al. Venous air embolism during semi-sitting craniotomy evokes thrombocytopenia. *Anaesthesia.* 2011;66(1):25–30.

30. Pandia MP, Bithal PK, Dash HH, et al. Comparative incidence of cardiovascular changes during venous air embolism as detected by transesophageal echocardiography alone or in combination with end tidal carbon dioxide tension monitoring. *J Clin Neurosci.* 2011;18(9):1206–1209.

31. Bithal PK, Pandia MP, Dash HH, et al. Comparative incidence of venous air embolism and associated hypotension in adults and children operated for neurosurgery in the sitting position. *Eur J Anaesthesiol.* 2004;21(7):517–522.

32. Sloan T. The incidence, volume, absorption, and timing of supratentorial pneumocephalus during posterior fossa neurosurgery conducted in the sitting position. *J Neurosurg Anesthesiol.* 2010;22(1):59–66.

33. Watanabe E, Schramm J, Schneider W. Effect of a subdural air collection on the sensory evoked potential during surgery in the sitting position. *Electroencephalogr Clin Neurophysiol.* 1989;74(3):194–201.

34. McAllister RG. Macroglossia–a positional complication. *Anesthesiology.* 1974;40(2):199–200.

35. Pandia MP, Bithal PK, Bhagat H, et al. Airway obstruction after extubation following use of transesophageal echocardiography for posterior fossa surgery in the sitting position. *J Clin Neurosci.* 2007;14(11):1139–1141.

36. Morandi X, Riffaud L, Amlashi SF, et al. Extensive spinal cord infarction after posterior fossa surgery in the sitting position: case report. *Neurosurgery.* 2004;54(6):1512–1515; discussion 1515–1516.

37. Jadik S, Wissing H, Friedrich K, et al. A standardized protocol for the prevention of clinically relevant venous air embolism during neurosurgical interventions in the semisitting position. *Neurosurgery.* 2009;64(3):533–538; discussion 538–539.

38. Sloan TB. General anesthesia for monitoring. In: Koht A, Sloan TB, Toleikis JR, eds. *Monitoring the Nervous System for Anesthesiologists and Other Health Care Professionals.* New York, NY: Springer; 2012:319–335.

39. Albin MS. Venous air embolism: a warning not to be complacent–we should listen to the drumbeat of history. *Anesthesiology.* 2011;115(3):626–629.

22

Air Embolism

Steven B. Edelstein

KEY POINTS

1. The position of the patient and the speed and dose of air entrainment are key determinants of the development of clinically significant consequences from venous air embolism (VAE).
2. Precordial Doppler has been determined to be the most sensitive noninvasive monitor for VAE detection.
3. Aspiration of air via multiorifice catheters has limited success.
4. Utilization of nitrous oxide in patients at high risk for VAE continues to be controversial.
5. Maintenance of right coronary perfusion pressure is key to the prevention of right heart failure due to VAE.

I. Definition

A. As the name would denote, venous air embolisms (VAEs) are embolic structures composed primarily of entrained air that enters into the venous system of a patient. The resulting emboli will lead to the central circulation and ultimately to a variety of highly vascular organs, predominately the lungs. Air entrainment occurs when there is a pressure gradient between the venous opening and the level of the heart, leading to a sump-like effect.

B. Pathophysiology. One of the most devastating consequences of air embolism is cardiovascular collapse. Multiple mechanisms are at work for this event to occur. These include an air lock obstruction to pulmonary blood flow, and intense pulmonary vasoconstriction leading to a rapid increase in right ventricular afterload, increase in right ventricular oxygen consumption, and ultimately failure.

C. Clinical symptoms. Multiple symptoms are noted with significant VAE. These include diffuse pulmonary wheezes, cyanosis, hypotension, arrhythmias, a mill wheel murmur, and cardiac arrest [1].

TABLE 22.1 Risk factors and procedures at risk for venous air embolism		
Elevated position (wound higher than heart), e.g., lumbar laminectomy, cervical laminectomy, posterior fossa cranial surgery in sitting position	Numerous noncompressed venous channels	Gravitational threat (thoracotomy, urologic procedures in Trendelenburg)
Laparoscopic surgery	Cesarean section (during uterine repair/exteriorization)	Vascular access procedures (central-line insertion or removal)
Epidural catheter insertion with loss of air technique	Intra-aortic balloon pump	Kyphoplasty/vertebroplasty
Pressurized fluid delivery systems	Red cell transfusions (fluid warmers without air trapping or dysfunctional air trapping devices)	Others: Radical neck dissections, upright shoulder surgery, hypophysectomy

Adapted from: Mirski MA, Lele AV, Fitzsimmons L, et al. Diagnosis and treatment of vascular air embolism. *Anesthesiology.* 2007;106(1):164–177.

II. Potential risk factors

A. There are multiple factors that play a role in the development of VAE. A list of these factors may be found in Table 22.1, described in an extensive review by Mirski et al. [2], but the table is by no means inclusive. *The major risk factor associated with VAE is the final position of the patient,* with an elevated position of wound higher than the heart being the position most at risk.

B. *Sitting or semi-sitting craniotomy is the classic procedure associated with VAE.* This is the result of having not only an elevated position of surgery, but also due to the fact that there are noncompressible structures such as dural sinuses that may enhance air entrainment. Jadik et al. [3], have described three potential pressure situations which may affect the likelihood of development of VAE during semi-sitting craniotomy:

   1. Low risk. Pressure proximal and distal to the injured vessel is under constant pressure and bleeding site is relatively easy to find.

   2. Intermediate risk. Pressure is constantly negative, bleeding of injured vessel and source of entrainment are absent or difficult to find (moderate jugular compression may assist in identification).

   3. High risk. Positive pressure in the injured sinus of vein during the inspiration of mechanical ventilation and negative pressure during expiration leads to large entrainment.

C. During particular procedures such as kyphoplasty/vertebroplasty, the prolonged uncapping of the needle can lead to entrainment which is similarly seen in central-line insertions [4]. It is important to note that *the standard prone position of the procedure results in a position higher than the heart,* and may lead to venous pooling and a decrease in venous pressure within vertebral elements. This may ultimately increase the risk of air entrainment.

D. There are some smaller risk procedures such as cesarean section, hypophysectomy, and upright shoulder surgery, which have reportedly been associated with VAE [5].

CLINICAL PEARL The major risk factor associated with VAE is the position of the surgical/procedural site in relation to the heart. Though the sitting or semi-sitting craniotomy is the classic procedure associated with VAE, a VAE can occur in any procedure where venous disruption is above the level of the heart.

III. Incidence

A. The *overall incidence of VAE is unclear as a result of a variety of detection techniques that* make the observation of emboli relatively easy. These specific techniques will be discussed later in this chapter, but clinically significant VAE events appear to be a relatively rare event.

TABLE 22.2   Four grades of intensity of venous air embolus (VAE)

Grade I	Characteristic changes in Doppler sounds
Grade II	Changes in the Doppler sound, fall of $EtCO_2 > 0.4\%$
Grade III	Changes in Doppler sounds, fall of $EtCO_2$ concentration, plus aspiration of air through the atrial catheter
Grade IV	Combination of above signs with arterial hypotension over 20% and/or arrhythmia or other pathologic ECG changes

$EtCO_2$, end-tidal carbon dioxide.
Adapted from: Matjasko J, Petrozza P, Cohen M, et al. Anesthesia and surgery in the seated position: Analysis of 554 cases. *Neurosurgery*. 1985;17:695–702.

B. O'Quin and Lakshminarayan [6] reported an observed rate for VAE in the operative setting to be approximately 21% to 40% in sitting neurosurgical or otolaryngologic procedures (namely, neck dissections) with a subsequent study revealing an overall incidence of 25% to 60% in procedures where the surgical site was higher than the level of the heart [7]. A recent investigation by Jadik et al. [3] revealed a rate of 50% in semi-sitting position craniotomies.

C. Syymons et al. [8] also reported a rate which was more widespread, from a low of 1.6% to a high of 93% with subsequent mortality rates of 0% to 73%.

D. It appears that the *sensitivity of the detection device is the key feature in identifying the presence or absence of venous air.*

CLINICAL PEARL   The overall incidence of VAE is unclear as the sensitivity of the detection device is the key feature in identifying the presence or absence of venous air. While clinically significant VAEs are rare, they can be associated with significant hemodynamic changes and potential morbidity.

IV. **Grading scale**

A. There are numerous ways in which VAEs are classified, but most are a variation of one another, many based on the initial work of Matjasko et al. [9], whose team described four major grades based on changes in precordial Doppler sounds, changes in end-tidal carbon dioxide ($EtCO_2$), ability to aspirate air, and hemodynamic instability (Table 22.2). Perhaps the most extensive description scale comes from Girard et al. [10] that incorporates detection devices such as precordial Doppler, $EtCO_2$, and blood pressure measurements (Table 22.3).

B. The utilization of transesophageal echocardiography (TEE) has also increased the degree of identification of venous air, thus increasing the reported incidence rate. However, clinically significant VAE remains low [11] (Table 22.4).

V. **Dose required for significant events**

A. It is important to note that *there is a dose requirement associated with VAE to create a hemodynamically significant event.* Determination of this number has been under constant investigation

TABLE 22.3   Girard scale for venous air embolism

Grade I	Positive precordial Doppler signal without hemodynamic alterations
Grade II	Positive precordial Doppler signal, increase in systolic pulmonary artery pressure (PAP) >5 mm Hg, and/or decrease of end-tidal CO_2 ($EtCO_2$) ≥3 mm Hg
Grade III	Arterial blood pressure decreases >20% or >20% increase in heart rate, plus one positive Grade II criteria
Grade IV	Arterial blood pressure decreases >40% or >40% increase in heart rate, plus one positive Grade II criteria
Grade V	Cardiocirculatory collapse in the presence of one positive Grade II criteria

Adapted from: Girard F, Ruel M, McKenty S, et al. Incidences of venous air embolism and patent foramen ovale among patients undergoing selective peripheral denervation in the sitting position. *Neurosurgery*. 2003;53:316–319.

TABLE 22.4   Scale for venous air embolism utilizing TEE

Grade I	Single gas bubble in right atrium (RA), right ventricle (RV), and right ventricular outflow tract (RVOT)
Grade II	Gas bubbles filling < half the diameter of RA, RV, and RVOT
Grade III	Gas bubbles filling > half the diameter of RA, RV, and RVOT
Grade IV	Gas bubbles completely filling the diameter of the RA, RV, and RVOT

Adapted from: Schmandra TC, Mierdl S, Bauer H, et al. Transesophageal echocardiography shows high risk of gas embolism during laparoscopic hepatic resection under carbon dioxide pneumoperitoneum. *Br J Surg*. 2002;89:870–876.

with many initial studies utilizing dog or swine models to determine lethal doses (LDs). Early investigations revealed that the LDs associated with air was 40 to 50 mL in a small dog and 100 to 200 mL in a larger animal. Early determinations noted that the LD amount required was 7.5 mL/kg with a human range of 200 to 300 mL [12], while others determined the mean cumulative dose for VAE associated with circulatory collapse in the swine model was 4.5 mL/kg [13].

B. One of the very few human case reports has come from Toung et al. [12], whose team described a patient with a history of heart failure who underwent pneumopericardiography in which 200 mL of air was injected over 3 to 5 seconds. This led to restlessness, apnea, ST depression on electrocardiography (ECG), and a varying degree of atrioventricular (AV) block. Overall, *the consensus is that the adult lethal dose is approximately 200 to 300 mL or 3 to 5 mL/kg.*

C. It is also important to note that it is not just the volume involved, but also the *speed of injection that plays a vital role.* It has been mentioned that the LD of 200 to 300 mL in humans can be exceeded if the air is entrained slowly, allowing for hemodynamic compensation [8,14].

D. The more rapid speed of injection of air results in a lower dose of air required for a lethal event. A bolus of air tends to lead to an increase in central venous pressure (CVP), a decrease in pulmonary artery pressure (PAP), ST segment depression, and shock that is thought to be related to an air lock in the right ventricle. On the contrary, a slow infusion of air results in an increase in CVP/PAP and with a decrease in systemic vascular resistance (SVR) with a compensatory increase in cardiac output [15].

E. As the *volume of entrainment increases, a variety of clinical effects can be seen.* These effects vary from changes in oxygen saturation, decrease in EtCO$_2$, electrocardiographic effects, and cardiovascular collapse (Table 22.5).

CLINICAL PEARL   The volume associated with VAE to create a hemodynamically significant event is related to both the volume and rate of air entrainment. However, the threshold of a lethal adult dose is in the range of 200 to 300 mL or 3 to 5 mL/kg.

VI. **Complications associated with VAE**
A. **Hypoxia/sympathetic reflex vasoconstriction.** The development of hypoxia and increase in pulmonary vascular resistance (PVR) are some of the key complications associated with

TABLE 22.5   Entrainment dose of air embolism and clinical effects

Small < 0.5 mL/kg	Decreased EtCO$_2$, increased EtN$_2$, oxygen desaturation, altered mental status, wheezing
Medium 0.5–2 mL/kg	Breathlessness, wheezing, hypotension, right heart strain, electrocardiographic evidence (ST-segment changes and peaked P-waves), pulmonary hypertension, pulmonary vasoconstriction, jugular venous distension, myocardial ischemia, bronchoconstriction, cerebral ischemia, and altered mental status
Large > 2 mL/kg	Chest pain, right heart failure, cardiovascular collapse

EtCO$_2$, end-tidal carbon dioxide; EtN$_2$, end-tidal nitrogen.
Adapted from: Mirski MA, Lele AV, Fitzsimmons L, et al. Diagnosis and treatment of vascular air embolism. *Anesthesiology*. 2007;106(1):164–177.

TABLE 22.6 Complications associated with VAE

Sympathetic reflex vasoconstriction
Hypoxia due to increase in physiologic dead space
Release of endothelial/humoral mediators
Air lock
Right ventricular failure
Thrombocytopenia
Cerebral ischemia/embolization

VAE. Essentially, the *air embolus lodges into the pulmonary vasculature and results in a rapid increase in sympathetic reflex vasoconstriction* leading to ventilation–perfusion abnormalities with increase in the physiologic dead space. These events result in decreased EtCO$_2$, increased partial pressure of carbon dioxide (PaCO$_2$), and hypoxemia [16,17].

B. Role of microbubbles and humoral/neurogenic factors. A significant number of effects of VAE are a result of the interaction of microvascular air bubbles with elements within the circulation and are known to *activate the release of endothelial mediators* that result in an excessive complement production, cytokine release, and production of reactive oxygen species (ROS) [18]. Microbubbles also lead to an obstruction of blood flow with an increase in PAP as well as a resultant trigger in platelet and neutrophil activation. The neutrophils can also release superoxide anions leading to pulmonary microvascular damage [16].

    1. Humoral mediators. A thorough review of the subject has revealed that multiple mediators play a role in the induction of damage associated with the VAE. These include serotonin (which results in intense vasoconstrictor of pulmonary vasculature), adenosine diphosphate (ADP), thrombin, catecholamines, leukotrienes, bacterial toxins, cytokines, ROS, angiotension II (AT-II), endothelin-1 (ET-1), platelet-derived growth factor (PDGF), platelet activating factor (PAF) [19]. Ultimately these mediators also lead to a reduction in lung compliance due to increased permeability, interstitial edema, and airway resistance.

    2. Neurogenic mediators. It is also known that embolism will trigger a *serotonin-induced von Bezold–Jarisch reflex* possibly via J-receptors, pulmonary irritant receptors, and pulmonary c-fibers. This stimulation results in the apnea, bradycardia, and hypotension routinely seen with massive embolism [19].

C. Right ventricle failure/air lock. In the case of massive VAE the generation of an air lock may occur. This air lock is essentially a complete outflow obstruction leading to no forward blood flow, increased wall tension in the right ventricle (RV), increased myocardial oxygen consumption of the RV, RV ischemia, and ultimately cardiovascular collapse. More modest volumes may still result in significant right ventricular outflow obstruction [2] that can also trigger the humoral agents' release of inflammatory mediators, bronchoconstriction, increase in ventilation/perfusion mismatch, and reflex vasoconstriction previously mentioned [20].

D. Thrombocytopenia

    1. The mechanism for VAE-induced thrombocytopenia is unknown, but may be related to the direct binding and activation of platelets when they encounter microbubbles. This activation will lead to a *formation of air–platelet conglomerates* that ultimately liberate more mediators leading to further platelet aggregation [21]. It has been suggested that the formation of platelet–air conglomerates adversely affects air reabsorption, and may lead to a prolonged increase in right ventricular afterload and aggravation of the cardiopulmonary complications associated with VAE [22].

    2. Platelet activation results in the release of humoral factors (both procoagulant and vasoconstrictor in nature) that contribute to the pathophysiology of VAE. The release of thromboxane-A2 leads to pulmonary vasoconstriction and a proaggregatory effect on platelets that results in even further release of thromboxane-A2, as well as serotonin, a substance that also has pulmonary vasoconstrictive properties [19,23].

E. **Cerebral air (cerebral edema and capillary leak as well as ischemia).** Another catastrophic complication associated with VAE is the entrainment of venous air into the arterial circulation with a resultant embolic event, notably cerebral in nature [24]. Notably, this situation occurs when air transverses a patent foramen ovale (PFO) which is a defect that can be found in approximately 25% of the adult population [25]. Cerebral air embolism *results in local ischemia and cerebral edema that results in a capillary leak syndrome induced by the ischemic event.* Manipulation of central venous catheters, utilization of extracorporeal circulation, arteriography, and hemodialysis are the procedures most at risk. Though there is no conclusive consensus regarding patients with pre-existing PFOs and subsequent neurosurgical procedures, an extensive review by Fathi et al. [26] suggests that screening for the presence of PFO may be warranted. The presence of the structural anomaly would potentially alter the neurosurgical approach to the procedure (i.e., changing from sitting to horizontal) or allow for a surgical repair of the defect prior to the definitive procedure.

CLINICAL PEARL   There are numerous physiologic responses associated with a VAE. An air embolus lodges into the pulmonary vasculature and results in a rapid increase in sympathetic reflex vasoconstriction leading to ventilation–perfusion abnormalities. If a larger air embolus occurs, an air lock in the right ventricle can cause a complete outflow obstruction leading to cardiovascular collapse.

VII. Detection. In order to prevent and treat VAE, it is important to recognize the event. As such, a multitude of techniques for detection have been proposed. A summary of these techniques along with their sensitivity and limitations can be seen in Table 22.7. Some of these techniques include *echocardiography, precordial Doppler, changes in PAP/CVP, EtCO$_2$ tension, or end-tidal nitrogen.* Echocardiography, a method that is highly sensitive for micro- and macroemboli, typically is not routinely utilized due to its highly invasive nature and the degree of expertise required.

A. **Precordial Doppler**

   1. As mentioned previously, echocardiography is a very invasive, labor-intensive monitoring device. As such there has been a strong desire to have a noninvasive device that is effective

TABLE 22.7   Methods of detection for venous air embolism

Method	Sensitivity (mL/kg)	Limitation
Intracardiac TEE[26]	Extremely high, most sensitive	High technical expertise required, limited availability, highly invasive
TEE	High (0.02)	Expertise required, expensive, invasive, not quantitative
Precordial Doppler	High (0.05)	Obese patients, intravenous mannitol can mimic air embolism, electrocautery interference
Pulmonary artery catheter	High (0.25)	Fixed distance, small orifice
Transcranial Doppler	High	Expertise
EtN$_2$	Moderate (0.5)	N$_2$O, hypotension
EtCO$_2$	Moderate (0.5)	Pulmonary disease, nonspecific, other causes (e.g., low cardiac output)
Oxygen saturation	Low	Late changes
Direct visualization	Low	No physiologic data
Esophageal stethoscope	Low (1.5)	Late changes
Electrocardiography	Low (1.25)	Late changes

TEE, transesophageal echocardiography; EtN$_2$, end-tidal nitrogen; EtCO$_2$, end-tidal carbon dioxide.
Adapted and modified from: Mirski MA, Lele AV, Fitzsimmons L, et al. Diagnosis and treatment of vascular air embolism. *Anesthesiology.* 2007;106(1):164–177.

2

for determining the presence of VAE. The precordial Doppler, a device that is placed along the sternal border to detect signals from the right ventricular outflow tract, has been determined to be the most sensitive noninvasive monitor (detects as little as 0.05 mL/kg or 0.015 to 0.020 mL/kg/min of air).

2. Placement of the device is not without controversy. Typically it is recommended to place the probe over the right sternal border between the second and fourth intercostal space, or between the right scapula and spine [27]. However, it has been concluded that a Doppler signal can be obtained *more reliably at the left parasternal than at the right parasternal border*, but left lateral precordial probe placement frequently fails to detect intravascular bubbles [28].

3. The Tinker test, in which the injection of 5 mL to 10 mL of air-agitated saline via a peripheral or central venous catheter results in an erratic high-pitched roar can confirm placement [29]. As air entrainment occurs, the observer detects a "drum-like" or "mill wheel" murmur. However, a limitation of the device is that it needs to be louder than ambient noise of the operating room and can be affected by electrocautery, prone/lateral positioning, and obesity [2].

B. **End-tidal nitrogen and end-tidal carbon dioxide.** It has been noted that the monitoring for the presence of end-tidal nitrogen is the most sensitive gas detection device for VAE. When air is present in concentrations as low as 0.04%, end-tidal nitrogen gives a positive reading. The problem, however, is that this gas sensor is rarely available and can be affected by the utilization of nitrous oxide [2]. $EtCO_2$ typically is a later and less sensitive monitor. *An acute decrease in $EtCO_2$ is the result of an acute change in dead-space ventilation* (ventilation without perfusion) and may be the result of not only emboli, but also hypotension or cardiovascular collapse.

VIII. **Treatment**

A. **Treatment options.** When a VAE occurs in the perioperative environment, there are several options that are available to the provider. These may be quite simple and relatively intuitive, such as *notification of the surgeon, flooding of the field, closure of the entrainment source, and compression venous structures such as jugular compression* (Table 22.8).

B. **Aspiration of air via multiorifice catheter**

1. A more controversial and invasive treatment option includes the aspiration of air to improve hemodynamics. Though routinely taught (and felt to be the gold standard by some practitioners), *the recovery of air from the heart has been noted not to be a major factor in improving hemodynamics as compared to the packing of the site of air entry* [16,30].

2. Several multiorifice catheters exist on the market and some of these catheters have the ability to allow electrocardiographic guidance to ensure proper location in the right atrium (observation of biphasic P-waves). The ideal location for maximum recovery of air is 2 cm distal to the junction of superior vena cava and atrial chamber at an inclination of 80 degrees [31].

3

3. However there is ample *evidence that air aspiration is noneffective*. In a recent animal study, data revealed that significant right ventricular air was present within 5 seconds of air entrainment and was thus unreachable when using atrial catheters for aspiration [13]. This may explain why success rates of air aspiration have been reported to be as low as 6% to 16% with Swan–Ganz catheters to as high as 30% to 60% with a Bunegin–Albin

TABLE 22.8 Treatment options
Notification of surgeon
Flooding of surgical field/closure of entrainment source
Compression of cerebral venous structures (jugular compression)
Aspiration of entrained air via multiorifice catheter
Partial left lateral positioning with Trendelenburg tilt (Durant maneuver)
Turn off nitrous oxide if utilizing
Institution of hemodynamic support
Hyperbaric oxygen therapy

multiorifice catheter (Cook Critical Care, Bloomington, IN). As such there is *no role for the emergent insertion of these catheters* in the setting of an acute VAE.

> **CLINICAL PEARL** Primary treatment for an AE includes notification of the surgeon, flooding of the field, closure of the entrainment source, and manual compression venous structures such as jugular vein. A multiorifice right atrial catheter aspiration may remove a small volume of air from the heart. However, aspiration is not a major factor in improving hemodynamics as compared to the packing of the site of air entry.

C. **Partial left lateral position (Durant maneuver)/Trendelenburg.** Changing patient position is one of the first maneuvers performed after the detection of VAE. The *change in position is performed to remove the gradient that exists between the surgical site and the heart.* However, many times the alteration of position is in response to the catastrophic hemodynamic effects associated with the event. The Durant maneuver (partial left lateral decubitus) is felt to assist in the removal of an air lock; but this is still controversial since numerous dog studies do not substantiate its value [2]. In a swine model, Schafer et al. [13] revealed that the right atrial and ventricular disappearance times for air were faster in the supine position. As such, the group recommended that maintaining the sitting position prolonged the duration of air in the heart and the time available to aspirate air. One caveat is that this study was performed in a swine model and relied on the placement and utilization of right ventricular catheters.

D. **Discontinuation of nitrous oxide**
1. The utilization of nitrous oxide in patients at high risk for VAE continues to be controversial. If the patient developed a VAE, due to differences in solubility, the air bubble could expand in the presence of nitrous oxide; thus it has been recommended that if nitrous oxide is to be used, it should be discontinued immediately upon detection of VAE [32].
2. Theoretically, the use of nitrous oxide could potentially improve the initial detection of VAE by its expansion of the air embolus. However, Lossaso et al. [33] could find no evidence that nitrous oxide increased the incidence of detection of VAE or perceived volume of VAE.

E. **Hyperbaric oxygen therapy**
1. The role of hyperbaric oxygen (HBO) therapy has been described extensively, most notably in the presence of cerebral air embolism. It is important to note that the spontaneous absorption of air bubbles can take up to 15 hours [34].
2. The value of HBO is that the descent to a level of six atmospheres of pressure significantly reduces the bubble size by favoring nitrogen diffusion and relieves obstruction to blood flow. The high levels of hemoglobin saturation and partial pressure of oxygen (PaO_2) created by HBO improve tissue oxygen delivery and relieve the ischemic insult [16].

F. **Hemodynamic support**
1. It is essential during a VAE event to support the hemodynamics of the patient thus ensuring end-organ perfusion. *The value of catecholamine utilization is to restore the oxygen supply to demand ratio for the right ventricle.* Right ventricular (RV) pressure overload increases wall tension, thus increasing oxygen consumption. Systemic hypotension subsequently leads to a decrease in right coronary artery (RCA) perfusion and ultimately ischemia of the RV, decreased RV output and RV failure. *Thus maintenance of RCA perfusion pressure is paramount.*
2. It is important to note that the *sympathomimetics have effects on the pulmonary circulation.* The following has been observed [19]:
   a. Epinephrine: Constricts normal baseline PAP and dilates increased baseline PAP
   b. Norepinephrine: Constricts normal baseline; constricts and dilates increased baseline PAP
   c. Phenylephrine: Constricts normal; constricts/dilates increased
   d. Acetylcholine: Constricts, dilates normal, dilates increased baseline

3. Some *key elements regarding the administration of catecholamines* must also be kept in mind [19]:

   a. With the exception of norepinephrine, all vasoactive catecholamines increase PVR when PAP is elevated.

   b. Phenylephrine, in the presence of RV failure associated with constant RV afterload as seen in VAE, increases RCA perfusion pressure.

IX. Summary. VAEs and their complications can be ameliorated by several maneuvers, namely awareness, vigilance, and preparedness. A heightened awareness regarding the procedure and which patients are at risk allows for the appropriate interventions required for these cases. The utilization of precordial Doppler and EtCO$_2$ monitoring appears to be of value as well as maneuvers to support right ventricular function during periods of air entrainment.

REFERENCES

1. Buckland RW, Manners JM. Venous air embolism during neurosurgery—a comparison of various methods of detection in man. *Anaesthesia.* 1976;31:633–643.
2. Mirski MA, Lele AV, Fitzsimmons L, et al. Diagnosis and treatment of vascular air embolism. *Anesthesiology.* 2007;106(1):164–177.
3. Jadik S, Wissing H, Friedrich K, et al. A standardized protocol for the prevention of clinically relevant venous air embolism during neurosurgical interventions in the semi-sitting position. *Neurosurgery.* 2009;64:533–539.
4. White JB, Thielen KR, Kallmes DF. Putative risk of substantial venous air embolism during vertebroplasty. *Spine.* 2009;34:1526–1529.
5. Black S, Cucchiara RF, Nishimura RA, et al. Parameters affecting the occurrence of paradoxical air embolism. *Anesthesiology.* 1989;71:235–241.
6. O'Quin RJ, Lakshminarayan S. Venous air embolism. *Arch Intern Med.* 1982;142:2173–2176.
7. Gottdiener JS, Papdemetriou V, Notargiacomo A, et al. Incidence and cardiac effects of systemic venous air embolism: Echocardiographic evidence of arterial embolization via noncardiac shunt. *Arch Intern Med.* 1988;148:795–800.
8. Syymons NLP, Leaver HK. Air embolism during craniotomy in the seated position: a comparison of methods for detection. *Can Anaesth Soc J.* 1985;32:174–177.
9. Matjasko J, Petrozza P, Cohen M, et al. Anesthesia and surgery in the seated position: Analysis of 554 cases. *Neurosurgery.* 1985;17:695–702.
10. Girard F, Ruel M, McKenty S, et al. Incidences of venous air embolism and patent foramen ovale among patients undergoing selective peripheral denervation in the sitting position. *Neurosurgery.* 2003;53:316–319.
11. Schmandra TC, Mierdl S, Bauer H, et al. Transesophageal echocardiography shows high risk of gas embolism during laparoscopic hepatic resection under carbon dioxide pneumoperitoneum. *Br J Surg.* 2002;89:870–876.
12. Toung TJ, Rossberg MI, Hutchins GM. Volume of air in a lethal venous air embolism. *Anesthesiology.* 2001;94:360–361.
13. Schafer ST, Lindemann J, Neumann A, et al. Cardiac air transit following venous air embolism and right ventricular air aspiration. *Anaesthesia.* 2009;64:754–761.
14. Flanagan JP, Gradisar IA, Gross RJ, et al. Air emboli: a lethal complication of subclavian venipuncture. *N Engl J Med.* 1969;281:488–489.
15. Adornato DC, Gildenberg PL, Ferrario CM. Pathophysiology of intravenous air embolism in dogs. *Anesthesiology.* 1978;49:120–127.
16. Orebaugh SL. Venous air embolism: clinical and experimental considerations. *Crit Care Med.* 1992;20:1169–1177.
17. Muth CM, Shank ES. Gas embolism. *N Engl J Med.* 2000;342:476–482.
18. Lam KK, Hutchinson RC, Gin T. Severe pulmonary oedema after venous air embolism. *Can J Anaesth.* 1993;40:964–967.
19. Stratmann G, Gregory GA. Neurogenic and humoral vasoconstriction in acute pulmonary thromboembolism. *Anesth Analg.* 2003;97:341–354.
20. Naulty JS, Meisel LB, Datta S, et al. Air embolism during radical hysterectomy. *Anesthesiology.* 1982;47:420–422.
21. Schafer ST, Sandalcioglu IE, Stegen B, et al. Venous air embolism during semi-sitting craniotomy evokes thrombocytopenia. *Anaesthesia.* 2011;66:25–30.
22. Barak M, Katz Y. Microbubbles: pathophysiology and clinical implications. *Chest.* 2005;128:2918–2932.
23. Schafer ST, Neumann A, Lindemann J, et al. Venous air embolism induces both platelet dysfunction and thrombocytopenia. *Acta Anaesthesiol Scand.* 2009;53:736–741.
24. Blanc P, Boussuges A, Henriette K, et al. Iatrogenic cerebral air embolism: importance of an early hyperbaric oxygenation. *Intensive Care Med.* 2002;28:559–563.
25. Hagen PT, Scholz DG, Edwards WD. Incidence and size of patent foramen ovale during the first 10 decades of life: An autopsy study of 965 normal hearts. *Mayo Clin Proc.* 1984;59:17–20.
26. Fathi AR, Eshtehardi P, Meier B. Patent foramen ovale and neurosurgery in sitting position: a systematic review. *Br J Anaesth.* 2009;102:588–596.
27. Schafer ST, Lindemann J, Brendt P, et al. Intracardiac transvenous echocardiography is superior to both precordial Doppler and transesophageal echocardiography techniques for detecting venous air embolism and catheter-guided air aspiration. *Anesth Analg.* 2008;106:45–54.
28. Schubert A, Deogaonkar A, Drummond JC. Precordial Doppler probe placement for optimal detection of venous air embolism during craniotomy. *Anesth Analg.* 2006;102:1543–1547.

29. Tinker JH, Gronert GA, Messick JM, et al. Detection of air embolism, a test for positioning of right atrial catheter and Doppler probe. *Anesthesiology.* 1975;43:104–105.

30. Bedford RF, Marshall WK, Butler A, et al. Cardiac catheters for diagnosis and treatment of venous air embolism. *J Neurosurg.* 1981;55:610–614.

31. Albin MS. Venous air embolism: a warning not to be complacent—we should listen to the drumbeat of history. *Anesthesiology.* 2011;115:626–629.

32. Pasternak JJ, Lainer WL. Is nitrous oxide use appropriate in neurosurgical and neurologically at-risk patients? *Curr Opin Anaesthesiol.* 2010;23:544–550.

33. Lossaso TJ, Black S, Muzzi DA, et al. Detection and hemodynamic consequences of venous air embolism. Does nitrous oxide make a difference? *Anesthesiology.* 1992;77:148–152.

34. Dexter F, Hindman BJ. Recommendations for hyperbaric oxygen therapy of cerebral air embolism based on a mathematical model of bubble absorption. *Anesth Analg.* 1997;84:1203–1207.

23

Stroke and Brain Protection

John Dunford

KEY POINTS

1. Stroke is the third leading cause of death and the leading cause of serious, long-term disability in the United States.
2. The neuroanesthesiologist must have a fundamental knowledge of the pathophysiology of neuronal cell death and the appropriate measures, be physiologic or pharmacologic, to prevent and treat ischemic brain injury.
3. Cerebral ischemia results in a rapid uncontrolled increase in intracellular calcium, resulting in excitatory neurotransmitter release, the activation of lipases, proteases, endonucleases, free radical formation, fatty acid production, nitric oxide production, inflammation, and the production caspases. All of these can contribute to neuronal cell death.
4. In contrast to apoptosis (Type I cell death) and necrosis (Type III cell death), autophagy is described as Type II cell death. All three processes can be activated by cerebral ischemia.
5. Anesthetics generally decrease the cerebral metabolic rate by as much as 60% by decreasing neuronal functional activity on the electroencephalogram (EEG) and can increase the supply of oxygen by cerebral vasodilation.
6. Exposure to the brain by anesthetics either immediately or up to a few days prior to the induction of ischemia decreases ischemic brain injury. This is referred to as "preconditioning."
7. Anesthetics may cause cerebral protection by reduction in ischemia-induced glutamate release, increased GABA-A–mediated hyperpolarization, blockage of postsynaptic glutamate receptors, and increased levels of antiapoptotic proteins.
8. Anesthetic agents have shown cerebral protective effects in vitro and in vivo. The mechanism for cerebral protection by anesthetic agents is most likely multimodal. In vitro and animal studies support the neuroprotective properties of barbiturates, volatile anesthetics, propofol, ketamine, benzodiazepines, and lidocaine. Human clinical trials have been disappointing.

(continued)

9. Nonanesthetic agents including calcium channel blockers, magnesium, free radical scavengers, excitatory amino acid modulators, erythropoietin, trophic factors, cytokines, statins, and antiapoptotic agents all show potential for cerebral protection. However, with the exception of the use of statins in nonhemorrhagic stroke, more research needs to be performed before these classes of drugs will be found to be clinically useful.
10. Intravenous thrombolytics for ischemic embolic stroke and mild hyoothermia for both spontaneous circulation after out of hospital cardiac arrest and neonates with hypoxic-ischemic encephalopathy are associated with improved outcomes.

I. Introduction

A. Stroke is the third leading cause of death and the leading cause of serious, long-term disability in the United States [1,2].

1. Stroke is a dreaded perioperative complication. Cardiopulmonary bypass is associated with a 1.3% to 7.9% risk of focal neurologic deficit [3].
2. There is a 4.8% chance of stroke after the resection of head and neck tumors, and a 5.4% to 6.1% with carotid endarterectomy [4–6].
3. In the United States, the aggregate lifetime cost associated with an estimated 392,344 first-time strokes in 1990 was $40.6 billion dollars [7].
4. Therefore, the ability to provide perioperative cerebral protection both before and after cerebral ischemia would have obvious benefits.

B. Cerebral ischemia can be classified as either global or focal.

1. Global cerebral ischemia results from decreased global cerebral perfusion either from cardiogenic or noncardiogenic causes [8].
2. Focal cerebral ischemia results from small vessel occlusion, arterial emboli, cerebral vasospasm, and direct surgical vascular injury.
3. Focal ischemia is described as having an ischemic "core" and a larger variable zone that is called the "penumbra."
   a. In the core, the lack of blood supply results in rapid neuronal death.
   b. In the penumbra, the flow reduction is sufficient to result in an isoelectric EEG, but not severe enough to result in rapid cell loss. If the diminished blood flow to the penumbra continues, then cell death will follow. The opportunity to salvage neurons is greatest in the ischemic penumbra [9].

C. There has been a significant increase recently in our knowledge of the mechanisms of neuronal ischemic cell death particularly in the mechanisms of apoptosis. However, effective therapeutic modalities short of good hemodynamic control, hypothermia, thrombolytic therapy, and perhaps barbiturates have as of yet proved elusive.

II. Pathophysiology of cerebral ischemia

A. Histopathologic events

1. Neurons of different areas of the brain vary in their sensitivity to ischemia. This may be secondary to differences in blood supply.
2. In the cerebral cortex, the ischemic injury is often more severe in the parietal and the occipital lobes especially in the depths of the sulci.
3. Within seconds of cerebral ischemia, the brain interstitial space disappears. This is thought to be secondary to cell swelling and sodium influx.
4. At 10 minutes, there is clumping of nuclear material.
5. At 30 minutes, further swelling is seen within the astrocytes, with intracellular swelling of the mitochondria, disappearance of microtubules, and detachment of ribosomes from the endoplasmic reticulum.
6. After 2 hours, the mitochondria show flocculent densities suggesting calcium overload. Lysosomes are not involved at this stage and therefore catastrophic cell death is not yet seen. Lysosomes can be stable for up to 4 hours after an ischemic insult.
7. Therefore, lethal cell injury occurring with ischemia of less than 30 minutes duration is typically histopathologically thought secondary to damage of the mitochondria and ribosomes.

8. On typical histologic cadaveric preparations, the first visible change after cerebral ischemia typically occurs 12 to 24 hours after the ischemic cerebral insult. The affected neurons develop a very eosinophilic cytoplasm and a small pyknotic nucleus sometimes called a "red dead neuron."

9. This process is often widespread but not often completely uniform in the cerebral cortex with clusters of damaged cells being found next to unaffected cells, even in the same cortical layer.

10. After about 48 to 72 hours, there is softening and disintegration of the infarcted area with pronounced edema of both the infarcted tissue and adjacent tissue. This can cause herniation if the infarct is large enough.

11. Swelling of astrocytes can cause compression of cerebral capillaries. Histologically, there is an initial influx of polymorphonuclear leukocytes (PMNs) followed by macrophages invading and digesting the necrotic tissue. Fibroblasts are only located around blood vessels in the brain; therefore, a scar does not form. Rather, a cystic cavity with fibrillary gliosis is seen.

12. Glial cells respond to hypoxia. Astrocytes swell accumulating glycogen and cytoplasmic filaments. Oligodendrocytes are less affected and microglia participates in the phagocytosis of cellular debris.

3

B. Biochemical events

1. The EEG disappears within 20 seconds of ischemia in a normothermic brain. This is probably secondary to ATP depletion.

2. Within 5 minutes, high energy phosphate levels have been depleted and profound changes in cellular electrolyte balance begins to occur. Sodium and calcium ions enter the cell and potassium leaks out. Water follows the sodium intracellularly resulting in cellular swelling. This is particularly pronounced in the astrocytes.

3. Calcium has an extracellular gradient of 10,000 to 1. This gradient is maintained by the active pumping out of intracellular calcium.

4. Calcium pumps include an ATP-driven membrane pump, exchange for calcium for sodium in the sodium–potassium ATP-driven membrane pump, an ATP-driven sequestration of calcium in the mitochondria, and accumulation of calcium in the mitochondria by an oxidation-dependant mechanism. Three of these four mechanisms require ATP and will fail during ischemia. The resulting increase in mitochondrial calcium causes diminished oxidative phosphorylation resulting in a decrease in ATP production [10,11].

5. Elucidating the exact mechanisms of calcium toxicity and identifying the subcellular compartment playing the most important role in this pathologic process might help in the evaluation of strategies for specific therapeutic interventions.

C. Necrotic cell death

1. There is evidence that excitatory neurotransmitters that are released during ischemia play an important role in the etiology of neuronal ischemic injury. Ischemia increases intracellular levels of calcium and sodium, and the resulting nerve depolarization results in the release of excitatory amino acids, especially glutamate. The glutamate transporter protein pumps glutamate into the extracellular compartment when the neuron is ischemic. Glutamate activates alpha-amino-hydroxy-5-methyl-isoxazole propionic acid (AMPA) and N-methyl-d-aspartate (NMDA) receptors. NMDA receptor activation results in increasing intracellular calcium and the activation of metabotropic receptors via second messenger systems. Also, the glutamate-induced depolarization of the cell results in calcium entry into the cell from voltage-gated calcium channels and from the endoplasmic reticulum. These ionic and biochemical changes that occur in the brain due to increased glutamate are called excitotoxicity.

2. Increased cytoplasmic calcium is deleterious to the neuron. High calcium levels increase the activity of proteases and phospholipases. Phospholipases cause the production of free fatty acids including arachidonic acid from membrane lipids. Free fatty acids damage cell membranes and further decrease the cell's ability to pump out calcium. The fatty acid, arachidonic acid, causes the release of thromboxane and leukotrienes. Both of these can cause platelet aggregation, clotting, vasospasm, and edema with resultant further compromise of cerebral blood flow.

3. Lactic acidosis is associated with cerebral injury during ischemia. Increased levels of lactic acid result in decreased pH. Decreased pH can damage and inactivate mitochondria while lactic acid degradation of NADH (needed for ATP production) may decrease reperfusion ATP levels [12,13].

4. Free radicals are produced during cerebral ischemia [14,15]. Ischemia in the presence of increased intracellular calcium results in xanthine oxidase production. With reperfusion and the reintroduction of oxygen, in the presence of xanthine oxidase, super oxide anion (O_2^-), hydroxyl radical (OH^-), and free lipid radicals are produced. O_2^- is also released from the leukotriene-activated neutrophils. The resulting reoxygenation permits active uptake of calcium in an already calcium-enriched mitochondria with reperfusion resulting in extreme calcium overload and free radical release. These free radicals will damage proteins and lipids [16].

5. Neutrophil activation is thought to play a role in cerebral ischemia hours to days after the initial ischemic event [17]. PMNs have been implicated as a significant cause of pathology in cerebral ischemia. This is especially true with reperfusion injury. Their acute activation may be responsible for many of the effects of cerebral ischemia including loss of capillary integrity and loss of cerebral ultrastructure with cerebral reperfusion [18,19]. Activated polymorphonuclear cells can generate lots of hydrogen peroxide. This hydrogen peroxide along with myeloperoxide, also from activated PMNs, reacts with halides such as chloride and bromide to produce hypohalous acids. Chloride is the halide with the highest concentration. Therefore the molecule most produced by the reaction of the halide with hydrogen peroxide is hypochlorous acid (HClO). HClO is most commonly known as household bleach. HClO reacts with a wide variety of biomolecules including deoxyribonucleic acids (DNA), ribonucleic acids (RNA), fatty acid groups, cholesterol, and proteins.

6. Nitric oxide is typically released by vascular endothelium during cerebral ischemia thereby increasing cerebral blood flow. In contrast, neuronal nitric oxide produced cerebral ischemia, when combined with free radicals, results in the production of peroxynitrite which is harmful to neurons.

7. Necrotic neuronal cell death from ischemia results from decreased ATP production by oxidative phosphorylation in the mitochondria. The resulting inability for the neuron to run its membrane ion pumps results in an increase in intracellular calcium and the release of the excitatory neurotransmitter glutamate. Increased intracellular calcium results in the activation of proteases, phospholipases, free radical production, and mitochondrial damage. The resulting disintegration of the cell activates an immune response with the recruitment of macrophages. Macrophages cause increased free radical production, inflammation, and damage to adjacent neurons.

D. Apoptotic cell death

1. Another type of ischemic cell death, apoptosis, results in cell death without the breaking apart of the cell membrane [20]. Apoptosis is a normal phenomenon. There are between 50 and 70 billion cells that die each day due to apoptosis in an average human adult. When the neurons go through apoptosis, there is a lack of an inflammatory response and in contrast to necrotic cell death, no resulting death of adjacent neurons occurs.

2. Apoptosis, the process of programmed cell death, histologically manifests as blebbing, cell shrinkage, nuclear fragmentation, chromatin condensation, and chromosomal DNA fragmentations.

3. Apoptosis produces cell fragments called apoptotic bodies that phagocytic cells can engulf before the contents of the dying cell can leak out and cause inflammation.

4. Apoptosis is controlled by a diverse set of cell signals that have both intracellular and extracellular origins.

5. Dying cells that undergo the final stages of apoptosis display phagocytotic molecules. These molecules mark the cell for phagocytosis by cells possessing the appropriate receptors, such as macrophages.

6. Neuronal ischemia can affect the expression of genes that result in the production of apoptotic or antiapoptotic proteins. Antiapoptotic proteins which help prevent apoptosis include neuronal apoptosis inhibitory protein, heat shock proteins, and Bcl-2 type proteins.

Trophic factors can inhibit apoptosis while interleukin 1B and tumor necrosis factor can promote it.

7. Some types of mice with abnormal extrinsic signaling proteins (FasL) show a 93% reduction in infarct volume after experimental middle cerebral artery (MCA) occlusion suggesting a significant contribution of these receptors to cell death in cerebral ischemia [21].

E. Autophagy

1. Autophagy is a cellular process required for the recycling of proteins and damaged organelles. Typically, the part of the cell that is to be "autophaged" is surrounded by a membrane separating its contents from the rest of the cytoplasm. This resulting vesicle then attaches to the lysosome, and its contents are digested by lysosomal proteases. In contrast to apoptosis (Type I cell death) and necrotic cell death (Type III cell death), autophagy is described as Type II cell death.

2. Cerebral ischemia is associated with enhanced expression of the autophagy regulator Beclin 1 and subcellular redistribution of the autophagic marker LC3 in ischemic neurons.

3. Prolonged overaction of autophagy can lead to self-destruction of the cell [22].

F. Neurogenesis

1. Evidence suggests that new neurons are generated not only in the neonatal brain but also in the adult brain. The dentate gyrus and the subventricular zone are two areas in the adult brain in which neurogenesis has been identified. The newborn neurons are integrated into neuronal networks and make appropriate connections with target neurons. Exercise, trophic factors (brain-derived neurotrophic factor, epidermal growth factor, and fibroblast growth factor), and neurotransmitters affect proliferation of these neurons. Migrating neuroblasts from the subventricular zone are directed to areas of neuronal ischemic damage.

2. With both focal and global ischemia, neurogenesis significantly increases with peak proliferation between 7 and 10 days postinjury. The majority of the new neurons die. Therefore, their contribution to functional improvement after a stroke remains to be examined.

3. Transplantation of stem cells or their derivatives in animal models of cerebral ischemia can improve function by replacing the lost neurons and glial cells and by mediating remyelination and modulation of inflammation. Transplant cell therapy may work by providing trophic support to the injured tissue and brain fostering both neurogenesis and angiogenesis [23].

G. In summary, ischemia results in a rapid uncontrolled increase in intracellular calcium, resulting in excitatory neurotransmitter release, the activation of lipases, proteases, endonucleases, free radical formation, fatty acid production, nitric oxide production, inflammation, Beclin 1, and the production caspases. All of these can contribute to neuronal cell death [24].

III. Cerebral protection by anesthetic agents

A. Mechanism of action

1. Anesthetics affect the pathophysiology of cerebral ischemia in many different ways. Anesthetics generally decrease the cerebral metabolic rate by as much as 60% by decreasing neuronal functional activity on the EEG, and can increase the supply of oxygen by cerebral vasodilation. In addition, volatile anesthetics reduce ischemia-induced glutamate release, increase GABA-A–mediated *hyperpolarization*, antagonize postsynaptic glutamate receptors, and increase levels of antiapoptotic proteins [25,26]. Exposure to the brain by anesthetics, either immediately or up to a few days prior to the induction of ischemia, decreases ischemic brain injury. This is referred to as "preconditioning." Possible mechanisms for cerebral protection from preconditioning include activation of potassium (K+) channels, production of nitric oxide, activation of adenosine receptors, and activating prosurvival signaling cascades such as serine/threonine protein kinase B (PKB) now called AKT, protein kinase C (PKC), and p38 pathways [27,28].

CLINICAL PEARL Data on ischemic brain neuroprotection from anesthetics has been derived from animal stroke models make it more difficult to form conclusions about the role of inhalational anesthetics in human perioperative cerebral ischemia.

2. In spite of extensive work on the basic science of stroke injury mechanisms and countless hours spent on preclinical trial animal stroke models, we have yet to have a single chemical neuroprotection agent. A visit to the stroke trials center (www.strokecenter.org/trials) will show a summary of the clinical trials for stroke. There are no conclusive clinical successes from this list.

B. Barbiturates

1. The ability of barbiturates to provide cerebral protection in focal ischemia has been described in animal studies and one human clinical trial of postcardiopulmonary bypass patients utilizing very high barbiturate doses [29,30]. Another clinical trial did not show that the use of barbiturates in open heart surgery resulted in cerebral protection [31]. Studies have shown that barbiturate doses that are not sufficient to result in an isoelectric EEG are protective in focal ischemia [32].

2. Any combination of decreased cerebral metabolic requirements of oxygen ($CMRO_2$), reverse steal, free radical scavenging, redistribution of cerebral blood flow, blockage of sodium (Na+), potassium (K+), and calcium (Ca++) ion fluxes, scavenging free radicals, decreased intracranial pressure (ICP), and increased regional blood flow are suggested as possible mechanisms for cerebral protection by barbiturates. Studies of the use of barbiturates after cardiac arrest resulting in global ischemia have demonstrated no improvement in clinical outcomes [33]. Another variable to consider is the common drop in body temperature concurrent with the use of the barbiturate.

3. Therefore, barbiturates seem to be protective in models of focal ischemia and in one human clinical trial on cardiac patients.

C. Volatile anesthetics

1. Volatile anesthetics have been shown to be neuroprotective in animal models for focal, hemispheric, and near-complete cerebral ischemia [34,35]. Proposed mechanisms include activation of ATP-dependent potassium channels, upregulation of nitric oxide synthase, reduction of excitotoxic stressors, augmentation of peri-ischemic cerebral blood flow, and upregulation of antiapoptotic factors [36,37].

2. Rat organotypic hippocampus slices treated with isoflurane had substantially less damage when compared with controls [38–40]. In animal models, in rats subjected to hemispheric ischemia, comparing 2% sevoflurane with fentanyl–nitrous oxide (N_2O), the sevoflurane group had significantly less damage even out at 28 days [41]. In models in which ischemic brain was evaluated at 2 days postevent, a significant decrease in neuronal death was noted, however, if the ischemic brain was evaluated at 14 days, a reduction in cerebral injury was not observed [42]. This may be due to a lack of protection by volatile anesthetics against ongoing apoptosis. If caspase inhibitors are used along with isoflurane in a focal ischemic model of neuronal injury, sustained neuroprotection is noted [43,44]. The contradiction in the degree of cerebral protection described in these animal models may be secondary to the degree cerebral ischemia used in the model. It may be that cerebral protection in mature adult brains from volatile anesthetics is seen only with mild to moderate ischemia. However, with severe ischemia, cerebral protection by volatile anesthetics may not be possible.

3. Sevoflurane preconditioning for 45 minutes and 60 minutes prior to 1 hour of focal ischemia in a rat model showed a significant decrease in infarct volume, functional outcome, and evidence of apoptosis in the preconditioned animals [45].

4. Recent animal findings suggest that commonly used general anesthetics are damaging to developing neurons and cause significant neuronal deletion in vulnerable brain regions [46–48]. In addition, emerging animal and human data suggest an association between early exposure to general anesthesia and long-term impairment of cognitive development [49].

5. This information, in addition to the fact that most current experimental data on ischemic brain neuroprotection from volatile anesthetics has been derived from animal stroke models makes it more difficult to form conclusions about the role of inhalational anesthetics in human perioperative cerebral ischemia [35].

D. Nitrous oxide

1. Nitrous oxide has been shown to cause a vacuolar reaction, and prolonged exposure can result in neuronal cell death in animal models [46]. Its effect on vitamin B12 metabolism and its lack of effect on metabolic rate seem detrimental.

2. Nitrous oxide probably has a limited role in neuroprotection. Pasternak et al. [50], using the Induced Hypothermia for Aneurysm Surgery Trial (IHAST) database to review delayed ischemic neurologic deficits and 3-month postoperative neurologic or neuropsychological dysfunction in patients delivered nitrous oxide, found no evidence of adverse effects.

E. Propofol

1. Propofol reduces cerebral blood flow, maintains coupling with cerebral metabolic rate for oxygen, and decreases ICP. In vitro and in vivo studies of propofol have shown a neuroprotective effect of propofol in addition to its positive effects on cerebral physiology [51]. Propofol given prior to onset of ischemia, during ischemia, and 3 hours after ischemia, reduces infarct volumes and decreases apoptotic changes and the expression of apoptotic protein Bcl-2 in postperfusion neurons [52,53].

2. In anesthetized animals, propofol showed a similar infarct size when compared to pentobarbital [54]. High dose propofol during focal cerebral ischemia in an animal model when evaluated at 28 days resulted in decreased neurogenesis in comparison to focal cerebral ischemia without propofol [55]. Electroencephalographic burst suppression with propofol during cardiac valve replacement did not significantly reduce the incidence or severity of neurologic or neuropsychological dysfunction [56].

3. Although there is a lack of good clinical human data, animal data does show that propofol is neuroprotective.

F. Etomidate

1. Etomidate works by potentiating the effect of GABA on GABA-A receptors and like barbiturates and propofol can produce suppression of $CMRO_2$. In one model of temporary forebrain ischemia in comparison to 1.1 MAC of halothane and isoflurane or anesthesia with thiopental, there was no protective effect of etomidate seen in the cortex, reticular nucleus of the thalamus, and the striatum. There was some protection in the hippocampus [57,58]. In another investigation of temporary MCA occlusion, the volume of injury was not reduced in comparison to a 1.2 MAC halothane control group versus the etomidate group. In fact the size of volume of injury with etomidate was larger than the control group [57].

2. Etomidate may bind to nitric oxide resulting in decreased cerebral blood flow [57,59]. In patients who have temporary arterial occlusion, administration of etomidate resulted in greater tissue hypoxia and acidosis than equivalent doses of desflurane [60].

3. There is little evidence that etomidate provides cerebral protection.

G. Ketamine

1. Ketamine is an NMDA receptor antagonist. Glutamate excitotoxicity is in part caused by activation on NMDA receptors therefore it is possible that ketamine could provide neuroprotection.

2. Clinical trials with noncompetitive and competitive NMDA receptor antagonists in patients with stroke have shown that these patients develop adverse effects, particularly psychomimetic effects such as hallucinations and agitation [61].

3. In the normal brain, NMDA receptor antagonism results in increased neuronal proliferation. However, in the ischemic brain, NMDA receptor antagonism results in decreased neurogenesis.

4. In both in vitro and animal models of both focal and global ischemia, ketamine has been found to be neuroprotective [62].

5. In a human trial, Nagels et al. [63] could not demonstrate that S(+)-ketamine resulted in greater neuroprotective effects compared with remifentanil during cardiopulmonary bypass procedures when both were combined with propofol.

   6. Although there is a lack of good clinical human data, animal data suggest that ketamine is neuroprotective.
H. Benzodiazepines
   1. Midazolam is commonly used in anesthesia practice. It works by potentiating the effect of GABA on GABA-A receptors. In animal studies, midazolam has improved neuronal recovery after anoxic and ischemic injuries. High doses of midazolam reduce cerebral metabolic rate and cerebral blood flow. This effect is reversed by flumazenil, a benzodiazepine antagonist [64].
   2. Flumazenil has been shown to increase ICP, cerebral blood flow, and cerebral metabolic rate. These facts plus its pro epileptic properties suggest that flumazenil should, as a general rule, be avoided in neurosurgical patients.
I. Lidocaine
   1. Lidocaine is a sodium channel blocker. The neuronal depolarization that occurs during cerebral ischemia results in the large flux of sodium into the cell. Lidocaine's ability to block the sodium channel decreases depolarization and results in a delay in the drop in ATP during cerebral ischemia [65]. Lidocaine also decreases the cerebral metabolic rate for oxygen and inhibits white cell activation to inflammation. Both of these effects may be neuroprotective.
   2. In animal models of focal cerebral ischemia, lidocaine reduced infarct size and has shown improved neurologic outcome following focal cerebral ischemia [66,67]. In addition, administration of lidocaine after a 45-minute delay after ischemia resulted in improved survival of neurons in the ischemic penumbra. Lidocaine administered 30 minutes before ischemia and up to 60 minutes after ischemia improved the survival of pyramidal neurons after temporary global ischemia. This enhanced survival was seen at both 1 week and 4 weeks after the ischemic insult [67].
   3. Small clinical studies have found improved cognitive outcomes following cardiac surgery in patients to whom lidocaine was administered during their cases. In a follow-up double-blinded intention to treat trial, 158 cardiac surgery patients received a 12-hour infusion of lidocaine started at induction and referenced to a control group. Lidocaine was not found to result in improved scores on neurocognitive examinations at 10 and 25 weeks postanesthesia [68].
   4. Lidocaine is probably neuroprotective. Its clinical utility is under investigation.
IV. Cerebral protection by nonanesthetic agents
A. Calcium channel blockers
   1. Voltage-gated calcium channels have a central role in dendritic development, neuronal survival, synaptic plasticity, activation of gene transcription, and are essential to convert electrical activity to biochemical processes in the brain.
   2. Neurons express at least nine types of voltage-gated calcium channels specialized for different functions [69]. Some studies of dihydropyridine, phenylalkylamine, and benzothiazepine calcium channel blockers in both in vitro and animal models of cerebral ischemia have shown neuronal protection. However, this data is variable [70,71]. Nimodipine, a dihydropyridine which blocks L-type calcium channels, has been shown to increase recovery after subarachnoid hemorrhage [72]. In contrast, it has been demonstrated that prolonged exposure by cultured neurons to various antagonists of L-type voltage-gated calcium channels can induce apoptosis. In fact, activating L-type voltage-gated calcium channels, in vitro and in animal model studies of neuronal ischemia have actually reduced neuronal injury [71].
   3. A large clinical trial of the use of nimodipine after stroke was discontinued due to higher mortality in the nimodipine group [73]. With the exception of nimodipine for subarachnoid hemorrhage, calcium channel blockers do not seem clinically useful in ischemic neuroprotection.
B. Magnesium
   1. Magnesium blocks various voltage-gated and transmitter-activated channels. The NMDA receptor is normally blocked by magnesium ions and will only respond to glutamate when

this magnesium-induced block is removed on depolarization [74–76]. Magnesium blocks the influx of calcium and other ions.

2. In animal models of focal ischemia, magnesium has been shown to decrease levels of proapoptotic proteins [77].

3. Magnesium crosses the blood–brain barrier poorly and therefore has limited access to the central nervous system in the adult. Animal models have not reproducibly shown a reduction in infarct volume [78,79]. A clinical trial showed no improvement in outcome with the intravenous use of magnesium as therapy after stroke [80]. In addition, a human study of magnesium given before very preterm birth to protect the infant brain did not yield significant improvement with magnesium treatment [81].

4. Magnesium infusion has been shown to improve outcome when used in a postnatal fashion in term neonates with severe perinatal asphyxia [79].

5. At this point, there seems limited efficacy in the use of magnesium after cerebral ischemia except, perhaps, in the neonate.

C. Free radical scavengers

1. Both necrotic and apoptotic cell damage are thought to be secondary to free radical damage secondary to cerebral ischemia. Tirilazad, NXY-059, alpha-tocopherol, and N-tert-alpha-phenyl-butyl nitrone have been shown in animal studies to improve outcome after cerebral ischemia.

2. Tirilazad is a nonglucocorticoid, 21-aminosteroid that inhibits lipid peroxidation. Studies in experimental models of ischemic stroke had suggested that tirilazad had neuroprotective properties.

3. NXY-059 is a free radical trapping agent that is neuroprotective in animal models of stroke.

4. Tirilazad and NXY-059 did not show improved outcome in reproducible clinical trials after cerebral ischemia [82–84].

D. Excitatory amino acid modulators

1. Drugs that modulate glutamate action either by inhibiting its release or by blocking postsynaptic receptors could be neuroprotective agents [85].

2. Gavestinel (GV-150,526) is a drug which acts as an NMDA antagonist, binding selectively to the glycine site on the NMDA receptor complex. It is neuroprotective in animal studies and progressed to Phase II clinical trials in humans before being dropped for lack of efficacy [86].

3. Lubeluzole acts as an indirect NMDA antagonist. It inhibits the release of glutamate, inhibits nitric oxide synthesis, and blocks calcium- and sodium-gated ion channels. At high doses, Lubeluzole increases the Q–T interval therefore limiting its dose. Lubeluzole was not efficacious in clinical trials [85].

E. Trophic factors, erythropoietin, and cytokines

1. Neurons have receptors for trophic factors such as brain-derived growth factor and nerve growth factor. These are required for neuron survival. They phosphorylate amino acids via receptors that inhibit apoptosis. Ischemia can cause a reduction in the production of trophic factors and therefore trigger apoptosis.

2. In addition to its effect on erythropoiesis, erythropoietin may protect neurons from ischemia by acting as a trophic factor, activating antiapoptotic pathways, promoting angiogenesis, and decreasing inflammation. Erythropoietin crosses the blood–brain barrier poorly and therefore its ability to enter the brain may be dose dependent. In animal models for focal cerebral ischemia, systemic administration of erythropoietin has decreased infarct size [87,88]. Clinical trials using erythropoietin in the early postnatal period in very low birth weight infants have been associated with improved long-term neurologic and cognitive outcomes [89,90]. Erythropoietin has been shown to be safe and effective in clinical trials [91]. However, a recent double-blinded controlled randomized German multicenter stroke trial found no favorable effects with the use of erythropoietin. In addition, they found an increased death rate in the erythropoietin-treated group especially when the stroke patients were pretreated with thrombolytics [92,93].

3. Cytokines, such as tumor necrosis factor and interleukin 1B are immune system activators and can affect ischemic neuronal damage [94,95]. More research needs to be done in this area.

F. Statins

1. Statins are either synthetic- or fermentation-derived HMG-CoA reductase inhibitors. There is evidence that statins have beneficial effects within the cerebral circulation and the brain parenchyma during ischemic stroke and reperfusion. Statins upregulate endothelial nitric oxide synthase, attenuate inflammatory cytokine nitric oxide synthase, and possess antioxidant properties.

2. Human trials have shown a 16% reduction in strokes if treated with statins within the prior 1 to 6 months in patients with no known cardiac disease [96]. Studies have demonstrated that unlike those with prior ischemic stroke or transient ischemic attack (TIA), patients with prior hemorrhagic stroke had no statin-associated reductions in either recurrent stroke or major cardiovascular events. In fact, an increased risk of hemorrhagic stroke, particularly in patients treated with thrombolytics has been described [97,98].

3. Therefore, the use of statins must be used with caution after hemorrhagic stroke.

> **CLINICAL PEARL**   Human trials have shown a reduction in strokes if treated with statins within the prior 1 to 6 months in patients with no known cardiac disease.

G. Preconditioning

1. Preconditioning can be defined as presenting a stressful but nondamaging stimulus to cells to induce an endogenous adaptive response which would help cells to tolerate subsequent severe stresses. Preconditioning can be divided into two types: Early preconditioning that lasts between 4 and 6 hours and late preconditioning, involving *de novo* protein synthesis, that lasts from a few days to weeks [99].

2. Ischemia, hyperoxia, oxidative stress, prolonged hypoperfusion, hypothermia, hyperthermia, inflammatory cytokines, erythropoietin, metabolic inhibitors, deferoxamine, and inhalational anesthesia have all been associated with preconditioning.

3. Preconditioning has been demonstrated in animal models undergoing both global and focal ischemia as seen in in vitro brain slice preparations and cultured primary neurons. Preconditioning is also seen in humans after TIAs [100]. Retrospective clinical trials comparing stroke patients with and without TIAs prior to their stroke found that a TIA prior to a stroke is associated with significantly less severe stroke on admission and significantly smaller ischemic lesions after stroke utilizing examination with magnetic resonance imaging (MRI) [101,102].

4. The preconditioning of one part of the body can protect cells in another part of the body. Using this process of remote preconditioning in animal models, it has been demonstrated that cycles of short ischemic insult to a limb can protect the brain from a subsequent ischemic insult [103,104]. More work needs to be done to make ischemic preconditioning clinically useful.

H. Antiapoptotic agents

1. Caspases play a pivotal role in apoptotic ischemic cell death. Therefore it would make sense that caspase inhibitors would be neuroprotective. Indeed, if caspase inhibitors are used along with isoflurane in a focal ischemic model of neuronal injury, sustained neuroprotection can be noted [43,105].

2. Preconditioning may cause neurons to synthesize antiapoptotic proteins.

3. Specific blockers of caspases and modulators of apoptosis have been shown to improve neuron survival in vitro and in animal stroke models. However, caspase inhibitors do not demonstrate a reduction in infarct size in all models. This might be due to the severity of the ischemia, upregulation of caspase-independent apoptotic cell-death pathways, or failure to prevent necrotic cell death.

> **CLINICAL PEARL** In spite of extensive work on the basic science of stroke injury mechanisms and countless hours spent on preclinical trial animal stroke models, we have yet to have a single clinically useful chemical neuroprotection agent. A visit to the stroke trials center (www.strokecenter.org/trials) will show a summary of the clinical trials for stroke. There are no conclusive clinical successes from this list.

V. Effective current treatments for cerebral ischemia: Reperfusion and hypothermia

10

   A. The prompt restoration of spontaneous cerebral perfusion after embolic stroke by the administration of thrombolytic agents (TPA) has proven to be the most successful method for improving clinical recovery [106–108]. The risk of a devastating cerebral hemorrhage with this therapy is very possible. Therefore, computed tomography is important to rule out an intracranial hemorrhage prior to thrombolytic treatment. The treatment with thrombolytic therapy within 180 minutes of the onset of symptoms is the goal [109]. Direct intra-arterial introduction of TPA after unsuccessful treatment with intravenous TPA has shown a trend toward infarct reduction [110]. Mechanical removal of the clot is also possible. The Merci and the Penumbra systems are FDA-approved intra-arterial methods of removing clot [111]. The Penumbra system can provide safe revascularization up to 8 hours after the onset of symptoms [112,113]. Both intra-arterial thrombolysis and mechanical removal of clot should be performed only at specialist centers and under clinical trials. The Diffusion and Perfusion Imaging Evaluation for Understanding Stroke Evolution (DEFUSE) trial demonstrated the benefit of administering IV t-PA within 3 to 6 hours of stroke onset in patients with small ischemic cores on diffusion-weighted MRI and larger perfusion abnormalities (large ischemic penumbras) [114,115]. The Desmoteplase In Acute Ischemic Stroke (DIAS) trial similarly demonstrated the benefit of administering desmoteplase in patients within 3 to 9 hours of onset of acute stroke in patients with a significant mismatch (>20%) between perfusion abnormalities and ischemic core on diffusion-weighted MRI [116,117]. The European Cooperative Acute Stroke Study (ECASS 3) was a randomized trial comparing t-PA treatment with placebo in 821 stroke patients presenting 3 to 4.5 hours after symptom onset. ECASS 3 demonstrated clinical improvement with t-PA without increasing the risk of intracranial hemorrhage when compared with patients treated at less than 3 hours [118]. The Safe Implementation of Thrombolysis in Stroke Monitoring Study compared 11,865 patients treated with t-PA within 3 hours and those who received treatment from 3 to 4.5 hours. No differences between the less than 3 hour and the 3 to 4.5-hour cohort were noted in respect to symptomatic intracranial hemorrhage, mortality, or clinical improvement [119]. In 2009, the AHA/ASA issued a science advisory that extended the treatment window with t-PA to 4.5 hours with some additional exclusion criteria [120]. Therefore, the current widely used treatment for ischemic embolic stoke without evidence of hemorrhage and no other contraindication is treatment with thrombolytic agents within the first 3 hours with an extension to 4.5 hours in some patients.

   B. Following studies in 2003 demonstrating improved survival in patients treated with mild hypothermia after out-of-hospital cardiac arrest, The International Liaison Committee of Resuscitation recommended that "unconscious adult patients with spontaneous circulation after out-of-hospital cardiac arrest should be cooled to 32° to 34°C for 12 to 24 hours when the initial rhythm is ventricular fibrillation" [121–125]. In addition, clinical improvement with mild hypothermia has been shown to improve outcome in neonates of greater than 36 weeks of gestational age with hypoxic-ischemic encephalopathy when treated within 6 hours of delivery [126,127]. Although there are many animal studies in both in vitro and in vivo that demonstrate the protective effects of moderate hypothermia on focal ischemia, the clinical trials to demonstrate improved clinical outcome from their use in focal ischemia are lacking [128,129]. Studies have not shown improvement in patients cooled to 33°C during aneurysm surgery (IHAST) [130]. Clinical studies for the treatment of traumatic brain injury with mild hypothermia are conflicting with short-term mild hypothermia of 24 to 48 hours showing no clinical benefit [131–133], while others showing significant improvement with "long-term" cooling to 5 days [134,135]. Profound hypothermia to a temperature of 27°C or lower with the use of cardiopulmonary bypass has been shown to provide cerebral protection against irreversible brain injury. However, there are many systemic complications and technical difficulties that significantly limit its utilization to that of induced circulatory arrest in the operating room for major vascular surgery [136]. Animal models have demonstrated cerebral protection from hypothermia from as little as a 1°C drop in temperature [137]. Therefore, the neuroprotection from hypothermia seen in these patients is clearly not completely due to a depression of the supply/demand metabolism. Perhaps, antiapoptotic mechanisms are also responsible for this neuroprotection [138].

CLINICAL PEARL Cooling adult patients with spontaneous circulation after out-of-hospital cardiac arrest, and cooling neonates with hypoxic-ischemic encephalopathy is recommended.

C. In animal models, focal ischemic cerebral infarct size can be nearly tripled by increasing brain temperature by an average of 1.2°C [125]. Even mild postischemic hyperthermia having an onset of 24 hours after reperfusion from focal ischemic injury can worsen neurologic damage [139,140]. Therefore, hyperthermia can result in neuronal damage and must be avoided during periods of cerebral ischemia.

CLINICAL PEARL In animal models, focal ischemic cerebral infarct size can be nearly tripled by increasing brain temperature by an average of 1.2°C.

D. Hyperglycemia adversely affects the outcome after stroke. In a rat model of cerebral ischemia, hyperglycemia is associated with increased infarct volume. In stroke patients, patients who have glucose levels above 144 mg/dL have a 3-fold increase in mortality and a higher degree of disability. Possible etiologies include an increase in neutrophil infiltration, an exaggerated leukocyte–endothelial cell adhesion, and an increase in catalytic enzymes may all contribute to worsening outcome. Hyperglycemia should be avoided in neurosurgical patients [141,142].

CLINICAL PEARL In stroke patients, patients who have glucose levels above 144 mg/dL have an increase in mortality and a higher degree of disability.

VI. Summary
A. Cerebral ischemia activates numerous pathophysiologic events. Especially noted with an increase in intracellular calcium, which is associated with both necrotic and apoptotic cell death.
B. Control of physiologic variables and avoidance of both hyperthermia and hyperglycemia are important to prevent cerebral ischemia.

CLINICAL PEARL Thrombolytics after embolic stroke, mild hypothermia after cardiac arrest, and high dose barbiturates during cardiopulmonary bypass have been associated with improved clinical outcomes.

C. The role of ischemic preconditioning is being evaluated.
D. Anesthetic agents have shown cerebral protective effects in vitro and in vivo. The mechanism for cerebral protection by anesthetic agents is most likely multimodal. In vitro and animal studies support the neuroprotective properties of barbiturates, volatile anesthetics, propofol, ketamine, benzodiazepines, and lidocaine. Human clinical trials have been disappointing.

The emerging animal and human data suggesting an association between exposure to general anesthesia and long-term impairment of cognitive development needs to be further evaluated. Etomidate and perhaps nitrous oxide should be avoided in patients at risk for cerebral ischemia. There is no definitive evidence that one anesthetic agent is more protective than another.

E. Nonanesthetic agents including calcium channel blockers, magnesium, free radical scavengers, excitatory amino acid modulators, erythropoietin, trophic factors, cytokines, statins, and anti-apoptotic agents all show potential for cerebral protection. However, with the exception of the use of statins in nonhemorrhagic stroke, more research needs to be performed before these classes of drugs will be found to be clinically useful.

REFERENCES

1. Minino AM, Heron MP, Murphy SL, et al. Deaths: final data for 2004. *Natl Vital Stat Rep.* 2007;55:1–119.
2. Ng JL, Chan MT, Gelb AW. Perioperative stroke in noncardiac, nonneurosurgical surgery. *Anesthesiology.* 2011;115:879–890.
3. Tarakji KG, Sabik JF III, Bhudia SK, et al. Temporal onset, risk factors, and outcomes associated with stroke after coronary artery bypass grafting. *JAMA.* 2011;305:381–390.
4. Selim M. Perioperative stroke. *N Engl J Med.* 2007;356:706–713.
5. Nosan DK, Gomez CR, Maves MD. Perioperative stroke in patients undergoing head and neck surgery. *Ann Otol Rhinol Laryngol.* 1993;102:717–723.
6. Dahl T, Aasland J, Romundstad P, et al. Carotid endarterectomy: time-trends and results during a 20-year period. *Int Angiol.* 2006;25:241–248.
7. Taylor TN, Davis PH, Torner JC, et al. Lifetime cost of stroke in the United States. *Stroke.* 1996;27:1459–1466.
8. Harukuni I, Bhardwaj A. Mechanisms of brain injury after global cerebral ischemia. *Neurol Clin.* 2006;24:1–21.
9. Paciaroni M, Caso V, Agnelli G. The concept of ischemic penumbra in acute stroke and therapeutic opportunities. *Eur Neurol.* 2009;61:321–330.
10. Tymianski M, Tator CH. Normal and abnormal calcium homeostasis in neurons: a basis for the pathophysiology of traumatic and ischemic central nervous system injury. *Neurosurgery.* 1996;38:1176–1195.
11. Szydlowska K, Tymianski M. Calcium, ischemia and excitotoxicity. *Cell Calcium.* 2010;47:122–129.
12. Siesjo BK, Katsura KI, Kristian T, et al. Molecular mechanisms of acidosis-mediated damage. *Acta Neurochir Suppl.* 1996;66:8–14.
13. Rothman SM, Olney JW. Glutamate and the pathophysiology of hypoxic–ischemic brain damage. *Ann Neurol.* 1986;19:105–111.
14. Fisher M, Levine PH, Cohen RA. A 21-aminosteroid reduces hydrogen peroxide generation by and chemiluminescence of stimulated human leukocytes. *Stroke.* 1990;21:1435–1438.
15. Globus MY, Busto R, Lin B, et al. Detection of free radical activity during transient global ischemia and recirculation: effects of intraischemic brain temperature modulation. *J Neurochem.* 1995;65:1250–1256.
16. Lewen A, Matz P, Chan PH. Free radical pathways in CNS injury. *J Neurotrauma.* 2000;17:871–890.
17. Wang Q, Tang XN, Yenari MA. The inflammatory response in stroke. *J Neuroimmunol.* 2007;184:53–68.
18. Beray-Berthat V, Croci N, Plotkine M, et al. Polymorphonuclear neutrophils contribute to infarction and oxidative stress in the cortex but not in the striatum after ischemia-reperfusion in rats. *Brain Res.* 2003;987:32–38.
19. Hartl R, Schurer L, Schmid-Schonbein GW, et al. Experimental antileukocyte interventions in cerebral ischemia. *J Cereb Blood Flow Metab.* 1996;16:1108–1119.
20. Broughton BR, Reutens DC, Sobey CG. Apoptotic mechanisms after cerebral ischemia. *Stroke.* 2009;40:e331–e339.
21. Niu FN, Zhang X, Hu XM, et al. Targeted mutation of Fas ligand gene attenuates brain inflammation in experimental stroke. *Brain Behav Immun.* 2012;26:61–71.
22. Puyal J, Vaslin A, Mottier V, et al. Postischemic treatment of neonatal cerebral ischemia should target autophagy. *Ann Neurol.* 2009;66:378–389.
23. Gopurappilly R, Pal R, Mamidi MK, et al. Stem cells in stroke repair: current success & future prospects. *CNS Neurol Disord Drug Targets.* 2011;10:741–756.
24. Unal-Cevik I, Kilinc M, Can A, et al. Apoptotic and necrotic death mechanisms are concomitantly activated in the same cell after cerebral ischemia. *Stroke.* 2004;35:2189–2194.
25. Bickler PE, Buck LT, Feiner JR. Volatile and intravenous anesthetics decrease glutamate release from cortical brain slices during anoxia. *Anesthesiology.* 1995;83:1233–1240.
26. Bickler PE, Warner DS, Stratmann G, et al. gamma-Aminobutyric acid-A receptors contribute to isoflurane neuroprotection in organotypic hippocampal cultures. *Anesth Analg.* 2003;97:564–571, table of contents.
27. Kaneko T, Yokoyama K, Makita K. Late preconditioning with isoflurane in cultured rat cortical neurones. *Br J Anaesth.* 2005;95:662–668.
28. Zhao P, Zuo Z. Isoflurane preconditioning induces neuroprotection that is inducible nitric oxide synthase-dependent in neonatal rats. *Anesthesiology.* 2004;101:695–703.
29. Nussmeier NA, Arlund C, Slogoff S. Neuropsychiatric complications after cardiopulmonary bypass: cerebral protection by a barbiturate. *Anesthesiology.* 1986;64:165–170.
30. Lanier WL. Basic principles of cerebral protection in humans. *Liver Transpl Surg.* 1999;5:347–349.
31. Zaidan JR, Klochany A, Martin WM, et al. Effect of thiopental on neurologic outcome following coronary artery bypass grafting. *Anesthesiology.* 1991;74:406–411.

32. Warner DS, Takaoka S, Wu B, et al. Electroencephalographic burst suppression is not required to elicit maximal neuroprotection from pentobarbital in a rat model of focal cerebral ischemia. *Anesthesiology*. 1996;84:1475–1484.
33. Cattaneo AD. [Cerebral protection]. *Minerva Anestesiol*. 1993;59:403–417.
34. Yu Q, Wang H, Chen J, et al. Neuroprotections and mechanisms of inhalational anesthetics against brain ischemia. *Front Biosci (Elite Ed)*. 2010;2:1275–1298.
35. Kitano H, Kirsch JR, Hurn PD, et al. Inhalational anesthetics as neuroprotectants or chemical preconditioning agents in ischemic brain. *J Cereb Blood Flow Metab*. 2007;27:1108–1128.
36. Wang JK, Yu LN, Zhang FJ, et al. Postconditioning with sevoflurane protects against focal cerebral ischemia and reperfusion injury via PI3K/Akt pathway. *Brain Res*. 2010;1357:142–151.
37. Zhao P, Peng L, Li L, et al. Isoflurane preconditioning improves long-term neurologic outcome after hypoxic-ischemic brain injury in neonatal rats. *Anesthesiology*. 2007;107:963–970.
38. Popovic R, Liniger R, Bickler PE. Anesthetics and mild hypothermia similarly prevent hippocampal neuron death in an in vitro model of cerebral ischemia. *Anesthesiology*. 2000;92:1343–1349.
39. Liniger R, Popovic R, Sullivan B, et al. Effects of neuroprotective cocktails on hippocampal neuron death in an in vitro model of cerebral ischemia. *J Neurosurg Anesthesiol*. 2001;13:19–25.
40. Bickler PE, Zhan X, Fahlman CS. Isoflurane preconditions hippocampal neurons against oxygen-glucose deprivation: role of intracellular Ca2+ and mitogen-activated protein kinase signaling. *Anesthesiology*. 2005;103:532–539.
41. Pape M, Engelhard K, Eberspacher E, et al. The long-term effect of sevoflurane on neuronal cell damage and expression of apoptotic factors after cerebral ischemia and reperfusion in rats. *Anesth Analg*. 2006;103:173–179, table of contents.
42. Du C, Hu R, Csernansky CA, et al. Very delayed infarction after mild focal cerebral ischemia: a role for apoptosis? *J Cereb Blood Flow Metab*. 1996;16:195–201.
43. Inoue S, Drummond JC, Davis DP, et al. Combination of isoflurane and caspase inhibition reduces cerebral injury in rats subjected to focal cerebral ischemia. *Anesthesiology*. 2004;101:75–81.
44. Michenfelder JD, Sundt TM, Fode N, et al. Isoflurane when compared to enflurane and halothane decreases the frequency of cerebral ischemia during carotid endarterectomy. *Anesthesiology*. 1987;67:336–340.
45. Codaccioni JL, Velly LJ, Moubarik C, et al. Sevoflurane preconditioning against focal cerebral ischemia: inhibition of apoptosis in the face of transient improvement of neurological outcome. *Anesthesiology*. 2009;110:1271–1278.
46. Jevtovic-Todorovic V, Beals J, Benshoff N, et al. Prolonged exposure to inhalational anesthetic nitrous oxide kills neurons in adult rat brain. *Neuroscience*. 2003;122:609–616.
47. Nikizad H, Yon JH, Carter LB, et al. Early exposure to general anesthesia causes significant neuronal deletion in the developing rat brain. *Ann N Y Acad Sci*. 2007;1122:69–82.
48. Jevtovic-Todorovic V, Hartman RE, Izumi Y, et al. Early exposure to common anesthetic agents causes widespread neurodegeneration in the developing rat brain and persistent learning deficits. *J Neurosci*. 2003;23:876–882.
49. Jevtovic-Todorovic V. Developing brain and general anesthesia - is there a cause for concern? *F1000 Med Rep*. 2010;2:68.
50. Pasternak JJ, McGregor DG, Lanier WL, et al. Effect of nitrous oxide use on long-term neurologic and neuropsychological outcome in patients who received temporary proximal artery occlusion during cerebral aneurysm clipping surgery. *Anesthesiology*. 2009;110:563–573.
51. Adembri C, Venturi L, Tani A, et al. Neuroprotective effects of propofol in models of cerebral ischemia: inhibition of mitochondrial swelling as a possible mechanism. *Anesthesiology*. 2006;104:80–89.
52. Li J, Han B, Ma X, et al. The effects of propofol on hippocampal caspase-3 and Bcl-2 expression following forebrain ischemia-reperfusion in rats. *Brain Res*. 2010;1356:11–23.
53. Chen L, Xue Z, Jiang H. Effect of propofol on pathologic time-course and apoptosis after cerebral ischemia-reperfusion injury. *Acta Anaesthesiol Scand*. 2008;52:413–419.
54. Pittman JE, Sheng H, Pearlstein R, et al. Comparison of the effects of propofol and pentobarbital on neurologic outcome and cerebral infarct size after temporary focal ischemia in the rat. *Anesthesiology*. 1997;87:1139–1144.
55. Lasarzik I, Winkelheide U, Stallmann S, et al. Assessment of postischemic neurogenesis in rats with cerebral ischemia and propofol anesthesia. *Anesthesiology*. 2009;110:529–537.
56. Roach GW, Newman MF, Murkin JM, et al. Ineffectiveness of burst suppression therapy in mitigating perioperative cerebrovascular dysfunction. Multicenter Study of Perioperative Ischemia (McSPI) Research Group. *Anesthesiology*. 1999;90:1255–1264.
57. Drummond JC, Cole DJ, Patel PM, et al. Focal cerebral ischemia during anesthesia with etomidate, isoflurane, or thiopental: a comparison of the extent of cerebral injury. *Neurosurgery*. 1995;37:742–748.
58. Sano T, Patel PM, Drummond JC, et al. A comparison of the cerebral protective effects of etomidate, thiopental, and isoflurane in a model of forebrain ischemia in the rat. *Anesth Analg*. 1993;76:990–997.
59. Drummond JC, McKay LD, Cole DJ, et al. The role of nitric oxide synthase inhibition in the adverse effects of etomidate in the setting of focal cerebral ischemia in rats. *Anesth Analg*. 2005;100:841–846, table of contents.
60. Hoffman WE, Charbel FT, Edelman G, et al. Comparison of the effect of etomidate and desflurane on brain tissue gases and pH during prolonged middle cerebral artery occlusion. *Anesthesiology*. 1998;88:1188–1194.
61. Loscher W, Wlaz P, Szabo L. Focal ischemia enhances the adverse effect potential of N-methyl-D-aspartate receptor antagonists in rats. *Neurosci Lett*. 1998;240:33–36.
62. Reeker W, Werner C, Mollenberg O, et al. High-dose S(+)-ketamine improves neurological outcome following incomplete cerebral ischemia in rats. *Can J Anaesth*. 2000;47:572–578.
63. Nagels W, Demeyere R, Van HJ, et al. Evaluation of the neuroprotective effects of S(+)-ketamine during open-heart surgery. *Anesth Analg*. 2004;98:1595–1603, table of contents.
64. Artru AA. Flumazenil reversal of midazolam in dogs: dose-related changes in cerebral blood flow, metabolism, EEG, and CSF pressure. *J Neurosurg Anesthesiol*. 1989;1:46–55.

65. Niiyama S, Tanaka E, Tsuji S, et al. Neuroprotective mechanisms of lidocaine against in vitro ischemic insult of the rat hippocampal CA1 pyramidal neurons. *Neurosci Res.* 2005;53:271–278.

66. Lei B, Cottrell JE, Kass IS. Neuroprotective effect of low-dose lidocaine in a rat model of transient focal cerebral ischemia. *Anesthesiology.* 2001;95:445–451.

67. Lei B, Popp S, Capuano-Waters C, et al. Effects of delayed administration of low-dose lidocaine on transient focal cerebral ischemia in rats. *Anesthesiology.* 2002;97:1534–1540.

68. Mitchell SJ, Merry AF, Frampton C, et al. Cerebral protection by lidocaine during cardiac operations: a follow-up study. *Ann Thorac Surg.* 2009;87:820–825.

69. Catterall WA. Structure and regulation of voltage-gated Ca2+ channels. *Annu Rev Cell Dev Biol.* 2000;16:521–555.

70. Horn J, de Haan RJ, Vermeulen M, et al. Nimodipine in animal model experiments of focal cerebral ischemia: a systematic review. *Stroke.* 2001;32:2433–2438.

71. Li XM, Yang JM, Hu DH, et al. Contribution of downregulation of L-type calcium currents to delayed neuronal death in rat hippocampus after global cerebral ischemia and reperfusion. *J Neurosci.* 2007;27:5249–5259.

72. Petruk KC, West M, Mohr G, et al. Nimodipine treatment in poor-grade aneurysm patients. Results of a multicenter double-blind placebo-controlled trial. *J Neurosurg.* 1988;68:505–517.

73. Horn J, de Haan RJ, Vermeulen M, et al. Very Early Nimodipine Use in Stroke (VENUS): a randomized, double-blind, placebo-controlled trial. *Stroke.* 2001;32:461–465.

74. Lyden P, Wahlgren NG. Mechanisms of action of neuroprotectants in stroke. *J Stroke Cerebrovasc Dis.* 2000;9:9–14.

75. Muir KW. Magnesium for neuroprotection in ischaemic stroke: rationale for use and evidence of effectiveness. *CNS Drugs.* 2001;15:921–930.

76. Kang SW, Choi SK, Park E, et al. Neuroprotective effects of magnesium-sulfate on ischemic injury mediated by modulating the release of glutamate and reduced of hyperreperfusion. *Brain Res.* 2011;1371:121–128.

77. Huang CY, Liou YF, Chung SY, et al. Role of ERK signaling in the neuroprotective efficacy of magnesium sulfate treatment during focal cerebral ischemia in the gerbil cortex. *Chin J Physiol.* 2010;53:299–309.

78. Zhu HD, Martin R, Meloni B, et al. Magnesium sulfate fails to reduce infarct volume following transient focal cerebral ischemia in rats. *Neurosci Res.* 2004;49:347–353.

79. Bhat MA, Charoo BA, Bhat JI, et al. Magnesium sulfate in severe perinatal asphyxia: a randomized, placebo-controlled trial. *Pediatrics.* 2009;123:e764–e769.

80. Muir KW, Lees KR, Ford I, et al. Magnesium for acute stroke (Intravenous Magnesium Efficacy in Stroke trial): randomised controlled trial. *Lancet.* 2004;363:439–445.

81. Harrison V, Fawcus S, Jordaan E. Magnesium supplementation and perinatal hypoxia: outcome of a parallel group randomised trial in pregnancy. *BJOG.* 2007;114:994–1002.

82. Tirilazad mesylate in acute ischemic stroke: A systematic review. Tirilazad International Steering Committee. *Stroke.* 2000;31:2257–2265.

83. Lees KR, Zivin JA, Ashwood T, et al. NXY-059 for acute ischemic stroke. *N Engl J Med.* 2006;354:588–600.

84. Diener HC, Lees KR, Lyden P, et al. NXY-059 for the treatment of acute stroke: pooled analysis of the SAINT I and II Trials. *Stroke.* 2008;39:1751–1758.

85. Muir KW, Lees KR. Excitatory amino acid antagonists for acute stroke. *Cochrane Database Syst Rev.* 2003;CD001244.

86. Warach S, Kaufman D, Chiu D, et al. Effect of the Glycine Antagonist Gavestinel on cerebral infarcts in acute stroke patients, a randomized placebo-controlled trial: The GAIN MRI Substudy. *Cerebrovasc Dis.* 2006;21:106–111.

87. Yuen CM, Leu S, Lee FY, et al. Erythropoietin markedly attenuates brain infarct size and improves neurological function in the rat. *J Investig Med.* 2010;58:893–904.

88. Minnerup J, Heidrich J, Rogalewski A, et al. The efficacy of erythropoietin and its analogues in animal stroke models: a meta-analysis. *Stroke.* 2009;40:3113–3120.

89. He JS, Huang ZL, Yang H, et al. [Early use of recombinant human erythropoietin promotes neurobehavioral development in preterm infants]. *Zhongguo Dang Dai Er Ke Za Zhi.* 2008;10:586–588.

90. Wang YJ, Pan KL, Zhao XL, et al. [Therapeutic effects of erythropoietin on hypoxic-ischemic encephalopathy in neonates]. *Zhongguo Dang Dai Er Ke Za Zhi.* 2011;13:855–858.

91. Ehrenreich H, Hasselblatt M, Dembowski C, et al. Erythropoietin therapy for acute stroke is both safe and beneficial. *Mol Med.* 2002;8:495–505.

92. Ehrenreich H, Weissenborn K, Prange H, et al. Recombinant human erythropoietin in the treatment of acute ischemic stroke. *Stroke.* 2009;40:e647–e656.

93. Jia L, Chopp M, Zhang L, et al. Erythropoietin in combination of tissue plasminogen activator exacerbates brain hemorrhage when treatment is initiated 6 hours after stroke. *Stroke.* 2010;41:2071–2076.

94. Meistrell ME III, Botchkina GI, Wang H, et al. Tumor necrosis factor is a brain damaging cytokine in cerebral ischemia. *Shock.* 1997;8:341–348.

95. Potrovita I, Zhang W, Burkly L, et al. Tumor necrosis factor-like weak inducer of apoptosis-induced neurodegeneration. *J Neurosci.* 2004;24:8237–8244.

96. Tsai NW, Lin TK, Chang WN, et al. Statin pre-treatment is associated with lower platelet activity and favorable outcome in patients with acute non-cardio-embolic ischemic stroke. *Crit Care.* 2011;15:R163.

97. O'Regan C, Wu P, Arora P, et al. Statin therapy in stroke prevention: a meta-analysis involving 121,000 patients. *Am J Med.* 2008;121:24–33.

98. Gomis M, Ois A, Rodriguez-Campello A, et al. Outcome of intracerebral haemorrhage patients pre-treated with statins. *Eur J Neurol.* 2010;17:443–448.

99. Barone FC. Endogenous brain protection: models, gene expression, and mechanisms. *Methods Mol Med.* 2005;104:105–184.

100. Bhuiyan MI, Kim YJ. Mechanisms and prospects of ischemic tolerance induced by cerebral preconditioning. *Int Neurourol J.* 2010;14:203–212.

101. Weih M, Kallenberg K, Bergk A, et al. Attenuated stroke severity after prodromal TIA: a role for ischemic tolerance in the brain? *Stroke.* 1999;30:1851–1854.

102. Wegener S, Gottschalk B, Jovanovic V, et al. Transient ischemic attacks before ischemic stroke: preconditioning the human brain? A multicenter magnetic resonance imaging study. *Stroke.* 2004;35:616–621.

103. Ren C, Gao X, Steinberg GK, et al. Limb remote-preconditioning protects against focal ischemia in rats and contradicts the dogma of therapeutic time windows for preconditioning. *Neuroscience.* 2008;151:1099–1103.

104. Dave KR, Saul I, Prado R, et al. Remote organ ischemic preconditioning protect brain from ischemic damage following asphyxial cardiac arrest. *Neurosci Lett.* 2006;404:170–175.

105. Zhang Y, Zhen Y, Dong Y, et al. Anesthetic propofol attenuates the isoflurane-induced caspase-3 activation and Aβ oligomerization. *PLoS One.* 2011;6:e27019.

106. Kwiatkowski TG, Libman RB, Frankel M, et al. Effects of tissue plasminogen activator for acute ischemic stroke at one year. National Institute of Neurological Disorders and Stroke Recombinant Tissue Plasminogen Activator Stroke Study Group. *N Engl J Med.* 1999;340:1781–1787.

107. Wardlaw JM, Warlow CP, Counsell C. Systematic review of evidence on thrombolytic therapy for acute ischaemic stroke. *Lancet.* 1997;350:607–614.

108. Tissue plasminogen activator for acute ischemic stroke. The National Institute of Neurological Disorders and Stroke rt-PA Stroke Study Group. *N Engl J Med.* 1995;333:1581–1587.

109. Adams HP Jr, Adams RJ, Brott T, et al. Guidelines for the early management of patients with ischemic stroke: A scientific statement from the Stroke Council of the American Stroke Association. *Stroke.* 2003;34:1056–1083.

110. Sen S, Huang DY, Akhavan O, et al. IV vs. IA TPA in acute ischemic stroke with CT angiographic evidence of major vessel occlusion: a feasibility study. *Neurocrit Care.* 2009;11:76–81.

111. Frendl A, Csiba L. Pharmacological and non-pharmacological recanalization strategies in acute ischemic stroke. *Front Neurol.* 2011;2:32.

112. Menon BK, Hill MD, Eesa M, et al. Initial experience with the Penumbra Stroke System for recanalization of large vessel occlusions in acute ischemic stroke. *Neuroradiology.* 2011;53:261–266.

113. The penumbra pivotal stroke trial: safety and effectiveness of a new generation of mechanical devices for clot removal in intracranial large vessel occlusive disease. *Stroke.* 2009;40:2761–2768.

114. Marks MP, Olivot JM, Kemp S, et al. Patients with acute stroke treated with intravenous tPA 3-6 hours after stroke onset: correlations between MR angiography findings and perfusion- and diffusion-weighted imaging in the DEFUSE study. *Radiology.* 2008;249:614–623.

115. Hacke W, Kaste M, Bluhmki E, et al. Thrombolysis with alteplase 3 to 4.5 hours after acute ischemic stroke. *N Engl J Med.* 2008;359:1317–1329.

116. Dafer RM, Biller J. Desmoteplase in the treatment of acute ischemic stroke. *Expert Rev Neurother.* 2007;7:333–337.

117. Hacke W, Albers G, Al-Rawi Y, et al. The Desmoteplase in Acute Ischemic Stroke Trial (DIAS): a phase II MRI-based 9-hour window acute stroke thrombolysis trial with intravenous desmoteplase. *Stroke.* 2005;36:66–73.

118. Bluhmki E, Chamorro A, Davalos A, et al. Stroke treatment with alteplase given 3.0-4.5 h after onset of acute ischaemic stroke (ECASS III): additional outcomes and subgroup analysis of a randomised controlled trial. *Lancet Neurol.* 2009;8:1095–1102.

119. Wahlgren N, Ahmed N, Davalos A, et al. Thrombolysis with alteplase for acute ischaemic stroke in the Safe Implementation of Thrombolysis in Stroke-Monitoring Study (SITS-MOST): an observational study. *Lancet.* 2007;369:275–282.

120. Del Zoppo GJ, Saver JL, Jauch EC, et al. Expansion of the time window for treatment of acute ischemic stroke with intravenous tissue plasminogen activator: a science advisory from the American Heart Association/American Stroke Association. *Stroke.* 2009;40:2945–2948.

121. Bernard SA, Smith K, Cameron P, et al. Induction of therapeutic hypothermia by paramedics after resuscitation from out-of-hospital ventricular fibrillation cardiac arrest: a randomized controlled trial. *Circulation.* 2010;122:737–742.

122. Bernard SA, Gray TW, Buist MD, et al. Treatment of comatose survivors of out-of-hospital cardiac arrest with induced hypothermia. *N Engl J Med.* 2002;346:557–563.

123. Nolan JP, Morley PT, Hoek TL, et al. Therapeutic hypothermia after cardiac arrest. An advisory statement by the Advancement Life support Task Force of the International Liaison committee on Resuscitation. *Resuscitation.* 2003;57:231–235.

124. Soar J, Perkins GD, Abbas G, et al. European Resuscitation Council Guidelines for Resuscitation 2010 Section 8. Cardiac arrest in special circumstances: Electrolyte abnormalities, poisoning, drowning, accidental hypothermia, hyperthermia, asthma, anaphylaxis, cardiac surgery, trauma, pregnancy, electrocution. *Resuscitation.* 2010;81:1400–1433.

125. Kammersgaard LP, Jorgensen HS, Rungby JA, et al. Admission body temperature predicts long-term mortality after acute stroke: the Copenhagen Stroke Study. *Stroke.* 2002;33:1759–1762.

126. Shankaran S, Laptook AR, Ehrenkranz RA, et al. Whole-body hypothermia for neonates with hypoxic-ischemic encephalopathy. *N Engl J Med.* 2005;353:1574–1584.

127. Shankaran S. Neonatal encephalopathy: treatment with hypothermia. *J Neurotrauma.* 2009;26:437–443.

128. Huh PW, Belayev L, Zhao W, et al. Comparative neuroprotective efficacy of prolonged moderate intraischemic and postischemic hypothermia in focal cerebral ischemia. *J Neurosurg.* 2000;92:91–99.

129. Ridenour TR, Warner DS, Todd MM, et al. Mild hypothermia reduces infarct size resulting from temporary but not permanent focal ischemia in rats. *Stroke.* 1992;23:733–738.

130. Todd MM, Hindman BJ, Clarke WR, et al. Mild intraoperative hypothermia during surgery for intracranial aneurysm. *N Engl J Med.* 2005;352:135–145.

131. Clifton GL, Miller ER, Choi SC, et al. Lack of effect of induction of hypothermia after acute brain injury. *N Engl J Med.* 2001;344:556–563.

132. Clifton GL, Valadka A, Zygun D, et al. Very early hypothermia induction in patients with severe brain injury (the National Acute Brain Injury Study: Hypothermia II): a randomised trial. *Lancet Neurol.* 2011;10:131–139.

133. Davies AR. Hypothermia improves outcome from traumatic brain injury. *Crit Care Resusc.* 2005;7:238–243.

134. Jiang JY, Lyeth BG, Clifton GL, et al. Relationship between body and brain temperature in traumatically brain-injured rodents. *J Neurosurg.* 1991;74:492–496.

135. Qiu WS, Liu WG, Shen H, et al. Therapeutic effect of mild hypothermia on severe traumatic head injury. *Chin J Traumatol.* 2005;8:27–32.

136. Alam HB, Duggan M, Li Y, et al. Putting life on hold-for how long? Profound hypothermic cardiopulmonary bypass in a Swine model of complex vascular injuries. *J Trauma.* 2008;64:912–922.

137. Wass CT, Lanier WL, Hofer RE, et al. Temperature changes of > or = 1 degree C alter functional neurologic outcome and histopathology in a canine model of complete cerebral ischemia. *Anesthesiology.* 1995;83:325–335.

138. Yenari MA, Iwayama S, Cheng D, et al. Mild hypothermia attenuates cytochrome c release but does not alter Bcl-2 expression or caspase activation after experimental stroke. *J Cereb Blood Flow Metab.* 2002;22:29–38.

139. Kim Y, Busto R, Dietrich WD, et al. Delayed postischemic hyperthermia in awake rats worsens the histopathological outcome of transient focal cerebral ischemia. *Stroke.* 1996;27:2274–2280.

140. Baena RC, Busto R, Dietrich WD, et al. Hyperthermia delayed by 24 hours aggravates neuronal damage in rat hippocampus following global ischemia. *Neurology.* 1997;48:768–773.

141. Martin A, Rojas S, Chamorro A, et al. Why does acute hyperglycemia worsen the outcome of transient focal cerebral ischemia? Role of corticosteroids, inflammation, and protein O-glycosylation. *Stroke.* 2006;37:1288–1295.

142. Capes SE, Hunt D, Malmberg K, et al. Stress hyperglycemia and prognosis of stroke in nondiabetic and diabetic patients: a systematic overview. *Stroke.* 2001;32:2426–2432.

24

Anesthetic-induced Neurotoxicity

Andreas W. Loepke and Mary Ellen McCann

KEY POINTS

1. Prolonged exposure to most general anesthetics and sedatives administered to young mammals, including NMDA inhibitors (ketamine, nitrous oxide) and GABAA agonists (volatile anesthetics, barbiturates, benzodiazepines, propofol), has produced neurotoxic effects.
2. Detrimental effects have been observed on neuronal survival, neuro- and gliogenesis, dendrite formation, and long-term neurocognitive function.
3. Deleterious consequences are dose dependent and most often occur following prolonged or repeated exposures to general anesthetics.
4. Prolonged opioid exposure early in life can mimic many of the deleterious effects of general anesthetics; however, the comparative toxic potency remains unclear.
5. These abnormal findings peak during very early stages of brain development. The equivalent developmental state of the human brain remains controversial, complicating easy human translation of animal studies.
6. Several human epidemiologic studies have shown a link between anesthetics before the age of 4 years, and developmental and behavioral abnormalities later in childhood.

(continued)

> **7** At this point in time, there is not enough evidence for general anesthetic neurotoxicity in humans to recommend any changes in clinical practice.

I. Introduction. General anesthetics have been used for more than 160 years to facilitate surgery and to mitigate distress during painful procedures. Thus, millions of children worldwide are exposed to these agents every year. However, animal studies have uncovered potentially deleterious effects of prolonged anesthetic exposure on the developing brain [1,2]. While translation of these animal studies to pediatric anesthesia practice remains very difficult, the findings have led to serious concerns regarding the safe use of anesthetics in small children.

II. Effects of exposure to anesthetics, sedatives, and analgesics on the developing animal brain

1

  A. Deleterious effects of anesthetic exposure. Thus far, over 250 studies in immature animal models, including chicks, mice, rats, guinea pigs, pigs, and nonhuman primates, have shown exposure to anesthetic drugs and sedatives, such as desflurane, enflurane, halothane, isoflurane, sevoflurane, nitrous oxide, chloral hydrate, clonazepam, diazepam, ketamine, midazolam, pentobarbital, phenobarbital, and propofol may be deleterious (reviewed in [3]).

2

   1. Apoptotic cell death (and long-term viability). Apoptosis, or programmed cell death, which is a normal part of mammalian development, is increased following exposure to anesthesia in many immature animals.

   a. Normal neuroapoptosis eliminates up to 70% of all brain cells during development.

   b. The period of maximum susceptibility to anesthetic-induced neuroapoptosis is species specific, but generally corresponds to early stages of brain development.

   c. The window of vulnerability can be quite narrow. For example, rat pups younger than 1 day of age or older than 10 days are seemingly unaffected by anesthetic-induced neuroapoptosis in several forebrain structures [4].

3

   d. Anesthetic-induced neuroapoptosis is dose- and exposure time-dependent.

   e. The long-term effects of anesthetic-induced neurotoxic injury on subsequent neuronal density is controversial. One rat study showed a permanent decrease in neuronal density in adult rats, but another study showed no diminution, suggesting species- or drug-specific variability.

   f. Long-term neurocognitive impairment has been observed in several animal studies, while other studies did not detect neurologic abnormalities. Furthermore, most of the studies showing impairment have demonstrated neurocognitive deficits in discrete domains of testing, especially hippocampal learning, rather than global deficits.

2

   2. Neurogenesis and gliogenesis

   a. Abnormalities in neurogenesis—both reductions in neuronal stem cells and decreases in neuronal proliferation— have been observed in immature rats following prolonged exposure to isoflurane.

   b. Exposure to 24 hours of 3% isoflurane has been shown to impair growth and to delay maturation of astrocytes.

2

   3. Dendritic architectural alterations

   a. Ketamine, midazolam, propofol, desflurane, isoflurane, and sevoflurane can alter dendritic branching and synaptic density.

   b. Exposure to anesthesia during the first 2 weeks of life decreases synaptic and dendritic spine density whereas exposure after 2 weeks increases the number of dendritic spines in rodents [5].

   c. The functional significance of these findings and their permanence are unknown, with some studies showing no lasting effects later in life.

4

  B. Effects of opioid exposure on brain development. One study comparing an isoflurane-based anesthetic with a high-dose fentanyl anesthetic in newborn piglets found a dramatically reduced rate of neuroapoptotic cell death using the opioid versus isoflurane [6]. However, while not as widely studied as anesthetics, prolonged opioid exposure in immature animals can also lead to neurologic abnormalities.

1. **Opioid-induced apoptotic cell death.** Exposure to opioid receptor agonists in immature neurons can lead to several abnormalities (see [3] for details), including mitochondrial dysfunction, diminished neuronal viability, increased apoptosis, and DNA fragmentation. Moreover, apoptotic cell death has also been observed in neurons and microglia, but not astrocytes in human fetal brain cell cultures.

2. **Long-term neurologic functional impairments.** Several studies have observed long-term learning impairment in adult animals following prolonged morphine exposure early in life. Moreover, altered pain responses in adulthood were linked to exposure to the opioid agonists morphine, fentanyl, or methadone, early in life.

3. **Abnormal alterations in neurotrophic factors.** Similar to anesthetics, opioid receptor agonists, including buprenorphine and methadone, have also been found to decrease nerve growth factors in the immature brain.

4. **Alterations in opioid receptor density.** Diminished μ-receptor densities have been demonstrated immediately following prolonged morphine exposures in immature rats, and have been found to extend into adulthood.

C. **Anesthesia-induced neuroprotection**

1. Many general anesthetics (propofol, ketamine, isoflurane, sevoflurane, and xenon) have been shown to have protective effects in neuronal preservation in the setting of hypoxia and brain ischemia in adult animals.

2. Several studies using immature brain ischemia models have shown an improvement in neuronal survival by anesthetics [7,8].

CLINICAL PEARL   It is important to remember that untreated pain also causes neurologic abnormalities in animals and humans, demanding adequate anesthesia and analgesia in young children undergoing painful procedures.

III. **Effects of untreated pain and stress on the newborn animal brain.** Extensive evidence from laboratory and clinical studies has demonstrated that unopposed pain and stress can initiate deleterious effects in the developing brain that may be long lasting.

A. **Deleterious effects of noxious stimulation.** Painful stimulation and separation stress have been found to not only cause short-term alterations in the immature brain, but also to carry long-term effects into adulthood. Moreover, administration of anesthetics/analgesics may be able to diminish some of these deleterious effects caused by pain.

1. **Apoptotic cell death.** Immediately following repeated painful injections, extensive neuronal cell death was observed in neonatal rats [9]. Preemptive analgesia with small doses of ketamine ameliorated the deleterious effects of unopposed pain [9].

2. **Long-term neurologic consequences**

a. Repetitive painful skin lacerations can lead to long-term, local sensory hyperinnervation.

b. Inflammatory pain early in life resulted in hyperalgesia and lasting changes in nociceptive circuitry of the adult dorsal horn. Moreover, rat pups receiving repeated painful injections into the paw subsequently developed a generalized thermal hypoalgesia.

c. Altered behavior and cognitive function, decreased pain thresholds, increased vulnerability to stress and anxiety disorders or chronic pain syndromes have all been observed in adult animals exposed to painful stimulations early in life.

d. In addition to pain, adverse emotional experiences early in life can also induce long-lasting abnormalities, such as imbalances of the inhibitory nervous system, impairment of normal development of the nociceptive system, long-term behavioral changes, and persistent learning impairment.

IV. **Possible mechanisms of anesthetic-induced neuronal cell death.** Several hypotheses have been proposed to explain the neurotoxic effects of anesthetics, especially neuroapoptosis. Apoptotic cell death is vital to brain development to rid the organism of abnormal or superfluous cells and to prevent tumor formation. Numerous pathways, both promoting and preventing apoptosis, need to be balanced to promote cellular survival; anesthetics may interfere with several of these pathways, thereby altering this equilibrium and ultimately leading to cell death.

A. Abnormal neuronal inhibition. The most commonly advanced hypothesis for the mechanism of anesthetic neurotoxicity is that of an anesthesia-induced inhibition at the NMDA receptor and/or stimulation at the GABAA receptor leading to abnormal inhibition in immature neurons during a vulnerable developmental period, thereby triggering the cell's inherent apoptotic cell death machinery [10]. Incidentally, both GABA and NMDA receptor-mediated activities are essential during brain development. However, while NMDA-antagonist xenon and hypothermia increase the depth of anesthesia and thereby neuronal inhibition, they do not increase neuronal cell death, but may actually protect from the neurotoxic effects of other anesthetics [11,12].

B. Excitotoxicity

1. Another theory posits that an upregulation of NMDA receptor expression during a prolonged exposure to an NMDA antagonist, such as ketamine, exposes neurons to excitotoxic injury by endogenous glutamate immediately following the anesthetic's withdrawal [13].

2. In the immature brain, GABA is an excitatory rather than inhibitory neurotransmitter. Accordingly, GABA-ergic agents may cause excitation and even seizures due to the elevated intracellular chloride concentration resulting from the immature chloride transporter NKCC1, which produces chloride efflux leading to cell depolarization. GABA switches to its inhibitory mode once expression of the mature chloride transporter KCC2 intercedes.

C. Interference with trophic factors. The trophic factor BDNF is integral to neuronal survival, growth, and differentiation. Isoflurane-induced apoptosis in newborn mice has been found to be triggered by interference with BDNF formation [14].

D. Re-entry into cell cycle. Some experimental models of neurodegeneration have implicated the re-entry of postmitotic neurons into the cell cycle in contributing to cell death. Accordingly, ketamine exposure has been found to induce aberrant cell cycle re-entry, leading to apoptotic cell death in the developing rat brain.

E. Mitochondrial function. Anesthetics have recently been found to impair mitochondrial morphogenesis, to decrease mitochondrial density, and to lead to long-lasting disturbances in inhibitory synaptic transmission following a combined exposure to midazolam, nitrous oxide, and isoflurane in newborn rats.

F. Cytoskeletal integrity. Cytoskeletal destabilization as well as neuronal and astroglial depolymerization of actin, a major component of the cytoskeleton of all eukaryotic cells that participates in important cellular processes, such as cell signaling, cellular division, and motility as well as dendrite formation, have been detected in immature rodents following isoflurane exposure and may play a role in the observed apoptotic brain cell death.

V. Potential mitigating strategies. Since all currently routinely used anesthetics have demonstrated neurotoxic properties, extensive research efforts have been spent on finding alternative agents or mitigating treatments.

A. Preconditioning. Anesthetics, including isoflurane, can diminish cellular injury when administered briefly prior to an ischemic insult. This concept, called preconditioning, was also demonstrated by a short preconditioning exposure to isoflurane in rat's primary cortical neurons 4 hours prior to a prolonged exposure, which protected from the deleterious effects of the subsequent prolonged anesthetic exposure.

B. Protective drug therapy. Several drugs and endogenous hormones have been tested in conjunction with anesthetics to examine their protective properties for anesthesia-induced neurotoxicity.

1. **Caffeine.** In order to provide respiratory and neurologic stimulation during anesthetic exposure, caffeine has been studied as a protective agent during isoflurane exposure in newborn mice. However, preliminary results suggest that caffeine augmented, rather than ameliorated, the isoflurane-induced neuroapoptosis and also promoted neuronal cell death when administered by itself, questioning its role as a protective agent.

2. **L-carnitine.** L-carnitine was able to attenuate neuronal apoptosis caused by a 6-hour exposure to isoflurane and nitrous oxide in 7-day-old rat pups.

3. **β-estradiol.** The deleterious effects of a prolonged exposure to midazolam, isoflurane, and nitrous oxide on neuronal survival were successfully treated with β-estradiol supplementation. Similarly, phenobarbital-induced neuroapoptosis was significantly reduced by coadministration of β-estradiol in young rats.

4. **Melatonin.** Administration of the natural hormone melatonin was able to protect from the deleterious effects of the combination exposure to midazolam, isoflurane, and nitrous oxide in newborn rats.

5. **Jasplakinolide or TAT-Pep5.** Inhibition of the RhoA receptor or prevention of cytoskeletal depolymerization with either jasplakinolide or TAT-Pep5 has been found to attenuate isoflurane- or propofol-mediated neuroapoptosis.

6. **Lithium.** A protective strategy successfully tested in mouse pups exposed to ketamine or propofol was lithium, which abolished the anesthetic-induced neuroapoptosis in cortex and caudate/putamen. However, lithium has been labeled harmful to the human fetus and may cause neurocognitive impairment in young children.

7. **Pilocarpine.** Preliminary results in neonatal mice seem to suggest that pilocarpine may reduce neuroapoptosis induced by isoflurane and midazolam, while augmenting neurotoxicity caused by the NMDA-antagonist phencyclidine. However, pilocarpine's safety in young children is questionable due to its proconvulsant activity observed in animal studies.

8. **tPA, plasmin, p75NTR inhibition.** In the context of increasing the trophic factor BDNF, the coadministration of tissue-plasminogen activator, plasmin, or the pharmacologic inhibition of the neurotrophic receptor p75NTR during isoflurane exposure has been successfully studied to prevent isoflurane's neurotoxic effects [16].

9. **Xestospongin C.** In an in vitro study, the IP3 receptor-antagonist xestospongin C significantly ameliorated isoflurane cytotoxicity in primary cortical neurons.

10. **Bumetanide.** The diuretic bumetanide significantly decreased seizures in immature rats and caused a significant decrease in expression of activated caspase-3, a marker for apoptosis.

C. **Hypothermia.** Whole-body hypothermia of less than 30°C may protect from the neuroapoptotic ramifications of isoflurane or ketamine in neonatal mice. There are, however, significant difficulties in administering hypothermia to human infants including increased blood loss, prolonged postanesthetic recovery, and increased risk of surgical site infections.

D. **Alternative anesthetics/sedatives**

1. **Xenon.** The NMDA-antagonist xenon has been studied regarding its neurotoxic potential and has been found to only hold limited toxic potency [12]. Moreover, when administered in conjunction with isoflurane, xenon was able to mitigate some of the volatile anesthetic's toxic effects [12]. However, xenon has limited anesthetic potency compared with volatile anesthetics and due to its scarcity, remains very expensive.

2. **Dexmedetomidine.** The α_2-agonist dexmedetomidine has sedative properties and has been investigated regarding its toxic and protective properties in the developing brain. The encouraging finding from thus far limited in vitro and in vivo studies has been that repetitive injections of dexmedetomidine did not cause any neuroapoptosis and inhibited isoflurane-induced neuroapoptosis [15]. Moreover, dexmedetomidine also prevented memory impairment caused by isoflurane. However, because of its limited anesthetic potency, dexmedetomidine cannot be used as a sole anesthetic agent.

3. **Ketamine.** When given in large doses, or repeatedly over a prolonged period of time, ketamine is associated with marked apoptotic neuronal cell death. However, in lower analgesic doses, this NMDA antagonist ameliorated the immediate neuroapoptotic response to repetitive inflammatory pain and prevented subsequent pain-induced neurocognitive deficits [9]. Moreover, ketamine as well as other anesthetics have also been found to promote prosurvival cell proteins and to protect neurons exposed to ischemic stresses.

VI. Human applicability of animal data. The human applicability of the disturbing findings of anesthetic neurotoxicity in animal models remains unclear. Several differences exist between animal studies and pediatric anesthesia practice.

A. Experimental versus clinical conditions. Experimental conditions deviate from clinical practice in a variety of factors. Thus far, no animal model has been developed that completely replicates conditions during pediatric surgery and anesthesia.

1. Airway management. A majority of animal models rely on spontaneous breathing with a natural airway and not the instrumented airway, and controlled ventilation used during pediatric surgery, predisposing animals to adverse respiratory events.

2. Physiologic monitoring. Continuous physiologic monitoring, including electrocardiography, pulse oximetry, capnography, as well as temperature and blood pressure measurements are not routinely performed during animal studies, especially not in small rodent models. Several animal studies have shown abnormal blood gas analyses such as metabolic and respiratory acidosis.

3. Exposure times. Exposure times in animal studies are often protracted exposures of up to 24 hours. These studies may be more relevant to human intensive care sedation practices rather than the operating room.

B. Exposure time relative to biologic events

1. Relative life expectancies. Some suggestions exist that expressing the anesthetic exposure time as a fraction of the organism's life span would approximate a 6-hour anesthetic exposure in mice to an anesthetic lasting more than 2 weeks in humans. However, this argument is probably an oversimplification, given the fact that the rate of cellular processes is more closely related among species.

2. Comparative duration of brain development. However, since human brain development occurs at a much slower pace than in any other species, similar exposure times could have different effects on potential susceptibility and ability for postexposure repair among species. For example, the brain reaches adult size at 20 days of age in rats, 3 years of age in rhesus monkeys, 7 years of age in chimpanzees, and not until 15 years of age in humans. Accordingly, given the dramatic plasticity of the developing brain, it seems conceivable that slower growth rates may leave the brain more time for repair.

3. Cell cycle duration. Even on a cellular level, significant differences exist between humans and animals; during cortical neurogenesis, cell cycle duration is approximately 17 hours in mice, 28 hours in macaque monkeys, and 36 hours in humans. It therefore seems an oversimplification to equate anesthetic exposure times 1:1 between humans and animals.

C. Equivalency of anesthetic drug doses

1. Inhalational anesthetic doses used in animal research are mostly comparable between animals and humans.

2. Injectable drug doses are typically 3- to 12-fold higher in animals to achieve similar planes of anesthesia. The dose of ketamine needed to anesthetize a rhesus monkey infant is more than 10 times of what is needed to anesthetize a human infant. Accordingly, plasma levels of drugs are much higher in the animal studies, possibly exaggerating the neurotoxic effects of intravenous anesthetics.

D. Comparative brain developmental states. The potentially vulnerable period for anesthetic-induced neuroapoptosis during human development has not been identified. Rapid brain growth occurs in humans between the third fetal trimester and the first 24 months of life. Neuroinformatic approaches for predicting human vulnerability based on animal data suggest that the human brain may be most susceptible before birth.

1. Small rodents. Peak vulnerability for several forebrain structures in rodents centers on postnatal day 7, equating to 20 to 22 weeks of gestation in human fetuses.

2. Nonhuman primates. Susceptibility to ketamine-induced neurotoxicity has been observed in macaques at 122 days of gestation and at postnatal day 5, but not in 35-day-old animals [13]. The brain maturational state in early postnatal monkeys is closer to the term and early postnatal human neonate and studies in these animals may therefore be more applicable to pediatric anesthesia than current rodent studies [17].

E. **Assessment of neurocognitive outcomes**
   1. Assessment of neurocognitive performance in animal models largely relies on hippocampal-dependent memory tasks.
   2. There, currently, is no evidence to suggest these same domains are affected in children exposed to general anesthesia.

CLINICAL PEARL The choice of timing of surgery should depend on the child's medical condition, the projected surgical outcomes and the immediate anesthetic concerns rather than theoretic concerns about anesthetic neurotoxicity. If parents or practitioners seek to delay truly elective surgery, unfortunately no safe duration for postponing the procedure can be rationally recommended based on the currently available data.

VII. **Outcome in children exposed to surgery with anesthesia**

6

A. **Cohort studies of prenatal exposure**
   1. One study in 159 Japanese full-term infants exposed to nitrous oxide during the last stages of delivery demonstrated subtle neurologic abnormalities on postnatal day 5, such as weaker habituation to sound, stronger muscular tension, fewer smiles, and resistance to cuddling, compared with unexposed infants.
   2. Two smaller case-control studies by another group examined the effects of unspecified general or local anesthetic exposure during pregnancy and found abnormal visual pattern preference during the first week of life and vocabulary IQ scores at a 4-year follow-up. However, less than 15 patients were available for follow-up.
   3. However, a more recent, large epidemiologic study based on a birth cohort of over 5,000 babies from Olmstead County in Minnesota found that children exposed to general anesthesia for cesarean section were not more likely to develop learning disabilities later in life, compared with those born by vaginal delivery [18]. Interestingly, the risk of learning disabilities was lowest in children born by cesarean section with regional anesthesia. However, a separate study using this same database subsequently found no impact of neuraxial labor analgesia on the incidence of childhood learning disabilities.

B. **Cohort studies of neonatal and early childhood exposure**
   1. **Difficulties with cohort studies**
      a. Outcome of interest in most studies was surgery rather than anesthesia
      b. Confounders for these studies include the following:
         (1) Perioperative effects of surgery including adjunctive-inspired oxygen or the surgical inflammatory response may be neurotoxic.
         (2) Premorbid pathology: It is likely that sicker babies were treated surgically rather than medically for some conditions (necrotizing enterocolitis, patent ductus arteriosus).
   2. The Victorian Infant Collaborative Study group, in a case control study, found that infants born less than 27 weeks postconception suffered from an increased incidence of neurologic abnormalities, including cerebral palsy, blindness, deafness, and abnormal intelligence following surgery for ligation of a patent ductus arteriosus, inguinal hernia repair, laparotomy, neurosurgery, or tracheotomy.
   3. Another large study involving almost 4,000 extremely low birth weight infants found that those treated surgically for necrotizing enterocolitis rather than peritoneal drainage fared worse with a higher incidence of cerebral palsy and lower scores in the Bayley Scales of Infant Development 2 [19]. These findings have generally been corroborated by other, smaller studies.
   4. In contrast, a study examining children following neonatal repair of an isolated tracheoesophageal fistula did not observe abnormal intelligence quotient measurements compared with the general population in late childhood. A majority of the infants in this study were born at term, however, which may have impacted the observed incidence of developmental delays.

5. Several outcome studies in children who underwent neonatal cardiac surgeries have demonstrated an increased incidence of neurobehavioral abnormalities, including cerebral palsy, diminished intelligence, speech and language impairments, and motor dysfunction (see [20] for review). A prospective randomized trial comparing total circulatory arrest versus low flow cardiopulmonary bypass for the arterial switch operation followed 155 patients and performed neurologic assessments at 1, 2.5, 4, and 8 years of age. This study found that, although the mean scores for most outcomes were within normal limits, neurodevelopmental status of the cohort as a whole to be below expectations for academic achievement, fine motor function, visual spatial skills, working memory, hypothesis generating and testing, sustained attention, and higher order language skills.

C. **Epidemiologic studies specifically examining anesthetic exposure**

1. Studies demonstrating a positive correlation with anesthesia exposure and neurodevelopmental deficits

   a. In a large retrospective cohort study of 5,357 children, 593 children were identified as having received one or more general anesthetics before the age of 4 years [21]. Significant reading, written language, and math learning abnormalities were found in children who had been exposed to two or more general anesthetics, but not if they had only received a single exposure. The risk of learning disabilities also increased with the cumulative duration of the exposure. Limitations of this study included the lack of pulse oximetry monitoring and the predominant use of halothane, a volatile gas associated with cardiac depression and no longer utilized in pediatric anesthesia. Using the same population cohort, similar results were recently reported for children undergoing anesthesia before the age of 2 years.

   b. In a study comparing over 5,000 matched controls with 383 patients who underwent inguinal herniorrhaphy using a database developed from New York State Medicaid billing codes, an almost twofold increase in developmental and behavioral abnormalities was observed, even after controlling for gender and low birth weight. Another epidemiologic study from this same data set compared neurologic outcomes of 304 children with no risk factors for neurodevelopmental difficulties exposed to anesthesia before the age of 3 years with a cohort of 10,146 siblings and found a 60% greater incidence of developmental or behavioral problems in children exposed to general anesthesia [22]. However, when siblings were matched with their twins to correct for environmental and genetic factors, there was no association between anesthesia and developmental and behavioral issues [22].

   c. A pilot study to test the feasibility of using a validated child behavior checklist for parents in 314 children who had urologic surgery determined that there was more disturbed neurobehavioral development, albeit statistically non-significant, in children who underwent surgery prior to 24 months, compared with those who underwent surgery after 24 months of age.

2. Studies demonstrating no correlation with anesthesia exposure and neurodevelopmental deficits

   a. A study comparing the academic performance of 2,689 children who had undergone inguinal herniorrhaphy in infancy to a randomly selected, age-matched population control of 14,575 children derived from the Danish Civil Registration System from 1986 to 1990 found that after adjusting for known confounders, there was no statistically significant difference between exposure and the control group [23]. These results may not come as a surprise given the fact that several other epidemiologic studies were unable to detect any effect following a single anesthetic exposure.

   b. Similarly, using the Dutch Twin Registry, Bartels et al. [24] did not find any difference in the educational achievement of monozygotic twins who were discordant in their exposure to general anesthesia, meaning one twin was exposed to anesthesia, while the other was not. Importantly, the fact that concordantly unexposed twin pair fared better in this study would suggest an underlying genetic predisposition to adverse outcomes following surgery with anesthesia.

c. A recent, prospective follow-up study in 95 children undergoing neonatal cardiac surgery found no effects between anesthetic exposure and cumulative doses of perioperative anesthetics and sedatives on mental, motor, or vocabulary abilities at 18 to 24 months of age [25]. However, in their analysis, the authors were unable to use neurodevelopmental assessment as a continuous variable, which may have impacted the sensitivity of the assessment tool.

> **CLINICAL PEARL** Limiting exposure to general anesthesia in infants can be achieved by an increased use of regional techniques. Pain management postoperatively is often facilitated in young infants by these techniques. Light general anesthetics augmented by single-shot caudal techniques can help limit the dose of volatile anesthetics in procedures involving the lower extremities, pelvis, and lower abdomen. When possible, multiple procedures should be combined during a single exposure.

VIII. **Future research.** Clinical outcome studies examining this topic need to be performed and are currently underway in many areas of the world.
   A. Feasibility studies have been completed for the Pediatric Anesthesia NeuroDevelopmental Assessment (PANDA) study. The ambidirectional cohort study will compare neurocognitive functions in sibling pairs, one of whom had previous exposure to anesthesia during inguinal hernia surgery before 3 years of age (exposed) and the other one who was not exposed to anesthesia or surgery during the first 3 years of life (unexposed).
   B. A multisite randomized controlled trial, the GAS study, assesses regional versus general anesthesia for inguinal hernia repair before 60 weeks of postmenstrual age regarding their effects on neurodevelopmental outcome and apnea in infants. This multinational study's enrollment began in 2007 and is almost complete. The equivalence trial, which involves seven countries and 10 sites within the United States, tests the primary hypothesis that neurocognitive outcomes tested at the age of 5 years will be the same for both types of anesthesia. Enrollees in this trial return at the ages of 2 and 5 years to undergo extensive neurocognitive testing including Bayley-3 and Wechsler Preschool and Primary Scales of Intelligence.

IX. **Conclusion.** There is sufficient evidence from numerous animal studies to raise concern about the safety of general anesthetics in young infants. It seems conceivable that prolonged exposure to general anesthetics and sedatives may affect the developing human brain. However, a myriad of questions persist, including the potential susceptible age, the injurious doses, the potentially affected neurobehavioral domains, and the differences between clinical and laboratory settings, that preclude the direct translation from animal studies to humans. Further complicating this topic is the fact that epidemiologic evidence for neurologic abnormalities in clinical anesthesia practice is contradictory. Moreover, since the overwhelming majority of surgical procedures in neonates and infants is not elective, but rather performed to save lives or improve quality of life, and neurodegenerative effects have been found for all currently used anesthetics, there currently do not exist any viable alternatives to alleviate pain and distress during surgery. Accordingly, the U.S. Food and Drug Administration in conjunction with the International Anesthesia Research Society has stated that "*Currently, there is no scientific basis for delaying essential surgery.*" (http://www.smarttots.org/familyResourceCenter.html, accessed February 1, 2012.) In addition, the "*... dangers to infants and children from anesthesia remain unproven at this point.*" (http://www.smarttots.org/familyResourceCenter.html, accessed February 1, 2012.)

However, anesthesia providers should remain educated regarding this controversy and should avoid unnecessary exposure to anesthesia. If questions regarding the safety of pediatric anesthesia are raised, they must reassure patients, parents, pediatricians, and surgeons, but not hurriedly dismiss any stated concerns. Future research will hopefully provide more insight into this important concern for child health.

REFERENCES

1. Ikonomidou C, Bosch F, Miksa M, et al. Blockade of NMDA receptors and apoptotic neurodegeneration in the developing brain. *Science*. 1999;283:70–74.
2. Jevtovic-Todorovic V, Hartman RE, Izumi Y, et al. Early exposure to common anesthetic agents causes widespread neurodegeneration in the developing rat brain and persistent learning deficits. *J Neurosci*. 2003;23:876–882.
3. Loepke AW, Soriano SG. Impact of Pediatric Surgery and Anesthesia on Brain Development. In: Gregory GA, Andropoulos DB, eds. *Pediatric Anesthesia*. 5th ed. Oxford, UK: Wiley-Blackwell Publishing; 2012:1183–1218.
4. Yon JH, Daniel-Johnson J, Carter LB, et al. Anesthesia induces neuronal cell death in the developing rat brain via the intrinsic and extrinsic apoptotic pathways. *Neuroscience*. 2005;135:815–827.
5. Briner A, Nikonenko I, De Roo M, et al. Developmental Stage-dependent persistent impact of propofol anesthesia on dendritic spines in the rat medial prefrontal cortex. *Anesthesiology*. 2011;115:282–293.
6. Rizzi S, Ori C, Jevtovic-Todorovic V. Timing versus duration: Determinants of anesthesia-induced developmental apoptosis in the young mammalian brain. *Ann N Y Acad Sci*. 2010;1199:43–51.
7. Kurth CD, Priestley M, Watzman HM, et al. Desflurane confers neurologic protection for deep hypothermic circulatory arrest in newborn pigs. *Anesthesiology*. 2001;95:959–964.
8. Loepke AW, Priestley MA, Schultz SE, et al. Desflurane improves neurologic outcome after low-flow cardiopulmonary bypass in newborn pigs. *Anesthesiology*. 2002;97:1521–1527.
9. Anand KJ, Garg S, Rovnaghi CR, et al. Ketamine reduces the cell death following inflammatory pain in newborn rat brain. *Pediatr Res*. 2007;62:283–290.
10. Olney JW, Young C, Wozniak DF, et al. Anesthesia-induced developmental neuroapoptosis. Does it happen in humans? *Anesthesiology*. 2004;101:273–275.
11. Ma D, Williamson P, Januszewski A, et al. Xenon mitigates isoflurane-induced neuronal apoptosis in the developing rodent brain. *Anesthesiology*. 2007;106:746–753.
12. Cattano D, Williamson P, Fukui K, et al. Potential of xenon to induce or to protect against neuroapoptosis in the developing mouse brain. *Can J Anaesth*. 2008;55:429–436.
13. Slikker W Jr, Zou X, Hotchkiss CE, et al. Ketamine-induced neuronal cell death in the perinatal rhesus monkey. *Toxicol Sci*. 2007;98:145–158.
14. Lemkuil BP, Head BP, Pearn ML, et al. Isoflurane neurotoxicity is mediated by p75NTR-RhoA activation and actin depolymerization. *Anesthesiology*. 2011;114:49–57.
15. Sanders RD, Sun P, Patel S, et al. Dexmedetomidine provides cortical neuroprotection: impact on anaesthetic-induced neuroapoptosis in the rat developing brain. *Acta Anaesthesiol Scand*. 2010;54:710–716.
16. Head BP, Patel HH, Niesman IR, et al. Inhibition of p75 neurotrophin receptor attenuates isoflurane-mediated neuronal apoptosis in the neonatal central nervous system. *Anesthesiology*. 2009;110:813–825.
17. Clancy B, Finlay BL, Darlington RB, et al. Extrapolating brain development from experimental species to humans. *Neurotoxicology*. 2007;28:931–937.
18. Sprung J, Flick RP, Wilder RT, et al. Anesthesia for cesarean delivery and learning disabilities in a population-based birth cohort. *Anesthesiology*. 2009;111:302–310.
19. Hintz SR, Kendrick DE, Stoll BJ, et al. Neurodevelopmental and growth outcomes of extremely low birth weight infants after necrotizing enterocolitis. *Pediatrics*. 2005;115:696–703.
20. Loepke AW, Soriano SG. An assessment of the effects of general anesthetics on developing brain structure and neurocognitive function. *Anesth Analg*. 2008;106:1681–1707.
21. Wilder RT, Flick RP, Sprung J, et al. Early exposure to anesthesia and learning disabilities in a population-based birth cohort. *Anesthesiology*. 2009;110:796–804.
22. DiMaggio C, Sun L, Li G. Early childhood exposure to anesthesia and risk of developmental and behavioral disorders in a sibling birth cohort. *Anesth Analg*.2011;113:1143–1151.
23. Hansen TG, Pedersen JK, Henneberg SW, et al. Academic performance in adolescence after inguinal hernia repair in infancy: A nationwide cohort study. *Anesthesiology*. 2011;114:1076–1085.
24. Bartels M, Althoff RR, Boomsma DI. Anesthesia and cognitive performance in children: No evidence for a causal relationship. *Twin Res Hum Genet*. 2009;12:246–253.
25. Guerra GG, Robertson CM, Alton GY, et al. Neurodevelopmental outcome following exposure to sedative and analgesic drugs for complex cardiac surgery in infancy. *Paediatr Anaesth*. 2011;21:932–941.

25

Neurosurgery in the Pregnant Patient

Cristina Wood and Brenda Bucklin

KEY POINTS

1. Intracranial and subarachnoid hemorrhages are leading causes of indirect maternal mortality and are frequently associated with hypertensive disorders.
2. Intracranial lesions do not have an increased incidence in pregnancy but some lesions grow more rapidly secondary to increases in blood volume and hormonal changes.
3. Pregnancy is associated with a 30% to 40% decrease in anesthetic requirements. It is also associated with increased cardiac output, heart rate and blood volume, decreased functional residual capacity, and an increased risk of aspiration.
4. Uterine blood flow is not autoregulated and solely dependent on maternal blood pressure. Phenylephrine is the vasopressor of choice to maintain blood pressure within 20% of baseline.
5. Fetal exposure to perioperative medications can result in fetal hemodynamic changes and teratogenic effects. No anesthesia medications are known teratogens but desflurane, nitrous oxide, and ketamine have been shown to be teratogenic in animal models.

I. **Incidence and epidemiology**

A. **Subarachnoid hemorrhage (SAH)** is a leading cause of indirect maternal mortality, occurring in 5 to 17 per 100,000 deliveries. It is involved in 4% of all pregnancy-related in-hospital deaths with half-occurring postpartum. Independent risk factors include certain ethnicities (African, American, and Hispanic), hypertension, coagulopathy, drug abuse (tobacco, alcohol, illicit drugs), and venous thrombosis [1].

1. **Aneurysm/arteriovenous malformation**

   a. **Epidemiology.** Found in 0.01% to 0.05% of all pregnancies, similar to the general population (7 vs. 5 per 100,000 person years). The incidence of aneurysm to arteriovenous malformation (AVM) is 3:1. Hemorrhage has been reported to be fivefold higher in pregnancy in some studies and most commonly occurs late in pregnancy, at delivery or postpartum. This increase is possibly due to hemodynamic changes seen in pregnancy [1,2]. It should be noted that it is unclear if the increase in hemorrhage seen in some studies is related to etiologies of SAH other than aneurysm or AVM. Mortality is similar to the nonpregnant population at 35% while fetal mortality is 17%. Both are improved with surgical intervention versus conservative management.

   b. The risk of rupture from vaginal versus cesarean delivery may not be increased; therefore, guidelines against vaginal delivery may not be warranted [2].

   c. There is a wide differential diagnosis including pituitary apoplexy, cerebral venous thrombosis, intracranial arterial occlusion, migraines, postdural puncture headache, preeclampsia, and mass lesions.

   d. Treatment includes watchful waiting, clipping and/or resection in the operating room, or embolization in the interventional radiology suite.

2. **Cerebral venous/arterial thrombosis**

   a. **Epidemiology.** Seventy-five percent of adult cases are pregnant women and commonly found in the cortical veins (12 per 100,000 deliveries). Cases are seen more frequently in the last trimester and 2 to 3 weeks postpartum. Thrombosis may also occur secondary to trauma (i.e., compromise of the endothelial lining during the second stage of labor), or due to the hypercoagulable state of pregnancy [3].

   b. Treatment may involve anticoagulation, thrombolytic therapy, or embolic therapy, depending on location and symptomology.

3. **Hypertension**

   a. **Epidemiology.** Occurs in 40% of SAHs in the peripartum period [1].

   b. The most common causes of mortality in hypertensive disorders of pregnancy are eclampsia and proteinuric hypertension (83%). Others include chronic hypertension, HELLP (hemolysis, elevated liver enzymes, low platelets), liver rupture, and acute fatty liver disease [4].

   c. Systolic blood pressure greater than (160 mm Hg) should be treated during the peripartum period. Medications should lower the blood pressure in a smooth fashion (lowered by 30 mm Hg over a 60-minute period) [4].

4. **Vertebral artery dissection.** This is a very uncommon cause of SAH and only a few case reports occurring in pregnancy are found in the literature, one resulting in a fatality. Medical management has been the treatment in most cases [5].

5. **Moyamoya.** This disease results in stenotic arteries, mainly the internal carotids, and can result in hemorrhage, albeit a rare cause of SAH in pregnancy. Parturients can either deliver by cesarean or vaginal delivery with this diagnosis, as long as the hemodynamics are controlled. The goal is for adequate blood pressure control in the peripartum period to prevent intracranial hemorrhage.

B. **Maternal intracranial hemorrhage**

1. **Epidemiology.** Occurs in approximately 6 per 100,000 deliveries, which is similar to SAH, but mortality may be twice that of SAH (20% vs. 10%) [1].

2. Intracranial hemorrhage has similar risk factors and likely similar etiologies as seen in SAH.

C. **Ventriculoperitoneal shunt**
1. **Epidemiology.** Initial placement during pregnancy is usually indicated for elevated intracranial pressure (ICP) secondary to hemorrhage or obstruction from mass effect. Of those parturients that become pregnant with a shunt in place, 58% of those will develop shunt malfunction, usually due to the increased intra-abdominal pressure related to the gravid uterus [6].
2. **Treatment** may include diuretics or shunt revision. Care must be taken if revision includes placement into the abdomen, given the risk of inducing premature labor.

D. **Trauma**
1. **Epidemiology.** Trauma occurs in approximately 7% of pregnancies, with a small percentage of these related to intracranial traumas [7].
2. Most will likely undergo some form of craniotomy.

E. **Benign and malignant lesions**
1. **Epidemiology.** The incidence (3.6 per million live births) of these lesions does not appear to be greater in the pregnant than in the nonpregnant patient [8].
2. The treatment may involve biopsy, resection via craniotomy, or radiation during pregnancy. This all depends on the gestational age, type of tumor, growth rate, and associated symptoms (e.g., signs of elevated ICP or focal neurologic signs).
3. Some lesions appear to grow more rapidly during pregnancy, likely secondary to sodium and water retention and an increase in blood volume. In addition, hormone sensitivity may accelerate growth. Progesterone receptors are located on some lesions (meningiomas) which explain the direct effect hormones can illicit on these tumors [9].

II. **Physiologic changes relevant to the pregnant patient undergoing neurosurgery**
A. **Neurologic**
1. The minimum alveolar concentration (MAC) of inhalational anesthetics is reduced by 30% to 40% in the parturient. This reduction is likely secondary to progesterone, which is increased 10- to 20-fold late in pregnancy and can cause central nervous system depression. Also, increased plasma endorphin levels may have a synergistic effect with inhalational anesthetics [10].
2. Local anesthetic action is enhanced during pregnancy. This enhancement is likely due to both mechanical and hormonal factors.
   a. The volume of the intrathecal space is reduced secondary to the engorgement of epidural veins. This results from mechanical compression of the inferior vena cava by the gravid uterus and from increases in blood volume.
   b. Hormonally, pregnant animal models have shown neuronal conduction blockade that does not appear to be anatomically mediated, but related to progesterone and other hormonal mediators [11].
   c. In addition, the pH of cerebrospinal fluid of parturients is higher secondary to the hypocapnia seen in pregnancy. This may allow for increased movement of the nonionized form of local anesthetics across nerve membranes [12].

B. **Cardiac**
1. Blood volume increases by approximately 40% (approximately 1.5 L) during pregnancy starting by 6 weeks of gestation and plateaus during the third trimester [13,14]. A physiologic anemia develops as the plasma expands more than the red blood cells, normal HCT is 30% to 35%. Heart rate also increases from 10% to 20%. The combination of these results in a 30% to 60% increase in cardiac output seen as early as the first trimester. The vascular circulation compensates by decreasing peripheral vascular resistance, resulting in an overall decrease in systemic blood pressure (see Table 25.1).
2. Aortocaval compression occurs at approximately 20 weeks of gestation when the parturient is positioned supine and the gravid uterus compresses both the aorta and inferior vena cava. This makes it paramount to position the pregnant patient with left uterine displacement (LUD), or lateral position to maintain effective preload [15].
3. Oxygen consumption increases from 40% to 60% from prepregnancy values secondary to the enlarged uterus, the placenta, and fetus.
4. ECG changes are common in pregnancy, given the elevation of the diaphragm by the uterus resulting in a leftward axis. However, depending on the gestational age, there can

TABLE 25.1 Physiologic changes in pregnancy

Measurement	Percentage change
Blood volume	+40
Plasma volume	+55
Red blood cell volume	+30
Heart rate	+15
Cardiac output	+30–60
Peripheral systemic resistance	−20

be an axis deviation in either direction, which is normal. In addition, premature atrial contractions and sinus tachycardia are commonly observed.

C. Respiratory

1. Pregnant women have increased airway mucosal edema secondary to increased blood volume [16], which contributes to the eightfold increase in failed intubation seen in parturients. In addition, there is concern for tissue friability and nasal intervention is discouraged.

2. The elevation of the diaphragm as the uterus enlarges results in decreased functional residual capacity (FRC) of up to 40% at term. However, closing capacity does not change; therefore in the supine position, small airway closure and shunting occur resulting in arterial desaturation. During periods of apnea, clinically significant desaturation can occur quickly in the supine position. In a study evaluating desaturation (SaO_2 < 90%), after a period of apnea following 99% denitrogenation, desaturation occurred after 4 minutes of apnea for parturients and 7.5 minutes for nonparturients [17].

3. Increased minute ventilation occurs in parturients, likely secondary to progesterone sensitization of the central respiratory centers. This results in an increase in respiratory rate (15%) and tidal volume (40%). Normal CO_2 in pregnancy is about 32 mm Hg versus 40 mm Hg in the nonpregnant patient. There is increased renal excretion of sodium bicarbonate to compensate for this hypocapnia, resulting in a minimal increase in pH (7.41 to 7.44) [17].

D. Gastrointestinal

1. Gastric emptying does not decrease throughout pregnancy, but it is slowed with painful contractions and during opioid administration.

2. The placenta produces gastrin, which in theory can result in increased secretions and decreased pH. However, studies have shown that gastrin levels are actually reduced in pregnancy [18].

3. Progesterone and estrogen cause relaxation of smooth muscle tone, including lower esophageal sphincter (LES) tone [19]. Also, the gravid uterus causes rotation of the stomach, resulting in decreased compliance of the LES.

4. The risk of aspiration pneumonia is increased in the pregnant patient, given the increased gastric secretions, decreased gastric pH, and compromised LES tone. All pregnant patients undergoing surgery should receive aspiration prophylaxis, including an H_2 blocker, promotility agent, and nonparticulate antacid prior to induction of anesthesia, as well as a rapid sequence induction (RSI).

E. Renal

1. Renal blood flow is increased by 75% and GFR is increased by 60% during pregnancy, resulting in a BUN and creatinine decrease by 50% to 60% from prepregnancy values [20].

2. There is a reduction in glucose and bicarbonate tubular reabsorption, possibly resulting in diabetes mellitus (gestational diabetes) and compensatory metabolic acidosis in response to the respiratory alkalosis.

3. Primary peripheral vasodilation causes increased aldosterone levels resulting in increased sodium and water retention. This can cause increased edema in intracranial lesions, leading to worsening of symptoms.

F. Hepatic

1. There is no increase in blood flow to the liver during pregnancy.

2. The clearance of drugs is reduced secondary to the increased volume of distribution associated with the increase in blood volume.
3. There is an increase in the splanchnic, portal, and esophageal venous pressure, which results in esophageal varices in 60% of parturients [20].
4. Serum albumin decreases up to 60% due to an increase in plasma volume [20].
5. Transaminases remain normal, with elevations in alkaline phosphatase, due to increased placental production.
6. During pregnancy, pseudocholinesterase levels are mildly decreased, but no documented cases of prolonged paralysis have been noted following succinylcholine administration [21].

G. Hematologic

1. A dilutional anemia of pregnancy is normal, with the hematocrit decreasing to 30% to 35%.
2. Gestational thrombocytopenia is observed in a small number of parturients (90,000 to 100,000). There is no associated platelet dysfunction or increased risk of bleeding complications.
3. There is an increase in coagulation factors I, VII, VIII, and X, a decrease in protein S, and inhibition of fibrinolysis. These changes result in a prothrombic state [22].

III. Uterine blood flow and perfusion

A. Uterine blood flow (UBF) is not autoregulated; therefore it is dependent solely on maternal perfusion pressure.

1. UBF is about 700 cc/min (approximately 10% to 15% of cardiac output).
2. Hypovolemia, vasodilators, anesthesia medications, positive pressure ventilation, sympathetic blockade, aortocaval compression, uterine hypertonicity (due to oxytocin or α-adrenergic stimulation) can all cause decreases in UBF.
3. Excessive hyperventilation and hypocapnia should be avoided during general anesthesia in order to prevent placental vasoconstriction and fetal compromise.

B. Vasopressors

1. Ephedrine and phenylephrine are both acceptable for use in pregnancy, but phenylephrine has been shown to result in less fetal acidosis and crosses the placenta with less efficacy. It is therefore the vasopressor of choice. Ephedrine appears to stimulate fetal metabolism, resulting in acidosis [23].
2. Vasopressin receptors (V1) are present on the human uterus and administration of vasopressin for hypotension should be avoided, as this can induce uterine contractions [24].
3. Epinephrine is a suitable third-line agent (after phenylephrine and ephedrine) for treatment of hemodynamic instability. Epinephrine will cross the placenta and can cause a dose-dependent decrease in UBF from vasoconstriction. In addition, epinephrine has an effect on β-adrenergic receptors. As a tocolytic, it can be used to decrease uterine contractions [25].

IV. Pharmacology

A. Placental transfer of water and solutes

1. Movement is dependent on hydrostatic, osmotic pressure gradients, and concentration gradients.
2. Transporter-mediated transport and endocytosis occur at the plasma membrane and may be faster than simple diffusion.
3. The higher the lipid solubility, the increased ease of transfer across the placenta.
4. Molecular weight can limit transfer. Five hundred Daltons seem to be the upper limit in order for complete placental transfer.
5. The maternal cytochrome P450 system is induced during pregnancy, resulting in a decreased fraction of free drug [26].

B. Placental transfer of anesthesia drugs

1. Inhalational agents freely cross the placenta, are of low molecular weight and extremely lipophilic.
2. Opioids freely cross the placenta, are lipophilic and of low molecular weight.
3. Induction agents (propofol, thiopental, etomidate) also freely cross the placenta, but first pass maternal hepatic metabolism reduces fetal exposure.
4. Neuromuscular blocking and reversal agents are highly ionized making placental transfer minimal.

TABLE 25.2 Magnesium toxcity

Magnesium plasma level (mEq/L)	Side effects
1.5–2	None
4–8	Therapeutic
5–10	PR prolongation, wide QRS
10	Reduced deep tendon reflexes, respiratory depression
15	Respiratory arrest, conduction defects
25	Cardiac arrest

5. **Additional medications**
   a. **Anticholinergics.** Glycopyrrolate has minimal transfer due to ionization resulting from its quaternary ammonium structure. Atropine and scopolamine freely pass as they are minimally ionized and are tertiary amines.
   b. **Anticoagulation.** Coumadin (<500 Daltons) crosses the placenta freely as it is minimally ionized and small. Heparin is ionized and does not cross the placenta. If the parturient has taken coumadin, the fetus is anticoagulated as well. Unfortunately, there is not a mechanism for fetal reversal of this anticoagulation until after delivery.
   c. **Antihypertensives.** All β-blockers, hydralazine, nitroprusside, and nitroglycerin cross the placenta. It should be noted that β-blockers can cause a transient fetal bradycardia, but may be necessary to decrease maternal blood pressure or heart rate. Angiotensin-converting enzyme (ACE) inhibitors are contraindicated in the second and third trimesters secondary to teratogenic effects [27], so they are not typically used.
   d. **Magnesium sulfate** is used for seizure prophylaxis in preeclampsia and for neuroprotection. This medication can cause hypotension, uterine atony, and hypotonia. The side effects of magnesium are listed in Table 25.2.
   e. **Mannitol** is used in neurosurgical procedures to assist with reduction of ICP. However, this drug accumulates in the fetus, resulting in a hyperosmolar state, reduced urinary blood flow and lung fluid production. Individual case reports demonstrate that doses of 0.25 to 0.5 mg/kg appear to be safe [28].

V. Fetal effects
  A. Medications
   1. All inhalational agents have been shown to have neuroprotective effects in adult animal models and are used in neurosurgical anesthesia cases; however, they must be administered at less than 1 MAC (preferably at <0.7 MAC) to reduce cerebral vasodilation and minimize increases in ICP. Isoflurane or sevoflurane is recommended for neurosurgical procedures because they also reduce cerebral metabolic rate and have a lesser effect on ICP. In rodent neonatal models, when compared to sevoflurane and isoflurane, desflurane resulted in increased neuroapoptosis, so there may be a reason to avoid this inhalational agent in parturients [29].
   2. Benzodiazepines do not appear to cause any teratogenic effects [30], even when used in the first trimester.
   3. Nitrous oxide is a weak teratogen in rodents [31,32]. Even though nitrous oxide inhibits methionine synthase (and therefore DNA synthesis), neurologic symptoms cannot be corrected with the coadministration of folic acid. The etiology of the teratogenicity is likely multifactorial and its use is not recommended during pregnancy.
   4. When mannitol is administered, there is concern for fetal dehydration (oligohydramnios), increased osmolarity and electrolyte concentrations. Individual case reports show that doses of 0.25 to 0.5 mg/kg appear to be safe [28].
   5. β-blockers cross the placenta and can place the fetus at risk for fetal bradycardia, as well as neonatal bradycardia, hypoglycemia, and respiratory depression [33]. Atenolol and metoprolol cross the placenta more readily than labetolol (100% vs. 40% respectively). Although there is minimal placental transfer of esmolol (20%), there have been reports of profound fetal bradycardia requiring emergency cesarean delivery [34]. β-blockers are

useful to blunt the hemodynamic changes of intubation and extubation; therefore labetalol is the best option for the parturient.

6. Steroids are routinely used in neurosurgery to decrease the perifocal edema seen with intracranial mass lesions. The use of dexamethasone or betamethasone has decreased the risk of respiratory distress syndrome, intraventricular hemorrhage, and neonatal death in premature infants. However, recent studies have shown that repeat doses of antenatal steroids over time have resulted in decreased placental size and neonatal birth weight [35]. The use of steroids for maternal benefit during neurosurgical procedures is probably not harmful though and may decrease neonatal morbidity and mortality if the fetus is delivered within several days of the surgical intervention.

7. All anticonvulsants cross the placenta and have the potential to cause neural tube, orofacial, cardiovascular and digital malformations, as well as fetal coagulopathies. Valproate, phenytoin, carbamazepine, phenobarbital, and topiramate all have been associated with congenital malformations [36]. Most structural abnormalities will occur with use in the first trimester; however, the research is focused on chronic use and little is known about acute use of anticonvulsive agents. Levetiracetam (Keppra) is commonly used in neurosurgical procedures, and in one recent study from Australia, there were no malformations seen in parturients taking Keppra [37].

8. Hyperventilation is frequently used during neurosurgery to reduce ICP; however, excessive hypocapnia can result in uteroplacental vasoconstriction increasing the risk for fetal compromise ($ETCO_2 < 25$).

B. **Radiation exposure**
1. Ionizing radiation exposure could result in spontaneous abortion, congenital malformation, or fetal cerebral injury depending on the dose and the timing of exposure. Exposure during the first 15 weeks of development places the fetus at greatest risk for injury and declines by a factor of 4 after 15 weeks of gestation, likely due to organogenesis. After 26 weeks of gestation, the risks are minimal. The American College of Obstetricians and Gynecologists (ACOG) recommend that exposure not exceed 5 rad (radiation absorbed dose). The parturient should be shielded with lead in the anterior and posterior position during any exposure to minimize risk. For reference, a computed tomography (CT) of the chest results in fetal exposure of up to 0.1 rad and a chest x-ray results in exposure of <0.001 rad [38].
2. Radiopaque agents used in CT scans can contain iodine and cross the placenta, potentially resulting in fetal hypothyroidism. These agents should be used if the benefit outweighs the risk to the fetus [39].
3. The safety of paramagnetic contrast agents (gadolinium) has not been established in humans, but they do cross the placenta and should be used only if the benefit outweighs the risk [39].

VI. **Anesthetic considerations specific to the parturient**
A. **General considerations**
1. For all anesthetic procedures, all pregnant patients should receive a nonparticulate acid, an H_2 blocker, and a gastric motility agent.
2. An rapid sequence induction is recommended.
3. When the gestational age is >20 weeks, left uterine displacement should be maintained.
4. Parturients should wear sequential compression devices when nonambulatory, given the hypercoagulable state of pregnancy.
5. Agents that increase ICP should be avoided, as in any craniotomy for the nonpregnant patient (e.g., ketamine). Succinylcholine may produce transient increases in ICP. However, those increases may be abolished with IV lidocaine, adequate depth of anesthesia, hyperventilation, or a defasciculating dose of a nondepolarizing paralytic [40].

B. **Blood pressure monitoring**
1. **In such cases, an arterial line should be utilized.** The blood pressure should be maintained within 20% of baseline, with a mean arterial pressure of >70 mm Hg. During aneurysm clipping, there may be a need to induce hypotension acutely, but this should be avoided if possible.
2. Sodium nitroprusside can be used to lower blood pressure, but it crosses the placenta and may cause fetal cyanide toxicity (keep infusions to less than 0.5 mg/kg/h).

3. Nitroglycerin can also be used to control blood pressure without adverse fetal effects, although experimentally, nitroglycerin is metabolized to nitrites, causing methemoglobinemia.

4. Inhalation agents like isoflurane can also be used to lower blood pressure and even at greater than 1 MAC, uteroplacental perfusion is maintained as long as maternal blood pressure is maintained [41].

C. **Fetal monitoring.** ACOG recommends the following:

1. Any fetus termed viable (approximately 24 weeks) should have minimum Doppler fetal heart tones and tocometer analysis immediately prior to and after an operation. Continuous intraoperative monitoring should be performed if (1) there is an obstetrical physician or nurse qualified to interpret the fetal tracing; (2) monitoring is possible during the surgery; and (3) an emergency cesarean delivery could be performed without compromising the parturient's safety. Neurosurgery should take place in a facility that has obstetrical, pediatric, and neonatal expertise readily available. The operating room should be equipped for an emergency cesarean section should the need arise [42].

2. Any fetus termed previable should have Doppler confirmation of fetal heart rate prior to and immediately after the surgical procedure. Continuous intraoperative fetal monitoring for a previable fetus should be performed to optimize placental blood flow in cases of fetal bradycardia and on a case-by-case basis [42].

3. Blood pressure should be maintained within 20% of maternal baseline and should be increased if fetal bradycardia ensues.

4. Loss of beat-to-beat variability is normal during general anesthesia. However in awake patients, it can be a sign of fetal compromise. Fetal heart rate decelerations are abnormal and should be corrected with increased blood pressure, increased oxygenation, or a change in position.

D. **Tocolytics.** Tocolytics may be needed if uterine contractions are detected on the tocometer during surgery.

1. Inhalational agents are potent tocolytics, but can cause increases in ICP at MAC greater than 0.7 to 1, so their use in neurosurgical procedures is limited.

2. Calcium channel blockers (nicardipine and nifedipine) and intravenous hydration are frequently used to prevent preterm contractions. However, calcium channel blockers can cause hypotension. Hydration must be balanced with the maternal risk of cerebral edema.

3. Alternatives are terbutaline and NTG, but one should be aware that both of these can result in maternal hypotension. In addition, terbutaline can result in maternal and fetal tachycardia as well as maternal pulmonary edema.

4. Magnesium has not been shown to prevent preterm labor when compared with placebo, but has shown benefit in fetal neuroprotection [43].

VII. **Anesthetic induction**

A. **Induction agents**

1. We recommend using either thiopental 5 to 7 mg/kg (if available), or propofol 2 mg/kg as induction agents, as both may have neuroprotective effects in the setting of mild cerebral ischemia [44]. It should be noted that these medications do not appear to have neuroprotective effects in situations of severe ischemia in humans. Ketamine is controversial because of its potential effects on ICP and should be used with caution [45]. In addition, ketamine has been associated with increased fetal neuroapoptosis in the rhesus monkey model. However, any animal data should be interpreted with caution when extrapolating to human subjects [46]. Etomidate has been favored in the past for its hemodynamic stability when used as an induction agent. However, it has been associated with adrenal suppression in trauma and critically ill patients, even in one dose [47].

2. Opioids readily cross the placenta and are appropriate for induction to blunt the hemodynamic response of laryngoscopy. However if a cesarean is performed, the neonatal team should be aware of the fetal exposure and likely respiratory depression. Remifentanil is an acceptable option for use during intubation and throughout the case. Studies have shown that neonates delivered to parturients who have received remifentanil have minimal respiratory depression that is usually self-limited [48].

3. All parturients should undergo rapid sequence intubation using either rocuronium 1.2 mg/kg or succinylcholine 1 mg/kg.

4. Parturients have increased airway edema, weight gain, increased breast tissue, and decreased FRC, making intubation more difficult. Studies have suggested that the incidence of failed intubation in the obstetric population is approximately 1:300, which is eight times higher than that of the general surgical population [49]. Emergency airway equipment should be immediately available for such cases, given the increased risk of failed intubation. In addition, we suggest "ramping" the patient to align the external auditory meatus with the sternal notch, in order to align the oral, pharyngeal, and laryngeal axes to improve intubating conditions.

VIII. **Anesthetic maintenance**

A. **Total intravenous anesthesia (TIVA) versus inhalational agents.** TIVA is preferred if neuromonitoring will be performed during the surgery since inhalational agents can result in decreased amplitude and increased latency of the electrical signals recorded. If inhalational agents are used, sevoflurane and isoflurane may be preferred over desflurane for reasons discussed above. Inhalational agents should be maintained at no more than 0.7 MAC in order to minimize increases in cerebral blood flow and thus reduce ICP. Also, remember MAC is reduced by 30% to 40% in parturients.

B. **Paralytics.** There are no fetal effects, as these drugs do not cross the placenta. Any paralytic agent can be utilized for maintenance of paralysis during the surgical intervention, unless there are maternal contraindications.

C. **Glucose management.** Maintaining euglycemia intraoperatively is beneficial to both the mother and the fetus. The fetus is dependent on maternal glucose for metabolic oxidative processes and fetal glucose levels are usually about 20 mg/dL less than maternal levels. Fetal metabolic derangements will occur if the fetus becomes hypo- or hyperglycemic, and can result in cardiac dysrhythmias and seizures. Maternal glucose levels are important as well, as hypo- or hyperglycemia in neurosurgery has been associated with adverse outcomes, including increased mortality. The optimal glucose concentration is difficult to determine, but in general, glucose levels of 110 to 150 mg/dL are recommended.

IX. **Anesthetic emergence**

A. **General considerations.** It is paramount on emergence of most neurosurgical procedures (for pregnant and nonpregnant patients) that (1) the patient awakens quickly for neurologic assessment; (2) hemodynamic alternations are minimized; and (3) a smooth extubation performed to limit increases in ICP or stress on the cranial vasculature. In addition, the patient must meet the criteria for extubation, including following commands, full reversal from paralytics, adequate oxygenation, and hemodynamic stability. In the parturient, these should be balanced with attempts to maintain adequate placental perfusion as dictated by fetal monitoring and maternal baseline blood pressure. We recommend elevating the head of bed (or using reverse Trendelenburg) during emergence to minimize increases in ICP, as well as decreasing the effects of the gravid uterus on the thoracic cavity.

B. **Pharmacologic interventions.** Smooth emergence can be accomplished using several pharmacologic interventions (antisympathetic and antinociceptive) listed below.

1. Lidocaine is utilized topically or intravenously as an antinociceptive agent to prevent straining and coughing on the endotracheal tube. Lidocaine is not known to have any teratogenic effects.

2. β-blockers are useful in blunting the hemodynamic changes seen on extubation. See discussion above for details, but labetalol is the β-blocker of choice in pregnancy.

3. Venodilators such as NTG, nitroprusside, and hydralazine all cross the placenta easily and can cause uterine hypoperfusion if systemic blood pressure is too low. NTG and nitroprusside can be useful in reducing elevated blood pressures and are easily titratable, given their short half-lives. Hydralazine has a half-life of several hours and is not as easily titratable.

X. **Breastfeeding.** The current recommendation from the American Academy of Pediatrics is exclusive breastfeeding for approximately the first 6 months of life. The mother should be encouraged to breastfeed her infant prior to surgical intervention and the mother may express and store her breast milk in the possibility that she is unable to breastfeed postoperatively. After general anesthesia, current opinion recommends breastfeeding as soon as the patient is physically and mentally able to do so, as there does not appear to be infant complications from the standard medications used in a single maternal anesthetic. However, production of breast milk may be decreased after pituitary intervention if the neurohypophysis axis is disrupted, decreasing the production of oxytocin.

XI. Conclusion. Pregnancy creates unique challenges for the anesthesiologist due to the physiologic changes seen in pregnancy and concern for fetal well-being. Intracranial pathologies do not appear to occur more frequently in pregnancy, but these patients can be at higher risk for hemorrhage and growth due to the physiologic changes in pregnancy. Maintaining hemodynamic stability is critical as UBF is not autoregulated, and dependent on maternal blood pressure. Most anesthetic drugs appear safe in pregnancy; however, animal models have shown possible teratogenic effects. Fetal monitoring should be utilized based on gestational age and availability of surgical intervention.

REFERENCES

1. Bateman BT, Olbrecht VA, Berman MF, et al. Peripartum subarachnoid hemorrhage: nationwide data and institutional experience. *Anesthesiology.* 2012;116:324–333.
2. Dias MS, Sekhar LN. Intracranial hemorrhage from aneurysms and arteriovenous malformations during pregnancy and the puerperium. *Neurosurgery.* 1990;27:855–865; discussion 865–866.
3. Stam J. Thrombosis of the cerebral veins and sinuses. *N Engl J Med.* 2005;352:1791–1798.
4. Moodley J. Maternal deaths due to hypertensive disorders in pregnancy. *Best Pract Res Clin Obstet Gynaecol.* 2008;22: 559–567.
5. Tuluc M, Brown D, Goldman B. Lethal vertebral artery dissection in pregnancy: a case report and review of the literature. *Arch Pathol Lab Med.* 2006;130:533–535.
6. Wisoff JH, Kratzert KJ, Handwerker SM, et al. Pregnancy in patients with cerebrospinal fluid shunts: report of a series and review of the literature. *Neurosurgery.* 1991;29:827–831.
7. Ikossi DG, Lazar AA, Morabito D, et al. Profile of mothers at risk: an analysis of injury and pregnancy loss in 1,195 trauma patients. *J Am Coll Surg.* 2005;200:49–56.
8. Haas JF, Janisch W, Staneczek W. Newly diagnosed primary intracranial neoplasms in pregnant women: a population-based assessment. *J Neurol Neurosurg Psychiatry.* 1986;49:874–880.
9. Lee LS, Chi CW, Chang TJ, et al. Steroid hormone receptors in meningiomas of Chinese patients. *Neurosurgery.* 1989;25: 541–545.
10. Chan MT, Mainland P, Gin T. Minimum alveolar concentration of halothane and enflurane are decreased in early pregnancy. *Anesthesiology.* 1996;85:782–786.
11. Popitz-Bergez FA, Leeson S, Thalhammer JG, et al. Intraneural lidocaine uptake compared with analgesic differences between pregnant and nonpregnant rats. *Reg Anesth.* 1997;22:363–371.
12. Hirabayashi Y, Shimizu R, Saitoh K, et al. Acid-base state of cerebrospinal fluid during pregnancy and its effect on spread of spinal anaesthesia. *Br J Anaesth.* 1996;77:352–355.
13. Lund CJ, Donovan JC. Blood volume during pregnancy. Significance of plasma and red cell volumes. *Am J Obstet Gynecol.* 1967;98:394–403.
14. Pritchard JA. Changes in the blood volume during pregnancy and delivery. *Anesthesiology.* 1965;26:393–399.
15. Bamber JH, Dresner M. Aortocaval compression in pregnancy: the effect of changing the degree and direction of lateral tilt on maternal cardiac output. *Anesth Analg.* 2003;97:256–258.
16. Kodali BS, Chandrasekhar S, Bulich LN, et al. Airway changes during labor and delivery. *Anesthesiology.* 2008;108:357–362.
17. McClelland SH, Bogod DG, Hardman JG. Apnoea in pregnancy: an investigation using physiological modelling. *Anaesthesia.* 2008;63:264–269.
18. Murray FA, Erskine JP, Fielding J. Gastric secretion in pregnancy. *J Obstet Gynaecol Br Emp.* 1957;64:373–381.
19. Ulmsten U, Sundstrom G. Esophageal manometry in pregnant and nonpregnant women. *Am J Obstet Gynecol.* 1978;132: 260–264.
20. Paech MJ, Scott K. Liver and renal disease. In: *Obstetric Anesthesia and Uncommon Disorders.* Gambling D, Douglas MJ, McKay RSF, eds. Cambridge: Cambridge University Press; 2008:249–257.
21. Blitt CD, Petty WC, Alberternst EE, et al. Correlation of plasma cholinesterase activity and duration of action of succinylcholine during pregnancy. *Anesth Analg.* 1977;56:78–83.
22. Stirling Y, Woolf L, North WR, et al. Haemostasis in normal pregnancy. *Thromb Haemost.* 1984;52:176–182.
23. Ngan Kee WD, Khaw KS, Tan PE, et al. Placental transfer and fetal metabolic effects of phenylephrine and ephedrine during spinal anesthesia for cesarean delivery. *Anesthesiology.* 2009;111:506–512.
24. Maggi M, Del Carlo P, Fantoni G, et al. Human myometrium during pregnancy contains and responds to V1 vasopressin receptors as well as oxytocin receptors. *J Clin Endocrinol Metab.* 1990;70:1142–1154.
25. Segal S, Csavoy AN, Datta S. The tocolytic effect of catecholamines in the gravid rat uterus. *Anesth Analg.* 1998;87:864–869.
26. Anderson GD. Pregnancy-induced changes in pharmacokinetics: a mechanistic-based approach. *Clin Pharmacokinet.* 2005;44:989–1008.

27. Cooper WO, Hernandez-Diaz S, Arbogast PG, et al. Major congenital malformations after first-trimester exposure to ACE inhibitors. *N Engl J Med.* 2006;354:2443–2451.
28. Tuncali B, Aksun M, Katircioglu K, et al. Intraoperative fetal heart rate monitoring during emergency neurosurgery in a parturient. *J Anesth.* 2006;20:40–43.
29. Kodama M, Satoh Y, Otsubo Y, et al. Neonatal desflurane exposure induces more robust neuroapoptosis than do isoflurane and sevoflurane and impairs working memory. *Anesthesiology.* 2011;115:979–991.
30. Wikner BN, Kallen B. Are hypnotic benzodiazepine receptor agonists teratogenic in humans? *J Clin Psychopharmacol.* 2011;31:356–359.
31. Mazze RI, Fujinaga M, Rice SA, et al. Reproductive and teratogenic effects of nitrous oxide, halothane, isoflurane, and enflurane in Sprague-Dawley rats. *Anesthesiology.* 1986;64:339–344.
32. Fujinaga M, Mazze RI, Baden JM, et al. Rat whole embryo culture: an in vitro model for testing nitrous oxide teratogenicity. *Anesthesiology.* 1988;69:401–404.
33. Witter FR, King TM, Blake DA. Adverse effects of cardiovascular drug therapy on the fetus and neonate. *Obstet Gynecol.* 1981;58:100S–105S.
34. Ducey JP, Knape KG. Maternal esmolol administration resulting in fetal distress and cesarean section in a term pregnancy. *Anesthesiology.* 1992;77:829–832.
35. Sawady J, Mercer BM, Wapner RJ, et al. The National Institute of Child Health and Human Development Maternal-Fetal Medicine Units Network Beneficial Effects of Antenatal Repeated Steroids study: impact of repeated doses of antenatal corticosteroids on placental growth and histologic findings. *Am J Obstet Gynecol.* 2007;197:281. e281–e288.
36. Werler MM, Ahrens KA, Bosco JL, et al. Use of antiepileptic medications in pregnancy in relation to risks of birth defects. *Ann Epidemiol.* 2011;21:842–850.
37. Vajda FJ, Graham J, Roten A, et al. Teratogenicity of the newer antiepileptic drugs–the Australian experience. *J Clin Neurosci. Official Journal of the Neurosurgical Society of Australasia.* 2012;19:57–59.
38. Groen RS, Bae JY, Lim KJ. Fear of the unknown: ionizing radiation exposure during pregnancy. *Am J Obstet Gynecol.* 2012; 206:456–462.
39. ACOG Committee Opinion. Number 299, September 2004 (replaces No. 158, September 1995). Guidelines for diagnostic imaging during pregnancy. *Obstet Gynecol.* 2004;104:647–651.
40. Kovarik WD, Mayberg TS, Lam AM, et al. Succinylcholine does not change intracranial pressure, cerebral blood flow velocity, or the electroencephalogram in patients with neurologic injury. *Anesth Analg.* 1994;78:469–473.
41. Dahlgren G, Tornberg DC, Pregner K, et al. Four cases of the ex utero intrapartum treatment (EXIT) procedure: anesthetic implications. *Int J Obstet Anesth.* 2004;13:178–182.
42. ACOG Committee on Obstetric Practice. ACOG Committee Opinion No. 474: Nonobstetric surgery during pregnancy. *Obstet Gynecol.* 2011;117:420–421.
43. King JF. Tocolysis and preterm labour. *Curr Opin Obstet Gynecol.* 2004;16:459–463.
44. Schifilliti D, Grasso G, Conti A, et al. Anaesthetic-related neuroprotection: intravenous or inhalational agents? *CNS Drugs.* 2010;24:893–907.
45. Mayberg TS, Lam AM, Matta BF, et al. Ketamine does not increase cerebral blood flow velocity or intracranial pressure during isoflurane/nitrous oxide anesthesia in patients undergoing craniotomy. *Anesth Analg.* 1995;81:84–89.
46. Brambrink AM, Evers AS, Avidan MS, et al. Ketamine-induced neuroapoptosis in the fetal and neonatal rhesus macaque brain. *Anesthesiology.* 2012;116:372–384.
47. Hildreth AN, Mejia VA, Maxwell RA, et al. Adrenal suppression following a single dose of etomidate for rapid sequence induction: a prospective randomized study. *J Trauma.* 2008;65:573–579.
48. Ngan Kee WD, Khaw KS, Ma KC, et al. Maternal and neonatal effects of remifentanil at induction of general anesthesia for cesarean delivery: a randomized, double-blind, controlled trial. *Anesthesiology.* 2006;104:14–20.
49. Barnardo PD, Jenkins JG. Failed tracheal intubation in obstetrics: a 6-year review in a UK region. *Anaesthesia.* 2000;55: 690–694.

26

Electrophysiologic Monitoring (EEG and Evoked Potentials)

Tod B. Sloan and Francesco Sala

KEY POINTS

1. The EEG is a recording of the synaptic activity in the cortical pyramidal cells.
2. The loss of EEG activity may represent cortical ischemia.
3. The EEG is the method used to locate the focus of a seizure in the brain.
4. Anesthesia agents exert their influence on the nervous system through interactions with synaptic function.
5. Prolonged "trains" of EMG activity usually represent injurious events.
6. EMG monitoring is one of the most effective methods of monitoring nerve roots in cervical and lumbosacral spine surgery.
7. The SSEP monitors the posterior column pathway of proprioception and vibration.
8. The ABR can be used to monitor the brainstem as well as the auditory nerve and cochlea.
9. MEP monitors the corticospinal tract.
10. Immaturity of the central and peripheral nervous systems limits MEP monitoring in very young children.

I. Intraoperative electrophysiologic monitoring (IOM) is commonly used because these techniques monitor the functional status of neural pathways rather than physiologic monitors (e.g., blood pressure and oxygenation) which only measure parameters that are supportive of function. Some of these techniques monitor spontaneous electrical activity and others monitor evoked activity. In general, multiple techniques are usually used together (multimodality monitoring) during surgery to provide the optimal surveillance of the nervous system. IOM has become an essential tool for some surgeries and a standard of care in others. Although not a replacement for an awake neurologic examination, intraoperative neurophysiologic monitoring can detect an unfavorable surgical or physiologic environment that may allow surgical or physiologic maneuvers that can reduce operative morbidity. [1]

II. Electroencephalography

A. History. The human electroencephalography (EEG) was first recorded by Berger in 1924 after having been measured in animals since 1875 (Richard Caton). Since that time a large number of diagnostic and monitoring applications have developed (especially with regards to epilepsy).

B. Anatomy

1. The EEG is generated in pyramidal cells oriented perpendicular to the dura in cortical layers 3, 5, and 6. The EEG is produced at the thousands of synaptic connections to these pyramidal cells from other neurons.

2. Neural cells maintain an electronegative "resting" membrane potential (about −60 mV) by maintaining concentration gradients of electrolytes (primarily sodium, potassium, and chloride). Neurotransmitters produce a postsynaptic potential (PSP). These can be inhibitory and hyperpolarize the membrane or be excitatory raising the transmembrane potential toward zero. The EEG represents the summation of these tiny PSP currents. If the change in voltage reaches the depolarization threshold, an action potential occurs which does not normally contribute to the EEG.

C. Technique of recording

1. The EEG is measured as the electrical difference between the activities at a pair of electrodes (termed a bipolar montage). A differential amplifier is used so that the difference between the active and reference electrodes is amplified and the electrical activity at a third ground electrode is removed. Occasionally the EEG is recorded by comparing each electrode to a reference set of other electrodes (referential montage).

2. Each electrode records the spontaneous activity of a spherical region below the electrode of about 2 to 3 cm in diameter.

3. The most common method of describing the location of scalp electrodes is the International 10–20 system. The locations are defined by a grid which is spaced at 10% and 20% of the distance from the nasion to the inion, and between the left and right aural tragus. The middle location from these landmarks is termed the "vertex" and is designated Cz. Other locations are designated by a letter (i.e., C, central; F, frontal; P, parietal; T, temporal) and a number indicating the side and relative distance from the midline (Z, midline).

4. A diagnostic EEG is usually recorded using a large number of electrodes (e.g., 16) in order to identify the location of abnormal activity across the entire cortex. Monitoring is usually done with a smaller number of electrodes to focus on specific areas of the brain that may be at risk; often a single pair is used on the forehead when examining anesthetic drug effect.

5. The electrical signal at scalp electrodes includes the activity of the heart (electrocardiogram [ECG]), muscle activity (electromyography [EMG]), and the electrical activity resulting from the movement of the eye (electrooculography [EOG]). Most of the activity of the EEG occurs in a frequency range of 0.5 to 40 Hz which allows filtration to separate the EEG from some of this other activity.

6. Direct recording of the EEG from the surface of the brain is termed electrocorticography (ECoG) and is often used to locate seizure foci.

7. During direct cortical stimulation (DCS) to localize eloquent areas, ECoG is also important to detect afterdischarges as these represent subclinical seizure-like electrical activity that can mimic the effect of DCS (e.g., a muscle motor response or a speech arrest). It

TABLE 26.1 Frequency bands of the EEG

Band	Frequencies (Hz)
Delta	0–4
Theta	4–8
Alpha	8–12
Beta	12–25
Gamma	25–100

is important to rule out the presence of afterdischarges to avoid misleading information during the localization of cortical functions.

8. Occasionally, EEG activity is recorded from the electrodes implanted deeper in the brain such as to determine the focus of seizure activity in temporal lobe epilepsy.

D. EEG interpretation and processed EEG. EEG interpretation involves visual inspection of the frequency content, distribution of activity across the cortex, and recognition of specific patterns of activity. To simplify interpretation, computerized methods have been developed to enhance detection of certain EEG features and allow a compressed display rather than yards of raw EEG paper printouts.

1. **Time domain**
   a. The EEG can be displayed as a simple tracing of voltage over time (referred to as the time domain).
   b. The EEG has been divided in frequency bands (Table 26.1).
   c. The basic frequency bands are thought to be rhythmic activity resulting from neural connections with the brainstem and thalamus (sometimes referred to as EEG pacemakers).
   d. Simple methods of computer processing include the average frequency and the average power (voltage squared) contained in the entire EEG or in each of the frequency bands.
   e. EEG spike activity and burst suppression are important features of the raw EEG.
      (1) EEG "spikes" or "sharp waves" occur when massive synchronized activity occurs with a seizure. Repetitive spikes are used in the diagnosis of epilepsy.
      (2) Burst suppression (intermittent electrical activity interspersed with periods of little or no electrical activity) indicates a reduction in synaptic activity associated with reduced cerebral metabolic activity. This can occur from several mechanisms (e.g., trauma, drugs, hypothermia, etc.). The Burst Suppression Ratio (BSR) is used to characterize this and is the fraction of time where the EEG is suppressed.

2. **Frequency domain.** Since the frequency content of the EEG changes with anesthesia and various brain states, computer processing methods to better quantify the EEG frequency content can be used.
   a. One of the most frequently used methods is a mathematical technique called Fourier series analysis developed by Baron Jean Baptiste Joseph Fourier. In this method, the EEG is assumed to be composed of a large number of individual waves of specific frequencies much like light is composed of a mix of different colors. The results of this analysis is termed frequency domain and allows a plot of power at each frequency.
      (1) There are two types of common frequency domain displays. The Compressed Spectral Array (CSA) presents the plot of power versus frequency with plots stacked in a third dimension showing changes over time. The Density Spectral Array (DSA) is similar except the amplitude of the power is shown in color or gray scale.
      (2) In the frequency domain a commonly derived parameter is the spectral edge frequency (SEF) (above which there is very little power; e.g., SEF95 is the frequency where 95% of the power is below).

E. Other mathematical processing techniques. A variety of other mathematical processing techniques have been employed. These include analyzing the relationship of different frequency components within the EEG with each other. [2] The bispectrum measures the correlation of phase between different frequency components. This analysis may describe the synchrony of different generators of the EEG. The degree of asynchrony or variability in the EEG has also been quantitated.

F. Anesthesia effects

1. EEG abnormalities appear rapidly when cerebral blood flow is reduced making the EEG useful to detect cerebral ischemia; generally an asymmetric drop in amplitude or reduction in frequency occurs with ischemia.

    a. The EEG becomes abnormal below 22 cc/min/100 g and absent below 15 cc/min/100 g (ischemic threshold). The EEG usually fails in 20 seconds following complete cessation of blood flow. This ischemia can eventually lead to cellular death; cell death is also a function of the duration of hypoperfusion. For example, cell death may take 3 to 4 hours when the cerebral blood flow is just below the blood flow where the EEG becomes abnormal. Infarction occurs after progressively shorter periods of time as the blood flow is reduced below this level.

    b. Regions that have the highest metabolic rate or are farthest from the major supply arteries (i.e., boundary regions) are most sensitive to hypoperfusion, making them among the best electrode locations to detect regional ischemia.

    c. EEG monitoring is used during surgery where there is a risk of stroke due to reduced blood flow such as during intracranial and extracranial vascular surgery (e.g., carotid endarterectomy, [CEA], intracranial aneurysm surgery).

    d. With vascular surgery the time to change in the EEG following cross-clamping has also been used to estimate the allowable ischemic time before irreversible neuronal injury occurs or to prompt the consideration for the use of a shunt. Of note with CEA, the EEG only monitors the surface of the brain and may miss ischemic insults deep in the brain. In addition, it may not detect the two-thirds of postoperative strokes in CEA that are thought to result from embolic events.

    e. The EEG can also be used during intracranial vascular surgery to determine the tolerance of the cortex for temporary cross-clamping. Rapid EEG loss indicates poor collateral flow and suggests that medical interventions such as induced hypertension should be considered to improve collateral flow.

2. Since approximately 40% to 50% of the resting energy utilization of the neurons is utilized by normal neuronal activity reflected in the EEG, the EEG has been used to monitor intentional metabolic suppression of the brain to improve the supply–demand relationship during the periods of reduced supply.

> **CLINICAL PEARL**   The EEG is a reflection of the 40% to 50% of the metabolic activity in the cortical neurons related to synaptic function.

    a. During surgical procedures

        (1) The reduction of EEG activity during metabolic suppression by anesthetics has allowed the EEG to be used to insure or guide suppression during procedures where cerebral blood flow may be compromised (e.g., repair of an aortic arch, CEA, intracranial vascular surgery).

        (2) This technique is used to monitor metabolic suppression in the intensive care unit (e.g., "barbiturate coma").

        (3) The EEG can also be used with hypothermia, which can reduce the entire cellular metabolism.

        (4) Burst suppression is used as the endpoint of drug-induced suppression as it represents near-maximal suppression of neuronal activity.

> **CLINICAL PEARL**   Burst suppression shows near-maximal neuronal depression.

        (5) The EEG can also detect the increased metabolism associated with seizure activity to prompt treatment which will reduce the excessive metabolic activity.

3. The ability to detect the electrical activity of seizures is a unique aspect of the EEG which is useful during surgery and in the intensive care unit.

   a. In the operating room this allows the EEG to be recorded directly from the cortex of the brain (electrocorticography or ECoG) to identify a seizure focus for tissue resection. When the abnormal foci is located near the eloquent cortex (near the speech or motor cortex), an awake craniotomy allows the identification of the cortex critical for speech or motor function so as to preserve these functions while resecting the seizure foci with a reasonable possibility of permanent seizure resolution.

   b. An awake craniotomy may not be essential when motor areas are involved, as nowadays motor evoked potential (MEP) monitoring as well as cortical and subcortical mapping represent safe and reliable methods to protect these functions in patients under general anesthesia. Yet, awake craniotomies remain the gold standard when language and other cognitive functions are at risk during surgery because there are no techniques yet that can assess the functional integrity of these functions in an asleep patient.

   c. EEG, in the form of ECoG, can also be used to detect evoked seizures (the so-called afterdischarges) during electrical stimulation of the brain when it is used to detect the speech centers by interruption of clinical function during stimulation. It can also detect seizure activity when stimulation of the cortex is used to map the motor cortex (about 25% of cases have induced seizures when a 50- to 60-Hz monopolar stimulator device [Penfield technique] is used for the stimulation).

   d. If a clinical seizure is induced intraoperatively by cortical stimulation, before the administration of any antiepileptic or neuroprotective drug that may interfere with the result of mapping, it is advisable to irrigate the cortex with cold (4°C) Ringer's solution. This suffices, most of the time, to arrest the seizure without compromising further neurophysiologic testing; if needed, a small dose of propofol will terminate the seizure.

   e. EEG is useful for seizure detection in the intensive care unit, particularly when patients are pharmacologically paralyzed such that the motor component is not observable. It will also detect seizures that are not associated with motor activity (this occurs in 4% to 14% of traumatic brain-injured patients).

   f. In ICU patients, EEG monitoring has also been used to determine brain death (cessation of EEG activity in the absence of hypothermia or medications known to depress the EEG).

4. Anesthesia effects on the EEG appear to be mediated by drug effects on synaptic function. Differences between anesthetic agents relate to the spectrum of synaptic receptors altered and the effect on a multitude of receptor subtypes throughout the nervous system. [3,4]

   a. A general pattern of drug effects is common among many anesthetics; however, not all drugs follow the same pattern.

   b. The general changes in the EEG when anesthetics are added to the awake state include the following: (1) An initial excitatory stage with increased power in the faster alpha and beta frequencies that is prominent in the frontal regions, (2) prominent activity in the alpha frequencies which develops in the more posterior regions, (3) the faster frontal region activity moves posterior while the posterior alpha activity moves forward, (4) a reduction in the variability across the brain with a marked increase in the global cortical synchrony and an uncoupling or disruption of the interaction between right and left frontal and parietal regions, (5) a general reduction in high-frequency activity with increases in slower frequencies (theta and delta), (6) a general reduction in EEG amplitude after an initial increase in amplitude, and (7) some agents will stop all activity at higher doses (metabolic suppression).

CLINICAL PEARL A decrease in EEG amplitude and frequency usually occurs with deeper anesthesia.

   (1) Currently used volatile anesthetic agents (sevoflurane, desflurane, and isoflurane) cause a progressive and profound depression of the EEG at higher doses. At deep surgical anesthetic concentrations, burst suppression occurs at approximately 1.5 times

the minimal alveolar concentration (MAC). Higher concentrations produce electrocerebral silence.

(2) Intravenous anesthetic drugs (propofol, barbiturates, etomidate, benzodiazepines) at higher doses produce the typical EEG anesthetic depression pattern described above.

(3) Nitrous oxide, as well as the intravenous agent ketamine, can produce EEG excitation with the increase of higher frequencies. Ketamine has been reported to provoke seizure activity in patients with epilepsy but not in normal subjects.

(4) The opioids produce a dose-related decrease in frequency of the EEG until it is in the delta range while maintaining amplitude. Since the opioids do not produce marked suppression of the EEG, they are frequently used during ECoG in surgery for seizure focus identification and ablation.

(5) Dexmedetomidine does not produce burst suppression and produces an EEG which is very similar to slow-wave sleep.

(6) Some anesthetics can produce both depression and enhancement of synaptic activity. With excitement, the EEG has increased amplitude and frequency that can become epileptiform. In small doses these agents (methohexital and etomidate) can be used to enhance epileptic foci during ECoG to assist in identifying native seizure foci. Only enflurane and sevoflurane of the volatile anesthetics can, in high concentrations with hyperventilation, cause epileptiform spikes or electrographic seizures.

CLINICAL PEARL   Methohexital and etomidate can be used to enhance recording of a native seizure focus.

    c. Monitoring anesthetic agent effect can be done by visual inspection of the EEG as well as using a variety of processed EEG devices. In each case, mathematical tools are used to derive a parameter associated with the degree of anesthetic drug effect.

III. Electromyography is the recording of the electrical activity of muscles and has been known since Francesco Redi's observations in 1666. Clinical diagnostic uses evolved between the 1920s and 1950s with its major intraoperative use starting in the 1960s to preserve facial nerve function during brainstem surgery for acoustic neuroma (vestibular schwannoma). Additional interest emerged to assess nerve roots during spinal surgery in the 1990s [5,6].

    A. Overview. Similar to the EEG, the EMG is the observation of spontaneous activity. When a person is awake, the muscle activity of the EMG has characteristic activity; under anesthesia the EMG is normally quiet allowing it to show abnormal activity in the muscles or the nerves which innervate the muscle being monitored (termed "free run" monitoring). In addition, the EMG can be used for the detection of stimulation of the motor nerves (intentional or unintentional).

CLINICAL PEARL   The EMG is normally quiet (inactive) under anesthesia.

    B. Recording techniques. EMG recording can be recorded from muscles innervated by both peripheral and cranial nerves

      1. Cranial nerve monitoring is of particular interest since they are susceptible to damage intraoperatively due to their small size, limited epineurium, and complicated course. They also may be intertwined in tumors placing them at risk during tumor resection. Damage occurs from either trauma (surgical disruption, manipulation) or ischemia, and this leads to paresis or paralysis (with subsequent disability or deformity) and possibly pain [7].

      2. Monitoring can be accomplished from all cranial nerves which have motor components. The most frequently monitored cranial nerve is the facial nerve which is commonly monitored using the orbicularis oculi and orbicularis oris muscles ipsilateral to the side of surgery (Table 26.2).

TABLE 26.2 Muscles for cranial nerve monitoring

Cranial nerve	Muscles monitored
III	Oculomotor: Inferior or superior rectus muscle
IV	Trochlear: Superior oblique muscle
V	Trigeminal: Masseter muscle and/or temporalis muscle
VI	Abducens: Lateral rectus muscle
VII	Facial: Orbicularis oculi muscle and/or orbicularis oris muscle
IX	Glossopharyngeal: Stylopharyngeus muscle (posterior soft palate)
X	Vagus: Vocal folds, cricothyroid muscle
XI	Spinal accessory: Sternocleidomastoid muscle and/or trapezious muscle
XII	Hypoglossal: Genioglossus muscle (tongue)

3. EMG techniques have been used with peripheral nerves, most notably to assess nerve roots with spinal corrective surgery (Table 26.3) [8].

C. **Responses**

1. The EMG is recorded by electrode pairs placed in (especially for diagnostic applications) or near (typically for monitoring) the muscles of interest. The difference in electrical activity between the two electrodes is displayed similar to EEG techniques. The activity can also be played in a loudspeaker to give audible feedback.

2. Three types of abnormal spontaneous activities are usually seen during monitoring.

   a. Continuous low-amplitude activity seen in multiple muscles is often due to light anesthesia. The audible sound is often continuous noise.

   b. Neurotonic bursts are high-frequency intermittent or continuous bursts from nerve irritation such as mechanical stimulation (e.g., nearby dissection, ultrasonic aspiration, or drilling), nerve retraction, thermal irritation (e.g., heating from irrigation, lasers, drilling, or electrocautery), and chemical or metabolic insults. Bursts usually last less than 200 msec with single or multiple motor unit potentials firing at 30 to 100 Hz. The audible sound is often a short "blurp." Typically, these bursts last only for a short time after the mechanical stimulation of the nerve has stopped, and usually are not of concern unless they are of high amplitude or sustained.

   c. Long neurotonic trains of activity may be indicative of neural injury and are causes for concern and alarm. They are commonly associated with impending nerve injury (nerve compression, contusion, sustained traction, stretching, or ischemia of the nerve); the more sustained the activity, the greater the likelihood of nerve damage. Their audible

TABLE 26.3 Muscles typically monitored for peripheral nerve monitoring

C2–C4	Trapezoids, sternocleidomastoid
C5–C6	Biceps, deltoid
C6–C7	Flexor carpi radialis
C8–T1	Adductor pollicis brevis, abductor digiti minimi
T5–T6	Upper rectus abdominis
T7–T8	Middle rectus abdominis
T9–T11	Lower rectus abdominis
T12	Inferior rectus abdominis
L2	Adductor longus
L2–L4	Vastus medialis
L4–S1	Tibialis anterior
L5–S1	Peroneus longus
S1–S2	Gastrocnemius
S2–S4	Anal sphincter

sounds have a more musical quality and have been likened to the sound of an outboard motor boat engine, swarming bees, popping corn ("popcorn"), or an aircraft engine ("bomber") potentials.

d. Recently, a specific pattern of neurotonic discharges, called A train, have been identified in the spontaneous activity of the facial nerve during surgery for vestibular schwannomas. Unlike other patterns of EMG activity, these trains and their duration seem to represent a reliable prognostic indicator of postoperative facial nerve palsy [9].

e. Often multiple muscles are monitored so as to identify activity in different branches of a nerve or so that the responses from one nerve and muscle are not confused with the response of a different nerve and a nearby muscle. For example, recordings from the orbicularis oris or orbicularis oculi might show EMG thought to be from stimulation of the facial nerve, but may actually be recordings of activity from the nearby masseter (CN V) or temporalis muscles (CN VII) when nearby cranial nerves are stimulated.

f. Multiple peripheral muscles may be monitored because they are often innervated through multiple nerve roots.

g. Cutting a nerve may not result in an EMG response.

3. EMG as a result of stimulation of a cranial or peripheral nerve can be used to locate the nerve or identify its integrity during surgery (this evoked EMG response is often termed a compound muscle action potential [CMAP]).

a. Searching with high-intensity stimulation can find the general vicinity of a nerve. Lower-intensity stimulation can locate the nerve. In this way, it is possible to identify regions of a tumor where there is no motor component of a cranial nerve present so that large portions of the tumor can be quickly resected with a low risk of causing permanent neurologic injury.

b. Continual stimulation with electrified instruments during surgery can assist a surgeon in operating with warning when they may be encroaching on the nerve.

c. The amplitude of the CMAP response of the facial nerve has been correlated with immediate and long-term muscle function.

d. Overall, the recording of free-running EMG activity remains a valuable and very common method to monitor cranial nerve function. Yet, one of the limitations of this methodology is due to the variety of stimuli that can influence the pattern of discharge. With the exception of facial nerve monitoring in cerebellopontine surgery, the reliability of EMG activity to monitor the function of other cranial motor nerves is still debated due to the existence of false-negative and especially false-positive responses. Paradoxically, a cranial nerve can be cut with no changes in the EMG activity. Vice versa, sustained activity may not necessarily result in postoperative deficits.

e. For these reasons, other techniques to assess the functional integrity of cranial motor nerves have been explored. Corticobulbar techniques are less commonly used methods to continuously assess the facial nerve by stimulation of the brain similar to the MEP technique described below. This allows a continual evoked assessment of the neural pathway rather than intermittent assessment using stimulation mapping techniques during brainstem surgery (see below).

D. Applications of EMG monitoring. Applications of EMG monitoring provide useful information in a large array of surgical situations including posterior fossa, head and neck, spine, and major joint surgery.

1. EMG is frequently utilized during brainstem surgery to monitor cranial nerve integrity.

a. EMG monitoring of the facial nerve is particularly helpful with vestibular schwannoma (acoustic neuroma) where monitoring increases the likelihood that the anatomic integrity of the nerve will be maintained during surgery. In these cases, over 60% of patients with intact nerves at the conclusion of surgery will regain at least partial function several months postoperatively. An NIH consensus panel has established this use as a standard of care [10].

b. Some authors suggest that a very low threshold (<0.05 mA) for stimulation of the facial nerve at the brainstem, after the removal of a vestibular schwannoma, indicates good motor outcome. Yet, this has been recently questioned due to the low negative and positive predictive values of such a test.

c. Monitoring of the lower cranial nerve nuclei (IX to XII) can help prevent complications of dyspnea, severe dysphagia, and aspiration requiring tracheostomy.

d. EMG monitoring is used in surgery with hyperactive cranial nerves and cranial nerve compression syndromes including trigeminal neuralgia (V), hemifacial spasm (VII), and vagoglossalpharyngeal neuralgia (IX, X).

2. EMG has been frequently utilized during spinal surgery where it is considered more sensitive for detecting radiculopathy than the somatosensory evoked potential (SSEP); the SSEP pathway traverses multiple nerve roots such that the SSEP cortical responses may be unaffected if only one nerve root is injured.

a. Spontaneous ("free run") EMG is used to identify unfavorable stretch or impending injury to nerve roots during approaches to the spine (e.g., lateral approach to the lumbar spine which traverses the lumbar plexus).

b. EMG monitoring has been used to reduce the risk of nerve injury secondary to misplaced pedicle screws (as frequent as 15% to 25%). In this case the pilot hole or screw is stimulated and the current necessary to activate the EMG from the nerve root or spinal cord is measured. If the current is low, then the screw may need to be repositioned as it may have broached the pedicle wall and may be too near to the neural elements so as to cause irritation.

c. EMG during surgery on the cauda equina has proven essential to differentiate neural tissue from nonfunctioning tissue structures tethering the spinal cord which would be cut. It is especially useful to identify nerve roots to the anal and urethral sphincters to maintain bowel or bladder control (S2–S4) [9,11].

d. EMG is useful to identify nerve rootlets during dorsal rhizotomy for sacrifice to reduce incapacitating spasticity (often seen with cerebral palsy). Here, EMG recording is used to identify the most hyperactive rootlets by observing the spread of activity to adjacent myotomes when the rootlets are stimulated (usually between L2 and S2). As with surgery in the cauda equina, EMG recording is also the key preserving rootlets to the anal sphincter and urogenital system.

3. EMG Monitoring has been found to be useful in a variety of other surgeries.

a. Recording of vagal nerve EMG activity is typically done using electrodes in the vocalis muscle or with an endotracheal tube with attached electrodes which are able to make contact with the vocal cords. This is used in surgery on the anterior neck (e.g., thyroidectomy, neck dissection, anterior spine surgery) to identify and prevent damage to the recurrent laryngeal nerve.

b. EMG recordings from the facial musculature can also be used during facial surgery (such as surgery on the parotid gland) to reduce the risk of facial nerve injury.

c. EMG responses have been used to detect unfavorable stretch of peripheral nerves in orthopedic joint surgery. For example, hip replacement or hip arthroscopy can cause nerve stretch where the EMG would signal caution.

d. Identification of the motor cortex can be done by stimulation of the cortex and recording EMG of muscles activated by the stimulation. This can be helpful to preserve motor function during resection of nearby cerebral pathology.

E. **Anesthesia effects.** Anesthesia considerations concern the use of muscle relaxation. If relaxation must be used, the amplitude of the EMG response will be reduced which may make spontaneous activity undetectable. For stimulated activity, CMAP activity can generally be detected when train-of-four (TOF) testing produces only one twitch or with 75% suppression of the single twitch. However, having more than one twitch is desirable, since the amplitude of the CMAP is reduced by muscle relaxants and small CMAPs may be missed. Pedicle screw thresholds may be falsely elevated with greater than 75% blockade.

CLINICAL PEARL Muscle relaxants should be avoided when electromyographic (EMG) recording is being done.

IV. **Somatosensory evoked potentials** are a method to assess a normally quiet sensory pathway by stimulating the pathway and recording the evoked response (much like stimulated EMG). Because of the small size of the cortical response to peripheral nerve stimulation, the development of the SSEP required signal averaging and the development of digital computers in the 1970s and 1980s. Applications in IOM became common when Nash and Brown in the 1970s found an application in reducing the risk of paralysis in scoliosis correction.

A. **Overview.** The SSEP response has wide clinical utility because of the length of its neural pathway and the various neural risks associated with surgery along that pathway.

B. **Anatomy.** The SSEP is a sensory-evoked response which involves stimulation of a peripheral sensory nerve and recording the response of the sensory cortex.

1. Although any sensory nerve could be used, large, mixed motor and sensory nerves are usually stimulated electrically. The nerves usually utilized for IOM tend to be the median (component roots C6–T1), ulnar (C8–T1), posterior tibial (L4–S2), and occasionally the common peroneal nerve (L4–S1).

2. Peripheral nerve stimulation activates the large diameter, fast conducting Ia muscle afferent and group II cutaneous nerve fibers producing both sensory transmission giving rise to the monitored response and transmission through the motor fibers giving rise to muscle contraction.

3. The evoked sensory response follows the pathway of proprioception and vibration (Fig. 26.1) that enters the spinal cord via several posterior nerve roots in the brachial or

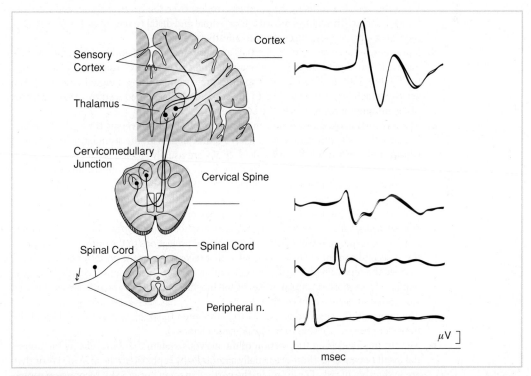

FIGURE 26.1 Pathway of the somatosensory evoked potential. The SSEP is produced by stimulation of a peripheral nerve (*arrow*). The electrical activity enters via the dorsal nerve root and ascends the spinal cord via the dorsal column pathway of proprioception and vibration. It synapses at the cervicomedullary junction and crosses the midline ascending in the medial lemniscus to the ventromedial nucleus of the thalamus where it has a second synapse. From there it ascends to the sensory cerebral cortex for the limb stimulated. SSEP recordings can be made along the pathway; shown are the responses from the peripheral nerve, spinal cord, cervical spine, and cerebral cortex. (Reproduced from Jameson LC, Janik DJ, Sloan TB. Electrophysiologic monitoring in neurosurgery. *Anesthesiol Clin.* 2007;25:605–630, with permission.) [12]

lumbar plexus and ascends the spinal cord via the ipsilateral dorsal column. It makes its first synapse near the nucleatus cuneatus (upper extremity) and nucleatus gracilis (lower extremity), crosses the midline near the cervicomedullary junction, ascending through the brainstem via the contralateral medial lemniscus. It makes a second synapse in the ventroposterolateral nucleus of the thalamus and then continues to the contralateral sensory cortex. The upper extremity cortical region is in the parietal lobe and that for the lower extremity is along the interhemispheric fissure.

4. The middle cerebral artery provides blood flow to the cortex generating the upper extremity SSEP and the anterior cerebral artery (ACA) provides the blood flow to the cortex of the lower extremity response.

C. **Recording techniques**

1. **Basic method**

    a. Traditionally, the nerves are stimulated using repetitive (2 to 5 Hz) electrical stimuli delivered peripherally (e.g., at the wrist or ankle). Each limb is stimulated separately so as to allow observation of each limb's pathway. The intensity is usually set above the motor threshold, so hand and foot motion signals successful stimulation. Occasionally an ECG or pulse oximetry artifact of stimulation is seen.

    b. The response is recorded using a differential amplifier with one electrode near the tissue generating the response and another reference electrode to remove noise similar to that used for EEG and EMG.

    c. Recording electrodes can be placed at numerous locations along the neural pathway. For example, the posterior tibial nerve SSEP can be recorded at the popliteal fossa, along the spinal cord using epidural electrodes, over the cervical spine, and over the sensory cortex. This allows recordings proximal and distal to the surgical site as well as recordings that are less susceptible to anesthetic effects.

    d. Since these evoked electrical potentials are very small (less than 10 μV), signal averaging is used to resolve them from the much larger EEG and ECG activity. A large number (100 to 200) of time-locked responses are summed using a digital computer. The activity which is not time locked to the stimulus (noise) is reduced by the square root of the number of responses in the average.

    e. The recorded evoked response consists of a plot of voltage versus time. This typically has an artifact of stimulation at time zero (coincident with the stimulation) and then a subsequent series of peaks and valleys. Peaks are usually labeled by the polarity (positive [P] or negative [N]) followed by the time in milliseconds from stimulation. Hence the cortical N_{20} of the median or ulnar nerve SSEP is a negative peak occurring about 20 msec after stimulation and the cortical peak of the posterior tibial nerve is labeled P38 for a positive cortical peak at about 38 msec.

    f. Several peaks can be identified in high-quality diagnostic recordings. The most commonly monitored response is that of the thalamocortical projections to the primary sensory cortex. A second commonly recorded peak is that recorded over the posterior cervical spine (termed the cervicomedullary or "subcortical" response). The response recorded from the popliteal fossa (posterior tibial nerve) or the brachial plexus (Erb's point) can also be used with spinal surgery to confirm that the evoked volley has been generated.

    g. The information recorded is usually the amplitude (peak to adjacent trough) and the time from the stimulation to the peak (called latency).

    h. Monitoring focuses on the portion of the nervous system that best reflects the potential insult of concern. These are usually anatomically cephalad to the area of risk or they are in the area of risk. For example, the cortical median nerve SSEP response is cephalad with spinal surgery and also the area of risk with middle cerebral artery surgery.

    i. Monitoring consists of acquiring baseline responses before surgery and then repeatedly rechecking the response. As a general principle, amplitude reduction of 50% or latency increase of 10% of cortical SSEPs is considered significant, although smaller changes may indicate impending compromise.

    j. If significant changes occur, then a search for the cause is made to prevent neural injury. Generally speaking, the causative event is likely technical, physiologic, anesthetic, or patient related (e.g., positioning or related to surgery). Often checking the SSEP in other limbs and other IOM modalities allows identification of the possible etiology [1].

D. Applications. Applications of the SSEP are many because its pathway traverses a large number of anatomic and vascular territories at risk during surgeries.

1. One of the biggest applications is during spinal cord surgery where it can identify mechanical or ischemic insults and reduce neural morbidity by 50% to 80% [13]. The utility of the SSEP in spinal surgery for scoliosis was shown in an analysis conducted by the Scoliosis Research Society (SRS) and European Spinal Deformities Society [14]. They evaluated the results of monitoring during correction of spinal deformity in 51,263 cases (scoliosis, kyphosis, fractures, and spondylolisthesis) by 173 surgeons. In these cases, the overall injury incidence was 0.55% (1 in 182 cases), well below the 0.7% to 4% historical average expected for instrumentation without monitoring. The incidence of definite false-negative response (i.e., in which the patient sustained a major neurologic injury without SSEP warning) was 0.063% (about 1 case in 1,500 procedures), indicating that the dissociation of motor loss with the SSEP was rare. The economic impact of monitoring was assessed by Nuwer, who estimated that the cost of monitoring enough cases (200 cases) to prevent one major, persistent neurologic deficit is small compared to the cost of lifelong medical care [15]. This has made monitoring during scoliosis correction a virtual standard of care. It should be noted that the SRS study was done at a time when MEP monitoring was not available and that the occurrence of a motor deficit in spite of preserved SSEP is a rare but possible event also in scoliosis surgery. Currently it is recommended to combine SSEP and MEP monitoring during spine procedures where the spinal cord is at risk, scoliosis surgery included.

2. The SSEP may be used to identify physiologic insults (e.g., hypotension) or positioning problems. Fast losses (with minimal latency change) may be due to mechanical injury or localized ischemia, especially in gray matter.

3. The SSEP is responsive to ischemia, but not as sensitive to cortical ischemia as the EEG. A 50% loss in cortical SSEP amplitude correlates with a regional cerebral blood flow of 14 to 16 cc/min/100 g, a level of blood flow above that which produces irreversible injury [16].

4. The SSEP can also detect inadequate spinal cord perfusion of the white matter tracts of the posterior columns. This has made it useful in surgery that can compromise the blood supply to the spinal cord such as with the repair of thoracoabdominal aneurysms [17]. In these surgeries the SSEP has been used to identify inadequate distal perfusion of the spinal cord from bypass techniques. Changes have also been used to identify when the patient is critically dependent on a radicular artery that may need to be reimplanted.

5. SSEP monitoring is frequently utilized during surgery on the posterior fossa to assess the integrity of the brainstem. When combined with auditory brainstem response (ABR) monitoring (below), they can monitor the functional integrity of about 20% of the brainstem.

6. The SSEP has also been used during craniotomy to localize the gyrus separating the motor and sensory strip (rolandic fissure). Here the location of a phase reversal of the response as measured by electrodes placed on the cortical surface identifies the sulcus (the phase reversal occurs because the generator is located deep in the sulcus).

7. The SSEP has been used to identify cortical ischemia during CEA and during retractors placed during craniotomies. In addition to specific vascular occlusion, combinations of surgical actions (e.g., retractor pressure, hypotension, temporary clipping, hyperventilation, and vasospasm) can combine to produce unexpected neuronal ischemia.

8. In supratentorial vascular surgery (e.g., intracranial arteriovenous malformation [AVM], intracranial aneurysm surgery, and interventional neuroradiologic procedures), the SSEP has been used to detect cortical ischemia. Among the most common applications is during aneurysm surgery of the anterior circulation. For ACA aneurysms, the lower extremity SSEP is most useful due to the vascular territory involved, whereas upper extremity SSEP is used with middle cerebral artery aneurysms and those of the internal carotid artery. Monitoring of both upper and lower extremities may be useful if perforating arteries are at risk.

E. Effects of anesthesia

1. With respect to anesthesia, the cortical SSEP shows decreased amplitude and increased latency in a dose-related manner by inhalational agents. However, it can usually be obtained in most neurologically normal patients with 0.5 MAC of a volatile anesthetic supplemented by intravenous medications (usually opioids or intravenous hypnotics) [16,18,19].

> **CLINICAL PEARL**   Anesthesia tends to affect the amplitude of the SSEP more than the latency.

2. Total intravenous anesthesia (TIVA) is used when inhalational agents must be removed to acquire responses such as in patients with significant preoperative neurologic findings. This is typically a propofol–opioid infusion.

3. Most intravenous sedative/hypnotic agents (e.g., propofol) produce minimal depression of cortical amplitude unless high doses are used.

4. Opioids have minimal effect except for transient decreases in cortical amplitude with bolus administration.

5. Etomidate and ketamine have been shown to increase rather than decrease cortical amplitude at lower doses.

6. Complete muscle relaxation may improve the responses recorded near muscles (such as over the cervical spine); however, relaxation may not be acceptable if EMG or MEPs are also being monitored.

7. The anesthetic effects are markedly less on recordings from the cervical spine, epidural space, or over peripheral nerves.

V. Dermatomal evoked potentials are an evoked sensory response that has the potential to assess individual nerve roots. In this technique the skin dermatome of interest is stimulated and the cortical response is recorded like the SSEP. The specific anatomic paths stimulated by the DEP are unknown, but the amplitude of the cortically recorded response appears to be related to the somatotopic representation of the dermatome with regions such as the hands and feet having larger responses. Unfortunately, the use of DEP is limited because of controversy surrounding the exact dermatome distribution in some regions (e.g., L_5), poor amplitude of responses in areas of regions with small cerebral representation (such as thoracic region), and substantial anesthetic effects.

VI. Auditory brainstem response is a second widely used sensory evoked response [20]. Also known by the terms brainstem auditory evoked response (BAER), and brainstem auditory evoked potential (BAEP), it has been known since 1967 with the development of applications in the 1970s. Like the SSEP, it requires signal averaging so that the availability of digital computers markedly facilitated its development.

A. Overview. The use of ABR in IOM is important because the cochlear nerve, which is responsible for hearing and has been termed one of the most fragile cranial nerves, is frequently involved in tumors of the posterior fossa.

B. Anatomy and physiology

1. The neural pathway of the ABR appears to follow that of normal hearing (Fig. 26.2).

2. Stimulation is accomplished by sound which activates the cochlea after transmission through the external and middle ear.

3. The resulting nerve impulse travels to the brainstem via the eighth cranial nerve. It traverses the brainstem auditory pathway via the acoustic relay nuclei and lemniscal pathways to activate neurons in the auditory cortex.

4. Seven peaks are identified and named by roman numerals in the first 10 msec after stimulation. Peaks I, III, and V are most reliably seen and used during monitoring.

5. Wave I is produced by the extracranial portion of CN VIII, wave III by the cochlear nucleus and tracts deep in the midline of the lower pons, and wave V by the lateral lemniscus and inferior colliculus in the contralateral pons. Occasionally, wave II (auditory nerve) and wave IV (midline pons near the superior olivary complex) are seen; wave IV may blend with wave V.

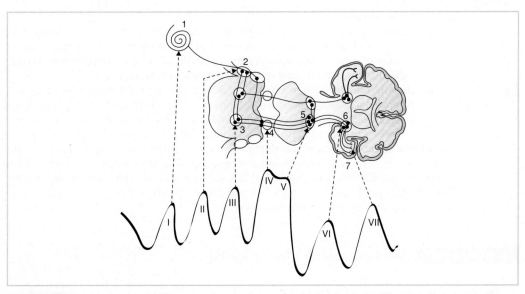

FIGURE 26.2 Pathway of the auditory brainstem response. The first seven peaks of the ABR are produced near the structures in the brainstem as described in the text. (Reproduced from Aravabhumi S, Izzo KL, Bakst BL, et al. Brainstem auditory evoked potentials: intraoperative monitoring technique in surgery of posterior fossa tumors. *Arch Phys Med Rehab*. 1987;68:142, with permission.) [21]

6. The auditory pathways in the brainstem represent components that are bilateral; however, waves I, II, and III are from structures primarily ipsilateral to the ear stimulated, whereas waves IV and V are primarily contralateral.

7. The neural signal continues to the auditory cortex where it can be recorded (termed the middle latency auditory evoked response).

C. **Recording technique**

1. The stimulation used for the ABR is the "clicks" delivered by headphones or insert earphones with broad frequency content with significant stimulation in the 1,000- to 4,000-Hz range. Other types of sound have also been used for stimulation, including short pure tone bursts, which have more defined frequency content.

2. The intensity of the sound is measured in decibels. The decibels peak equivalent sound pressure level (dB-PeSPL) is the physical sound pressure level. Occasionally the intensity is measured as decibels normal hearing level (dB-NHL) relative to the average normal adult hearing threshold level for the stimulus.

3. One ear is usually stimulated at a time, in order to focus on the neural pathway from that ear. Bone-conducted sound may also stimulate the contralateral cochlea, so "white" noise may be delivered to that ear to mask the bone-conducted sound.

4. The response is usually measured by recording electrodes near the ear and referenced to the top of the head (vertex). Since the ABR is of small amplitude, thousands (1,000 to 2,000) of responses must be signal averaged to acquire an adequate average similar to the technique used for the SSEP.

5. Because of the need for signal averaging, alternate recording locations have been used that require less averaging time. Cochlear microphonics are the recordings directly from an electrode placed in the inner ear near the cochlear capsule and from the electrodes in the lateral recess of the fourth ventricle (near the cochlear nucleus) or from the exposed intracranial portion of the eighth cranial nerve (cochlear nerve action potentials).

D. **Applications.** Applications are made more effective because the presence of several peaks from different anatomic locations help identify the anatomic location of intraoperative neural insults.

1. Posterior fossa

    a. Among the most common IOM applications of the ABR is to monitor for hearing preservation such as with acoustic neuroma, cerebellopontine tumor resection, decompression of space occupying defects in the cerebellum, removal of cerebellar vascular malformations, and vertebral and basilar artery aneurysm clipping.

    b. The ABR has been used to monitor the general viability of the brainstem such as during procedures for microvascular decompression for relief from hemifacial spasm, trigeminal neuralgia, or glossopharyngeal neuralgia. It is also used in conjunction with procedures to relieve tinnitus and disabling positional vertigo.

E. Anesthesia effects. In general, anesthetic effects on the ABR are minimal. Small shifts in latency may be seen as the concentration of inhalational agent increases. Nitrous oxide has little effect unless it causes increases in middle ear pressure from a blocked Eustachian tube. Some changes can be seen with shifts in body temperature and will be most dramatic if cold irrigation fluids are applied into the brainstem.

CLINICAL PEARL   Anesthesia has little effect on the ABR.

VII. Visual evoked potentials (VEPs) have been known since the response evoked in the EEG from light stimulation was noticed by Adrian and Matthew in 1934. Similar to other sensory responses, the development for diagnostic applications occurred in the 1970s. This has not been used as extensively in IOM as the SSEP or ABR [22].

A. Technique. Light flashes to the eye initially trigger a response by activating the photoreceptors in the retina. This response travels via the optic nerve to the optic chiasm and onward bilaterally, via the optic tracts to the lateral geniculate nucleus of the thalamus which then projects via the optic radiations to the visual cortex. It is important to note that the optic pathways cross at the chiasm such that monocular or binocular flash stimuli used in monitoring will produce bilateral activation behind the chiasm unless a means of hemivisual field stimulation can be done (as can be done in awake subjects).

B. Limitations. Technical problems with devices that provide the light flashes to the eye have limited the IOM applications of the VEP.

    1. Stimulation for diagnostic applications utilizes high-contrast stimuli such as a reversing checkerboard screen. Under anesthesia the patient is not able to focus on such a screen and the cornea must be protected from dehydration. Hence flash stimuli (often from light-emitting diodes) are delivered through closed eyelids or techniques such as scleral caps are used to mount a stimulator and also protect the eye.

    2. The response of the retina can be recorded near the eye. Termed the electroretinogram (ERG), the responses of the rods and cones can be separated by manipulating the color and intensity of the stimulus.

    3. The traditional VEP is measured using electrodes over the occipital visual cortex. One major peak is identified: N70 from IOM flash stimulation or P100 from checkerboard diagnostic stimulus in awake individuals.

    4. Since the correlation of visual acuity and flash-evoked responses is poor, the visual pathway monitored with the VEP may not be the pathway of useful vision.

C. Applications. Although diagnostic applications have been developed, IOM techniques are currently limited.

D. Anesthesia effects. Both the ERG and VEP are highly susceptible to anesthesia and physiologic effects.

    1. In general it appears that opioid and ketamine or propofol-based anesthetic techniques (TIVA), along with those employing low-dose volatile anesthetics without nitrous oxide, seem to facilitate intraoperative recording of VEPs.

    2. Concerns have been raised about the constriction of the pupils by opioids; however, this does not appear to be a problem that limits IOM.

VIII. Spinal stimulation techniques have been of interest because the anesthetic effects are markedly less than that on the SSEP and MEP.

  A. Epidural to epidural recording. Epidural to epidural recording involves two electrodes in the epidural space; one for stimulating and the other for recording the evoked response (spinal to spinal EPs). The pathway monitored is not clearly known and may include both sensory and motor tracts.

  B. Neurogenic motor evoked potentials (NMEP). One popular spinal cord stimulation technique was termed neurogenic motor evoked potentials (NMEPs). In this technique, stimulating electrodes are placed percutaneously near the vertebral bodies at adjacent levels cephalad to the level of surgery and recording electrodes are placed near a peripheral nerve distal to the surgical site, such as the sciatic nerve. Studies suggest this clearly has sensory components mediating the response and may not specifically monitor motor pathways.

  C. These techniques have largely been replaced by MEP.

IX. Motor evoked potentials have been developed because motor function is often considered more important clinically than sensory function. The pioneering work of Barker and of Merton and Morton in the 1980s led to the ability to stimulate the motor cortex transcranially through the scalp and record motor pathway responses in the spinal cord and muscle. The current technique became widely utilized in IOM in 2002 when it was approved by the Food and Drug Administration of the United States [23].

  A. Anatomy. Activation of the motor pathway is done by stimulation of the pyramidal cells of the motor cortex which results in a wave of depolarization that involves 4% to 5% of the corticospinal tract (Fig. 26.3). When this is recorded by electrodes in the epidural space, it is termed the "D" (direct) wave. Additional transsynaptic activation of internuncial pathways in the cortex results in a series of smaller waves called "I" (indirect) waves that follow the D wave. The motor pathway descends in the corticospinal pathway from the motor cortex, crossing the midline in the lower lateral brainstem and descending in the ipsilateral and anterior funiculi of the spinal cord. The electrical activity of the D and I waves summate in the anterior horn cell resulting in activation of the peripheral nerve which produces a CMAP.

  B. MEP techniques

  1. Stimulation can be accomplished by magnetic or electrical means.

  a. Magnetic stimulation is done using a coil held over the motor cortex which delivers a brief magnetic field (about 2 Tesla). This is a painless technique usable in awake individuals; however, some forms of magnetic stimulation preferentially activate the motor cortex transsynaptically. The CMAP produced is more susceptible to anesthesia and is difficult to record in the operating room because the presence of the coil over the motor cortex may interfere with surgery and a sustained stimulation can cause overheating of the coil. For these reasons, magnetic stimulation has been abandoned for intraoperative use.

  b. Electrical stimulation can be accomplished by application of a painful high-voltage (100 to 400 V) impulse to the scalp over the motor cortex. A single brief pulse (50 to 500 μsec) is useful to produce a single D wave that can be monitored in the epidural space. Unfortunately, single-pulse techniques (as with the magnetic technique) are less useful for IOM using muscle responses due to anesthesia effects at the spinal cord.

  c. The technique used most commonly at present is electrical stimulation using a high-frequency (approximately 500 Hz) train of 5 to 7 impulses described above. The multiple stimuli produce a series of D waves that are more effective in overcoming the anesthetic effects. In some patients two of these burst trains (double-burst technique) are delivered such that the first primes the motor pathway and the second train is more effective in producing a response.

  d. Another technique to enhance the response is to use a sensory stimulus, similar to that used for the SSEP, just before the MEP stimulus to prime the motor pathway.

  e. For monitoring of the motor cortex, the intensity of the stimulus is important since all of these techniques have the capacity to activate the corticospinal tract deep in

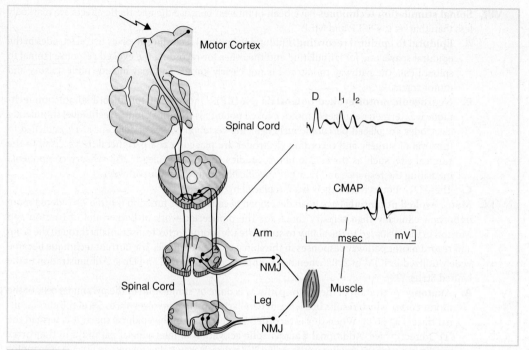

FIGURE 26.3 Pathway of the motor evoked potential. Motor evoked potentials (MEPs) are produced by stimulation of the motor cortex (*arrow*). The electrical activity descends following the corticospinal tract to the anterior horn of the spinal cord. After synapsing to the peripheral nerve and traversing the neuromuscular junction producing a muscle response. The MEP can be measured in the epidural space as D and I waves, or as a compound muscle action potential (CMAP). (Reproduced from Jameson LC, Sloan TB. Monitoring of the brain and spinal cord, *Anesthesiol Clin* 2006;24:777–792, with permission.) [24]

the brain (particularly at bends in the neural tracts) when the intensity is at higher levels. For this reason, direct stimulation of the cortex after craniotomy can be used to preferentially stimulate the motor cortex with low intensity (usually less than 20 mA) therefore reducing the risk of false-negative results (namely, a motor deficit in spite of intraoperatively preserved muscle MEPs) secondary to deep activation of the cortico-spinal tract.

f. Since the stimulation techniques involve stimulating the brain, concerns have been raised about cortical injury. Despite the theoretical concerns, the technique appears remarkably safe with the most common injury being tongue- or lip-bite injuries from jaw motion with stimulation (hence a good bite block is important). Controversy surrounds the contraindications to its use. Clearly implanted intracranial devices are a contraindication, but most other issues (e.g., seizure disorders, pacemakers, skull defects) are a balance between the benefits of IOM and the potentials risks of stimulation.

2. Recording

a. Epidural recording of the D wave can be done using epidural electrodes placed at surgery or percutaneously. IOM using this response has been favored during intramedullary surgery (e.g., spinal cord tumors) because the amplitude of the D wave is considered a semiquantitative assessment of the number of preserved fibers in the fast conducting fibers of the corticospinal tract and correlates better with long-term functional motor outcome than the muscle response (EMG) [25]. There are some disadvantages of epidural recordings. First, they likely represent activation of bilateral pathways, whereas recordings from muscles can differentiate unilateral changes and multiple segmental gray matter levels. Second, they cannot be used for lesion located at or caudally to the T10-T11 spine level, as most of the fibers have already left the spinal cord and the epidural recording would overlap the cauda equina rather than the spinal cord. Third, some multilevel spinal cord lesions D-wave recording may not be possible.

b. The more common recording technique is the measurement of the amplitude of the usually multipeaked CMAP (highest peak to lowest peak) and onset latency (time from stimulation to the beginning of the muscle response) using electrode pairs in muscles similar to the recording of EMG. Typically distal muscles with excellent corticospinal innervation are used (e.g., abductor pollicis brevis [component spinal levels C8–T1], anterior tibialis [L4–S1], and abductor hallucis [S1–S2]), but many other muscles can be used depending on the specific IOM concerns.

c. The D wave and CMAP responses are sufficiently large that signal averaging is not required which allows single pulse recording. This is advantageous since patient movement from stimulation may interfere with the surgery unless timed in coordination with the surgery. Hence stimulation is usually intermittent and coordinated with the surgeon.

d. Controversy surrounds the warning criteria for change in the CMAP responses primarily because the amplitude of the response is often variable. Loss of the response is universally accepted as concern; however, the degree of amplitude reduction, a change in morphology, and an increase in the stimulation voltage required (threshold) have also been suggested as signs of neural compromise.

3. Differences from SSEP make the MEP an important complementary technique in IOM. IOM of the motor tracts improves prediction of clinical motor outcome; the ability of the SSEP to predict most motor deficits probably results from mechanisms such as transverse mechanical insults which impact the entire spinal cord.

  a. The MEP traverses the anterior spinal cord, whereas the SSEP follows the posterior spinal cord. This can explain why an injury on one region may not be reflected in the other region.

  b. Second, although the MEP and SSEP pathways are white matter tracts, the MEP includes gray matter pathways in the anterior horn. Since the gray matter fails more quickly with ischemia, the MEP pathway is more effective in detecting spinal cord ischemia when it involves the gray matter of the muscles being monitored.

  c. The topographic difference is highlighted by the fact that the motor pathways are preferentially supplied by the anterior spinal artery and the SSEP pathways are supplied by the paired posterior spinal arteries.

  d. This difference in vascularity is also reflected in the vascular supply to these arteries. Hence compromise of radicular arteries, including the artery of Adamkiewicz (AA), makes the MEP more important in IOM with anterior spine surgery or procedures involving the thoracic aorta [17].

C. Applications. Surgical procedures where MEP is commonly used include corrective axial skeletal procedures, surgery on neural parenchymal disease (spinal cord tumor, brain tumor, neurovascular lesions), and procedures where spinal cord or cortical perfusion is at risk (thoracoabdominal aneurysms) [17].

1. Spinal corrective procedures commonly include MEP monitoring to warn of impending motor tract injury. The most frequent use of MEPs is in conjunction with SSEP and EMG monitoring. Because of the risk for damage to the spinal cord, both SSEP and MEP are usually monitored with surgery cephalad to the termination of the cord (L1–L2). Below this level the MEP is often omitted unless used to monitor the motor components of spinal roots. When the spinal cord may extend below the usual level (e.g., tethered cord), MEP is usually included.

2. MEP monitoring has been considered essential for intramedullary surgery [25]. As above, the D-wave amplitude decline has been considered an essential endpoint for stopping the surgery. In addition, stimulation within the spinal cord allows location of the corticospinal tract by producing a "collision" which blocks the D wave preventing a muscle response and thereby identifying the location of the tract.

3. MEP monitoring has also been useful during surgery where the vascular supply from the aorta is at risk. This includes surgical or interventional radiologic treatment for thoracoabdominal aneurysm and corrective anterior thoracic spine surgery.

4. MEP can be used to assess the general integrity of the brainstem structures near the surgical site or under retractors. With surgery close to the cerebral peduncles or the ventral medulla, injury to the corticospinal tracts is a concern and monitoring with MEP is important.

5. Monitoring MEPs of the face and hand musculature can assess the corticospinal and corticobulbar tracts, particularly for tumors in the posterior fossa. Corticobulbar MEPs for monitoring motor cranial nerve VII to XII have been introduced as an alternative to free-running EMG. The presence of these potentials at the end of surgery retains a good prognostic value for long-term motor outcome, while their disappearance well correlates with a postoperative deficit. However, discrepancies between monitoring data and clinical outcome exist and can be due to several reasons. First, corticobulbar MEPs cover only the efferent pathways of complex lower brainstem reflexes such as swallowing and coughing. If the sensory pathway is injured, this is not detectable with MEPs. Second, the amount of corticobulbar fibers monitored is variable and this may result in both false-positive or false-negative results depending on which fibers are monitored and which are injured.

6. Like the SSEP, MEP is useful in cortical vascular surgery. During middle and anterior cerebral aneurysm clipping, multiple portions of the motor pathway are at risk for ischemia (motor cortex, corticospinal tracts, internal capsule). With AVMs, the monitoring has allowed provocative testing of the vascular supply similar to that described above for spinal surgery to determine the safety of vessel sacrifice. MEP is also useful in intracranial aneurysm surgery where perforating arteries may be at risk to deep structures including the motor pathways in the corona radiata, internal capsule, cerebral peduncle, basis pontis, and pyramids.

7. Monitoring using MEP and SSEP has been used with tumors near the motor cortex, motor tracts (including in the brainstem), and insula (including cavernous angiomas) [26]. With surgery near the motor cortex, MEP using direct stimulation of the cortex can be used to identify the motor strip.

D. **Anesthesia effects.** Anesthesia effects on the MEP are among the most profound of all responses [16,19]. Although the epidural recording of the D wave is resistant to the effects, the CMAP response has a pattern of effects similar to the cortical SSEP except the effects are more dramatic.

1. As such, recording of the MEP often requires avoidance of inhalational agents since these significantly reduce the amplitude.

2. Intravenous agents such as benzodiazepines, etomidate, barbiturates, propofol, and dexmedetomidine can usually be used, but higher doses of these agents decrease the probability of generating a CMAP.

3. TIVA using propofol or propofol/ketamine mixture plus opioid are usually used to obtain an MEP muscle response.

CLINICAL PEARL TIVA is usually recommended for MEPs monitoring of muscle responses.

4. Similar to the cortical SSEP, ketamine increases the CMAP amplitude and decreases the threshold for the MEP response. Ketamine can therefore enhance the responses while reducing the amount of propofol needed for anesthesia (and its attendant depression) during TIVA.

CLINICAL PEARL Ketamine enhances the cortical amplitude of SSEP and the amplitude of MEP muscle responses, especially in children.

5. Neuromuscular blocking drugs must be avoided or their effects very carefully titrated as described above with EMG.

X. **Reflex pathway responses** are another method of monitoring the neural pathways which involves the utilization of reflex arcs in the central nervous system [27].

A. **The H-reflex.** The H-reflex involves a CMAP recorded from muscle which results from what is believed to be electrical activation of a monosynaptic spinal cord reflex.

1. The H-reflex can be monitored following stimulation of a peripheral nerve which produces a motor response (M wave) and a simultaneous centrally traveling volley of activity in the sensory and motor fibers of the nerve. The motor pathway response invades motor neurons in the ventral gray matter which are activated producing a second motor response (F wave). The activity traveling centrally along the sensory pathway activates reflex pathways in the spinal cord which results in activation of the anterior horn cell and a third motor response called the H-reflex. H-reflex responses can be recorded from several muscles in the adult; however, the reflex is most often acquired from the gastrocnemius muscle following stimulation of the tibial nerve at the popliteal fossa (primarily via S1).

2. In addition to monitoring the sensory and motor nerves, the H-reflex also monitors the spinal cord gray matter at the level of the reflex. In addition, it monitors the integrity of the more cephalad spinal cord because several descending pathways contribute to the excitability of the anterior horn cell and the reflex. Hence, a more proximal spinal cord injury produces a block of the reflex at lower levels ("spinal shock"). H-reflexes have been used when the MEP is not possible or contraindicated.

3. The H-reflex can usually be monitored using less than 0.5 MAC of any inhalational agent and a continuous infusion of an opioid. Similar to EMG and MEP, neuromuscular blocking agents can eliminate or reduce the amplitude of the response.

B. **Other reflex responses.** Other types of reflex responses can be monitored such as in posterior fossa surgery (blink reflex) and cauda equina (bulbocavernosis from pudendal nerve stimulation).

XI. **Consideration for IOM in pediatric patients**

A. **Overview.** The techniques described above are extensively used in adult surgery and, in principle, can be applied to children [28,29]. However, several issues make monitoring different in children when compared to adults. These include different pathology, changes in physical size, and changes in the nervous system as it matures. These have specific impacts on the different modalities. In some respects these are not an issue for monitoring since the patient serves as their own control; however, the ability to obtain recordings may be difficult and, when acquired, may appear abnormal compared to adults.

B. **Electroencephalography**

1. The pediatric EEG differs from the adult EEG because the electrical activity of the brain changes during growth and development. Therefore, children have different baseline EEG rhythms that are age specific.

2. In general, the normal pediatric EEG activity has more variation than adult EEG. Focal abnormalities are often normal. The EEG uniformly changes during different states of arousal.

3. The EEG has age-related changes in voltage, frequency, and morphology until it reaches stable levels at age 15 to 20 years. The most notable changes are in the dominant rhythm on the posterior/occipital area in the awake child. The dominant frequency increases with age (3 to 4 Hz at the age of 2 to 3 months, 5 Hz at 5 months, 6 to 7 Hz at 1 year, 8 Hz at the age of 2 years, 9 Hz at the age of 9 years, leveling at 10 Hz at the age of 13 years). The amplitude increases, peaking at the age of 2 years, with a steady decline thereafter, leveling off the age of 11 to 15 years.

4. The EEG is not frequently monitored in children except for epilepsy in older children. In these children a higher-stimulation voltage may be needed for identification of the eloquent cortex.

5. Penfield's technique—which accounts for a 50- to 60-Hz bipolar stimulation sustained for several seconds—has been extensively used in adults during epilepsy surgery and

brain tumor surgery. In children, due to the much lower incidence of gliomas, cortical mapping with Penfield's technique has been applied mainly in epilepsy surgery. There is some consistency across the literature in reporting limitations to elicit a motor response in younger children using this technique. Although failures to evoke motor activity in this population are likely due to the immaturity of the motor system, the kind of stimulation technique can play a role. Preliminary studies suggest a lower success rate of Penfield's technique versus the MEP short-train technique in performing DCS of the motor cortex in children [30].

6. Awake craniotomies for epilepsy surgery are not feasible in young children due to the lack of collaboration and the stressfulness of a surgical event at this age. Language and other cognitive functions, nevertheless, can be tested in children using a two-stage surgical strategy. On the first surgery, large cortical grids are implanted and can be used to study cortical function in the ward. The child then comes back to the operating room where surgery is tailored on the basis of the results of cortical testing. This approach is very popular in North America for epilepsy surgery but can certainly be applied also for the removal of tumors or other lesions, such as AVMs, in eloquent areas.

C. **Electromyography**

1. EMG recording is made difficult in children by a larger amount of subcutaneous fat. This obscures bony landmarks making it more difficult to identify muscles. In addition, longer needles may be needed to acquire adequate muscle responses.

2. Due to the myelination and maturation of the nervous system, nerve conduction and awake EMG activity will vary with age. Since peripheral myelination advances gradually for the first 3 to 5 years after birth, nerve conduction velocity in the very young will be about one-half of adult values and won't reach adult values until the age of 3 years.

3. Infants and newborns have an immature neuromuscular junction which may appear as a neuromuscular transmission defect.

4. The maturation process also affects the motor unit potential size and EMG amplitude. Hence the amplitude may be smaller in the very young than those found in older children and may resemble a patient with a myopathy.

5. EMG is commonly used during surgery for lumbosacral lipomas in children with occult spina bifida. Recording of CMAPs from lower extremity muscles and the sphincters prevents injuring functional rootlets encased in the fat tissue. In addition, it may help improve cord detethering as some of these rootlets, in spite of their anatomical appearance, are not functional and can be cut to improve cord release. Yet, before cutting any rootlet, it is of outmost importance to make sure that the functional information pertinent to that spinal cord level is carried on by other, preserved, rootlets.

6. To improve the localizing value of rootlet mapping in the cauda of young children, due to the small size of these neural structures and the fact that are packed in a very narrow space, it is advisable to use a handheld bipolar concentric rather than a monopolar electrode in order to limit current spreading.

D. **Somatosensory evoked potentials**

1. The developmental changes in the nervous system result in improved conduction velocity and reduced latency from birth to the age of 4 years. At that time, the growth of body size and nerve length results in prolonged latencies until adult values are obtained. The effect is more pronounced in the lower extremity response than in the upper extremity response. Since maturation proceeds at different rates in different regions (proceeding more slowly in central regions), the morphology of the SSEP changes from a wide cortical peak to the more defined peak of adulthood by 3 to 4 years.

2. In children under the age of 3 years, the effects of anesthesia may be more profound owing to the immaturity of the neural pathways. This effect is more profound in younger children and may require TIVA (often with ketamine to enhance the recordings). At the opposite end, a healthy adolescent may have excellent responses allowing more inhalational agent use than in an adult.

3. Especially in younger children, where the motor cortex and pathways are sometimes too immature for a successful motor mapping, the SSEP phase reversal technique may be the only way to identify the central sulcus and therefore, indirectly, the primary motor area.

E.   Auditory brainstem responses
1. The smaller size of the child's ear will necessitate smaller ear insert stimulators.
2. Chronic or acute middle ear infection may result in wave I prolongation or loss.
3. The myelination of the auditory nerve starts during postconceptual week 24 and progresses so that the nerve and brainstem tracts are incomplete at birth, although wave I has a normal adult latency at that time. Myelination is likely complete by the age of 3 years when peak V reaches adult latency values.

F.   Motor evoked potentials
1. The child's physical size may impact the muscle recordings as above with EMG.
2. In children under the age of 3 years the effects of anesthesia may be more profound owing to the immaturity of the neural pathways. Ketamine may be a helpful agent in these children, especially if propofol raises concerns about propofol infusion syndrome.
3. The D-wave was only anecdotally recorded in children younger than 21 months. This is likely due to the immaturity of the corticospinal fibers in younger children where incompletely myelinated fibers have variable conduction velocities resulting in desynchronization.
4. The immature motor pathways make acquiring MEP muscle responses difficult in very small children [30].
   a. Development of the motor pathways has a major impact on the ability to record MEPs in the child. Functional synaptic corticospinal projections to motoneurons and to spinal interneurons are established prenatally during the last trimester of pregnancy.
   b. Corticospinal pathways then develop throughout childhood, with motor stimulation threshold increasing over the first 3 months of life but then linearly decreasing until early adolescence when the adult motor threshold is reached.
   c. Although corticomotoneuronal connections reach sacral levels between 18 and 28 weeks postconceptional age, and are completed at birth, myelination of the lumbar spinal cord occurs between 1 and 2 years of age, with a slower development for lower extremities than for upper extremities. The neurophysiologic maturation of these pathways progresses throughout childhood and adolescence with myelogenesis and synaptogenesis that continues in to the second decade of life.
   d. The developing axons in the corticospinal tract develop such that their conduction velocity does not achieve adult levels until age 15 to 16 years.
   e. MEP stimulation is usually applied using corkscrew electrodes which guarantee low impedance, but these electrodes should be cautiously used in infants under 18 months with open fontanels and in children with ventricular shunt systems to avoid injury due to misplacement of the screw.
   f. Stimulating thresholds to elicit muscle MEPs may be elevated in children. However, this variable is counterbalanced by the thinner thickness of the skull which should facilitate motor cortex activation at lower intensities because of lower impedance. Stimulation threshold reaches adult levels by the age of 16 years.
   g. Double-train stimulation as well as spatial facilitation through peripheral stimulation have both been used to improve MEP monitoring in patients with impaired spinal cord function as well as in children.
5. As with EMG, maturation in the peripheral nervous system also impacts MEP, especially in the first 2 years of life. Yet, maturation of the peripheral nerves is faster than that of central pathways, suggesting that conduction velocity approach adult values by the age of 3 years.

CLINICAL PEARL   The effects of central nervous system maturation alter some IOM responses (particularly MEP) but usually reach adult levels during adolescence.

6. **Other considerations.** One of the principles of intraoperative neurophysiology is to always keep a control modality to exclude changes in evoked potentials not induced by surgery. As such, monitoring of the pathways not expected to be altered by surgery as controls are important. This policy is of paramount importance in younger children where the possibility of nonspecific changes in monitoring data is even bigger due to their sensitivity to environmental factors such as room temperature, the immaturity of the monitored pathways, and the limitations in the anesthesia management of these young patients.

REFERENCES

1. Koht A, Sloan T, Toleikis JR. *Neuromonitoring for the Anesthesiologist.* New York, NY: Springer-Verlag; 2012.
2. Rampil IJ. A primer for EEG signal processing in anesthesia. *Anesthesiology.* 1998;89:980–1002.
3. Jameson LC, Sloan TB. Using EEG to monitor anesthesia drug effects during surgery. *J Clin Monit Comp.* 2006;20:445–472.
4. Jäntti V, Sloan T. Anesthesia and intraoperative electroencephalographic monitoring. In: Nuwer M, ed. *Intraoperative Monitoring of Neural Function, Handbook of Clinical Neurophysiology.* New York, NY: Elsevier B.V.; 2008:77–93.
5. Holland NR. Intraoperative electromyography. *J Clin Neurophysiol.* 2002;19:444–453.
6. Slimp JC. Electrophysiologic intraoperative monitoring for spine procedures. *Phys Med Rehab Clin North Am.* 2004;15: 85–105.
7. Yingling C, Ashram YA. Intraoperative monitoring of cranial nerves in skull base surgery. In: Jackler RK, Brackmann D, eds. *Neurotology.* Philadelphia, PA: Elsevier-Mosby; 2005:258–293.
8. Campbell WW. Evaluation and management of peripheral nerve injury. *Clin Neurophysiol.* 2008;119:1951–1965.
9. Prell J, Rampp S, Romstock J, et al. Train time as a quantitative electromyographic parameter for facial nerve function in patients undergoing surgery for vestibular schwannoma. *J Neurosurg.* 2007;106:826–832.
10. National institute of health (NIH). Consensus development conference (held December 11–13, 1991). *Consensus statement.* 1991:9.
11. Khealani B, Husain AM. Neurophysiologic intraoperative monitoring during surgery for tethered cord syndrome. *J Clin Neurophysiol.* 2009;26:76–81.
12. Jameson LC, Janik DJ, Sloan TB. Electrophysiologic monitoring in neurosurgery. *Anesthesiol Clin.* 2007;25:605–630.
13. Pajewski TN, Arlet V, Phillips LH. Current approach on spinal cord monitoring: the point of view of the neurologist, the anesthesiologist and the spine surgeon. *Eur Spine J.* 2007;16(suppl 2):S115–S129.
14. Scoliosis Research Society. *Position Statement on Somatosensory Evoked Potential Monitoring of Neurologic Spinal Cord Function During Surgery.* Park Ridge, IL; 1992.
15. Nuwer MR, Dawson EG, Carlson LG, et al. Somatosensory evoked potential spinal cord monitoring reduces neurologic deficits after scoliosis surgery: Results of a large multicenter survey. *Electroencephalogr Clin Neurophysiol.* 1995;96:6–11.
16. Sloan TB, Jäntti V. Anesthesia and physiology and intraoperative neurophysiological monitoring of evoked potentials. In: Nuwer M, ed. *Handbook of Clinical Neurophysiology.* New York, NY: Elsevier B.V.; 2008:94–126.
17. Sloan TB, Jameson LC. Electrophysiologic monitoring during surgery to repair the thoraco-abdominal aorta. *J Clin Neurophysiol.* 2007;24:316–327.
18. Banoub M, Tetzlaff J, Schubert A. Pharmacologic and physiologic influences affecting sensory evoked potentials. *Anesthesiology.* 2003;99:716–737.
19. Sloan T, Jameson LC, Janik D. Evoked potentials. In: Cottrell J, Smith D, eds. *Anesthesia and Neurosurgery.* New York, NY: Elsevier; 2010:115–130.
20. Moller A. *Intraoperative Neurophysiological Monitoring.* New York, NY: Springer; 2011.
21. Aravabhumi S, Izzo KL, Bakst BL, et al. Brainstem auditory evoked potentials: intraoperative monitoring technique in surgery of posterior fossa tumors. *Arch Phys Med Rehab.* 1987;68:142.
22. Toleikis SC. VEP. In: Koht A, Sloan T, Toleikis JR, eds. *Monitoring the Nervous System for Anesthesiologists and Other Health Care Professionals.* New York, NY: Springer; 2012:69–94.
23. MacDonald D: Intraoperative motor evoked potential monitoring: overview and update. *J Monit Comp.* 2006;20:347–377.
24. Jameson L, Sloan TB. Monitoring of the brain and spinal cord. *Anesthesiol Clin.* 2006;24:777–792.
25. Kothbauer KF. Intraoperative neurophysiologic monitoring for intramedullary spinal-cord tumor surgery. *Neurophysiol Clin.* 2007;37:407–414.
26. Neuloh G, Pechstein U, Cedzich C, et al. Motor evoked potential monitoring with supratentorial surgery. *Neurosurgery.* 2004;54:1061–1070; discussion 1070–1072.
27. Leppanen RE. Intraoperative applications of the h-reflex and f-response: a tutorial. *J Clin Monit Comp.* 2006;20:267–304.
28. Sala F, Krzan MJ, Deletis V. Intraoperative neurophysiological monitoring in pediatric neurosurgery: why, when, how? *Child's Nerv Syst.* 2002;18:264–287.
29. Zamel, KM. Special considerations in pediatric surgical monitoring. In: Galloway GM, Nuwer MR, Lopez JR, eds. *Intraoperative Neurophysiologic Monitoring.* Cambridge: Cambridge University Press; 2010:163–171.
30. Sala F, Manganotti P, Grossauer S, et al. Intraoperative neurophysiology of the motor system in children: a tailored approach. *Child's Nerv Syst.* 2010;26:473–490.

27

Intracranial Pressure Monitoring

Jess W. Brallier

KEY POINTS

1. Traumatic brain injury (TBI) is the most common, primary cause of elevated ICP.
2. In spite of searching for less-invasive means of measuring ICP, ventriculostomy remains the "Gold Standard" among the available monitoring modalities.
3. ICP monitoring is used to diagnose intracranial pathology and direct treatment.
4. TBI is the most well-established indication for ICP monitoring.

I. **Introduction.** Since antiquity, raised intracranial pressure (ICP) has accompanied a number of pathologic states including brain tumors and traumatic brain injury (TBI). Furthermore, elevation in ICP with symptoms such as headache, vomiting and pupillary changes, and alteration in level of consciousness has been described in medical texts since the early part of the last century. Although the concept of intracranial hypertension and its deleterious consequences have long been established, monitoring ICP in order to gain diagnostic and treatment information is relatively new.

ICP monitoring was pioneered by Guillaume and Janny who used an electromagnetic transducer to measure ventricular fluid pressure signals in patients with various types of intracranial pathology [1,2]. Although this work was published in the early 1950s, it was really the research of Nils Lundberg [3] a decade later that established modern ICP monitoring. Not only did he institute intraventricular ICP cannulation as an acceptable and safe method for continuous monitoring, he also described the various wave patterns that are caused by different intracranial lesions.

In the 21st century, neurologic disease accompanied by raised ICP continues to be a significant source of morbidity and mortality. The potential value of continuous ICP monitoring lies in the ability to prevent and control increased ICP while executing medical interventions to optimize cerebral perfusion pressure (CPP). Although ICP monitoring is not without risk and its merits have often been questioned, it remains a recommended diagnostic and therapeutic tool in conditions such as TBI.

II. **Pathophysiology of elevated intracranial pressure**
   A. **Pathophysiology**
      1. The normal range for ICP varies with age, but accepted values for adults and older children are generally less than 10 to 15 mm Hg. The ranges for young children and infants are 3 to 7 mm Hg and 1.5 to 6 mm Hg, respectively [4]. Although the definition of intracranial hypertension depends on the age of the individual and the type of pathology present, ICP values greater than 20 to 25 mm Hg require treatment in most instances, while sustained ICP values of greater than 40 mm Hg represent severe, life-threatening intracranial hypertension [4].

2. The adult brain is enclosed in a rigid, nonexpendable skull. According to the Munro–Kellie doctrine, its contents, namely, brain tissue, cerebrospinal fluid (CSF), and blood must therefore remain unchanged if ICP is to remain stable. In order for ICP to remain constant, an increase in the volume of one of the components of the intracranial cavity requires a concomitant decrease in another. This allows for minimal changes in ICP demonstrating the compensatory reserve of the cranial space. Brain tissue has very minimal compressibility, so any increase in ICP due to brain swelling initially results in extrusion of CSF and venous blood from the intracranial cavity. This is a phenomenon known as "spatial compensation." CSF can be expelled from the intracranial cavity into the "reservoir" of the spinal theca making it the largest contributor to spatial compensation [5]. However, this reserve is finite and when the compensatory capacity of the brain is exhausted, further increases in intracranial volume will lead to abrupt and dangerous increases in ICP [6–8]. The dynamic relationship between ICP and intracranial volume is described by the pressure–volume curve that is composed of three parts (Fig. 27.1). The initial (flat) portion of the curve reflects what occurs when compensatory reserves are adequate and ICP remains low despite increase in intracerebral volume (A–B). The second (steep) part of the curve illustrates what happens when compensatory mechanisms become exhausted and intracranial elastance ($\Delta P/\Delta V$) (often referred to as compliance which is $\Delta V/\Delta P$) is critically reduced. At this point, the pressure–volume curve turns upward exponentially because small increases in intracerebral volume cause a substantial increase in ICP (B–C). As a side note, it is important to understand the difference between elastance and compliance. The term "compliance" is often used when discussing the ICP changes that accompany increases in intracranial volume. However, this nomenclature is incorrect [9]. Compliance ($\Delta V/\Delta P$) is actually the inverse of elastance ($\Delta P/\Delta V$) and, thus,

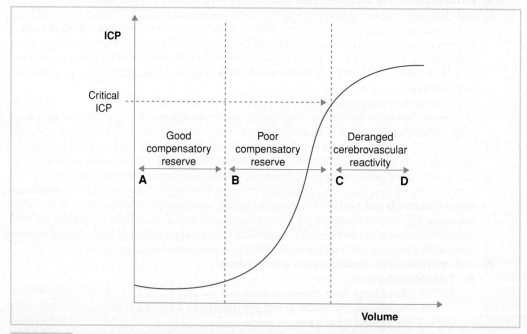

FIGURE 27.1 Intracranial pressure (ICP)–volume curve. The curve has three parts: A flat part representing good compensatory reserve (**A–B**), an exponential part representing reduced compensatory reserve (**B–C**), and a final flat part representing terminal derangement of cerebrovascular responses at high ICP (**C–D**). (Reproduced from Smith M. Monitoring intracranial pressure in traumatic brain injury. *Anesth Analg.* 2008;106:240–248, with permission.)

inaccurate in this context. At critically high levels of ICP, the cerebrovasculature's ability to dilate in response to reduced CPP becomes exhausted resulting in a plateaued curve (C–D). At this point, the ability of the brain to autoregulate its blood flow is lost and cerebral perfusion becomes dependent on the systemic blood pressure.

3. In order to appreciate the utility behind ICP monitoring, an understanding of the negative consequences of elevated ICP and its relationship to CPP should to be understood.

   a. CPP is dependent on mean arterial pressure (MAP) and ICP as represented by the following equation:

$$CPP = MAP - ICP$$

   b. According to this relationship, CPP can be reduced from an increase in ICP, a decrease in blood pressure, or a combination of both. As CPP is reduced below the lower threshold of autoregulation (usually below 60 to 70 mm Hg), CBF drops precipitously as the autoregulatory ability is lost (see Chapter 1).

   c. Due to the relative inflexibility of the cranial vault, increased ICP causes a critical reduction in CPP and cerebral blood flow (CBF) leading to secondary ischemic injury. If left untreated, sustained elevations in ICP also generate pressure gradients within the cranial cavity that can lead to herniation of brain tissue through the tentorial hiatus or foramen magnum. In the case of foramen magnum herniation, pressure on the brainstem results in a Cushings response (bradycardia, hypertension), and if left untreated, respiratory depression and death. This makes the recognition and treatment of elevated ICP critical [1,5].

CLINICAL PEARL   Increased ICP causes a critical reduction in CPP and cerebral blood flow (CBF) leading to ischemic injury.

4. **Several physiologic factors influence ICP.** These include arterial carbon dioxide (CO_2) reactivity, metabolic coupling with CBF, and blood pressure autoregulation.

   a. Carbon dioxide directly affects vascular tone which in turn changes ICP (see Chapter 1). As CO_2 tension in the blood increases, the cerebral vasculature vasodilates increasing CBF and hence ICP. Similarly, as the $PaCO_2$ decreases, CBF and ICP do so in a proportional manner. Hyperventilation has historically been utilized to lower ICP but has lost favor in recent years due to a concomitant risk of precipitating cerebral ischemia (see Chapter 1). Evidence suggests that hyperventilation should only be employed in the case of emergent management of intracranial hypertension [10].

   b. Decreasing cerebral metabolic oxygen consumption ($CMRO_2$) also has the potential to decrease ICP since the normal brain adjusts arterial blood flow to metabolic demand (see Chapter 1). Although this mechanism is not always preserved, decreasing $CMRO_2$ theoretically reduces CBF [1,11].

   c. The effect of blood pressure on ICP is more complex and depends on whether or not CBF autoregulation is preserved. When this mechanism is intact and blood pressure is raised within the autoregulatory range, CBF remains constant due to a reduction in arteriole diameter and an increase in cerebrovascular resistance. However, when cerebral autoregulation is impaired, these same vessels dilate passively and increase ICP by increasing intracerebral blood volume. In addition, the increase in blood pressure is transmitted to the capillary bed worsening intercapillary hydrostatic pressure and worsening edema. Adding to the complexity is the fact that autoregulation may not be simply preserved or absent but rather has varying degrees of autoregulatory capacity [1].

B. **Etiology**

1. TBI is the most common primary cause of elevated ICP. Other etiologies include intracranial hemorrhage, ischemic infarction, and intracranial neoplasms (Table 27.1). A number of mechanisms are responsible for the changes in intracranial volume that subsequently lead to elevation in ICP. In the case of TBI, traumatic hematomas may collect in the intracerebral, subarachnoid, subdural, or extradural spaces creating pressure

TABLE 27.1   Causes of elevated ICP

Intracranial (primary)	Extracranial (primary)
Traumatic brain injury (cerebral contusions, epidural and subdural hematomas)	Hypoxia
Brain tumor	Hypercarbia
Intracranial hemorrhage (nontraumatic)	Hypertension
Ischemic stroke	Hyponatremia
Hydrocephalus	Hyperpyrexia
Infection	Seizures
Status epilepticus	Hepatic failure
Idiopathic	Drugs and toxins
Postoperative (hemorrhage, edema, CSF disturbances)	Jugular venous obstruction High-altitude cerebral edema

gradients within the cranium leading to brain shifts. Cerebral edema, hyperemia, and hydrocephalus also contribute to this increase in intracranial volume [1].

2. **ICP waveforms** (see Figs. 27.2–27.5 below)

   a. ICP waveform analysis is complex but can yield valuable insight into the pathophysiology of raised ICP. The normal ICP waveform is a result of small pulsations transmitted from the systemic blood pressure to the intracranial cavity that are superimposed on slower oscillations caused by the respiratory cycle [4]. Pathologic waveforms include A, B, and C types, all described by Lundberg in the 1960s [4]. "A" waves, also known as plateau waves, occur in any number of conditions and reflect an increase in ICP from normal to moderately elevated to gross intracranial hypertension. They occur in patients whose autoregulatory ability is intact and are due to intense vasodilation in response to decreased cerebral perfusion. ICP rises to between 50 and 100 mm Hg and lasts from 5 to 20 minutes. They are always pathologic and should raise concern as their presence may be associated with early signs of brain herniation such as bradycardia and hypertension. Furthermore, they lead to the development of a vicious cycle causing decreases in CPP leading to more "A" waves and further reductions in CPP and eventually irreversible cerebral ischemia [3,5,12,13]. "B" waves occur at a frequency of 0.5 to 2 waves/min with elevations in ICP 20 to 30 mm Hg above baseline. These waves reflect changes in vascular tone that occur when CPP is at the lower limit of pressure autoregulation. "C" waves occur simultaneously with ABP at a frequency of 4 to 8/min with smaller amplitude than "B" waves. They reflect changes in systemic vasomotor tone and have little pathologic significance [5].

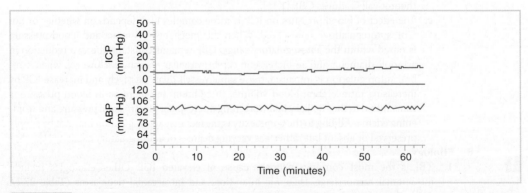

FIGURE 27.2 Normal ICP waveform. Mean arterial blood pressure (ABP) is plotted along the lower panel. (Reproduced from Czosnyka M, Pickard JD. Monitoring and interpretation of intracranial pressure. *J Neurol Neurosurg Psychiarty.* 2004;75(6):813–821, with permission.)

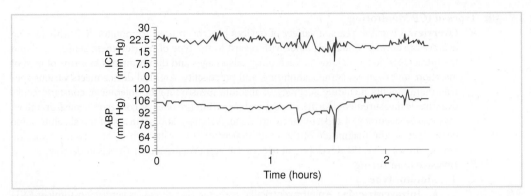

FIGURE 27.3 Represents stable and elevated ICP. This waveform is seen the majority of time in head injury patients. (Reproduced from Czosnyka M, Pickard JD. Monitoring and interpretation of intracranial pressure. *J Neurol Neurosurg Psychiarty.* 2004;75(6):813–821, with permission.)

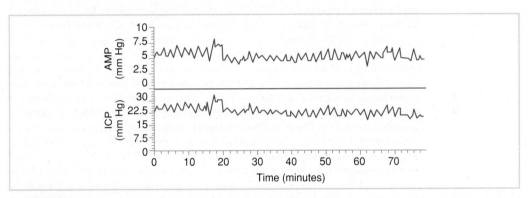

FIGURE 27.4 "B" waves of ICP. These waves reflect changes in vascular tone that occur when CPP is at the lower limit of pressure autoregulation. (Reproduced from Czosnyka M, Pickard JD. Monitoring and interpretation of intracranial pressure. *J Neurol Neurosurg Psychiarty.* 2004;75(6):813--821, with permission.)

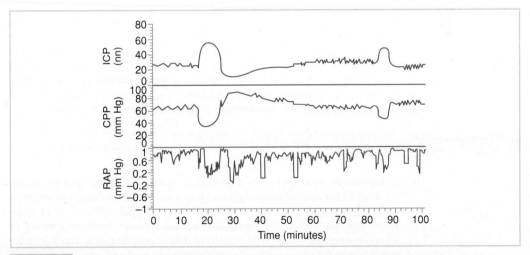

FIGURE 27.5 "A" waves, also known as plateau waves, occur in any number of conditions and reflect an increase in ICP from normal to moderately elevated to gross intracranial hypertension. They are always pathologic. (Reproduced from Czosnyka M, Pickard JD. Monitoring and interpretation of intracranial pressure. *J Neurol Neurosurg Psychiarty.* 2004;75(6):813–821, with permission.)

III. Types of ICP Monitoring

A. Overview. Over the years, a variety of devices have been used to monitor ICP with varying degrees of success. Modalities differ with regard to the type of measurement sensor used and the intracranial location chosen. Each offers advantages and disadvantages in terms of ease of insertion, invasiveness, complication rate, and practicality. An ideal device meets various specific requirements including accuracy of absolute measurements (tolerance), constant values over timely measurements (drift), low dependency from previous or consecutive measurements (hysteresis), accuracy of repeated measurements (validity), and accuracy of the absolute value dependent on the magnitude of the value (linearity) [14]. Although most currently available devices are invasive, the development of accurate, noninvasive alternatives is underway.

B. Invasive monitoring

   1. Monitor type

   a. Intraventricular. An intraventricular catheter, also known as ventriculostomy or EVD is considered the gold standard for monitoring ICP and is therefore the method to which all others are compared. A ventriculostomy is an open-ended conduit placed directly into the CSF of the lateral ventricle. Once in place, it is connected to a standard pressure transducer via fluid-filled catheter, and zero referenced at the external auditory meatus. In addition to continuous monitoring of ICP, these devices, with the addition of a 3-way stopcock, can be used to drain CSF for diagnostic and therapeutic purposes. Although this is considered advantageous, it is important to realize that draining CSF and measuring ICP simultaneously leads to inaccurate recordings that underestimate actual ICP. Therefore, performing these two functions separately is conducive to accurate monitoring. These catheters can also be used to administer drugs such as antibiotics and thrombolytic agents, and have the added advantage of periodic external recalibration. Disadvantages include difficult placement, particularly when raised ICP causes compression or shifting of the ventricles leading to bleeding and inaccurate recordings. Fluid leaks, air bubbles, blood clots, and brain tissue can all lead to erroneous ICP readings by interfering with pressure wave conduction from the ventricles to the external transducer. Also, in order to obtain accurate ICP readings, the transducer must be re-zeroed each time the level of the patient's head is altered. Perhaps the biggest disadvantage to this system is that the ventricular catheter pierces the meninges and brain, potentially leading to serious infection [14]. CSF sepsis is the most serious of these with infection rates ranging from 0% to 45% [15]. This complication leads to increased morbidity and mortality as well as longer hospital stays and higher hospital costs, and can be significantly reduced with careful attention to aseptic technique when placing and managing the catheter [15]. The development of antibiotic-impregnated catheters has further lowered the incidence of infection [16]. As mentioned, intraventricular catheterization remains the gold standard method of ICP monitoring and the initial modality chosen in most instances where ICP monitoring is necessary. However, risks related to infection, hemorrhage, obstruction, and misplacement have led to the development of alternative methods of ICP monitoring.

CLINICAL PEARL Ventriculostomy is considered the gold standard for monitoring ICP.

   b. Intraparenchymal. After intraventricular catheters, intraparenchymal devices are the most widely applied methods of measuring ICP and are gaining relative priority in selected cases [14]. Two types of intraparenchymal monitors are in widespread use. The first is a wire system containing a microtransducer at the tip of a flexible wire. The second type consists of thin fiber optic cables with a pressure transducer at the tip requiring a microprocessor to read and interpret the signal. The advantage of the wire system is that it is compatible with standard bedside monitors and is less expensive than the fiberoptic design. Regardless of the system used, both are introduced into the brain parenchyma via a hollow screw inserted into the skull. Intraparenchymal devices have a high degree of accuracy (second only to a ventriculostomy) and can be easier to place than intraventricular catheters. Furthermore, infection and hemorrhage rates are low and the device only need to be calibrated once regardless of changes in head position. There is also very little zero-drift so that measurements remain relatively constant over time. Disadvantages include the inability to drain CSF and decreased accuracy compared to intraventricular system [5,14,17].

  c. **Subarachnoid.** The subarachnoid "bolt" or "screw" was developed in the 1970s as an alternative to ventriculostomy. In this system, a small bolt is threaded through a burr hole with the tip placed 1 mm under the dura. The screw is connected to a stopcock assembly via a saline-filled extension tube connected to a transducer. The system is zero-balanced at the level of the screw in the subarachnoid space and a calibrated ICP is recorded. Like intraventricular catheters, these devices can also be used to drain CSF [18]. Although these systems are easier to place than a ventriculostomy and have low infection and hemorrhage rates, in most instances their unacceptable inaccuracy trumps any possible advantage to their use and are, therefore, rarely used [19].

  d. **Epidural.** The epidural space has also been used to monitor ICP. Theoretical advantages to using the epidural space are ease of placement and low infection and hemorrhage rates. However, experience demonstrates that these monitors are unreliable due to system malfunction, misplacement, and baseline drift [14]. A recent study demonstrated that epidural ICP monitors consistently yielded artificially high ICP values unrelated to the sensor but rather the specific characteristics of the epidural intracranial space [20].

  e. A number of different monitors and spaces have been used to invasively measure ICP. Each offers their own advantages and disadvantages with regard to infection and hemorrhage rate, accuracy, and overall management (see Table 27.2).

C. Noninvasive monitoring

  1. Invasive techniques for monitoring ICP remain the gold standard. However, the complications inherent to invasive monitoring (infection, hemorrhage, device malfunction) have led to the search for less invasive means of recording ICP.

  2. **Tympanic membrane displacement.** Specific changes in tympanic membrane displacement are indicative of high or low ICP [21]. The degree of displacement can be recorded using a measuring probe that is placed into the external auditory meatus. The probe measures the transmission of ICP waves via the cochlear duct to the inner ear and then via the oval window to the auditory ossicles of the middle ear which are firmly attached to the tympanic membrane. The resulting pressure waves then characteristically distort the tympanic membrane allowing one to make inferences regarding ICP measurements (see Fig. 27.6 below). Unfortunately, this modality has been shown to provide unreliable

TABLE 27.2 Types of invasive ICP monitors and their associated advantages and disadvantages

	Summary of invasive ICP monitors	
Monitor	**Advantages**	**Disadvantages**
Intraventricular (ventriculostomy)	"Gold standard" modality, allows for re-zeroing, ability to drain CSF and administer drugs, measures global ICP	Most invasive modality, high infection rate, placement can be difficult
Intraparenchymal (microtransducer and fiberoptic)	Low rate of infection and hemorrhage, ease of placement, very little zero-drift	Decreased accuracy compared to ventriculostomy, inability to drain CSF
Subarachnoid (subarachnoid bolt)	Low rate of infection and hemorrhage, ability to drain CSF	Unreliable accuracy
Epidural	Low rate of infection and hemorrhage, ability to drain CSF	Unreliable accuracy

A

a)

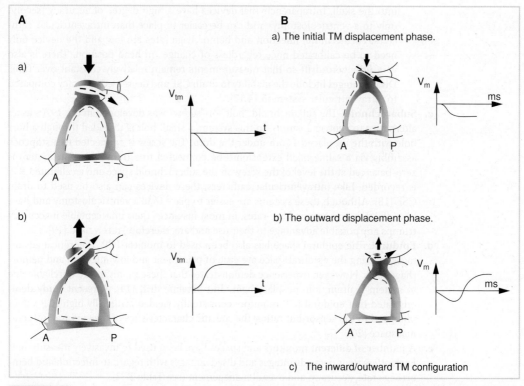

b)

B

a) The initial TM displacement phase.

b) The outward displacement phase.

c) The inward/outward TM configuration

FIGURE 27.6 A: Schematic drawings and graphs showing TMD in cases of raised (**a**) and low (**b**) ICP. In instances of raised ICP, the TM is displaced inwardly, resulting in a negative graph as the stapes footplate is displaced medially on acoustic stimulation of the stapedius (**a**). In instances of low ICP the graph is positive as the stapes footplate is displaced laterally on acoustic stimulation of the stapedius (**b**). **B:** Schematic drawings and graphs displaying the initial TM displacement phase (**a**) and the outward displacement phase (**b**). The TM displacement is bidirectional in cases of normal or low ICP because the stapes footplate rests centrally at the oval window. This is described as the inward/outward TM configuration (**c**). A, anterior; P, posterior. (Reproduced from Samuel M, Burge DM, Marchbanks RJ. Tympanic membrane displacement testing in regular assessment of intracranial pressure in eight children with shunted hydrocephalus. *J Neurosurg.* 1998;88(6):983–995, with permission.)

measures of ICP in patients with hydrocephalus [22] but may prove valuable as a screening tool in patients suspected of having intracranial hypertension [21].

3. **Ultrasonography.** Ultrasonography of the optic nerve sheath diameter (ONSD) is another noninvasive modality that has been investigated and suggested as a possible indicator of elevated ICP. It has been demonstrated that changes in CSF pressure causes changes in ONSD reflecting changes in ICP [23]. Although the use of ultrasound as an ICP monitoring modality is appealing due to its relatively low cost and wide availability, results are mixed. One study examining the use of ONSD in trauma patients revealed this modality to be inaccurate and unreliable [24]. Another review and meta-analysis of six studies involving 231 patients showed that ultrasonography of ONSD showed a good level of diagnostic accuracy for detecting intracranial hypertension. Although it is not accurate or reliable enough to replace invasive monitoring techniques, its use may be valuable in cases where invasive monitoring is contraindicated or in clinical settings where a neurosurgeon is not readily available. Furthermore, it may help physicians decide to transfer patients to specialized centers or to place an invasive device when specific recommendations for such placement do not exist [25].

4. **Transcranial Doppler.** This diagnostic modality has also been investigated as a means of monitoring ICP. In the ICU, investigators have found that a strong correlation exists between pulsatility index (PI) and ICP in patients with a variety of intracranial pathology [26] (see Chapter 4). Unfortunately, other studies have found this modality to be inaccurate and unreliable, making it a poor replacement for invasive monitoring [27,28].

TABLE 27.3   Types of noninvasive ICP monitors

Summary of noninvasive ICP monitors
Tympanic membrane displacement
Ultrasonography
Transcranial Doppler

5. To summarize, promise exists for the use of these noninvasive modalities as a means to diagnose and monitor elevated ICP. However, at this point, data suggest that these devices are not as robust as their invasive counterparts. They should be used for screening and in adjunctive roles but not as replacements for invasive ICP modalities (see Table 27.3).

IV. Indications for ICP monitoring

A. The adult patient

1. ICP monitoring has been applied to a wide range of pathology from intracerebral hemorrhage to hepatic encephalopathy. Despite its widespread application, supporting data from randomized controlled trials are lacking and indications for its use outside of TBI are ill-established. A large body of Class II evidence (moderate degree of clinical certainty) exists to support its application in TBI, but its value in other neurologic conditions is less conclusive.

2. **ICP monitoring in TBI**

   a. **Why monitor?** Deciding whether or not ICP monitoring is indicated requires an understanding of its potential value. Uncontrolled intracranial hypertension is the most frequent cause of death in victims of TBI. CPP is an indirect measure of cerebral perfusion and is dependent on two variables, mean arterial pressure (MAP) and ICP. Evidence shows that CPP values below 50, systemic hypotension, and intracranial hypertension are associated with deleterious outcomes. Therefore, the only reliable means by which to reliably determine CPP and cerebral hypoperfusion is to continuously monitor ICP and blood pressure [29]. Monitoring is initiated with the intention of introducing goal-directed therapy designed to lower critically high ICP (>20 mm Hg), to maximize cerebral perfusion and oxygenation, and to avoid secondary injury while the brain recovers [29,30]. On the other hand, some interventions that effectively lower ICP may worsen outcomes by altering the metabolic state of the brain and pro moting ischemia [31,32]. That is, continuous monitoring not only guides medical management but also prevents blind, prophylactic treatment of ICP avoiding the potential dangers that accompany such interventions. In addition, ICP monitoring also triggers prompt imaging and timely evacuation of space-occupying lesions, preventing surgical delays and secondary brain injury [30].

   b. **Is monitoring useful?** The next pertinent question is whether ICP monitoring is useful. According to the Brain Trauma Foundation (BTF), ICP can be used to predict outcome and worsening intracranial pathology, calculate and manage CPP, allow therapeutic CSF drainage when a ventriculostomy is in place, and restrict potentially deleterious ICP reduction therapies. ICP is a powerful predictor of outcome from TBI and threshold values for treatment are recommended [29]. Furthermore, ICP monitoring is often the first sign of worsening intracranial pathology and surgical mass lesions. This was demonstrated in a study following patients after traumatic subarachnoid hemorrhage. In 20% of the patients, ICP monitoring was the first indicator of an evolving intracranial lesion in patients with initially normal ICP [33].

3. The BTF [29] guidelines are the most widely accepted international guidelines for ICP monitoring in TBI, with the most recent BTF guidelines published in 2007. While Level 1 evidence to support a treatment standard for ICP monitoring is lacking, adequate Level II and III data exist to support its recommended use. According to BTF guidelines, "ICP monitoring should be performed in all salvageable patients with a severe TBI (Glasgow Coma Scale [GCS] score of 3 to 8 after resuscitation) and an abnormal computed tomography (CT) scan. An abnormal CT scan of the head is one that reveals hematomas,

contusions, swelling, herniation, or compressed basal cisterns." The guidelines also state that "ICP monitoring is indicated in patients with severe TBI with a normal CT scan if two or more of the following features are noted at admission: Age over 40 years, unilateral or bilateral motor posturing, or systolic blood pressure (BP) <90 mm Hg."

4. The strongest evidence-based indication for ICP monitoring is in patients at risk for intracranial hemorrhage (ICH) after TBI. Not only are ICP data useful in predicting outcome in patients who respond to ICP lowering therapies, but ICP monitoring also prevents potential, deleterious outcomes that can result from treating elevated ICP in a blind fashion.

B. **The pediatric patient**

1. Indications for ICP monitoring in the pediatric population are more opaque than they are in the adult. This is due to the fact that the available evidence base needed to direct ICP monitoring and treatment in children is much smaller causing much of the work published in adults with TBI to be extrapolated to children. Much of the pediatric literature comprises studies with small sample sizes and wide age ranges. For example, some studies extend their inclusion criteria to patients aged 18 to 21 years, making the median age of the patient older, creating a group of subjects more similar to adults in physiology. This is significant because children are different than adults in several important aspects relevant to TBI, including pathophysiology, pressure–volume intracranial dynamics, imaging interpretation, and the normative ranges for blood pressure and ICP which change depending on age [1].

2. Although the indications for ICP monitoring in children are less defined, elevated ICP is associated with poor outcomes [34–36]. Furthermore, ICP monitoring has a substantial influence on medical and surgical management of children with TBI and is considered to be safe with a low complication rate [37].

V. Complications

A. Although ICP monitoring is generally considered safe, the risk of complication accompanies any invasive procedure. The most common complications encountered with ICP monitoring include infection, hemorrhage, and device malfunction. Infection rates vary proportionately with the duration of monitoring and depend on the type of device inserted and the technique used. Infection and hemorrhage rates are highest with ventricular catheters than with other devices but are overall very low.

VI. Conclusions

A. Despite the complexities and controversies surrounding ICP monitoring, it remains a useful management modality particularly after TBI. In addition to yielding valuable information regarding ICP and CPP, continuous monitoring can offer insight into cerebral pathophysiology and treatment. Although noninvasive modalities are in the development phase, intraventricular and intraparenchymal devices remain the most accurate and widely used means of measuring ICP.

REFERENCES

1. Padayachy LC, Figaji AA, Bullock MR. Intracranial pressure monitoring for traumatic brain injury in the modern era. *Childs Nerv Syst*. 2010;26:441–452.
2. Guillaume J, Janny P. Continuous intracranial manometry; importance of the method and first results. *Rev Neurol (Paris)*. 1951;84(2):131–142.
3. Lundberg N, Troupp H, Lorin H. Continuous recording of the ventricular-fluid pressure in patients with severe acute traumatic brain injury. A preliminary report. *J Neurosurg*. 1965;22(6):581–590.
4. Rangel-Castillo L, Robertson CS. Management of intracranial hypertension. *Crit Care Clin*. 2007;22:713–732.
5. Smith M. Monitoring intracranial pressure in traumatic brain injury. *Anesth Analg*. 2008;106:240–248.
6. Kellie G. An account of the appearances observed in the dissection of two of the three individuals presumed to have perished in the storm of the third, and whose bodies were discovered in the vicinity of Leith on the morning of the 4th November 1821 with some reflections on the pathology of the brain. *Trans Med Chir Sci Edinburgh*. 1824;1:84–169.
7. Kellie G. On death from cold, and on congestions of the brain: an account of the appearances observed in the dissection of two of the three individuals presumed to have perished in the storm of 3rd November 1821; with some reflections on the pathology of the brain. *Trans Med Chir Sci Edinburgh*. 1824;1:84–169.
8. Monro A. *Observations on the Structure and Function of the Nervous System*. Edinburgh: Creech and Johnson; 1823.
9. Drummond JC. Elastance versus compliance. *Anesthesiology*. 1995;82(5):1309–1310.
10. Curley G, Kavanagh BP, Laffey JG. Hypocapnia and the injured brain: more harm than benefit. *Crit Care Med*. 2010;38(5):1348–1359.

11. Oertel M, Kelly DF, Lee JH, et al. Efficacy of hyperventilation, blood pressure elevation, and metabolic suppression therapy in controlling intracranial pressure after head injury. *J Neurosurg.* 2002;97(5):1045–1053.

12. Rosner MJ, Becker DP. Origin and evolution of plateau waves. Experimental observations and a theoretical model. *J Neurosurg.* 1984;60(2):312–324.

13. Czosnyka M, Smielewski P, Piechnik S, et al. Hemodynamic characterization of intracranial pressure plateau waves in head-injury patients. *J Neurosurg.* 1999;91:11–19.

14. Zhong J, Dujovny M, Park HK, et al. Advances in ICP monitoring techniques. *Neurol Res.* 2003;25:339–350.

15. Kitchen WJ, Singh N, Hulme S, et al. External ventricular drain infection: improved technique can reduce infection rates. *Br J Neurosurg.* 2011;25(5):632–635.

16. Zabramski JM, Whiting D, Darouiche RO, et al. Efficacy of antimicrobial-impregnated external ventricular drain catheters: a prospective, randomized, controlled trial. *J Neurosurg.* 2003;98:725–730.

17. Gambardella G, d'Avella D, Tomasello F. Monitoring of brain tissue pressure with a fiberoptic device. *Neurosurgery.* 1992;31(5):918–921.

18. Vries JK, Becker DP, Young HF. A subarachnoid screw for monitoring intracranial pressure. Technical note. *J Neurosurg.* 1973;39(3):416–419.

19. Miller JD, Bobo H, Kapp JP. Inaccurate pressure readings for subarachnoid bolts. *Neurosurgery.* 1986;19(2):253–255.

20. Poca MA, Sahuquillo J, Topczewski T, et al. Is intracranial pressure monitoring in the epidural space reliable? Fact and fiction. *J Neurosurg.* 2007;106(4):548–556.

21. Stettin E, Paulat K, Schulz C, et al. Noninvasive intracranial pressure measurement using infrasonic emissions from the tympanic membrane. *J Clin Monit Comput.* 2011;25:203–210.

22. Shimbles S, Dodd C, Banister K, et al. Clinical comparison of tympanic membrane displacement with invasive intracranial pressure measurements. *Physiol Meas.* 2005;26(6):1085–1092.

23. Liu D, Kahn M. Measurement and relationship of subarachnoid pressure of the optic nerve to intracranial pressures in fresh cadavers. *Am J Opthalmol.* 1993;116(5):548–556.

24. Strumwasser A, Kwan RO, Yeung L, et al. Sonographic optic nerve sheath diameter as an estimate of intracranial pressure in adult trauma. *J Surg Res.* 2011;170(2):265–271.

25. Dubourg J, Javouhey E, Geeraerts T, et al. Ultrasonography of optic nerve sheath diameter for detection of raised intracranial pressure: a systematic review and meta-analysis. *Intensive Care Med.* 2011;37:1059–1068.

26. Bellner J, Romner B, Reinstrup P, et al. Transcranial Doppler sonography pulsatility index (PI) reflects intracranial pressure (ICP). *Surg Neurol.* 2004;62(1):45–51.

27. Figaji AA, Zwane E, Fieggen AG, et al. Transcranial Doppler pulsatility index is not a reliable indicator of intracranial pressure in children with severe traumatic brain injury. *Surg Neurol.* 2009;72(4):389–394.

28. Behrens A, Lenfeldt N, Ambarki K, et al. Transcranial Doppler pulsatility index: not an accurate method to assess intracranial pressure. *Neurosurgery.* 2010;66(6):1050–1057.

29. Bratton SL, Chestnut RM, Ghajar J, et al. Guidelines for the management of severe traumatic brain injury. VI. Indications for intracranial pressure monitoring. *J Neurotrauma.* 2008;24(suppl 1):S37–S44.

30. Lavino A, Menon DK. Intracranial pressure: why we monitor it, how to monitor it, what to do with the number and what's the future? *Curr Opin Anesthesiol.* 2011;24:117–123.

31. Coles JP, Fryer TD, Coleman MR, et al. Hyperventilation following head injury: effect on ischemic burden and cerebral oxidative metabolism. *Crit Care Med.* 2007;35(2):568–578.

32. Yundt KD, Diringer MN. The use of hyperventilation and its impact on cerebral ischemia in the treatment of traumatic brain injury. *Crit Care Clin.* 1997;13(1):163–184.

33. Servadei F, Antonelli V, Giuliani G, et al. Evolving lesions in traumatic subarachnoid hemorrhage: prospective study of 110 patients with emphasis on the role of ICP monitoring. *Acta Neurochir Suppl.* 2002;81:81–82.

34. Cantais E, Paut O, Giorgi R, et al. Evaluating the prognosis of multiple, severely traumatized children in the intensive care unit. *Intensive Care Med.* 2001;27(9):1511–1517.

35. Catala-Temprano A, Claret Teruel G, Cambra Lasaosa FJ, et al. Intracranial pressure and cerebral perfusion pressure as risk factors in children with traumatic brain injuries. *J Neurosurg.* 2007;106(suppl 6):463–466.

36. Chambers IR, Jones PA, Lo TY, et al. Critical thresholds of intracranial pressure and cerebral perfusion pressure related to age in paediatric head injury. *J Neurol Neurosurg Psychiatry.* 2006;77(2):234–240.

37. Pople IK, Muhlbauer MS, Sanford RA, et al. Results and complications of intracranial pressure monitoring in 303 children. *Pediatr Neurosurg.* 1995;23(2):64–67.

28. Other Monitoring Techniques: Jugular Venous Bulb, Transcranial Doppler, and Brain Tissue Oxygen Monitoring

Benjamin Scott

KEY POINTS

1. Optimal prevention of secondary brain injury depends on real-time functional monitoring of cerebral physiology. The techniques described in this chapter represent several of the most robust modalities clinically available. Others will emerge. These monitoring techniques are best understood in clinical context and with reference to multimodal monitoring data. In other words, they should be used together, and rarely in isolation.

2. Jugular venous saturation monitoring, using continuous oximetric sampling of the venous drainage from the cerebral circulation, can guide therapeutic interventions that optimize cerebral oxygen delivery and minimize excess oxygen consumption.

3. The normal arteriojugular venous oxygen difference (AJVO$_2$) averages 4 to 8 mL O$_2$ per 100 mL blood corresponding to a normal saturation or SjVO$_2$ of 55% to 75%, and an SjVO$_2$ less than 50% represents inadequate cerebral blood flow/oxygen delivery.

4. SjVO$_2$ may have a role in guiding resuscitation, transfusion, and ventilator management in the patient with moderate to severe TBI.

5. Increases in cerebral oxygen extraction and low SjVO$_2$ may precede the clinical development of delayed ischemic neurologic deficits by up to 1 day and the AVDO$_2$ normalizes after successful treatment for vasospasm was initiated.

6. Transcranial Doppler does not calculate volumetric flow. However, the largest intracranial vessels maintain a constant caliber over a wide variety of conditions. If blood viscosity is stable, changes in flow velocity will be proportional to changes in blood flow.

7. In the setting of cerebral vasospasm, the best-validated vessel, the MCA, velocities between 120 and 200 cm/sec represent luminal narrowing of 25% to 50%, and velocities over 200 cm/sec are indicative of greater than 50% reduction in luminal diameter.

8. Changes in blood flow velocity through the major cerebral arteries, measured over time using transcranial Doppler ultrasound, may identify critical stenosis, cerebral vasoconstriction, and allow for real-time noninvasive assessment of cerebral autoregulation and intracranial pressure.

9. Brain tissue oxygen tension monitoring is a direct, focal measurement of the oxygen content of brain parenchyma. Therapeutic maintenance of adequate brain tissue oxygen levels shows promise in the management of acute brain injury.

(continued)

10. Small differences in cellular oxygen tension can have significant effects on cellular metabolism and treatment strategies aimed at maintaining $PbtO_2$ greater than 20 mm Hg may reduce secondary injury and improve outcomes in patients with acute brain injury. $PbtO_2$ values less than 20 mm Hg have been defined as *moderate* brain hypoxia and values less than 10 mm Hg as *severe* brain hypoxia.

I. Introduction: Other monitoring techniques

A. Prevention of secondary injury has assumed fundamental importance in the acute management of brain-injured patients. However, functional monitoring of the injured brain remains a challenge, particularly in the setting of focal or regional differences in metabolic demand, blood flow, and autoregulation.

B. Impaired autoregulation couples cerebral blood flow (CBF) to blood pressure, resulting in regional vulnerability to brain tissue ischemia on the one hand, and hyperemia on the other. Functional monitors attempt to measure the adequacy of CBF and oxygen supply in relation to demand, and to do so in real time.

II. Jugular venous oxygen saturation monitoring

A. Physiologic rationale: In much the same way that the mixed venous oxygen saturation (SVO_2), measured in the pulmonary artery, has been used to assess the balance between systemic oxygen supply and consumption, the jugular venous oxygen saturation ($SjVO_2$), measured in the jugular bulb, reflects a similar balance between cerebral oxygen supply and demand.

1. **Anatomy**

   a. The jugular bulb is a dilated portion of the jugular vein just below the skull base that receives venous drainage from the cerebral sinuses.

   b. Autopsy specimens suggest that subcortical areas of the brain tend to drain into the left lateral sinus, whereas cortical areas tend to drain into the right.

   c. Each jugular receives approximately 70% of its flow from the ipsilateral side and 30% from the contralateral side.

   d. Drainage is asymmetric and most often right-dominant.

> **CLINICAL PEARL** Venous drainage of the brain is asymmetric with most of the cortical areas of the brain draining into the right jugular vein.

2. **Physiology.** Oxygen saturation of venous blood in the jugular bulb reflects the global balance between oxygen delivery and consumption in the brain.

   a. Cerebral oxygen delivery (DO_2) is equal to the CBF multiplied by the cerebral arterial oxygen content (CaO_2).

   $$DO_2 = CBF \times CaO_2$$

   b. Cerebral oxygen consumption ($CMRO_2$) is defined as the difference between cerebral arterial and venous oxygen content, multiplied by CBF.

   $$CMRO_2 = CBF \times (CaO_2 - CjvO_2)$$

   c. In the equation above, $CaO_2 - CjvO_2$ can be thought of as the arteriojugular venous oxygen difference ($AJVO_2$) which represents the ratio of metabolic demand to oxygen supply.

3

    d. Normal $AJVO_2$ averages 4 to 8 mL O_2 per 100 mL blood, corresponding to a normal saturation or $SjVO_2$ of 55% to 75% (slightly lower than the systemic SVO_2) [1].

    e. If cerebral metabolic rate remains stable, a change in $SjVO_2$ therefore represents a change in perfusion. Conversely, if cerebral metabolic rate increases without a compensatory increase in CBF, more oxygen will be extracted and $SjVO_2$ will fall.

3

    f. Practically speaking, the most salient feature of this relationship is that a low $SjVO_2$ suggests inadequate CBF. Experimental data suggest that repeated $SjVO_2$ desaturations, or even a single desaturation to less than 50% are associated with worsened outcomes [2,3].

    g. Supranormal $SjVO_2$ may reflect increased perfusion or hyperemia, often in the setting of impaired autoregulation or diminished cerebral oxygen extraction, as in the setting of diffuse ischemia, trauma, or reperfusion injury.

B. **Indications.** Despite a clear and well-developed physiologic rationale for the use of $SjVO_2$ in the setting of cerebral injury, there are no robust outcome data from controlled trials demonstrating a benefit from $SjVO_2$ monitoring. Nevertheless, several decades of clinical experience with this modality have led to the following suggested indications for $SjVO_2$ monitoring:

    1. **Traumatic brain injury**

        a. $SjVO_2$ may be useful for early detection of ischemia in the setting of intracranial hypertension or low cerebral perfusion pressure (CPP).

        b. $SjVO_2$ may facilitate optimization of short-term hyperventilation and management of CPP and intracranial hypertension based on the detection of ischemia in the individual patient in contrast to traditional reliance on predetermined universal normal values for ICP, CPP, etc. [4,5].

4

        c. $SjVO_2$ may have a role in guiding resuscitation, transfusion, and ventilator management in the patient with moderate to severe traumatic brain injury (TBI) [6].

CLINICAL PEARL In contrast to global monitoring parameters of ICP and CPP, $SjVO_2$ may help optimize short-term hyperventilation and management of CPP and intracranial hypertension based on the detection of increased extraction and low saturation.

5

    2. **Detection of vasospasm after subarachnoid hemorrhage**

        a. In a small sample of patients with aneurysmal subarachnoid hemorrhage (SAH), Heran et al. [7] found that increases in cerebral oxygen extraction (measured as increased arterio-venous oxygen difference [$AVDO_2$] using serial jugular bulb samples) preceded the clinical development of delayed ischemic neurologic deficits by approximately 1 day. Furthermore, $AVDO_2$ normalized after treatment for vasospasm was initiated. In patients who did not develop vasospasm, there was no change in $AVDO_2$. Fandino et al. [8] documented rapid improvements in $SjVO_2$ after catheter-directed selective intra-arterial infusion of papaverine for the treatment of vasospasm.

        b. The use of transcranial Doppler (TCD) to predict postaneurysmal vasospasm by detecting increased cerebral arterial flow velocities has become widespread (see below). One of the weaknesses of TCD is its inability to differentiate increased flow velocity due to hyperemia from that due to vessel narrowing. Concomitant use of $SjVO_2$ monitoring may help differentiate flow impediment (low $SjVO_2$) from hyperemia (normal or high $SjVO_2$).

    3. **Ischemia monitoring during cardiothoracic or neurosurgical procedures**

        a. **Cardiopulmonary bypass (CPB).** Although the accuracy of $SjVO_2$ monitoring during hypothermia has not been definitively demonstrated, several studies have attempted to assess the utility of jugular venous oximetry during and after CPB [9–11]. Croughwell et al. [12] demonstrated that a significant minority (23%) of patients undergoing CPB had $SjVO_2$ desaturations under 50% and that the likelihood of desaturation increased with low mean arterial blood pressure, low hematocrit, and rapid rewarming. More importantly, in a subsequent study, patients with $SjVO_2$ desaturations during CPB had worse postoperative cognitive declines than those who did not [13]. Souter et al. [10] documented a high rate of desaturation in the immediate postoperative period as well. Although these small studies are intriguing and suggest a role for jugular oximetry during CPB, this practice has not become widespread.

   b. **Off-pump cardiac surgery.** Recently, $SjVO_2$ monitoring has also been explored during off-pump coronary bypass surgery. Miura et al. [14] found a significant incidence of jugular venous desaturation occurring primarily during surgical displacement of the heart.

   c. **Neurosurgical procedures**

   (1) Matta et al. [15] reviewed a series of 100 patients undergoing a wide range of neurosurgical procedures and found intraoperative $SjVO_2$ desaturations in 60% of aneurysm surgeries, 72% of intracerebral hematoma evacuations, and 50% of tumor resections. A majority of these desaturations occurred at a $PaCO_2$ greater than 25 mm Hg and in the absence of significant differences in hemoglobin concentration or $PaCO_2$ compared with patients who did not have a desaturation, suggesting an independent role for $SjVO_2$ monitoring as a means of ensuring adequate perfusion. However, because this study did not compare outcomes between groups, it remains unclear if the measured desaturations were clinically significant.

   (2) During intracranial aneurysm clipping, Moss et al. [16] described the use of $SjVO_2$ monitoring to estimate the minimum mean arterial blood pressure needed to maintain perfusion during clip application.

   (3) In a series of pediatric patients undergoing intracranial surgery, Sharma et al. [17] also documented a significant incidence of jugular venous desaturation and suggested that $SjVO_2$ monitoring may be useful in guiding management decisions during anesthesia.

   4. Monitoring and prognostication after cardiac arrest and therapeutic hypothermia: In a few small studies, elevated jugular venous saturations in survivors of cardiac arrest have been found to correlate with worse survival, suggesting either hyperemia or a reduced ability of the globally injured brain to extract oxygen [18–20]. It is worth noting that other studies have not found any association between $SjVO_2$ and outcome [21].

C. **Contraindications.** Relative contraindications to jugular bulb oximetry include the following:

   1 Known thrombosis or aberrant anatomy of the jugular veins

   2. Anterograde jugular catheter already in situ

   3. Coagulopathy or hypercoagulable state

   4. Presence of tracheostomy (increased risk of line infection)

   5. Unstable cervical spine injury or cervical collar that cannot be removed

D. **Technique**

   1. **Placement**

   a. Jugular venous sampling may be accomplished using intermittent phlebotomy from the superior portion of the internal jugular (IJ) vein, but in most instances a dedicated oximetric catheter is preferred, thereby allowing continuous monitoring in real time.

CLINICAL PEARL $SjVO_2$ monitoring can be performed by intermittent phlebotomy from the superior portion of the IJ vein, or by placing an oximetric catheter and obtaining continuous real-time monitoring.

---

   b. Available data suggest that there is typically little variation in saturation between the right and the left jugular bulb [22]. However, it is reasonable to suspect that major regional or hemispheric brain injury might result in more disparate values. Unfortunately, no outcome data are available to support the choice of one side over the other. Since most patients have right-dominant jugular venous drainage, some have advocated routine cannulation of the right IJ. Others have suggested using ultrasound or CT to identify the larger (dominant) side. When an ICP monitor is present, sequential compression of each IJ to see which results in the greatest ICP increase may demonstrate the side that drains the largest cerebral territory. In the setting of a known focal injury, some have advocated ipsilateral placement to maximize sensitivity to regional ischemia in the injured side [22].

c. Retrograde cannulation using a sterile, ultrasound-guided Seldinger technique should proceed in a similar fashion to IJ central line placement. The IJ may be accessed distally between the two heads of the sternocleidomastoid muscle or more proximally, at the level of the cricoid. Although positioning the patient in a head-down or horizontal position may simplify ultrasound-guided identification and cannulation of the jugular vein, this may not be feasible in a patient with intracranial hypertension, and cannulation can be accomplished in a head-up position [23]. The 4.5- to 5-French oximetric catheter should be inserted in a cephalad direction, 12 to 15 cm, until a slight increase in resistance is met, as the catheter reaches a small curve in the vessel that typically occurs at the skull base. The catheter is then withdrawn a few millimeters. Placement is confirmed most easily by obtaining an over-penetrated lateral cervical spine x-ray. Ideally, the tip of the catheter should be visualized above the C1–C2 disc. The use of a 5- to 6-French introducer catheter and a sterile cover (similar to those used for pulmonary artery catheters) allows repositioning of the oximetric catheter.

2. **Complications**

   a. Complications include those accompanying central line placement (hematoma, carotid puncture, thrombosis, infection, etc.). Like central lines, more generally, these risks appear to be low in the hands of conscientious and experienced operators. In one review of 44 patients with jugular bulb catheters, Coplin et al. [24] found complications rare and likely to be clinically insignificant when they did occur.

   b. **Effect on ICP.** Subclavian central venous access has traditionally been favored in neurosurgical and head-injured trauma patients due to concerns that thrombosis around an IJ catheter may increase ICP by limiting venous drainage from the head. However, there is little experimental data to support this fear. Coplin et al. [24] found that 8 of 20 patients with jugular bulb catheters (in situ for up to 6 days) had evidence of thrombosis on ultrasound examination, but none had occlusive or clinically significant clot. In a study of 37 consecutive pediatric patients undergoing jugular bulb catheterization, Goetting and Preston [25] found no evidence that the jugular bulb catheter increased ICP. However, Stocchetti et al. [26] has more recently suggested that *bilateral* jugular cannulation may worsen intracranial hypertension.

CLINICAL PEARL   There is no evidence that the jugular bulb catheter increases ICP. However, *bilateral* jugular cannulation (i.e., jugular bulb and IJ vein cannulation for a central line) may worsen intracranial hypertension.

---

   c. **Errors based on inaccurate interpretation.** As the complexity of monitoring increases, so do the risks that artifact or flawed interpretation of the monitoring data will lead to potentially harmful treatment or physiologic manipulation. This would include the use of vasopressors, sedative-hypnotics, fluid resuscitation, blood transfusion, and surgical procedures, each of which has potential side effects and risks.

E. **Interpretation and management**

   1. Low SjVO$_2$ reflects an increase in oxygen extraction and should prompt a search for either increased metabolic demand or decreased supply of oxygen (see Fig. 28.1). Treatable factors that increase metabolic demand include fever, seizure, and inadequate sedation or analgesia. On the other side of the equation, inadequate supply of oxygen may result from decreased CPP (either from arterial hypotension or intracranial hypertension), severe anemia, hypoxemia, or vasospasm.

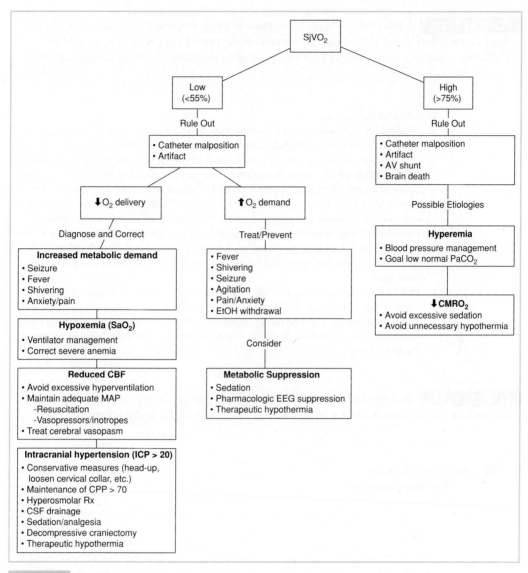

FIGURE 28.1 jVO$_2$ flow chart.

2. Elevated SjVO$_2$ is a marker of either luxuriant blood flow (or hyperemia) or diminished ability of the brain tissue to extract oxygen. Hyperemia is most often a result of loss of autoregulation or a restoration of normal flow to an area that was previously distal to a stenotic lesion. Cautious lowering of the arterial blood pressure may be beneficial recognizing that other areas of the brain may then be put at risk for inadequate flow. Elevated saturations may also represent the presence of an arteriovenous fistula. In cases of extreme intracranial hypertension, arterial blood may actually be shunted past the capillary beds into the venous circulation, thereby elevating the SjVO$_2$. Emergent management of intracranial hypertension is mandated in this case. Decreased oxygen extraction is the result of injury at the cellular level and remains difficult to treat.

> **CLINICAL PEARL**   A low SjVO$_2$ reflects an increase in oxygen extraction and should prompt a search for either increased metabolic demand or decreased supply of oxygen. A high SjVO$_2$ may represent excess blood flow (hyperemia) or shunting of arterial blood into the venous drainage.

3. **Pitfalls and limitations**
   a. **Artifact.** It may result from contamination by facial or other extra-CBF if the catheter is not sufficiently cephalad, so initial placement and interval reassessment of catheter position are crucial. Furthermore, most oximetric devices provide a measure of signal quality, which can be degraded by changes in pulsatility, hemodilution, adherent or adjacent thrombus, or contact with the vessel wall. Poor signal quality may be improved by flushing or repositioning the catheter. Fluctuations in serum hemoglobin concentration should also prompt manual recalibration of an indwelling catheter.
   b. **Focal or heterogeneous injury.** As a global monitor, SjVO$_2$ may be insensitive to focal pathology. Focal areas of increased or decreased supply on the one hand, or demand on the other, may end up mixing before the jugular bulb and result in a normal global saturation.
   c. **Bohr effect.** In the setting of alkalemia, a left shift of the hemoglobin dissociation curve may falsely elevate SjVO$_2$ readings.
   d. **Brainstem injury.** The neurologic importance of the brainstem far exceeds its contribution to venous outflow; therefore, jugular oximetry is of little utility in monitoring the brainstem.

> **CLINICAL PEARL**   As a global monitor, SjVO$_2$ can guide therapy designed to increase DO$_2$ and reduce excess demand, but it is insensitive to focal pathology and brainstem injury.

III. Transcranial Doppler
A. Physiologic rationale
   1. In the early 1980s, Aaslid et al. [27] demonstrated that ultrasound waves of 1 to 2 MHz generated by oscillating piezoelectric crystals could be directed through the temporal bone of the human skull and reflected off large intracranial blood vessels (and more specifically the echogenic erythrocytes coursing through them), returning to a microphone in the ultrasound probe and allowing calculation of depth and blood flow velocity using the principle of Doppler shift in wavelength between the original transmitted signal and its returning echoes.
   2. It is important to note that unlike duplex ultrasound (simultaneous two-dimensional b-mode and pulse-wave velocity) used in other parts of the body, TCD does not have the spatial resolution necessary to calculate volumetric flow. In fact, the diameter of the vessels of interest cannot be measured using this technique. However, across a wide variety of physiologic conditions, the largest intracranial vessels generally maintain a constant caliber and do not participate significantly in autoregulation [28,29]. If blood viscosity remains stable, changes in blood flow will be proportional to changes in flow velocity. TCD is thus a useful monitor for the identification of changes in blood flow over serial measurements.
   3. By utilizing m-mode (motion-mode), TCD can also record multiple overlapping velocities over a range of depths. Since both particulate emboli and gas bubbles within the blood have higher reflectivity than the surrounding erythrocytes, this mode can be used to make a semiquantitative assessment of the density of these emboli, referred to as high intensity transient signals (or HITS).

B. Indications

1. Detection of vasospasm after subarachnoid hemorrhage: Delayed ischemic deficits remain one of the most important sources of morbidity in patients after rupture of an intracranial aneurysm. Vasospasm is often initially asymptomatic, making early detection of significant clinical interest. Although its predictive value has recently been questioned [30], TCD is routinely used in many centers for the daily assessment of flow velocities in the major intracerebral arteries in patients recovering from aneurysmal SAH. Relevant flow velocities vary by vessel, but in the best-validated vessel, the middle cerebral artery (MCA), velocities between 120 and 200 cm/s represent luminal narrowing of 25% to 50%, and velocities over 200 cm/s are indicative of greater than 50% reduction in luminal diameter [31]. Intracerebral flow velocities must be considered in the context of overall blood flow. The Lindegaard ratio or index compares the mean flow velocity in the MCA with that in the ICA. A ratio of less than 3 is considered representative of hyperemia. A ratio of greater than 5 or 6 is associated with a significant risk of clinically significant cerebral ischemia [32,33].

2. **Intracranial vascular occlusion**
   a. **Carotid surgery.** TCD has the potential to rapidly detect MCA flow disruption during carotid endarterectomy. In a 2008 meta-analysis, Schnaudigel et al. [34] found that neuromonitoring-guided selective carotid shunting during endarterectomy was associated with a statistically significant reduction in postoperative infarcts when compared with obligate use of shunts. TCD represents a rapid and noninvasive modality that may help guide selective shunting.
   b. **Cardiac bypass and cerebral perfusion.** TCD has also been used to document cerebral perfusion during initiation of CPB for repair of aortic dissection, and to ensure flow during retrograde and selective antegrade cerebral perfusion in the setting of intraoperative circulatory arrest. Rapid identification of a low- or no-flow state allows repositioning of cannulae or relief cerebral outflow obstruction [35–38].
   c. **Acute ischemic stroke and thrombolysis.** TCD can be used to diagnose acute obstruction in the setting of large vessel ischemic stroke [39]. Recent evidence also supports an independent effect of TCD as an adjuvant therapeutic agent versus TPA alone [40,41].

3. **Assessment of cerebral autoregulation.** Using TCD to measure the effects of intentional alterations in MAP or $PaCO_2$ on cerebral blood flow velocity (CBFV) provides a dynamic test of cerebral autoregulation. TCD has also been used to derive an estimate of CPP in which CPP = (MAP × diastolic CBFV/mean CBFV) + 14 [42]. Continuous monitoring of CPP/MAP compared with time-averaged CBFV values has led to the development of a correlation coefficient known as the mean velocity index (Mx), which has been used as a measure of static autoregulation in conjunction with other multimodality monitoring data to target patient and context-specific optimal CPP [42]. Sorrentino et al. [43] have recently confirmed earlier studies suggesting worse outcomes in TBI patients with impaired autoregulation, and found that Mx less than 0.05 was associated with intact autoregulation whereas an Mx of greater than 0.3 implies significant impairment.

4. **Noninvasive ICP estimation.** Pulsatility index, defined as systolic CBFV – (diastolic CBFV/mean CBFV) has been used as a noninvasive approximation of ICP [43].

5. **Detection of shunt and embolism.** By providing semiquantitative detection of HITS (see above) in the intracranial circulation, TCD can facilitate the detection of intracardiac, intrapulmonary, or other right to left shunts, as well as ipsilateral microemboli in the setting to carotid or intracranial dissection, although it cannot reliably distinguish between these entities. TCD may also facilitate the rapid detection of massive intraoperative venous air embolism [44]. TCD-guided therapies have been noted to lessen the effects of embolization once recognized, for example, by encouraging less manipulation of the aorta or carotid [45], or by stimulating changes in surgical and perfusion techniques such as cardiotomy suction [46].

6. **Stroke risk in sickle cell anemia.** TCD has become a well-established screening tool in the management of sickle cell anemia. Strong evidence has accumulated that increased

flow velocities over 170 cm/sec are indicative of a need for transfusion to reduce elevated stroke risk, and in a randomized trial, use of this threshold was associated with a 92% absolute stroke risk reduction [47].

C. **Contraindications.** There are essentially no contraindications to TCD. Continuous, high-power ultrasonography may have effects on body tissues, but these have not been clearly identified and there is no significant evidence of risk to date.

D. **Technique**

1. Accurate insonation of the relevant cerebral vasculature requires the probe to be perpendicular to the vessel of interest at the appropriate depth, making TCD highly operator dependent. Nevertheless, interobserver agreement appears to be acceptable for skilled practitioners who perform frequent examinations [48].

2. In addition to the transtemporal approach, additional windows have been standardized including the transocular, foramen magnum, and retromandibular approach.

3. In most patients it is thus possible to monitor blood flow through the internal carotid, the carotid siphon, the anterior cerebral artery (ACA), MCA, the posterior cerebral artery (PCA), the basilar artery, and the vertebral arteries.

4. Examinations are generally performed in serial fashion. Although often impractical, continuous monitoring is possible.

5. Due to variations in skull and vessel anatomy, a significant number of patients will be missing one or more sonographic windows, making a full TCD examination impossible in these patients. Alternative insonation points may be available but may also exacerbate interobserver variability.

CLINICAL PEARL TCD is an appealing modality because it is noninvasive, real time, and has been applied to a wide range of clinical questions. In most patients, flow velocity can be monitored through the ACA, the MCA, the PCA, the basilar artery, and the vertebral arteries. Serial measurements can help to detect and treat alterations in flow velocity, an indicator of CBF.

E. **Interpretation.** TCD is an appealing modality because it is noninvasive, real time, and has been applied to a wide range of clinical questions. Nevertheless, interpretation of TCD data must be understood in terms of two of its limitations.

1. **TCD measures flow velocity, not flow.** In other words, although basal cerebral vessel diameter appears to change relatively little, certain conditions, such as severe acid–base disturbances, changes in blood viscosity, or significant hypercapnea may alter the relationship between velocity and flow. In these instances, a high-measured velocity may reflect either hyper- or hypoperfusion. Similarly, a low-measured velocity may represent vessel occlusion, low global flow, or a misplaced probe. In either case, alternative forms of investigation may be required.

2. **TCD does not identify cause.** Measurement of flow does not explain why the flow is high, normal, or low. The information TCD provides is best understood in context. For this reason, TCD is most often used in conjunction with additional diagnostic and monitoring modalities.

CLINICAL PEARL TCD is highly operator dependent and is not diagnostic of anything other than blood flow velocity. Since it measures flow velocity and not blood flow itself, its utility relies on simultaneous interpretation of alternative sources of clinical and imaging data.

IV. **Brain tissue oxygen monitoring**

A. **Physiologic rationale**

1. What does it measure? Brain tissue oxygen monitoring ($PbtO_2$) involves direct measurement of the partial pressure of oxygen in the interstitium of the brain. The

underlying physiology, however, has yet to be fully elucidated. Experimental evidence suggests that $PbtO_2$ depends, in part, on arterial oxygen tension (PaO_2) and CBF. Other factors influencing $PbtO_2$ include FiO_2, hemoglobin concentration, MAP, and CPP. $PbtO_2$ almost certainly reflects the balance between local oxygen delivery and cellular oxygen consumption [49]. But unlike the $SjVO_2$ it is also a more direct measure of local diffusion of oxygen, or the amount of oxygen available to the surrounding brain tissue [50]. Drawing on experimental oxygen, $PaCO_2$, and blood pressure challenges in a series of patients with TBI, Rosenthal et al. [51] have proposed that $PbtO_2$ is equal to the product of CBF and the arteriovenous oxygen tension difference ($AVTO_2$).

CLINICAL PEARL $PbtO_2$ reflects the balance between local oxygen delivery and cellular oxygen consumption. Thus it is useful in guiding changes in global factors to include FiO_2, hemoglobin concentration, MAP, and CPP.

2. **Normal values.** Mitochondrial function in the brain is dependent on an oxygen tension of approximately 1.5 mm Hg [52]. Physiologic studies indicate that this threshold corresponds to a measured $PbtO_2$ of 15 mm Hg to 20 mm Hg [50]. Estimates of normal brain tissue oxygen levels suggest a range of 25 mm Hg to 48 mm Hg [33,53]. Since small differences in cellular oxygen tension can have significant effects on cellular metabolism, it is biologically plausible that treatment strategies aimed at maintaining $PbtO_2$ greater than 20 mm Hg will reduce secondary injury and improve outcomes in patients with acute brain injury. $PbtO_2$ values less than 20 mm Hg have been defined as *moderate* brain hypoxia and values less than 10 mm Hg as *severe* brain hypoxia [54,55]. Alternatively, the Brain Trauma Foundation has proposed 15 mm Hg as a *critical* threshold for initiation of treatment aimed at increasing $PbtO_2$ [56].

3. **Evidence base.** Mounting evidence suggests an association between brain tissue hypoxia and worsened outcome [57–59]. Furthermore, this association appears to be independent of CPP and intracranial hypertension [60].

B. **Indications.** The vast majority of experimental and clinical experience involving brain oxygen monitoring has been related to management of TBI and aneurysmal SAH. In both cases, monitoring is most useful in comatose patients whose mental status cannot be followed using serial examination (Glasgow Coma Scale less than 8).

1. **Severe TBI.** Although no randomized controlled trials have been completed to date, a growing number of small prospective studies have demonstrated improved outcomes using $PbtO_2$-directed management strategies for patients with severe TBI [61–63]. Benefit may be limited to a subset of patients with correctable $PbtO_2$ abnormalities [64]. It is also important to note that not all studies have found improved outcomes when compared with traditional ICP/CPP management strategies [65]. In fact, Martini et al. [66] found worse outcomes among those who were managed using $PbtO_2$, presumably due to side effects and complications of a corresponding increase in the use of prolonged sedation, vasopressors, and hyperosmotic therapy.

CLINICAL PEARL   Evidence supporting the use of $PbtO_2$ in the management of severe TBI is mounting but randomized controlled trials are needed. It remains unclear if the association between reduced brain oxygen tension and poor outcome reflects reversible pathology or is primarily a reflection of injury severity.

2. **Poor-grade aneurysmal subarachnoid hemorrhage**
   a. As with TBI, randomized controlled trials are lacking. However, brain tissue hypoxia has been associated with increased mortality after SAH [67]. $PbtO_2$-derived indices have also been studied in SAH. A positive oxygen reactivity index (ORx, the correlation coefficient between $PbtO_2$ and CPP) has been found to predict delayed ischemia

in patients with poor-grade SAH, and may be helpful in guiding CPP management in these patients [68,69].

b. PbtO$_2$ has also been used to demonstrate that two of the mainstays of "Triple H" therapy, hypervolemia and hemodilution, are not helpful and may be harmful in the management of ruptured cerebral aneurysm [70]. Current recommendations favor induced hypertension alone for the management of delayed ischemia after SAH [71] (see chapter 9).

c. PbtO$_2$ has also shown promise in assessing the efficacy of interventional neuroradiology management of postaneurysmal cerebral vasospasm [72].

CLINICAL PEARL Experimental and clinical experience with PbtO$_2$ has been shown to be most useful in comatose patients whose mental status cannot be followed using serial examination (Glasgow Coma Scale less than 8).

---

3. Emerging indications. Although data are too limited to make summary judgments about the role of PbtO$_2$ in other kinds of brain injury, there is a great deal of interest in the use of this modality in both adult and pediatric ischemic stroke [73,74], intracerebral hemorrhage [75], infectious encephalitides [76], and during neurosurgical procedures [77].

C. Contraindications
  1. Absolute
    a. Infection at the desired insertion site
    b. Uncorrected coagulopathy
  2. Relative
    a. Thrombocytopenia (platelets 75,000 to 100,000)
    b. Conditions that predispose to coagulopathy such as advanced liver disease, renal failure, severe hypothermia

D. Placement
  1. Device. The most widely used device for direct measurement of brain oxygen tension is the Licox, a polarographic Clark-type electrode that measures oxygen content in an area 15 to 20 mm around the probe using the electrochemical properties of noble metals. The device is precalibrated, but requires postinsertion stabilization for 30 minutes to 2 hours. Values are temperature corrected using a thermometer at the tip of the catheter. Placement is via burr-hole craniotomy, similar to the approach used for other intraparenchymal brain monitors.

  2. Location. Placement is typically similar in location to ventriculostomy, and is directed at normal-appearing right frontal subcortical white matter, especially in the setting of diffuse or multifocal injury. However, there may be utility in placement of the catheter adjacent to an area of focal injury. Interestingly, one study suggested better correlation with outcome when the probe was placed in an area of injured brain [78]. Since injured tissue may have lower PbtO$_2$ values, some have worried that placement in these areas may confuse interpretation or prompt more aggressive treatment [50].

  3. Other considerations
    a. Oxygen challenge. Following the initial stabilization period, abnormally low values that are not consistent with the patient's pathophysiology should be evaluated using an oxygen challenge in which the FiO$_2$ is briefly raised to 100%, which should prompt an increase in PbtO$_2$ in a functional catheter.
    b. Transport. Since the monitors are stiff, protrude several inches from the patient's head, and are attached at all times to a series of long cables, they present a significant challenge during patient transfer and transport. Extreme care must be taken to prevent inadvertent dislodgement or damage to the monitor.

E. Complications. Complications are similar to those that accompany ventriculostomy or intraparenchymal ICP monitor placement and include scalp or intracerebral hematoma, inadvertent ventricular placement, and infection. In most studies, hematoma and infection combined occurred in only 1% to 2% of cases and the majority of these complications were not clinically significant [33,58].

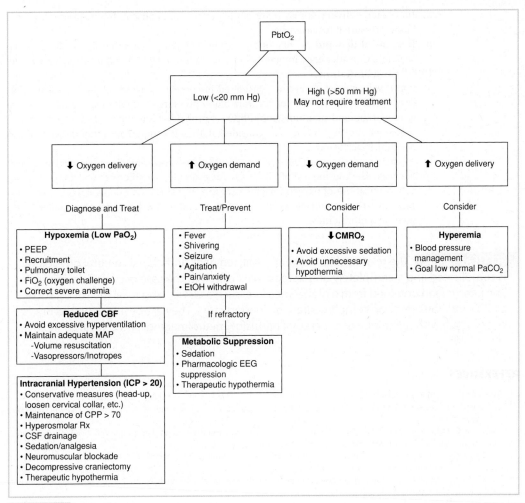

FIGURE 28.2 btO$_2$ flow chart.

F. Interpretation

1. **Low PbtO$_2$.** As discussed above, it is generally recommended that brain tissue hypoxia should be treated when PbtO$_2$ falls below 20 mm Hg (see Fig. 28.2). Treatment is generally directed toward minimizing increased oxygen demand on the one hand and impaired oxygen delivery on the other.

    a. **Increased oxygen demand.** Reversible factors that increase cerebral metabolic rate and thus oxygen demand include shivering, pain and agitation, fever, and seizures. Treatment with sedatives and analgesics, surface warming, antipyrrhetics, and anticonvulsants are thus important in the prevention of secondary injury.

    b. **Decreased oxygen delivery.** Reversible factors that decrease oxygen delivery to brain parenchyma include severe anemia, hypotension, hypovolemia, intracranial hypertension, and hypoxemia. Transfusion, vasopressors, fluid resuscitation, hyperosmotic therapy, and advanced modes of mechanical ventilation or administration of high FiO$_2$ may be necessary to normalize PbtO$_2$.

2. **High PbtO$_2$.** PbtO$_2$ greater than 50 mm Hg is uncommon. The significance of this finding is unclear and treatment may not be necessary. Possibilities include excessive oxygen delivery or reduced cerebral metabolic demand.

    a. Increased delivery. It may represent hyperemia or luxuriant flow. Consider lowering blood pressure if hypertensive.

    b. Decreased demand. It may occur during therapeutic hypothermia or during deep sedation. Consider lightening sedation, paralysis, or metabolic suppression if indicated.

3. **Pitfalls and limitations**

    a. $PbtO_2$ values must always be considered in context. Isolated values are not particularly useful in the absence of accurate blood pressure and ICP measurement, clinical examination, and neuroimaging. $PbtO_2$ is probably best utilized as part of a multimodal monitoring strategy that considers ICP, CPP, and perhaps other derived indices of cerebral perfusion.

    b. As discussed above, aggressive treatment of low $PbtO_2$ readings has clinical consequences. The routine use of high FiO_2, for example, may increase atelectasis and has a theoretical risk of oxygen toxicity. Excessive transfusion, prolonged use of vasopressors, invasive monitoring, over-resuscitation, and oversedation are all associated with their own morbidities.

CLINICAL PEARL The relationship between focal, regional, and global cerebral physiology is complicated and incompletely understood, particularly in the case of multifocal injury. The information obtained from a global measure, such as $SjVO_2$, and focal measures, such as TCD and $PbtO_2$ may be complimentary or contradictory. They are best interpreted in conjunction with other indices of cerebral perfusion, neuroimaging, and clinical context.

REFERENCES

1. Schell RM, Cole DJ. Cerebral monitoring: jugular venous oximetry. *Anesth Analg.* 2000;90(3):559–566.
2. Gopinath SP, Robertson CS, Contant CF, et al. Jugular venous desaturation and outcome after head injury. *J Neurol Neurosurg Psychiatry.* 1994;57(6):717–723.
3. De Deyne C, Decruyenaere J, Calle P, et al. Analysis of very early jugular bulb oximetry data after severe head injury: implications for the emergency management? *Eur J Emerg Med.* 1996;3(2):69–72.
4. Fandino J, Stocker R, Prokop S, et al. Cerebral oxygenation and systemic trauma related factors determining neurological outcome after brain injury. *J Clin Neurosci.* 2000;7(3):226–233.
5. Cruz J. The first decade of continuous monitoring of jugular bulb oxyhemoglobinsaturation: management strategies and clinical outcome. *Crit Care Med.* 1998;26(2):344–351.
6. Schaffranietz L, Heinke W. The effect of different ventilation regimes on jugular venous oxygen saturation in elective neurosurgical patients. *Neurol Res.* 1998;20(suppl 1):S66–S70.
7. Heran NS, Hentschel SJ, Toyota BD. Jugular bulb oximetry for prediction of vasospasm following subarachnoid hemorrhage. *Can J Neurol Sci.* 2004;31(1):80–86.
8. Fandino J, Kaku Y, Schuknecht B, et al. Improvement of cerebral oxygenation patterns and metabolic validation of superselective intraarterial infusion of papaverine for the treatment of cerebral vasospasm. *J Neurosurg.* 1998;89(1):93–100.
9. Anastasiou E, Gerolioliou K, Karakoulas K, et al. Reliability of continuous jugular venous bulb hemoglobin oxygen saturation during cardiac surgery. *J Cardiothorac Vasc Anesth.* 1999;13(3):276–279.
10. Souter MJ, Andrews PJ, Alston RP. Jugular venous desaturation following cardiac surgery. *Br J Anaesth.* 1998;81(2):239–241.
11. Trubiano P, Heyer EJ, Adams DC, et al. Jugular venous bulb oxyhemoglobin saturation during cardiac surgery: accuracy and reliability using a continuous monitor. *Anesth Analg.* 1996;82(5):964–968.
12. Croughwell ND, Frasco P, Blumenthal JA, et al. Warming during cardiopulmonary bypass is associated with jugular bulb desaturation. *Ann Thorac Surg.* 1992;53(5):827–832.
13. Croughwell ND, Newman MF, Blumenthal JA, et al. Jugular bulb saturation and cognitive dysfunction after cardiopulmonary bypass. *Ann Thorac Surg.* 1994;58(6):1702–1708.
14. Miura N, Yoshitani K, Kawaguchi M, et al. Jugular bulb desaturation during off-pump coronary artery bypass surgery. *J Anesth.* 2009;23(4):477–482.
15. Matta BF, Lam AM, Mayberg TS, et al. A critique of the intraoperative use of jugular venous bulb catheters during neurosurgical procedures. *Anesth Analg.* 1994;79(4):745–750.
16. Moss E, Dearden NM, Berridge JC. Effects of changes in mean arterial pressure on SjO_2 during cerebral aneurysm surgery. *Br J Anaesth.* 1995;75(5):527–530.
17. Sharma D, Siriussawakul A, Dooney N, et al. Clinical experience with intraoperative jugular venous oximetry during pediatric intracranial neurosurgery. *Paediatr Anaesth.* 2013;23(1):84–90.
18. Buunk G, van der Hoeven JG, Meinders AE. Prognostic significance of the difference between mixed venous and jugular bulb oxygen saturation in comatose patients resuscitated from a cardiac arrest. *Resuscitation.* 1999;41(3):257–262.

19. Takasu A, Yagi K, Ishihara S, et al. Combined continuous monitoring of systemic and cerebral oxygen metabolism after cardiac arrest. *Resuscitation.* 1995;29(3):189–194.

20. Zarzuelo R, Castaneda J. Differences in oxygen content between mixed venous blood and cerebral venous blood for outcome prediction after cardiac arrest. *Intensive Care Med.* 1995;21(1):71–75.

21. van der Hoeven JG, de Koning J, Compier EA, et al. Early jugular bulb oxygenation monitoring in comatose patients after an out-of-hospital cardiac arrest. *Intensive Care Med.* 1995;21(7):567–572.

22. Stocchetti N, Paparella A, Bridelli F, et al. Cerebral venous oxygen saturation studied with bilateral samples in the internal jugular veins. *Neurosurgery.* 1994;34(1):38–43; discussion 43–44.

23. Segal J. Percutaneous catheterization of the jugular bulb with a Doppler probe: technical note. *Neurosurgery.* 1993;33(1):151–153.

24. Coplin WM, O'Keefe GE, Grady MS, et al. Thrombotic, infectious, and procedural complications of the jugular bulb catheter in the intensive care unit. *Neurosurgery.* 1997;41(1):101–107; discussion 107–109.

25. Goetting MG, Preston G. Jugular bulb catheterization does not increase intracranial pressure. *Intensive Care Med.* 1991; 17(4):195–198.

26. Stocchetti N, Longhi L, Valeriani V. Bilateral cannulation of internal jugular veins may worsen intracranial hypertension. *Anesthesiology.* 2003;99(4):1017–1018.

27. Aaslid R, Markwalder TM, Nornes H. Noninvasive transcranial Doppler ultrasound recording of flow velocity in basal cerebral arteries. *J Neurosurg.* 1982;57(6):769–774.

28. Serrador JM, Picot PA, Rutt BK, et al. MRI measures of middle cerebral artery diameter in conscious humans during simulated orthostasis. *Stroke.* 2000;31(7):1672–1678.

29. Valdueza JM, Balzer JO, Villringer A, et al. Changes in blood flow velocity and diameter of the middle cerebral artery during hyperventilation: assessment with MR and transcranial Doppler sonography. *AJNR Am J Neuroradiol.* 1997;18(10): 1929–1934.

30. Carrera E, Schmidt JM, Oddo M, et al. Transcranial Doppler for predicting delayed cerebral ischemia after subarachnoid hemorrhage. *Neurosurgery.* 2009;65(2):316–323; discussion 323–324.

31. Tsivgoulis G, Alexandrov AV, Sloan MA. Advances in transcranial Doppler ultrasonography. *Curr Neurol Neurosci Rep.* 2009;9(1):46–54.

32. Rasulo FA, De Peri E, Lavinio A. Transcranial Doppler ultrasonography in intensive care. *Eur J Anaesthesiol Suppl.* 2008;42:167–173.

33. Messerer M, Daniel RT, Oddo M. Neuromonitoring after major neurosurgical procedures. *Minerva Anestesiol.* 2012;78(7):810–822.

34. Schnaudigel S, Groschel K, Pilgram SM, et al. New brain lesions after carotid stenting versus carotid endarterectomy: a systematic review of the literature. *Stroke.* 2008;39(6):1911–1919.

35. Edmonds Jr H. Monitoring of cerebral perfusion with transcranial Doppler ultrasound. In: Nuwer MR, ed. *Intraoperative Monitoring of Neural Function–Handbook of Clinical Neurophysiology.* London: Elsevier; 2008:909–923.

36. Ganzel BL, Edmonds HL Jr., Pank JR, et al. Neurophysiologic monitoring to assure delivery of retrograde cerebral perfusion. *J Thorac Cardiovasc Surg.* 1997;113(4):748–755; discussion 755–757.

37. Estrera AL, Garami Z, Miller CC 3rd, et al. Cerebral monitoring with transcranial Doppler ultrasonography improves neurologic outcome during repairs of acute type A aortic dissection. *J Thorac Cardiovasc Surg.* 2005;129(2):277–285.

38. Rodriguez RA, Cornel G, Semelhago L, et al. Cerebral effects in superior vena caval cannula obstruction: the role of brain monitoring. *Ann Thorac Surg.* 1997;64(6):1820–1822.

39. Camerlingo M, Casto L, Censori B, et al. Transcranial Doppler in acute ischemic stroke of the middle cerebral artery territories. *Acta Neurol Scand.* 1993;88(2):108–111.

40. Eggers J, Ossadnik S, Seidel G. Enhanced clot dissolution in vitro by 1.8-MHz pulsed ultrasound. *Ultrasound Med Biol.* 2009;35(3):523–526.

41. Alexandrov AV. Ultrasound enhancement of fibrinolysis. *Stroke.* 2009;40(3 suppl):S107–S110.

42. Radolovich DK, Aries MJ, Castellani G, et al. Pulsatile intracranial pressure and cerebral autoregulation after traumatic brain injury. *Neurocrit Care.* 2011;15(3):379–386.

43. Sorrentino E, Budohoski KP, Kasprowicz M, et al. Critical thresholds for transcranial Doppler indices of cerebral autoregulation in traumatic brain injury. *Neurocrit Care.* 2011;14(2):188–193.

44. Yeh T Jr., Austin EH 3rd, Sehic A, et al. Rapid recognition and treatment of cerebral air embolism: the role of neuromonitoring. *J Thorac Cardiovasc Surg.* 2003;126(2):589–591.

45. Borger MA, Taylor RL, Weisel RD, et al. Decreased cerebral emboli during distal aortic arch cannulation: a randomized clinical trial. *J Thorac Cardiovasc Surg.* 1999;118(4):740–745.

46. Brooker RF, Brown WR, Moody DM, et al. Cardiotomy suction: a major source of brain lipid emboli during cardiopulmonary bypass. *Ann Thorac Surg.* 1998;65(6):1651–1655.

47. Adams RJ, McKie VC, Hsu L, et al. Prevention of a first stroke by transfusions in children with sickle cell anemia and abnormal results on transcranial Doppler ultrasonography. *N Engl J Med.* 1998;339(1):5–11.

48. Shen Q, Stuart J, Venkatesh B, et al. Inter observer variability of the transcranial Doppler ultrasound technique: impact of lack of practice on the accuracy of measurement. *J Clin Monit Comput.* 1999;15(3–4):179–184.

49. Scheufler KM, Rohrborn HJ, Zentner J. Does tissue oxygen-tension reliably reflect cerebral oxygen delivery and consumption? *Anesth Analg.* 2002;95(4):1042–1048.

50. Maloney-Wilensky E, Le Roux P. The physiology behind direct brain oxygen monitors and practical aspects of their use. *Childs Nerv Syst.* 2010;26(4):419–430.

51. Rosenthal G, Hemphill JC 3rd, Sorani M, et al. Brain tissue oxygen tension is more indicative of oxygen diffusion than oxygen delivery and metabolism in patients with traumatic brain injury. *Crit Care Med.* 2008;36(6):1917–1924.

52. Siesjo BK, Siesjo P. Mechanisms of secondary brain injury. *Eur J Anaesthesiol.* 1996;13(3):247–268.

53. Pennings FA, Schuurman PR, van den Munckhof P, et al. Brain tissue oxygen pressure monitoring in awake patients during functional neurosurgery: the assessment of normal values. *J Neurotrauma.* 2008;25(10):1173–1177.

54. Longhi L, Pagan F, Valeriani V, et al. Monitoring brain tissue oxygen tension in brain-injured patients reveals hypoxic episodes in normal-appearing and in peri-focal tissue. *Intensive Care Med.* 2007;33(12):2136–2142.

55. van den Brink WA, van Santbrink H, Steyerberg EW, et al. Brain oxygen tension in severe head injury. *Neurosurgery.* 2000;46(4):868–876; discussion 876–878.

56. Bratton SL, Chestnut RM, Ghajar J, et al. Guidelines for the management of severe traumatic brain injury. X. Brain oxygen monitoring and thresholds. *J Neurotrauma.* 2007;24 (suppl 1):S65–S70.

57. Chang JJ, Youn TS, Benson D, et al. Physiologic and functional outcome correlates of brain tissue hypoxia in traumatic brain injury. *Crit Care Med.* 2009;37(1):283–290.

58. Maloney-Wilensky E, Gracias V, Itkin A, et al. Brain tissue oxygen and outcome after severe traumatic brain injury: a systematic review. *Crit Care Med.* 2009;37(6):2057–2063.

59. Eriksson EA, Barletta JF, Figueroa BE, et al. The first 72 hours of brain tissue oxygenation predicts patient survival with traumatic brain injury. *J Trauma Acute Care Surg.* 2012;72(5):1345–1349.

60. Oddo M, Levine JM, Mackenzie L, et al. Brain hypoxia is associated with short-term outcome after severe traumatic brain injury independently of intracranial hypertension and low cerebral perfusion pressure. *Neurosurgery.* 2011;69(5):1037–1045; discussion 1045.

61. Stiefel MF, Spiotta A, Gracias VH, et al. Reduced mortality rate in patients with severe traumatic brain injury treated with brain tissue oxygen monitoring. *J Neurosurg.* 2005;103(5):805–811.

62. Narotam PK, Morrison JF, Nathoo N. Brain tissue oxygen monitoring in traumatic brain injury and major trauma: outcome analysis of a brain tissue oxygen-directed therapy. *J Neurosurg.* 2009;111(4):672–682.

63. Nangunoori R, Maloney-Wilensky E, Stiefel M, et al. Brain tissue oxygen-based therapy and outcome after severe traumatic brain injury: a systematic literature review. *Neurocrit Care.* 2012;17(1):131–138.

64. Spiotta AM, Stiefel MF, Gracias VH, et al. Brain tissue oxygen-directed management and outcome in patients with severe traumatic brain injury. *J Neurosurg.* 2010;113(3):571–580.

65. Green JA, Pellegrini DC, Vanderkolk WE, et al. Goal directed brain tissue oxygen monitoring versus conventional management in traumatic brain injury: an analysis of in hospital recovery. *Neurocrit Care.* 2012 [Epub ahead of print].

66. Martini RP, Deem S, Yanez ND, et al. Management guided by brain tissue oxygen monitoring and outcome following severe traumatic brain injury. *J Neurosurg.* 2009;111(4):644–649.

67. Ramakrishna R, Stiefel M, Udoetuk J, et al. Brain oxygen tension and outcome in patients with aneurysmal subarachnoid hemorrhage. *J Neurosurg.* 2008;109(6):1075–1082.

68. Jaeger M, Schuhmann MU, Soehle M, et al. Continuous monitoring of cerebrovascular autoregulation after subarachnoid hemorrhage by brain tissue oxygen pressure reactivity and its relation to delayed cerebral infarction. *Stroke.* 2007;38(3): 981–986.

69. Radolovich DK, Czosnyka M, Timofeev I, et al. Reactivity of brain tissue oxygen to change in cerebral perfusion pressure in head injured patients. *Neurocrit Care.* 2009;10(3):274–279.

70. Muench E, Horn P, Bauhuf C, et al. Effects of hypervolemia and hypertension on regional cerebral blood flow, intracranial pressure, and brain tissue oxygenation after subarachnoid hemorrhage. *Crit Care Med.* 2007;35(8):1844–1851; quiz 1852.

71. Diringer MN, Bleck TP, Claude Hemphill J 3rd, et al. Critical care management of patients following aneurysmal subarachnoid hemorrhage: recommendations from the Neurocritical Care Society's Multidisciplinary Consensus Conference. *Neurocrit Care.* 2011;15(2):211–240.

72. Deshaies EM, Jacobsen W, Singla A, et al. Brain tissue oxygen monitoring to assess reperfusion after intra-arterial treatment of aneurysmal subarachnoid hemorrhage-induced cerebral vasospasm: a retrospective study. *AJNR Am J Neuroradiol.* 2012;33(7):1411–1415.

73. Cyrous A, O'Neal B, Freeman WD. New approaches to bedside monitoring in stroke. *Expert Rev Neurother.* 2012;12(8): 915–928.

74. Allen BB, Hoffman CE, Traube CS, et al. Continuous brain tissue oxygenation monitoring in the management of pediatric stroke. *Neurocrit Care.* 2011;15(3):529–536.

75. Hemphill JC 3rd, Morabito D, Farrant M, et al. Brain tissue oxygen monitoring in intracerebral hemorrhage. *Neurocrit Care.* 2005;3(3):260–270.

76. Puri VN, Pradeep K. The impact of brain tissue oxygenation (Pbto2) monitoring in a patient with West Nile Virus Encephalitis (Wnve): 264-T. *Crit Care Med.* 2005;33(12):A 179.

77. Cerejo A, Silva PA, Dias C, et al. Monitoring of brain oxygenation in surgery of ruptured middle cerebral artery aneurysms. *Surg Neurol Int.* 2011;2:70.

78. Ponce LL, Pillai S, Cruz J, et al. Position of probe determines prognostic information of brain tissue PO2 in severe traumatic brain injury. *Neurosurgery.* 2012;70(6):1492–1502; discussion 1502–1503.

29

Traumatic Brain Injury

Monica S. Vavilala and Deepak Sharma

KEY POINTS

1. Traumatic brain injury (TBI) should be considered in all children following trauma, particularly those with a suspicious mechanism of injury, loss of consciousness, multiple episodes of emesis, tracheal intubation, and extracranial injuries. Likewise, associated injuries (femur and pelvic fractures and intra-abdominal bleeding) should be managed concurrently.
2. The major goals of anesthetic management of TBI are to maintain age-appropriate CPP, treat increased ICP, and provide optimal surgical conditions.
3. Avoid secondary insults such as hypotension, hypoxemia, hyper- and hypocarbia, and hypo- and hyperglycemia.

INTRODUCTION

Pediatric neurotrauma is the leading cause of death in children more than 1 year of age and disability following pediatric neurotrauma is common with profound impact on functional long-term outcomes [1,2]. Traumatic brain injury (TBI) should be considered in all children following trauma, particularly those with a suspicious mechanism of injury, loss of consciousness, multiple episodes of emesis, tracheal intubation, and extracranial injuries.

I. Epidemiology. Each year about half a million children present to emergency departments (EDs) with TBI. The Centers for Disease Control and Prevention (CDC) in the United States reports TBI-related death rates for the different age groups as follows: 5.7/100,000 (0 to 4 years), 3.1/100,000 (5 to 9 years), and 4.8/100,000 (10 to 14 years) [3]. Fortunately, the majority of children (90%) suffers only from minor injuries and can be sent home after triage in the ED [1]. Nevertheless, 37,000 children with TBI require hospitalization, and up to 2,685 children with TBI per year do not survive their sustained injuries [1]. Boys and adolescents present more frequently to the ED for TBI with a male to female ratio of 3:2 [1]. Moreover, boys have a four times higher risk of fatal TBI compared to girls. Despite similar mortality rates, African-American children have a less favorable clinical and functional outcome after TBI likely as the result of differences in health care and/or health status [4,5].

II. Patterns and mechanisms of injury. Children are more susceptible to TBI because they have a larger head-to-body size ratio, thinner cranial bones providing less protection to the intracranial contents, and less myelinated neural tissue which makes them more vulnerable to damage [6]. Children have a greater incidence of diffuse injury, cerebral edema, and increased intracranial pressure (ICP) following TBI than adults [6]. Diffuse TBI is the most common type of injury and results in a range of injury severity from concussion to diffuse axonal injury (DAI) and permanent disability. Anatomically, the injury can be extra-axial (e.g., epidural hematoma [EDH], subdural hematoma [SDH], subarachnoid hemorrhage [SAH], and intraventricular hemorrhage [IVH]), intra-axial (e.g., DAI, cortical contusion, and intracerebral hematoma), or vascular (e.g., vascular dissection, carotid cavernous fistula, arteriovenous dural fistula, and pseudoaneurysm).

The observed types of TBI and mechanisms of injury differ with child age and development. According to the CDC, falls are the most common mechanism for TBI [1]. In toddlers, falls often result in direct contusions while older children increasingly suffer TBI from bicycle crashes or are hit by a car while walking, or while riding a bicycle, resulting in all types of TBI, especially diffuse, shearing injuries [1]. In adolescence, injuries resulting from automobile crashes increase dramatically and are the most common cause [1]. Sports-related head injuries can also be important in these older age groups and represent a unique type of repetitive mild injury that can have cumulative effects [1]. In an infant in a rear-facing child-safety seat, resultant injury causes skull fractures, brain contusion, and hemorrhage, whereas in a forward-facing front-seat child, injuries are not only confined to the cranium, but additional fractures or ligamentous injuries of the cervical spine are common [7,8].

Inflicted TBI, sometimes called nonaccidental trauma, is a unique, devastating category of TBI typically occurring in young children. Population-based studies estimate that 30/100,000 children younger than 1 year of age require hospitalization because of inflicted TBI per year [2]. In infants, inflicted trauma is a major cause of TBI and is associated with skull fractures, intracranial hemorrhage, DAI with or without cerebral edema, and delayed hypoxic-ischemic injury. Inflicted injuries are also age dependent with more DAI in neonates (due to the "shaken baby mechanism") and more focal lesions in older children when they are assaulted. In addition, strangulation or chest compression while shaking may result in additional hypoxic-ischemic injuries superimposed to the focal injuries. Children with inflicted TBI commonly present with altered consciousness, coma, seizures, vomiting, or irritability. Histories are often lacking and injuries out of proportion to history or developmental milestone should alert clinicians to consider this diagnosis.

III. Physiology and pathophysiology. The pathophysiology of TBI involves primary and secondary injuries to the brain. Primary injury is the damage caused by the initial trauma involving mechanical impact to the brain tissue and skull due to acceleration–deceleration or rotational forces, resulting in skull fracture, brain contusion, intracranial hematoma, or DAI. The primary injury then initiates inflammatory process, edema formation and excitotoxicity, resulting in further increase in ICP and reduced cerebral perfusion pressure (CPP), all leading to secondary injury to the brain. In addition, physiologic insults that develop over time after the onset of the initial injury cause further damage to the brain tissue worsening the outcome in TBI patients and are often referred to as the "secondary insults" or "second insults." Some of the common secondary insults include hypotension, hypoxemia, hypercarbia, hypocarbia, hyperglycemia, hypoglycemia, and hyperthermia. Modern management of TBI emphasizes avoidance of primary insult and minimizing secondary insults. Table 29.1 details the factors associated with poor outcome after pediatric TBI.

TABLE 29.1 Predictors of poor outcome after pediatric TBI

1. Age <4 yrs
2. Cardiopulmonary resuscitation
3. Multiple trauma
4. Hypoxia ($PaO_2 < 60$ mm Hg)
5. Hyperventilation ($PaCO_2 < 35$ mm Hg)
6. Hyperglycemia (glucose > 250 mg/dL)
7. Hyperthermia (temperature > 38°C)
8. Hypotension (SBP < 70 + 2 × age)
9. Intracranial hypertension (ICP > 20 mm Hg)
10. Poor rehabilitation

CLINICAL PEARL In-hospital treatment of TBI should focus on minimizing secondary insults to the injured brain due to hypotension, hypoxemia, hypercarbia, hypocarbia, hyperthermia, intracranial hypertension, seizures, hypoglycemia, and hyperglycemia.

A. **Cerebral metabolic rate, cerebral blood flow, and cerebral autoregulation.** Global cerebral metabolic rate (CMR) for oxygen and glucose is higher in children than in adults (oxygen 5.8 vs. 3.5 mL/100 g brain tissue/min and glucose 6.8 vs. 5.5 mL/100 g brain tissue/min respectively). Unlike in adults, cerebral blood flow (CBF) changes with age and may be higher in girls compared to boys. Following TBI, CBF and cerebral metabolic rate for oxygen ($CMRO_2$) may not be matched, resulting in either cerebral ischemia or hyperemia. The incidence of cerebral hyperemia is 6% to 10% and $CMRO_2$ may be normal, low, or high after TBI [6]. Metabolic failure is an integral component of the pathologic aftermath of TBI. In pediatric TBI patients, low oxygen extraction fraction (OEF)—a marker of metabolic dysfunction—correlates with the severity of injury and outcome [9]. Similar to adults, the incidence of impaired cerebral autoregulation is higher following severe compared to mild TBI and children with impaired cerebral autoregulation early after TBI may lead to cerebral ischemia and poor long-term outcome [10].

B. **Intracranial pressure.** In adults, normal ICP is between 5 and 15 mm Hg compared to 2 to 4 mm Hg in young children. Unlike the adult with relatively poor cranial compliance, the infant with open fontanelles may be able to accommodate slow and small increases in intracranial volume by expansion of the skull. However, rapid expansion of intracranial volume, small as it may be, can explain the not uncommonly encountered rapid deterioration in infants following TBI. Intracranial hypertension may be difficult to diagnose, is associated with poor neurologic outcomes and death, and may be present in children with open fontanelles and sutures.

CLINICAL PEARL TBI often leads to uncoupling between CBF and metabolism and leads to impairment of cerebral autoregulation. Hyperemia after pediatric TBI is relatively uncommon whereas cerebral ischemia is more common.

IV. **Imaging modalities.** The initial radiographic evaluation of the pediatric patient with TBI is performed using computed tomography (CT) imaging which can rapidly detect intracranial hematoma, contusion, skull fracture, cerebral edema, and obliteration of the basal cisterns indicating concern for elevated ICP. However, prior to transport to CT scanner, initial evaluation and resuscitation must be performed and appropriate monitoring must be instituted. Patients with DAI may initially have a normal CT scan despite significant neurologic findings and increased ICP; repeat CT scan often shows secondary injury due to cerebral edema [11]. In childhood, conventional MRI compared to CT scan has high sensitivity and specificity, better correlation with the outcome, and lack of radiation [12,13]. Although conventional MRI sequences are able to depict the precise anatomical location, extent, quality, and degree of TBI, functional MRI (fMRI) sequences give information about the microstructural (diffusion-weight imaging [DWI]/diffusion tensor imaging [DTI]), biochemical (magnetic resonance spectroscopy [MRS]), and hemodynamic perfusion-weighted imaging (PWI) short- and long-term consequences, and complications of TBI [12,13]. However, MRI is typically not obtained during the initial period because of its time-consuming imaging requirements. In addition, there are growing concerns about cumulative radiation exposure during CT scanning, and the current guidelines for the acute medical management of severe TBI in infants, children, and adolescents provide a level III recommendation that in the absence of neurologic deterioration or increasing ICP, obtaining a routine repeat CT scan >24 hours after the admission and initial follow-up study may not be indicated for decisions about neurosurgical intervention.

CLINICAL PEARL   Head CT imaging is often required to assess the extent and type of TBI. However, early MRI may be necessary to fully understand the extent of TBI. Routinely repeated head CT scanning is not advised due to ionizing radiation risks to the developing brain and other sensitive organs.

V. Indications for surgery. The major goal of surgery for TBI is to optimize the recovery of viable brain. Most operations deal with the removal of mass lesions for the purpose of preventing herniation, intracranial hypertension, or alterations in CBF. In general, unless small and venous, EDHs should be evacuated in comatose patients. SDHs that are associated with herniation, are greater than 10 mm thick, or produce a midline shift of >5 mm should be removed. Indications on intraparenchymal mass lesions include progressive neurologic deterioration referable to the lesion, signs of mass effect on CT, or refractory intracranial hypertension. Penetrating injury may often be managed with local debridement and watertight closure if not extensive and if there is minimal intracranial mass effect (as defined above). Patients with severe brain swelling as manifest by cisternal compression or midline shift on CT or intracranial hypertension by monitor are potential candidates for decompressive craniectomy. The relatively increased frequency of diffuse swelling in the pediatric population makes children more frequently candidates for such treatment.

VI. Anesthetic and perioperative management. The cornerstones of modern TBI management are field resuscitation, expeditious triage, emergent surgical evacuation of mass lesions, control of ICP, and support of CPP, multimodal monitoring and optimization of physiologic environment. Given the adverse impact of secondary insults on outcomes of TBI, the perioperative period may be particularly important in the course of TBI management. Despite the aggressive interventions to rapidly correct the secondary insults in the ED, it is not unusual for one or more of these complicating factors to persist or remain undetected as the patient is emergently transported to the operating room. Hence, perioperative period is an opportunity for the anesthesiologists to correct the pre-existing secondary insults. Moreover, surgery and anesthesia may predispose the patient to new onset secondary insults (such as intraoperative hypotension and new onset hyperglycemia), which are preventable/treatable. Therefore, the perioperative period may be a potential window to initiate interventions that may improve the outcome of TBI. Perioperative management involves rapid evaluation, continuation of cerebral and systemic resuscitation, early surgical intervention, intensive monitoring, and anesthetic planning.

CLINICAL PEARL   Surgery and anesthesia may predispose the patient to new onset secondary insults which are preventable/treatable. Anesthesiologists should anticipate and be prepared to rapidly treat these secondary insults.

A. Initial assessment. The initial approach to the traumatized child involves the primary and secondary surveys. Briefly, this involves rapid assessment of the airway, breathing, circulation, neurologic status, and associated injuries. The Glasgow Coma Scale (GCS) score (modified for children) is the most commonly used neurologic assessment (Table 29.2) and for grading the severity of TBI. A GCS score of 13 to 15 signifies mild TBI, 9 to 12 is moderate TBI, and 3 to 8 is severe TBI. Signs and symptoms of intracranial hypertension or impending herniation, such as altered level of consciousness, pupillary dysfunction, lateralizing extremity weakness, or Cushing's triad (hypertension, bradycardia, and irregular respirations) should alert the need for urgent interventions to control ICP including possible surgical decompression. Bruising around the mastoid ("Battle's sign") and in the periorbital area ("Raccoon eyes") and rhinorrhea indicate possible basilar skull fracture. The initial assessment and stabilization is usually achieved in the ED and resuscitation initiated before the patient is transported to CT scanner and then to the operating room. Nevertheless, it is important for the anesthesia team to perform another rapid assessment as the patient is received in the operating room. Associated

TABLE 29.2 Glasgow coma scale and modification for young children

Glasgow coma scale	Pediatric coma scale	Infant coma scale	Score
Eyes	*Eyes*	*Eyes*	
Open spontaneously	Open spontaneously	Open spontaneously	4
Verbal command	React to speech	React to speech	3
Pain	React to pain	React to pain	2
No response	No response	No response	1
Best verbal response	*Best verbal response*	*Best verbal response*	
Oriented and converses	Smiles, oriented, interacts	Coos, babbles, interacts	5
Disoriented and converses	Interacts inappropriately	Irritable	4
Inappropriate words	Moaning	Cries to pain	3
Incomprehensible sounds	Irritable, inconsolable	Moans to pain	2
No response	No response	No response	1
Best motor response	*Best motor response*	*Best motor response*	
Obeys verbal command	Spontaneous or obeys verbal command	Normal spontaneous movements	6
Localizes pain	Localizes pain	Withdraws to touch	5
Withdraws to pain	Withdraws to pain	Withdraws to pain	4
Abnormal flexion	Abnormal flexion	Abnormal flexion	3
Extension posturing	Extension posturing	Extension posturing	2
No response	No response	No response	1

thoracic, abdominal, spinal, and long bone injuries may be stable or evolve during the perioperative period and must be considered in differential diagnosis of new onset hypotension, anemia, hemodynamic instability, or hypoxemia during anesthesia and surgery. As the patient is transported to the operating room, all resuscitative measures should continue.

CLINICAL PEARL Initial assessment of pediatric TBI victim involves rapid assessment of the airway, breathing, circulation, GCS score, pupillary response, and associated injuries. Cushing's triad (hypertension, bradycardia, and irregular respirations) indicates impending herniation.

1. **Cervical spine immobilization.** In infants <6 months of age, the head and cervical spine should be immediately immobilized using a spine board with tape across the forehead, and blankets or towels around the neck. In infants ≥6 months of age, the head should be immobilized either in the manner described above or by using a small rigid cervical collar. Children >8 years of age require a medium-sized cervical collar. The use of rigid cervical collars is essential as it prevents cervical distraction during laryngoscopy. Since children under 7 years of age have a prominent occiput, a pad placed under the thoracic spine provides neutral alignment of the spine and avoids excessive flexion that may occur in the supine position. These two maneuvers are paramount in avoiding iatrogenic cervical spine injury.

2. **Airway management.** The most important therapy during the primary survey phase is to establish an adequate airway. The lucid and hemodynamically stable child can be managed conservatively but if the child has altered mental status, attempts should be made to establish the airway by suctioning the pharynx, chin-lift and jaw thrust maneuvers, or insertion of an oral airway. Children requiring surgery and those with a GCS score <9 require tracheal intubation for airway protection and management of increased ICP. Airway management in such circumstances is complicated by a number of factors including urgency of situation (because of pre-existing/worsening hypoxia), uncertainty of cervical spine status,

uncertainty of airway (due to presence of blood, vomitus, debris in the oral cavity or due to laryngopharyngeal injury or skull base fracture), full stomach, intracranial hypertension, and uncertain volume status. All TBI patients requiring tracheal intubation must be considered to have full stomach and airway management must account for possible underlying cervical spine injury. In the patients who arrive with an indwelling tracheal tube, adequate position of the tube must always be confirmed since the tube can possibly migrate during transport, leading to endobronchial intubation or even dislodgement.

The choice of technique for tracheal intubation is determined by urgency, individual expertise/skills, and available resources and generally incorporates rapid sequence orotracheal intubation with cricoid pressure and manual in-line stabilization. The anterior portion or cervical collar may be removed when manual in-line stabilization is established to allow greater mouth opening and facilitate laryngoscopy. Newer airway devices, particularly GlideScope video laryngoscope, have gained popularity in recent years for use in trauma victims and may be useful in difficult airway scenarios. However, recent studies show no difference in first-attempt success rates between video laryngoscopy and direct laryngoscopy in the newborn or infant simulators for pediatric emergency medicine providers although video laryngoscopy led to increased percentage of glottic opening (POGO) scores [14]. In any case, it is advisable to have a backup plan ready in case of difficult intubation, given the risk of intracranial hypertension resulting from increased cerebral blood volume (CBV) because of hypoxemia and hypercarbia during prolonged intubation attempts.

The choice of induction agents and muscle relaxants is important for successful uncomplicated airway management. Tracheal intubation is a noxious stimulus and can increase ICP. Hence, sodium thiopental (3 to 5 mg/kg), etomidate (0.2 to 0.6 mg/kg), or propofol (2 to 3 mg/kg) are often used to induce anesthesia before intubation in hemodynamically stable patients. All these agents decrease the systemic hemodynamic response to intubation, blunt increases in ICP, and decrease the $CMRO_2$. In addition, administration of lidocaine (1.5 mg/kg) and short-acting narcotic such as fentanyl (1 to 2 μg/kg) can decrease the catecholamine release associated with direct laryngoscopy. However, propofol and thiopental may cause cardiovascular depression leading to hypotension, especially in the presence of uncorrected hypovolemia. Etomidate (0.2 to 0.6 mg/kg) may be advantageous particularly in patients with unstable hemodynamic status due to little change in blood pressure during induction despite reduction of $CMRO_2$. Pediatric data on adrenal insufficiency following single-dose etomidate in TBI patients are lacking, although adrenal depression has been observed following etomidate use in children with sepsis [15]. Ketamine, which causes limited cardiovascular compromise, is often considered relatively contraindicated for intubating patients with risk for or pre-existing increased ICP for the fear of associated increased CBF and increased ICP. However, in mechanically ventilated pediatric patients with intracranial hypertension, ketamine has actually been shown to effectively decrease ICP and prevent untoward ICP elevations during potentially distressing interventions without lowering blood pressure and CPP [16]. In fact, ketamine may be a safe and effective drug for patients with TBI and intracranial hypertension and it can possibly be used safely in emergency situations. The choice of muscle relaxant for rapid sequence induction is between succinylcholine and rocuronium. While the clinical significance of the effect of succinylcholine on increasing ICP is questionable, increases in ICP secondary to hypoxia and hypercarbia are well documented and much more likely to be clinically important [17]. Hence, in patients with TBI, clinicians may not avoid using succinylcholine if difficult intubation is anticipated.

CLINICAL PEARL   Patients with GCS <9 require tracheal intubation to protect airway and to control ICP. Rapid sequence orotracheal intubation should be performed with cricoid pressure and manual in-line stabilization. Etomidate and ketamine may be used safely in TBI patients with unstable hemodynamics, if needed.

3. **Intravenous access and fluids.** Obtaining vascular access in the traumatized child can be very challenging. A well-functioning 20 gauge or larger peripheral intravenous catheter will suffice for induction of anesthesia. Saphenous veins are commonly used. A second intravenous line should be started after induction. In emergent cases, if peripheral access is unsuccessful after two attempts, an interosseous line should be placed. Central venous catheters should be inserted by experienced personnel and should not delay evacuation of expanding intracranial hematoma. Unlike adults, children can become hypovolemic from scalp injuries and isolated TBI. Isotonic crystalloid solutions are commonly used during the anesthetic and for cerebral resuscitation. Hypotonic crystalloids should be avoided and the role of colloids is controversial. The use of hydroxyethyl starch is discouraged because of its role in exacerbating coagulopathy. Nonglucose-containing warm, isotonic crystalloids are preferable for resuscitation and volume replacement in pediatric TBI.

> **CLINICAL PEARL** New power-driven intraosseous kits are available for children of all ages and should be attempted in a timely manner in the case of difficult intravenous access.

B. **Monitoring.** The current guidelines for the acute medical management of severe TBI in infants, children, and adolescents provide a level III recommendation that the use of ICP monitoring may be considered in infants and children with severe TBI (Table 29.3) [18]. This is based on the high incidence of intracranial hypertension in children with severe TBI, a widely reported association of intracranial hypertension and poor neurologic outcome, the concordance of protocol-based intracranial hypertension therapy and best-reported clinical outcomes, and improved outcomes associated with successful ICP-lowering therapies. In addition, intracranial hypertension may be difficult to diagnose, is associated with poor neurologic outcomes and death and may be present in children with open fontanelles and sutures. By contrast, ICP monitoring is not routinely indicated in children with mild or moderate TBI but may be instituted if serial neurologic examination is precluded by sedation, neuromuscular blockade, or anesthesia (e.g., for extracranial surgery in a child with TBI) [18]. Importantly, any pre-existing coagulopathy must be treated prior to monitor placement.

   Although many advanced technologies including cerebral microdialysis, thermal diffusion probes, transcranial Doppler, and near-infrared spectroscopy are increasingly being used for management of severe TBI, there are few systematic investigations specific to pediatric TBI, particularly pertaining to their use to guide therapy. Nevertheless, if brain oxygenation monitoring is used, maintenance of partial pressure of brain tissue oxygen ($PbtO_2$) ≥10 mm Hg may be considered based on a level III recommendation of the 2012 Pediatric Guidelines (Table 29.3) [18]. Pediatric patients requiring craniotomy or extracranial surgery for associated injuries should receive the standard American Society of Anesthesiologists monitoring, and invasive arterial blood pressure monitoring for beat-to-beat blood pressure monitoring, blood gas analysis, and blood glucose monitoring. Central venous pressure (CVP) may be useful, particularly for resuscitation and when vasopressors are administered. The internal jugular line may be safely placed and used without increasing ICP. However, it is advisable not to delay surgical evacuation of expanding intracranial hematoma because of institution of invasive monitoring. Jugular bulb oxygenation saturation monitoring can be useful to guide the degree of hyperventilation but is not standard of care.

> **CLINICAL PEARL** ICP monitoring is indicated in severe pediatric TBI. It is not routinely indicated in children with mild or moderate TBI but may be instituted if serial neurologic examination is precluded by sedation, neuromuscular blockade, or anesthesia. If brain oxygenation monitoring is used, $PbtO_2$ should be maintained ≥10 mm Hg. Reversal of coagulopathy is required prior to ICP monitor placement and ICP >20 mm Hg is considered intracranial hypertension.

TABLE 29.3 Summary of recommendations from the 2012 guidelines for the acute medical management of severe TBI in infants, children, and adolescents

Physiologic parameters	Recommendations
Intracranial pressure (ICP)	• Consider ICP monitoring in infants and children with severe TBI (level III) • Treatment of ICP may be considered at a threshold of 20 mm Hg (level III)
Cerebral perfusion pressure (CPP)	• A minimum CPP of 40 mm Hg may be considered in children with TBI (level III) • A CPP threshold 40–50 mm Hg may be considered with infants at the lower end and adolescents at the upper end of this range (level III)
Brain oxygenation (PbtO$_2$)	• If brain oxygenation monitoring is used, maintenance of PbtO$_2$ ≥ 10 mm Hg may be considered (level III)
Hyperosmolar therapy	• 3% hypertonic saline (0.1 and 1 mL/kg of body weight per h) should be considered for the treatment of intracranial hypertension (level III)
Hyperventilation	• Avoidance of prophylactic severe hyperventilation to a PaCO$_2$ <30 mm Hg may be considered in the initial 48 h after injury (level III) • If hyperventilation is used in the management of refractory intracranial hypertension, advanced neuromonitoring for evaluation of cerebral ischemia may be considered (level III)
Temperature control	• Moderate hypothermia (32°–33°C) beginning early after severe TBI for only 24 h duration should be avoided (level II) • Moderate hypothermia (32°–33°C) beginning within 8 h after severe TBI for up to 48 h duration should be considered to reduce intracranial hypertension (level II) • Rewarming at a rate of 0.5°C/h should be avoided (level II)
Cerebrospinal fluid (CSF) drainage	• CSF drainage through an external ventricular drain may be considered in the management of increased ICP (level III) • The addition of a lumbar drain may be considered in the case of refractory intracranial hypertension with a functioning external ventricular drain, open basal cisterns, and no evidence of a mass lesion or shift on imaging studies (level III)
Barbiturates	• High-dose barbiturate therapy may be considered in hemodynamically stable patients with refractory intracranial hypertension despite maximal medical and surgical management (level III) • When high-dose barbiturate therapy is used to treat refractory intracranial hypertension, continuous arterial blood pressure monitoring and cardiovascular support to maintain adequate cerebral perfusion pressure are required (level III)
Corticosteroids	• The use of corticosteroids is not recommended to improve outcome or reduce ICP for children with severe TBI (level II)
Analgesics, sedatives, and neuromuscular blockade	• Etomidate may be considered to control severe intracranial hypertension; however, the risks resulting from adrenal suppression must be considered (level III) • Thiopental may be considered to control intracranial hypertension (level III)
Antiseizure prophylaxis	• Prophylactic treatment with phenytoin may be considered to reduce the incidence of early posttraumatic seizures
Nutrition	• Do not use immune-modulating diet to improve outcome
Decompressive craniectomy	• Decompressive craniectomy (DC) with duraplasty may be considered for patients who are showing early signs of neurologic deterioration or herniation or are developing intracranial hypertension refractory to medical management during the early stages of their treatment

Level I recommendations are based on the strongest evidence for effectiveness and represent principles of patient management that reflect high degree of clinical certainty. Level II recommendations reflect a moderate degree of clinical certainty. For level III recommendations, the degree of clinical certainty is not established.

2

C. **Anesthetic technique, sedation, and analgesia.** The major goals of anesthetic management of TBI are to
1. maintain CPP;
2. treat increased ICP;
3. provide optimal surgical conditions;
4. avoid secondary insults such as hypotension, hypoxemia, hyper- and hypocarbia, hypo- and hyperglycemia; and
5. provide adequate analgesia and amnesia.

There are important pharmacodynamic and pharmacokinetic differences between intravenous and inhalational anesthetic agents. Intravenous agents including thiopental, propofol, and etomidate cause cerebral vasoconstriction and reduce CBF, CBV, $CMRO_2$, and ICP while opioids have no direct effects on cerebral hemodynamics in the presence of controlled ventilation. All inhaled anesthetic agents (isoflurane, sevoflurane, desflurane) decrease $CMRO_2$ and may cause cerebral vasodilation, resulting in increasing CBF and ICP. However, at concentration less than 1 minimum alveolar concentration (MAC), the cerebral vasodilatory effects are minimal and hence they may be used in low concentrations during craniotomy or extracranial surgery in patients with TBI. Nitrous oxide can increase $CMRO_2$ and cause cerebral vasodilation and increased ICP and should be avoided. Importantly, the effects of anesthetic agents (inhalation vs. total intravenous anesthesia) on the outcome of TBI have not been demonstrated. In the absence of conclusive evidence, either anesthetic technique may be employed judiciously. However, more importantly, the principles of anesthetic management should adhere to the current guidelines for the management of severe TBI.

Analgesics, sedatives, and neuromuscular blocking agents are often used in the severe pediatric TBI for purposes other than tracheal intubation and surgical anesthesia. Analgesics and sedatives are believed to favorably treat a number of important pathophysiologic derangements in severe TBI. Pain, stress, and the noxious stimuli associated with routine intensive care procedures such as tracheal suctioning and positioning markedly increase cerebral metabolic demands and can pathologically increase CBV and raise ICP besides causing significant hemodynamic stimulation [19]. By attenuating the cerebral and systemic responses to these stimuli, analgesic and sedative agents are believed to mitigate secondary brain damage. Moreover, they provide anticonvulsant and antiemetic benefits, prevent shivering, and attenuate the long-term psychological trauma of pain and stress. In addition, etomidate and thiopental may be considered for control of severe intracranial hypertension in the intensive care unit. While using etomidate for this purpose, the risks resulting from adrenal suppression must be considered. Continuous infusion of propofol for either sedation or the management of refractory intracranial hypertension in infants and children with severe TBI is not recommended by the Food and Drug Administration. Neuromuscular blocking agents may reduce ICP in intubated TBI patients in the intensive care units by reduction in airway and intrathoracic pressure with facilitation of cerebral venous outflow and by prevention of shivering, posturing, or breathing against the ventilator.

CLINICAL PEARL A balanced anesthetic technique involving low concentration of inhaled anesthetics with potent short-acting opioids and muscle relaxants is acceptable for pediatric TBI. Inhaled anesthetics are unlikely to cause brain swelling at <1 MAC. Etomidate and thiopental may be considered for control of severe intracranial hypertension. Avoid sevoflurane in the presence of seizures.

D. **Ventilation.** Ventilation should be adjusted to ensure adequate oxygenation and gas exchange. Inspired oxygen concentration should be adjusted to maintain PaO_2 >60 mm Hg. A recent study indicates association between discharge survivals with higher admission PaO_2 (301 to 500 mm Hg) but more evidence is needed before routine administration of higher inspired oxygen concentrations can be recommended. Monitoring arterial $PaCO_2$ is recommended since end-tidal CO_2 may not be reliable. Survival after severe pediatric TBI is associated with $PaCO_2$ 36 to 45 mm Hg, and both hypocarbia ($PaCO_2$ < 35 mm Hg) and hypercarbia ($PaCO_2$ >45 mm Hg) have been shown to be associated with increased discharge mortality and should be avoided [20]. Although controlled hyperventilation is an effective intervention to rapidly decrease elevated ICP, it must not be used indiscriminately because excessive hyperventilation may cause cerebral vasoconstriction leading to ischemia. Current pediatric guidelines provide level III recommendation for avoidance of prophylactic severe hyperventilation to a $PaCO_2$ <30 mm Hg in the initial 48 hours after injury (Table 29.3) [21]. If hyperventilation is used in the management of refractory intracranial hypertension, advanced neuromonitoring for evaluation of cerebral ischemia may be considered. In the intraoperative period, this may be accomplished by jugular venous oximetry and in the postoperative period by $PbtO_2$ or CBF monitoring (e.g., using transcranial Doppler ultrasonography). During craniotomy, hyperventilation should be used judiciously for short-term control of ICP and to facilitate surgical exposure and normocarbia should be restored before dural closure.

> **CLINICAL PEARL** Normocapnia should be targeted in pediatric TBI. Prophylactic hyperventilation to $PaCO_2$ <30 mm Hg should be avoided in the initial 48 hours after injury. Hyperventilation should be used judiciously for short-term control of ICP and to facilitate surgical exposure.

   E. **Systemic and cerebral hemodynamics.** CPP (mean arterial pressure minus the mean ICP) is the pressure gradient driving the CBF, which, in the healthy brain is autoregulated and coupled with CMR. Autoregulation and coupling between CBF and CMR may be disrupted following TBI, and a decrease in CPP may therefore lead to cerebral ischemia [10]. Hence, continuous monitoring of arterial blood pressure, ICP, and CPP with efforts to avoid systemic/cerebral hypotension is desirable. The 2012 Pediatric Guidelines recommend that a minimum CPP of 40 mm Hg may be considered in children with TBI (Table 29.3) [22]. A CPP threshold 40 to 50 mm Hg may be considered (Table 29.3) [22]. There may be age-specific thresholds with infants at lower end and adolescents at the upper end of this range. The presence of the Cushing's reflex and autonomic dysfunction might be the only indicators of increased ICP. While systolic blood pressure <5th percentile defines hypotension, in the absence of ICP monitoring and suspected increased ICP, supranormal systolic blood pressure may be needed to maintain CPP. At a minimum, MAP should not be allowed to decrease below values normal for age by using vasopressors.

> **CLINICAL PEARL** CPP threshold in pediatric TBI should be 40 to 50 mm Hg.

   F. **Management of intracranial hypertension**
      1. **Hyperosmolar therapy.** The 2012 Pediatric Guidelines recommend that treatment of ICP may be considered at a threshold of 20 mm Hg (Table 29.3) [23]. Intracranial hypertension can be initially managed through elevation of the head, sedation, analgesia and neuromuscular blockade, and hyperosmolar therapy. The 2012 Pediatric Guidelines cite class II evidence supporting the use of 3% hypertonic saline for the acute treatment of severe pediatric TBI associated with intracranial hypertension and class III evidence to support its use as a continuous infusion during the intensive care unit course (Table 29.3) [24]. Effective doses for acute use range between 6.5 and 10 mL/kg and as a continuous infusion of 3% saline range between 0.1 and 1 mL/kg of body weight per hour administered on a sliding scale. The minimum dose needed to maintain ICP <20 mm Hg should be used and serum osmolarity should be maintained <360 mOsm/L. The guidelines also indicate that there is insufficient evidence to support or refute the

use of mannitol, concentrations of hypertonic saline >3%, or other hyperosmolar agents for the treatment of severe pediatric TBI [24]. Clinicians are advised to weigh the value of long-standing clinical acceptance and safety of mannitol, which has no evidence to support its efficacy against hypertonic saline, for which there is less clinical experience but reasonably good performance in contemporary clinical trials.

Mannitol (0.25 to 1 g/kg) can reduce ICP by two distinct mechanisms [25]. The immediate effect results from a reflex vasoconstriction caused by viscosity reduction leading to improved microvascular perfusion in the presence of intact cerebral autoregulation, resulting in reduction of CBV and ICP. The effect of mannitol on blood viscosity is rapid but lasts <75 minutes. However, mannitol also reduces ICP by a more well-recognized osmotic diuretic effect, which develops relatively slowly over 15 to 30 minutes, persists up to 6 hours and requires an intact blood–brain barrier. Importantly, mannitol may accumulate in injured brain regions, where a reverse osmotic shift may occur, possibly causing a rebound increase in ICP. Hypertonic saline also has both the favorable rheologic and osmolar gradient effects involved in the reduction in ICP. Moreover, it may offer other beneficial effects including restoration of normal cellular resting membrane potential and cell volume, inhibition of inflammation, and enhancement of cardiac output.

CLINICAL PEARL　Initial management of intracranial hypertension should include elevation of the head, sedation, analgesia and neuromuscular blockade, and hyperosmolar therapy with 3% hypertonic saline.

2. **High-dose barbiturate therapy.** High-dose barbiturate therapy may be considered in hemodynamically stable patients with refractory intracranial hypertension and while doing so, continuous arterial blood pressure and cardiovascular support to maintain adequate CPP are required [26]. Refractory ICP can be treated with thiopental infusions, but volume loading and inotropic support may be needed to counter myocardial depression and hypotension (Table 29.3) [26]. High-dose barbiturates lower ICP by suppression of metabolism and alteration of vascular tone. Barbiturate therapy improves coupling of regional CBF to metabolic demands resulting in higher cerebral oxygenation with lower CBF and decreased ICP from decreased CBV.

3. **Cerebrospinal fluid drainage.** The 2012 Pediatric Guidelines recommend CSF drainage through an external ventricular drain (EVD) in the management of high ICP in children with severe TBI and also the addition of a lumbar drain in case of refractory intracranial hypertension with a functioning EVD, open basal cisterns, and no evidence of mass lesion or shift on imaging (Table 29.3) [27].

4. **Decompressive craniectomy for intracranial hypertension.** The 2012 Pediatric Guidelines recommend decompressive craniectomy with duraplasty in pediatric patients with TBI who are showing early signs of deterioration or herniation or are developing intracranial hypertension refractory to medical management during early stages of treatment [28]. It may consist of uni- or bilateral subtemporal decompressions, hemispheric craniectomies of varying sizes (from relatively small to quite expansive), circumferential craniectomy, or bifrontal craniectomy.

5. **Therapeutic hypothermia.** The 2012 Pediatric Guidelines recommend that moderate hypothermia (32° to 33°C) beginning early after severe TBI for 48 hours duration may be considered to reduce intracranial hypertension [29]. Following therapeutic hypothermia, rewarming at a rate of >0.5°C/h should be avoided [29]. The rationale for the use of therapeutic hypothermia is a reduction in mechanisms of secondary injury resulting from decreased cerebral metabolic demands, inflammation, lipid peroxidation, excitotoxicity, cell death, and acute seizures. In any case, fever and hyperthermia should be avoided in patients with TBI.

CLINICAL PEARL Treatment options for refractory intracranial hypertension in TBI include high-dose barbiturate therapy, CSF drainage, decompressive craniectomy, and possibly therapeutic hypothermia.

G. **Corticosteroids in TBI.** Steroid administration in severe pediatric TBI is not associated with improved functional outcome, decreased mortality, or reduced ICP. Instead, steroid use may cause suppression of endogenous cortisol levels and may increase the risk of pneumonia. Given the lack of evidence for benefit in children and the potential for harm from infectious complications and known suppression of the pituitary adrenal axis, routine use of steroids to lower ICP or improve functional outcomes or mortality is not recommended in children with TBI according to the 2012 Pediatric Guidelines (Table 29.3) [30].

H. **Glucose and nutrition.** The 2012 Pediatric Guidelines do not support the use of an immune-modulating diet for the treatment of severe TBI to improve outcome [31]. Multiple studies have shown that hyperglycemia occurs frequently in children with severe TBI and is associated with poor outcome. High glucose has been shown to be associated with longer pediatric intensive care unit length of stay and higher in-hospital mortality. Yet, there are no proven benefits of intensive glucose control strategies. In the absence of outcome data, the 2012 Pediatric Guidelines do not make any recommendation for glycemic control in infants and children with severe TBI. [31] Importantly, perioperative hyperglycemia is common and intraoperative hypoglycemia is not rare and regular intraoperative glucose sampling may be needed [32]. It is advisable to maintain glucose in the range of 80 to 180 mg/dL.

I. **Antiseizure prophylaxis.** The incidence of early posttraumatic seizures (occurring within 7 days of injury) in pediatric patients with TBI is approximately 10%. The 2012 Pediatric Guidelines recommend that prophylactic anticonvulsant therapy with phenytoin may be considered to reduce the incidence of early posttraumatic seizures after severe TBI (Table 29.3) [33]. Concomitant monitoring of drug levels is desirable.

VII. **Summary.** TBI is a major cause of morbidity and mortality in the pediatric age and results in large societal costs. Different trauma mechanisms compared to adults and their impact on the developing brain result in unique primary and secondary lesions. Modern TBI management emphasizes minimizing secondary insults to the injured brain. The perioperative period is an opportunity to optimize cerebral and systemic physiology, minimize secondary insults, and may be a potential window to initiate interventions that may improve the outcome of TBI. Anesthetic management should be based on the current guidelines for the acute medical management of severe TBI in infants, children, and adolescents.

REFERENCES

1. Heron M, Sutton PD, Xu J, et al. Annual summary of vital statistics: 2007. *Pediatrics.* 2010;125:4–15.
2. Keenan HT, Bratton SL. Epidemiology and outcomes of pediatric traumatic brain injury. *Dev Neurosci.* 2006;28:256–263.
3. Agran PF, Winn D, Anderson C, et al. Rates of pediatric and adolescent injuries by year of age. *Pediatrics.* 2001;108:E45.
4. Langlois JA, Rutland-Brown W, Thomas KE. The incidence of traumatic brain injury among children in the United States: differences by race. *J Head Trauma Rehabil.* 2005;20:229–238.
5. Haider AH, Efron DT, Haut ER, et al. Black children experience worse clinical and functional outcomes after traumatic brain injury: an analysis of the National Pediatric Trauma Registry. *J Trauma.* 2007;62:1259–1262; discussion 1262–1263.
6. Giza CC, Mink RB, Madikians A. Pediatric traumatic brain injury: not just little adults. *Curr Opin Crit Care.* 2007;13:143–152.
7. Newgard CD, Lewis RJ. Effects of child age and body size on serious injury from passenger air-bag presence in motor vehicle crashes. *Pediatrics.* 2005;115:1579–1585.
8. Marshall KW, Koch BL, Egelhoff JC. Air bag-related deaths and serious injuries in children: injury patterns and imaging findings. *AJNR Am J Neuroradiol.* 1998;19:1599–1607.
9. Ragan DK, McKinstry R, Benzinger T, et al. Depression of whole-brain oxygen extraction fraction is associated with poor outcome in pediatric traumatic brain injury. *Pediatr Res.* 2012;71(2):199–204.
10. Vavilala MS, Muangman S, Tontisirin N, et al. Impaired cerebral autoregulation and 6-month outcome in children with severe traumatic brain injury: preliminary findings. *Dev Neurosci.* 2006;28(4-5):348–353.
11. Le TH, Gean AD. Neuroimaging of traumatic brain injury. *Mt Sinai J Med.* 2009;76:145–162.
12. Pinto PS, Meoded A, Poretti A, et al. The unique features of traumatic brain injury in children. Review of the characteristics of the pediatric skull and brain, mechanisms of trauma, patterns of injury, complications, and their imaging findings–part 2. *J Neuroimaging.* 2012;22(2):e18–e41.

13. Pinto PS, Poretti A, Meoded A, et al. The unique features of traumatic brain injury in children. Review of the characteristics of the pediatric skull and brain, mechanisms of trauma, patterns of injury, complications and their imaging findings–part 1. *J Neuroimaging.* 2012;22(2):e1–e17.

14. Donoghue AJ, Ades AM, Nishisaki A, et al. Videolaryngoscopy versus direct laryngoscopy in simulated pediatric intubation. *Ann Emerg Med.* 2012 Oct 17. [Epub ahead of print]

15. Pizarro CF, Troster EJ, Damiani D, et al. Absolute and relative adrenal insufficiency in children with septic shock. *Crit Care Med.* 2005;33(4):855–859.

16. Bar-Joseph G, Guilburd Y, Tamir A, et al. Effectiveness of ketamine in decreasing intracranial pressure in children with intracranial hypertension. *J Neurosurg Pediatr.* 2009;4(1):40–46.

17. Brown MM, Parr MJ, Manara AR. The effect of suxamethonium on intracranial pressure and cerebral perfusion pressure in patients with severe head injuries following blunt trauma. *Eur J Anaesthesiol.* 1996;13(5):474–477.

18. Kochanek PM, Carney N, Adelson PD, et al. Guidelines for the acute medical management of severe traumatic brain injury in infants, children, and adolescents–second edition. Chapter 6. Advanced neuromonitoring. *Pediatr Crit Care Med.* 2012;13(suppl 1):S30–S32.

19. Kochanek PM, Carney N, Adelson PD, et al. Guidelines for the acute medical management of severe traumatic brain injury in infants, children, and adolescents–second edition. Chapter 15. Analgesics, sedatives and neuromuscular blockade. *Pediatr Crit Care Med.* 2012;13(suppl 1):S64–S67.

20. Ramaiah VK, Sharma D, Ma L, et al. Admission oxygenation and ventilation parameters associated with discharge survival in severe pediatric traumatic brain injury. *Childs Nerv Syst.* 2012 Dec 4. [Epub ahead of print].

21. Kochanek PM, Carney N, Adelson PD, et al. Guidelines for the acute medical management of severe traumatic brain injury in infants, children, and adolescents–second edition. Chapter 13. Hyperventilation. *Pediatr Crit Care Med.* 2012;13(suppl 1): S58–S60.

22. Kochanek PM, Carney N, Adelson PD, et al. Guidelines for the acute medical management of severe traumatic brain injury in infants, children, and adolescents–second edition. Chapter 5. Cerebral perfusion pressure thresholds. *Pediatr Crit Care Med.* 2012;13(suppl 1):S24–S29.

23. Kochanek PM, Carney N, Adelson PD, et al. Guidelines for the acute medical management of severe traumatic brain injury in infants, children, and adolescents–second edition. Chapter 4. Threshold for treatment of intracranial hypertension. *Pediatr Crit Care Med.* 2012;13(suppl 1):S18–S23.

24. Kochanek PM, Carney N, Adelson PD, et al. Guidelines for the acute medical management of severe traumatic brain injury in infants, children, and adolescents–second edition. Chapter 8. Hyperosmolar therapy. *Pediatr Crit Care Med.* 2012;13(suppl 1): S36–S41.

25. Bennett TD, Statler KD, Korgenski EK, et al. Osmolar therapy in pediatric traumatic brain injury. *Crit Care Med.* 2012;40(1):208–215.

26. Kochanek PM, Carney N, Adelson PD, et al. Guidelines for the acute medical management of severe traumatic brain injury in infants, children, and adolescents–second edition. Chapter 11. Barbiturates. *Pediatr Crit Care Med.* 2012;13(suppl 1):S49–S52.

27. Kochanek PM, Carney N, Adelson PD, et al. Guidelines for the acute medical management of severe traumatic brain injury in infants, children, and adolescents–second edition. Chapter 10. Cerebrospinal fluid drainage. *Pediatr Crit Care Med.* 2012;13(suppl 1):S46–S48.

28. Kochanek PM, Carney N, Adelson PD, et al. Guidelines for the acute medical management of severe traumatic brain injury in infants, children, and adolescents–second edition. Chapter 12. Decompressive craniectomy for treatment of intracranial hypertension. *Pediatr Crit Care Med.* 2012;13(suppl 1):S53–S57.

29. Kochanek PM, Carney N, Adelson PD, et al. Guidelines for the acute medical management of severe traumatic brain injury in infants, children, and adolescents–second edition. Chapter 9. Temperature control. *Pediatr Crit Care Med.* 2012;13(suppl 1): S42–S45.

30. Kochanek PM, Carney N, Adelson PD, et al. Guidelines for the acute medical management of severe traumatic brain injury in infants, children, and adolescents-second edition. Chapter 14. Corticosteroids. *Pediatr Crit Care Med.* 2012;13(suppl 1): S61–S63.

31. Kochanek PM, Carney N, Adelson PD, et al. Guidelines for the acute medical management of severe traumatic brain injury in infants, children, and adolescents–second edition. Chapter 16. Glucose and nutrition. *Pediatr Crit Care Med.* 2012;13(suppl 1):S68–S71.

32. Sharma D, Jelacic J, Chennuri R, et al. Incidence and risk factors for perioperative hyperglycemia in children with traumatic brain injury. *Anesth Analg.* 2009;108(1):81–89.

33. Kochanek PM, Carney N, Adelson PD, et al. Guidelines for the acute medical management of severe traumatic brain injury in infants, children, and adolescents-second edition. Chapter 17. Antiseizure prophylaxis. *Pediatr Crit Care Med.* 2012;13(suppl 1):S72–S82.

34. Kochanek PM, Carney N, Adelson PD, et al. Guidelines for the acute management of severe traumatic brain injury in infants, children and adolescents-second edition. *Pediatr Crit Care Med.* 2012;13:S1–82.

30

Intensive Care of Spinal Cord Injury in Adults

Linda S. Aglio and Grace Y. Kim

KEY POINTS

1. The initial treatment requires immobilization of the entire spine, cardiopulmonary resuscitation, stabilization of life-threatening injuries, assessment of the neurologic deficit, and transfer to the SCI center.
2. The pathophysiology of spinal cord injury (SCI) involves the cascade of inflammatory responses from spinal cord ischemia. Optimizing perfusion and oxygenation during this period is essential to minimize the secondary injury.
3. Dramatic changes in pulmonary mechanics often necessitate airway management and mechanical ventilatory support to maintain oxygenation and ventilation.
4. Loss of autonomic function causes cardiovascular dysfunction manifested as neurogenic shock. The goal is to maintain normal or slightly increased blood pressure with judicious use of fluids and inotropes.
5. Autonomic dysreflexia is common for SCI above T6 and should be treated promptly.
6. Prophylactic therapy for thromboembolism is initiated with a compression device in combination with low-dose heparin therapy.
7. Stress ulcer prophylaxis is necessary and early enteral feeding is recommended.
8. Urinary tract infection and stone formation are frequent complications of neurogenic bladder.
9. Prevention of decubitus ulcers is an important aspect of physical rehabilitation.

CLINICAL PEARLS High-dose steroid therapy in the first 48 hours after SCI is considered a treatment option, not a standard therapy.

It is prudent to perform elective intubation in a controlled setting instead of an emergent situation. In an emergent situation, the preferred technique is rapid sequence direct laryngoscopy with manual in-line stabilization of the neck. For nonurgent airway management, awake fiberoptic oral intubation is preferred. It is critical to anticipate hypotension and maintain perfusion pressure during airway management.

The breathing pattern for patients with SCI is shallow and rapid. Respiration is inefficient in gas exchange with a higher percentage of TV participating in dead space ventilation, gradually leading to hypoxemia and hypercarbia. Lung mechanics improve within 2 to 3 weeks after the injury. At this time, spinal shock resolves and the muscles in the chest and abdominal wall begin to develop spasticity.

A combination of PS with an SIMV mode is commonly used to prevent deconditioning of respiratory muscles. All SCI patients on mechanical ventilation should have positive end-expiratory pressure (PEEP), which prevents atelectasis and improves lung compliance.

Overzealous resuscitation can cause cardiogenic pulmonary edema in a heart without sympathetic innervation. In contrast, neurogenic pulmonary edema is noncardiogenic and can develop in the absence of fluid overload.

Preserving stroke volume is crucial in maintaining cardiac output in the absence of a compensatory increase in heart rate.

Before neurogenic shock is assumed as the cause of hypotension, other associated injuries must be ruled out.

For patients without cardiac dysfunction, norepinephrine or phenylephrine is commonly used for blood pressure support while either dopamine or epinephrine is used for patients with reduced cardiac function.

Fluid management should be guided by invasive lines if the fluid status is uncertain.

Since the baseline BP for patients with SCI above T6 is typically within the normal range, even a mild increase in BP requires immediate attention, and the precipitating stimuli for autonomic hyperreflexia must be sought after and eliminated.

The incidence of thromboembolic complication is high in SCI patients due to venous stasis and immobility. A mechanical device alone is not sufficient in preventing deep vein thrombosis (DVT) and must be used in combination with low-dose heparin.

H_2 blockers such as cimetidine, famotidine, and ranitidine, have been shown to reduce the risk of gastrointestinal hemorrhage. The major side effect of H_2 blockers is inhibition of cytochrome P450 system, causing delayed metabolism of other drugs using the same system.

In the acute phase of spinal shock, the flaccidity of the bladder muscles causes bladder distention and thus requires an indwelling Foley catheter. Colonization is common with catheter placement and prophylactic antibiotic coverage is not recommended.

Nutrition is an important aspect of critical care for SCI patients and should be considered early on. The main goal is to provide sufficient calories and to prevent nitrogen loss rather than restoring the nitrogen balance.

Prevention guidelines and frequent inspections of the skin are critically important in preventing the development of pressure sores.

I. Introduction. Spinal cord injury (SCI) is a life-threatening trauma with devastating long-term disability. Sudden loss of somatosensory, motor, and autonomic functions in acute SCI results in dramatic changes in respiratory and cardiovascular status, requiring multidisciplinary critical care in an intensive care unit (ICU). This chapter is primarily focused on traumatic SCI and its management. Neurologic, respiratory, cardiovascular, thromboembolic, gastrointestinal, urologic, nutritional, and integument complications are discussed. Anticipation, prevention, and early treatment of these problems are crucial in improving the mortality and morbidity of SCI.

A. Epidemiology. In the United States, approximately 262,000 people live with paralysis due to SCI, and each year there are 12,000 new SCIs [1]. The most common causes are motor vehicle accidents (MVAs), falls, violence, and sport activities [1]. The average age at the time of injury is 37.6 years old. In the younger age group, the most frequent cause of SCI is MVAs, whereas in the older age group, it is falls. The most common level of injury is cervical at 51%, while thoracic is at 34.3%, and lumbosacral at 10.7% [2]. The greatest risk is at the more mobile joints in the lower cervical spine (C4 to C6) and the thoracolumbar junction (T12 to L1) [2]. SCIs are often accompanied by traumatic brain injury. The best predictors of mortality for SCI are the level of injury, the Glasgow Coma Scale (GCS), and respiratory failure, while the most common causes of death are respiratory failure, cardiovascular insufficiency, and pulmonary embolism (PE) [3].

B. Types of spinal cord injury. The etiology of SCI includes traumatic, rheumatologic, neo-plastic, infectious, inflammatory, vascular, and metabolic causes [3]. The mechanism involves hyperflexion, hyperextension, compression, rotation, shear, avulsion, or a combination of the above [4]. SCI is considered complete when all somatosensory, motor, and autonomic functions are lost and incomplete when there is partial preservation of function below the injury level. For any patient with neurologic deficits, it is mandatory to perform frequent neurologic examinations using the American Spinal Injury Association (ASIA) clinical scoring system, which assesses motor strength in 10 muscle groups and sensory in 28 dermatomes. The ASIA system combines the extent of neurologic deficits and the status of completeness of the injury [3]. A patient with paralysis without distal sparing is considered to have complete injury. For this reason, rectal examination is important in determining the completeness of the neurologic injury [5].

C. Timing of surgery. Immediate realignment using mechanical traction with cranial tongs or halo offers stability for the injured spine prior to surgery. Although the best time for surgical fixation is not clearly known, it is generally believed that early surgical decompression, especially for bilateral locked facets with incomplete tetraplegia or unstable SCI with rapidly deteriorating neurologic condition, allows early mobilization and reduces the duration of ICU stay and postinjury complications [6,7]. For patients with stable neurologic examinations, the timing of surgery; however, remains controversial.

II. Pathophysiology

A. Primary injury. SCI is discussed in the context of primary and secondary injuries. Primary injury is caused by direct trauma or interruption of the blood supply to the spinal cord at the time of injury and is considered irreversible. When SCI occurs, the standard trauma protocol is instituted promptly with the primary goals being the immediate immobilization of the entire spine, organ support, and transfer to a level I trauma center, preferably to a specialized SCI center. Other associated life-threatening injuries must be identified and treated in a timely manner. In one study, 47% of spine trauma patients had other associated injuries: head (26%), chest (24%), or long bones (23%) [8].

B. Secondary injury. Secondary injury ensues within minutes after the primary injury and lasts for weeks to months. The understanding of the pathophysiology of spinal cord ischemia is essential for a good spinal cord protection strategy. The spinal cord is supplied by a single anterior spinal artery supplying the anterior two-thirds of the cord and two posterior spinal arteries supplying the posterior one-third. Below the level of the cervical cord, segmental or radicular arteries off the aorta provide additional blood supply to the cord. The most important of these is the artery of Adamkiewicz, which supplies the thoracolumbar region of the cord [4]. There are potential watershed areas in the boundaries between anterior and posterior portions and at the junction of the cervical/thoracic or thoracic/lumbar regions [3].

Hypoperfusion and hypoxia are the major causes of secondary injury. When the spinal cord is traumatized, autoregulation is lost [9]. In addition, the injured spinal cord is prone to hypoxic injury and no longer demonstrates responsiveness to carbon dioxide. As a result, hypotension and hypoxia can render the potentially viable areas nonviable. The mechanism of secondary injury is a cascade of inflammatory responses due to spinal cord ischemia. An ischemic spinal cord increases vascular permeability, thereby releasing inflammatory mediators, free radicals, and excitatory amino acids. These biochemical changes lead to cellular edema and apoptosis, thus creating a vicious cycle [10]. The spinal cord edema is maximal at 3 to 6 days after the injury [4]. The secondary injury phase offers a narrow window of therapeutic intervention. At present, there is no magic bullet to restore the injury. Instead, maintaining the physiologic parameters such as perfusion, cardiac output (CO), and oxygenation in the optimum range is the most effective treatment.

C. **Spinal shock.** Spinal shock is described by the loss of all forms of neurologic function below the level of injury including autonomic and reflex activities [11]. A patient with spinal shock develops hypotension, reflex bradycardia, paralysis of extremities, flaccid gastrointestinal tract, and bladder atony. The time course of spinal shock is variable. Spinal shock may last for up to 6 weeks although it usually resolves within 24 hours [10]. A four-phase spinal shock model has been proposed [11]. In this model, Phase I (1 day) is characterized by areflexia due to the loss of excitatory input from above, Phase II (1 to 3 days) by return of some reflexes when nerve endings develop supersensitivity, Phase III (3 days to 1 month) by hyperreflexia, and Phase IV (1 month to 1 year) by progressive spasticity. Classic autonomic dysreflexia develops during Phase IV in the spinal shock model [11].

III. **Neuroprotection strategy**

A. **Methylprednisolone.** Based on animal studies showing that corticosteroids decrease inflammation, edema, lipid peroxidation, and excitotoxicity of spinal injury [3], high-dose steroid therapy was studied in a prospective, randomized double-blind multicenter trial. In the National Acute Spinal Cord Injury Study (NASCIS II) in 1990, the high-dose methylprednisolone group failed to show neurologic benefits when compared to naloxone or placebo groups. The post-hoc subgroup analysis, however, demonstrated some neurologic benefits at 6 weeks and 6 months when high-dose methylprednisolone was given in the first 8 hours of injury and continued for 23 hours [12]. The subsequent study of NASCIS III involves an initial intravenous bolus of methylprednisolone of 30 mg/kg over 15 minutes followed by a 23-hour infusion of 5.4 mg/kg/h or a 47-hour infusion [13]. Although the high-dose methylprednisolone therapy failed to show clinical benefits when compared with the tirilazad group, the post-hoc subgroup analysis again showed the better neurologic outcome in the 48-hour methylprednisolone group at 6 weeks and 6 months when it was administered within 3 to 8 hours after SCI, compared with the 24-hour group. Unfortunately, the 48-hour methylprednisolone group demonstrated more severe sepsis and pneumonia than patients in the 24-hour group [13]. This study was limited by the lack of reproducibility, lack of a placebo group, and an underpowered post-hoc analysis for only a small subset of the patients. The minor improvement in motor scores appeared to be clinically insignificant and did not necessarily improve the quality of life. Overall, the beneficial effects were inconclusive, yet the potential harmful side effects were clearly demonstrated in the study. At present, high-dose steroid therapy in the first 48 hours after SCI is considered a treatment option, not a standard therapy.

B. **Hypothermia.** There is no prospective clinical trial assessing the effect of hypothermia on the outcome of SCI although animal studies have demonstrated beneficial effects of hypothermia. A small cohort study demonstrated that 43% of patients with complete cervical SCI showed improvement in American Spinal Injury Association (ASIA) and International Medical Society of Paraplegia Impairment Scale (AIS) scores after 48 hours of modest intravascular hypothermia (33°C) using a systemic cooling technique that appears to be safe [14]. At present, modest intravascular hypothermia remains as an experimental option to avoid secondary injury [15].

C. Cell transplantation. Human trials of pharmacologic neuroprotective agents including steroids have shown disappointing results. Currently, cell therapy using fetal stem cells or endogenous progenitor cells have demonstrated some promise in regenerating damaged neurons. These cell therapies, however, have serious side effects of tumor formation [16].

IV. Airway management

A. Cervical spine stabilization. Any trauma in proximity to the cervical spine should be suspected of having an unstable SCI unless proven otherwise. Immediate immobilization of the entire spine is mandatory. Although cervical spine immobilization is a priority, cervical spine clearance does not take precedence over other life-threatening injuries. Immobilization is achieved by placing sandbags on either side of the head and securing the head on a backboard with straps. A rigid cervical collar is used to keep the head in the neutral position. When the spine is unstable, closed reduction of the spine with a traction device is performed prior to surgery.

The cervical injuries are evaluated by cervical film, computerized tomography (CT), and magnetic resonance imaging (MRI). Typically anteroposterior, lateral, and odontoid (open mouth) views are required. If the cervical spine is not visualized from C1 to T1 and clinical suspicion remains high, CT is indicated to rule out bony injuries. MRI is superior in detecting soft tissue injuries such as ligamentous injury, cord edema, hemorrhage, and infarct. A small group of patients, however, present with SCI without any radiographic abnormality.

B. Intubation. Patients with SCI frequently require an artificial airway before the cervical spine is cleared. Cervical or high thoracic SCI, especially when it is accompanied by blunt chest trauma, frequently requires mechanical ventilation. It is prudent to perform elective intubation in a controlled setting instead of an emergent situation. Assessment of the mental status and fatigue level is important in the decision making process.

Airway management for patients with cervical SCI is challenging. The important goal is to secure the airway safely and rapidly. The general rule is to assume that the cervical spine is unstable. The blood or vomitus in the oropharynx, retropharyngeal edema, full stomach, and concomitant head injury can make intubation difficult. During direct laryngoscopy, the most significant movement occurs at the occipitoatlantal and atlantoaxial (C1 to C2) joints with minimal displacement at C2 to C5 [17]. Minimizing neck movement is crucial for a patient with unstable C1 or C2 injury. In an emergent situation, the preferred technique is rapid sequence direct laryngoscopy with manual in-line stabilization of the neck. This technique requires three people to perform manual in-line stabilization, intubation, and cricoid pressure simultaneously. It is the practical method applicable to emergent situations and uncooperative patients. Since the rigid cervical collar makes mask ventilation and intubation difficult, the front of the collar can be removed to open the mouth more easily. The technique using the GlideScope decreases cervical spine (C2 to C5) movement by 50% compared with using a Macintosh blade during intubation [18]. For nonurgent airway management, awake fiberoptic oral intubation is preferred because the technique does not require extension of the neck. However, there are no clinical outcome data to support that awake fiberoptic intubation is superior to rapid sequence direct laryngoscopy in patients with cervical SCI [19]. If the intubation or mask ventilation is challenging, a laryngeal mask airway is placed temporarily until a surgical airway is established.

The potential complications of airway management are many. The most feared one is cervical cord injury. It is critical to avoid neck movement at any time during intubation. Hypotension during intubation is common due to the pharmacologic effect of the sedatives, decreased sympathetic tone from resolving hypoxia and hypercarbia, positive pressure ventilation, and the lack of compensatory inotropic and chronotropic effects. It is critical to anticipate hypotension and maintain perfusion pressure during airway management. Succinylcholine is safe to use within the first 24 hours, but is contraindicated afterward because super-sensitive muscles with proliferated cholinergic receptors may release massive amounts of potassium.

C. **Tracheostomy.** Early tracheostomy is preferred for patients with high cervical SCI who require full mechanical support beyond 2 weeks. The benefits of tracheostomy include comfort, less dead space ventilation, and decreased incidence of laryngeal damage. The injury above C3 requires lifelong ventilator dependence because of complete paralysis of the diaphragm, accessory, and intercostal muscles. Patients with injury at C3 to C5 maintain some functions of the diaphragm and accessory muscles and may be weaned from a ventilator [4]. Due to the close proximity of tracheostomy to the surgical site, tracheostomy is usually placed after the spine surgery.

V. **Respiratory consideration.** Patients with cervical or high thoracic SCI are at high risk of pulmonary complications such as atelectasis, pneumonia, aspiration, neurogenic pulmonary edema, PE, and adult respiratory distress syndrome (ARDS). The respiratory complications remain the leading cause of mortality for SCI patients.

A. **Pulmonary mechanics.** Impaired pulmonary mechanics are present in all patients with cervical or upper thoracic SCI. The extent of respiratory dysfunction is directly proportional to the level of injury and the degree of respiratory muscle paralysis. A higher level of injury correlates with more dramatic changes in respiratory mechanics.

Respiration is coordinated by four muscle groups: diaphragm, intercostal, abdominal, and accessory muscles [20]. During inspiration, the diaphragm (C3 to C5) generates more than half of the forced vital capacity (FVC), and the accessory (C3 to C8) muscles assist inspiration further. During passive expiration, the abdominal muscles (T7 to L1) function as a major contributor while the intercostal muscles (T1 to T12) stabilize the chest wall. Cervical cord injury changes lung mechanics dramatically and affects the breathing patterns. When the diaphragm is paralyzed, the patient initially compensates for the loss of major respiratory function by using the accessory muscles, specifically the scalene muscle (C3 to C8) and the clavicular portion of the pectoralis major muscle (C5 to C7). However, the patient eventually becomes exhausted, thus leading to respiratory failure. As the pressure in the thoracic cavity becomes negative, the flaccid diaphragm moves upward along with the abdominal wall. The paralysis of the intercostal muscles (T1 to T12) causes a paradoxical inward movement of the rib cage during inspiration, similar to flail chest [20]. There is a dramatic reduction in the tidal volume (TV), FVC, and functional expiratory volume (FEV1), but the residual volume (RV) is increased [21]. It is recommended to get the baseline respiratory mechanics (VC, FEV1) and arterial blood gas early on to assess the later improvement [22].

The breathing pattern for patients with SCI is shallow and rapid. The chest wall compliance is reduced due to the rigid chest wall and the lung compliance is decreased due to atelectasis. As a result, the work of breathing is greater, and the exhausted respiratory muscles lead to alveolar hypoventilation. Respiration is inefficient in gas exchange with a higher percentage of TV participating in dead space ventilation, gradually leading to hypoxemia and hypercarbia. In addition, paralyzed intercostal and abdominal muscles prevent effective coughing, which results in atelectasis and mucus plugging.

As the edema in the cervical spinal cord worsens in the first few days after the injury, progressive respiratory failure ensues. The indications for mechanical ventilation are FVC < 15 mL/kg, hypercarbia, PaO_2 < 60 mm Hg, increased work of breathing, increased respiratory rate, and associated traumatic brain injury with GCS < 8 [3]. Lung mechanics improve within 2 to 3 weeks after the injury. At this time, spinal shock resolves and the muscles in the chest and abdominal wall begin to develop spasticity. Patients with cervical SCI breathe easier when they assume the supine position. This is because RV decreases when the abdominal muscles have less gravity effect. The postural dependence of RV is eliminated with the use of an abdominal binder [23].

B. **Ventilatory support.** The most common respiratory complications in the first 5 days after SCI are atelectasis, pneumonia, and ventilatory failure [24]. The goal of ventilation is to maintain adequate oxygenation and normocapnia. Since the patient may be able to maintain adequate $PaCO_2$ at the cost of rapid breathing and overuse of accessory muscles, observation of tachypnea and fatigue can guide the optimum time of intubation.

The mode of ventilatory support depends on lung mechanics, alertness, respiratory efforts, and the need for sedation. For noninvasive ventilation, continuous positive airway pressure (CPAP) improves compliance by increasing FRC and reduces the work of breathing. Bi-level noninvasive ventilation increases minute ventilation by assisting inspiration. For mechanical ventilation, volume-cycled ventilation modes, such as synchronized intermittent mandatory ventilation (SIMV) or assist control ventilation (ACV) modes, are frequently used. ACV is the preferred mode for a patient who is sedated or has minimum respiratory drive. However, ACV may not be useful for a patient with a high respiratory rate since all spontaneous respiratory initiatives are supported by full mechanical breaths. For those with sufficient respiratory drive, synchronized interactive mode such as SIMV or pressure support (PS) is commonly used. In SIMV mode, a preset number of breaths initiated by the patient are fully supported by the ventilator, while spontaneous breaths are allowed in between mandatory mechanical breaths. PS ventilation is useful to unload the work of breathing and minimize fatigue. A combination of PS with an SIMV mode is commonly used to prevent deconditioning of respiratory muscles.

All SCI patients on mechanical ventilation should have positive end-expiratory pressure (PEEP), which prevents atelectasis and improves lung compliance. Once atelectasis is developed, the best way to re-expand the collapsed lungs is early bronchoscopy. Frequent suctioning and vigorous pulmonary physiotherapy are recommended to avoid recurrent atelectasis.

VC and peak inspiratory pressure (PIP) reflect the respiratory muscle function and should be assessed periodically. For SCI patients, weaning from a ventilator can be a lengthy process and requires patience. The criteria for extubation include VC greater than 10 mL/kg, TV greater than 5 mL/kg, PIP greater than 20 cm H_2O, and a respiratory rate less than 30 breaths per minute [25]. Weaning is accomplished by decreasing the rate of mandatory mechanical breaths or the level of PS. In PS weaning, the level of PS is incrementally reduced until the patient is placed on CPAP. Weaning can be also accomplished by increasing the duration of a T-piece trial. Progressively less mechanical support and longer ventilator-free periods allow gradual training of the diaphragm. For either technique, the patient should be rested during the night.

C. **Pneumonia.** Pneumonia is the common etiology of morbidity and mortality among SCI patients, and its risk increases by 1% to 3% per day of mechanical ventilation [26]. The high incidence of pneumonia is explained by the inability to clear secretions, frequent episodes of atelectasis, ineffective coughing, risk of aspiration, and prolonged ventilator support. Pulmonary hygiene and frequent suctioning are important in preventing pneumonia. The classic signs of pneumonia include fever, productive sputum, worsening hypoxia, and infiltrates on the chest radiograph. The interpretation of the chest x-ray may be inconclusive in the setting of pulmonary edema, atelectasis, and lung contusion. Nosocomial pneumonia is a leading cause of sepsis and ARDS.

The antibiotic coverage begins with a broad spectrum and is tailored according to the Gram stain and microbiology culture results. The common pathogens for early-onset ventilator-associated pneumonia (VAP) in the first 4 days are mixed flora of the oropharynx including *Streptococcus pneumoniae* or *Haemophilus influenzae*, whereas the common pathogens for late-onset VAP after 4 days are *Pseudomonas aeruginosa*, methicillin-resistant *Staphylococcus aureus*, and *Acinetobacter baumannii* [27].

D. **Pulmonary edema.** Pulmonary edema occurs frequently in patients with SCI regardless of the fluid status. A typical patient with high cervical cord injury requires fluid resuscitation to maintain good perfusion. However, overzealous resuscitation can cause cardiogenic pulmonary edema in a heart without sympathetic innervation. In contrast, neurogenic pulmonary edema is noncardiogenic and can develop in the absence of fluid overload. Neurogenic pulmonary edema occurs in the central nervous system trauma, whether it involves the brain or spinal cord. Its mechanism is poorly understood, but it is associated with the overactive sympathetic tone at the time of injury.

VI. **Cardiovascular consideration**

A. **Neurogenic shock.** When the spinal cord is injured in an experimental model, the immediate response is severe hypertension for a few minutes due to massive sympathetic discharge [28].

This brief period of hypertension is followed by neurogenic shock, which is caused by the loss of sympathetic control of the cardiovascular system. Subsequent arterial and venous dilation result in relative hypovolemia, decreased preload, reduced CO, and hypotension. There is a significant correlation between the extent of hypotension and the injury level. In high SCI, the CO is dependent on the stroke volume (SV) because the cardiac accelerator fibers (T1 to T4) are paralyzed, and the patient is unable to increase heart rate. The loss of activity of the cardiac accelerator fibers causes myocardial dysfunction and bradycardia. Preserving SV is crucial in maintaining CO in the absence of a compensatory increase in heart rate. Since the sympathetic chains are present from T1 to L2, neurogenic shock is most commonly observed in patients with cervical or high thoracic injury.

It is important to note that neurogenic shock must be distinguished from hemorrhagic shock. Before neurogenic shock is assumed as the cause of hypotension, other associated injuries must be ruled out. When the spinal cord lesion is below T6, hypotension is more likely due to hypovolemia. Neurogenic shock occurs typically when the injured spinal cord has lost autonomic function. Profound hypotension may exacerbate the secondary injury. Maintaining BP in the normal or slightly higher range is critically important during this phase. Once intravascular volume is restored, vasopressors are considered if the patient remains hypotensive. Aggressive treatment of neurogenic shock with fluid and vasopressors is associated with better neurologic outcomes [29].

B. **Use of vasopressors and inotropes.** Optimizing patients in neurogenic shock requires continuous monitoring of electrocardiogram, BP, and central venous pressure. Although the optimal BP is unknown, it is believed that a mean arterial pressure (MAP) greater than 85 mm Hg in the first 7 days may improve neurologic outcome [29,30]. The hemodynamic parameters obtained from an invasive catheter can guide the vasopressor therapy. The ideal vasopressor should have an α-adrenergic response for vasoconstriction and a β-adrenergic response for chronotropic and inotropic effects. For patients without cardiac dysfunction, norepinephrine or phenylephrine is commonly used while either dopamine or epinephrine is used for patients with reduced cardiac function [3]. Norepinephrine in the dose of 0.1 to 0.2 μg/kg/min and dopamine in the range of 2 to 10 μg/kg/min increase peripheral vascular resistance and improve BP. Dobutamine augments CO, but is seldom used due to a risk of systemic hypotension. Phenylephrine, a pure α-agonist, effectively increases vascular tone and BP. However, it should be used with caution in patients with pre-existing bradycardia because of the potential risk for reflex bradycardia. Epinephrine is proarrhythmic and is seldom used. If the patient remains in neurogenic shock in spite of fluid resuscitation and vasopressor therapy, further assessment of cardiac function with echocardiogram should be considered.

C. **Arrhythmia.** After SCI, there is an imbalance of sympathetic and parasympathetic activities in the heart. Dysrhythmia is frequently observed and is caused by unopposed parasympathetic activity. The most common arrhythmia is bradycardia secondary to the paralysis of cardiac accelerator fibers (T1 to T4). Bradycardia is treated with atropine when it is accompanied with hypotension. A temporary pacemaker is considered in severe bradycardia with hemodynamic instability. Bradycardia resolves in the following 3 to 5 weeks after SCI, but may recur during stimulation [4].

D. **Fluid management.** In neurogenic shock, the effective circulating blood volume is insufficient, and fluid resuscitation is indicated. In high SCI patients, the response to fluid challenge may be absent because of the lack of compensatory sympathetic response. Fluid management should be guided by invasive lines if the fluid status is uncertain. The choice of fluid is isotonic saline, although hypertonic saline has shown to improve the blood flow in the spinal cord in an experimental model and may be considered [31]. Patients with SCI are prone to develop pulmonary edema regardless of the fluid status, and overzealous fluid administration should be avoided.

E. **Autonomic dysreflexia.** Patients with SCI above T6 have intact splanchnic innervation. In response to a stimulus below the lesion, the patient may develop sudden massive outflow from the uninhibited sympathetic nervous system. This phenomenon is called autonomic dysreflexia. It occurs most commonly for a lesion above T6 as early as 2 weeks, usually several months after the initial injury [4]. Autonomic dysreflexia is often precipitated by surgical stimulation or distention of a hollow viscus such as the bladder or the bowel. Autonomic dysreflexia must be monitored during rectal examination or urinary catheter placement. The patient develops vasoconstriction below the lesion and vasodilation above, accompanied by baroreceptor-mediated reflex bradycardia. Since the baseline BP for patients with SCI above T6 is typically within the normal range, even a mild increase in BP requires immediate attention, and the precipitating stimuli must be eliminated. The symptoms include paroxysmal hypertension, bradycardia, headache, and sweating. In severe cases, autonomic dysreflexia can result in life-threatening situations such as seizure, myocardial infarction, and cerebral hemorrhage. Hypertension is treated with short-acting agents with rapid onset. Potent direct-acting vasodilator or β-blockers are commonly used. General anesthesia and spinal anesthesia are also highly effective in blunting the hemodynamic response.

VII. **Thromboembolic consideration**

  A. **Deep vein thrombosis.** The incidence of thromboembolic complication is high in SCI patients due to venous stasis and immobility. It is as high as 100% and is highest during the first 3 months after injury [32]. The choice of prophylactic treatment options is based on risk benefit assessment. A standard therapy is a combination of mechanical compression device and anticoagulation with low-dose heparin. Mechanical devices such as an intermittent pneumatic device and compression stockings have little risk and should be used upon admission. However, a mechanical device alone is not sufficient in preventing deep vein thrombosis (DVT) and must be used in combination with low-dose heparin. Anticoagulation needs to be initiated as soon as the risk of bleeding is low. The initial treatment begins with low-dose heparin 5,000 units subcutaneous every 8 hours or low–molecular-weight heparin (LMWH) 1 mg/kg subcutaneous every 12 hours. Alternatively, adjusted-dose heparin can be used with a goal of obtaining a partial thromboplastin time (PTT) of 1.5 times control [25]. LMWH is the first choice for prophylaxis in most cases. Prophylactic treatment for DVT is recommended for 3 months [32].

The symptoms of DVT are leg swelling, pain, redness, and unexplained fever. The first workup for DVT is noninvasive duplex Doppler ultrasound. Its sensitivity and specificity are greater than 90% [33]. Invasive venography is considered a gold standard technique, but is seldom used because it involves contrast dye injection and travel to an angiography suite. It is usually reserved for patients with equivocal results of the duplex ultrasound or for patients with high clinical suspicions in spite of negative duplex ultrasound. D-dimer levels have high sensitivity but low specificity [34]. Once DVT is confirmed, full anticoagulation is achieved with intravenous heparin in the first 48 hours followed by warfarin for 3 to 6 months. The therapeutic level of 2 to 3 of international normalized ratio (INR) is a goal.

Anticoagulation is contraindicated in patients with intracranial bleeding, perispinal hematoma, or hemothorax [22]. If anticoagulation is contraindicated or the patient develops recurrent thromboembolic events in spite of therapeutic anticoagulation, the placement of a vena cava filter is highly recommended. The risks of a vena cava filter include filter migrations, caval perforation, and thrombosis. These complications are less likely with the use of a retrievable filter since the filter can be removed later when anticoagulation is safe [35]. Other prophylactic measures include the use of kinetic therapy with a rotating bed or electrical stimulation.

  B. **Pulmonary embolism.** PE is suspected in a patient with diaphoresis, tachypnea, tachycardia, pleuritic pain, acute change in arterial blood gases, and right heart strain ECG changes. The arterial blood gas may demonstrate low arterial oxygen and an increase in arterial carbon dioxide. The most commonly used diagnostic modality is a ventilation–perfusion scan or spiral CT. The use of spiral CT angiography has become more common because of its high sensitivity (94%) and specificity (96%) [36]. The treatment is full anticoagulation for 3 to 6 months with a goal of 2 to 3 of INR. A vena cava filter should be placed if recurrent PE develops in spite of adequate anticoagulation.

VIII. **Gastrointestinal consideration**

   A. **Gastric atony.** Due to interrupted sympathetic outflow, a patient with SCI frequently develops gastroparesis and ileus. Gastric distention can push the diaphragm upward and interfere with respiration. In addition, high residual volume from gastric atony causes vomiting and increases the risk of aspiration. Decompression with a nasogastric tube is recommended. Once enteral feeding has begun, the head of the bed should be elevated to 30° and the use of prokinetic agent such as metoclopramide may be considered. Gastric motility returns typically in the first few days.

   B. **Stress ulcer.** A stress ulcer is a serious complication during the acute phase of SCI. Increased vagal activity, high-dose steroid therapy, stress of trauma are believed to increase the risk of gastrointestinal ulcer and hemorrhage. The peak time for stress ulcers is 4 to 10 days after the injury and stress ulcer prophylaxis is recommended for 4 weeks [37]. H_2 blockers such as cimetidine, famotidine, and ranitidine have been shown to reduce the risk of gastrointestinal hemorrhage. The major side effect of H_2 blockers is inhibition of cytochrome P450 system, causing delayed metabolism of other drugs using the same system. These drugs include phenytoin, warfarin, and some antibiotics. Thus the drug levels must be monitored. Other side effects include thrombocytopenia, which may worsen bleeding complications of stress ulcer. Sucralfate improves mucosal regeneration and has the least side effects. Proton pump inhibitors are also used in combination with H_2 blockers. Antacids such as magnesium hydroxide or aluminum hydroxide neutralize gastric acid, but are less commonly used because they increase colonization of the gastrointestinal tract and increase the incidence of hospital-acquired pneumonia [38]. For any patient with a suspicion of gastrointestinal ulcer or hemorrhage, serial hemoglobin counts should be monitored and an endoscopic evaluation is warranted.

   C. **Bowel dysfunction.** Bowel dysfunction is a common cause of anxiety and embarrassment in many SCI patients. Unopposed vagal innervation impairs gastrointestinal motility and prolongs colonic transit time resulting in ileus and constipation. Intestinal motility is assessed by flatus and the frequency of bowel movement. Ileus and constipation, if untreated, can progress to bowel obstruction, fecal impaction, and occasionally life-threatening conditions such as toxic mega colon and perforation. The diagnosis of acute abdomen can be insidious because of the lack of pain sensation in the abdomen. Routine bowel regimen with adequate supply of fibers in diet, stool softener, and laxatives is crucial in preventing bowel dysfunction.

IX. **Urologic consideration**

   A. **Neurogenic bladder.** Initial resuscitation requires an indwelling urinary catheter until the patient is hemodynamically stable. In the acute phase of spinal shock, the flaccidity of the bladder muscles causes bladder distention and thus requires an indwelling Foley catheter. Once the patient recovers from spinal shock, the typical bladder hypotonia in the first 3 weeks is gradually replaced with progressive hypertonic dysfunction secondary to upper motor neuron dysfunction [39]. During this phase, bladder sphincter dyssynergia results in spasticity and incomplete emptying [25]. Urinary retention predisposes the patient to recurrent urinary tract infection (UTI), which is a leading cause of infectious complications in SCI patients. Its risk is directly related with the duration of catheterization. Colonization is common with catheter placement and prophylactic antibiotic coverage is not recommended. Since the patient lacks sensation in the area, symptoms of UTI are typically absent and a high index of suspicion must be maintained. The most common organisms are *Escherichia coli*, *Enterococci*, and commensal organisms in the perineum [40]. The development of resistant organisms is common. Intermittent clean straight catheterization or condom catheterization is the preferred method. Other urologic complications include bladder or kidney stones that may require surgical procedures.

X. **Nutrition**

   A. **Enteral feeding.** Nutrition is an important aspect of critical care for SCI patients and should be considered early on. The nutritional support is crucial in preserving muscle mass, improving immune function, and preventing stress ulcer. The nutritional status of patients with SCI is characterized by hypermetabolism and negative nitrogen balance due to significant loss of muscle mass from inactivity. The main goal is to provide sufficient calories and to prevent nitrogen loss rather than restoring the nitrogen balance. Nutritional status should be assessed within 48 hours after the injury. Indirect calorimetry is the best method to assess the caloric requirement after SCI [41]. Once the patient is no longer in a state of shock and has regained gastric motility, enteral feeding is initiated. Early feeding is considered to be safe during the acute phase of SCI [42]. The advantage of enteral feeding is to reduce the risk of stress ulcers and to prevent gut translocation by maintaining the structural and functional integrity of mucosa. It is important to place the patient in a semi-sitting position during enteral feeding. For a patient with a high cervical cord injury, the swallowing reflex should be evaluated. Once enteral feeding is begun, stress ulcer prophylaxis may increase the risk of pneumonia and is not necessary [43].

The route of administration is through nasogastric, orogastric, or nasojejunal tubes. Percutaneous endoscopic gastrostomy (PEG) is used for long-term feeding. Continual feeding is started at a rate of 20 to 30 mL/h and is increased to meet the goal, typically 30 to 40 kcal/kg/day. Intolerance to enteral feeding is manifested as high gastric aspirates, vomiting, and aspiration. If the patient does not tolerate gastric feeding, nasojejunal feeding is considered. The contraindications for enteral feeding are shock, bowel obstruction, and ileus.

B. **Total parenteral nutrition.** Total parenteral nutrition (TPN) is reserved for patients who are unable to tolerate enteral feeding. TPN is administered through a central line or peripherally inserted central catheter (PICC). The risk of line infection, duration of nutritional support, and the patient's clinical status should be considered in the benefit versus risk analysis of the need for TPN. Fluid and electrolytes are monitored closely in the first few days of infusion. Hyperglycemia is known to exacerbate ischemic neurologic injury and normoglycemia should be maintained in critically ill patients. For short-term nutritional support, parenteral nutrition can be provided at a lower osmolarity through a peripheral intravenous vein. The goal of peripheral parenteral nutrition (PPN) is to provide enough calories to avoid muscle breakdown.

XI. **Skin consideration.** Patients with SCI are unable to conserve heat by vasoconstriction or shivering. They are also unable to release heat by sweating. As a result, their body temperature is easily affected by the environmental temperature. Temperature monitoring is essential and appropriate measures should be taken to maintain normothermia.

Decubitus ulcers develop quickly from the initial immobilization of the spine. Lack of sensation and immobility predispose the dependent areas in particular to low tissue perfusion leading to eventual breakdown of the skin barrier. The most common sites are areas of bony prominence such as the sacrum, coccyx, ischial tuberosities, heels, and greater trochanter. Decubitus ulcers are frequent sources of cellulitis, osteomyelitis, gangrene, and even sepsis. The primary goal is prevention by frequent turning, foam padding, and vigilant inspections. Air flotation beds or rotational beds can be useful in relieving direct constant pressure in the dependent areas. Once decubitus ulcers are developed, the treatment is to relieve the pressure in the area and to consider early debridement. The prevention guidelines and frequent inspections of the skin are critically important in preventing the development of pressure sores. Contracture and chronic pain from spasticity frequently limit physical rehabilitation in patients with SCI.

XII. **Conclusion.** Acute traumatic SCI is a devastating injury with lifetime morbidity. The common problems and treatment options are summarized in Table 30.1 and Figure 30.1. The quality of life in SCI patients may improve when they receive timely critical care with a multidisciplinary approach during the acute phase.

TABLE 30.1 Common problems in spinal cord injury

	Problems	Considerations
Neurologic	Spinal shock	• Immobilization of the spine • Prevention of secondary injury • Surgical fixation
Respiratory	Airway protection	• Rapid and safe airway establishment • Avoidance of neck movement • Artificial airway placement • Tracheostomy
	Atelectasis	• Prevention of lung collapse • Use of PEEP • Chest physiotherapy • Incentive spirometry • Bronchoscopy
	Pneumonia	• Early treatment with antibiotics • Prevention of resistant organisms • Semi-sitting position
	Pulmonary edema	• Judicious administration of fluid to maintain euvolemia
Cardiovascular	Neurogenic shock	• Fluid resuscitation • Maintain normal or slightly higher BP than the baseline BP • Use of vasopressors and inotropes • Use invasive monitoring as needed
	Autonomic dysreflexia	• Maintenance of normal BP • Vasodilator • Removal of stimuli • High index of suspicion
Thromboembolic	• DVT • PE	• Anticoagulation prophylaxis for 3 months • Mechanical compression device • Vena cava filter placement • Maintenance of the therapeutic level
Gastrointestinal	Stress ulcer	• H_2 blockers • Proton pump inhibitors • Sucralfate • Early enteral feeding
	Gastroparesis	• Gastric decompression with a nasogastric tube • Prokinetic agents
	• Ileus • Fecal impaction • Occult peritonitis	• Healthy bowel regimen with fibers • Stool softeners • Laxatives • Enema
Urologic	• Atonic bladder • Neurogenic bladder UTI	• Prevention of urinary retention • Indwelling urinary catheter placement • Early detection • Prevention of resistant organisms • Clean straight catheterization
	Bladder/kidney stones	• Hydration • Lithotripsy
Nutrition	Nitrogen loss	• Prevention of nitrogen loss • Accurate assessment of caloric requirement • Early enteral feeding • PEG placement • TPN
Skin	Decubitus ulcer	• Early detection of pressure sores • Frequent turning • Foam padding • Rotating bed • Would debridement • Surgical reconstruction
	• Contracture • Spasticity	• Early physical therapy • Baclofen pump placement • Management of chronic pain

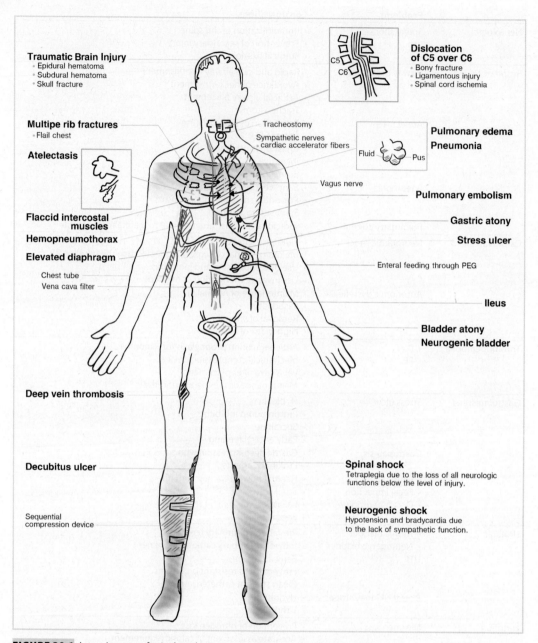

FIGURE 30.1 Intensive care of spinal cord injury

REFERENCES

1. The National SCI Statistical Center. SCI Facts and Figures at a Glance. *National Spinal Cord Injury Center.* Birmingham, Alabama; 2010.
2. Macias MY, Maiman DJ. Spinal cord injury. In: Torbey MT, ed. *Neurocritical Care.* New York, NY: Cambridge University Press; 2010:283–293.
3. Stevens RD. Spinal cord injury. In: Bhardwaj A, Mirski M, Ulatowski J, eds. *Handbook of Neurocritical Care.* Totowa, NJ: Humana Press; 2004:165–181.
4. Stier G, Gabriel C, Cole D. Neurosurgical diseases and trauma of the spine and spinal cord: Anesthetic considerations. In: Cottrell J, Young W, eds. *Cottrell and Young's Neuroanesthesia.* 5th ed. Philadelphia, PA: Mosby Elsevier; 2010:343–389.

5. Licina P, Nowitzke AM. Approach and considerations regarding the patient with spinal injury. *Injury*. 2005;36:SB2–SB12.
6. Fehlings MF, Perrin RG. The role and timing of early decompression for cervical spinal cord injury: update with a review of recent clinical evidence. *Injury*. 2005;36:S13–S26.
7. Fehlings MG, Perrin RG. The timing of surgical intervention in the treatment of spinal cord injury: A systematic review of recent clinical evidence. *Spine*. 2006;31:S28–S35.
8. Saboe LA, Reid DC, Davis LA, et al. Spine trauma and associated injuries. *J Trauma*. 1991;31(1):43–48.
9. Guha A, Tator CH, Rochon J. Spinal cord blood flow and systemic blood pressure after experimental spinal cord injury in rats. *Stroke*. 1989;20:372–377.
10. Hunt K, Laing R. Spinal cord injury. In: Gupta AK, Gelb AW, eds. *Essentials of Neuroanesthesia and Neurointensive Care*. Philadelphia, PA: Saunders Elsevier; 2008:211–216.
11. Ditunno JF, Little JW, Tessler A, et al. Spinal shock revisited: a four-phase model. *Spinal cord*. 2004;42(7):383–395.
12. Bracken MB, Shepard MJ, Collins WF, et al. A randomized, controlled trial of methylprednisolone or naloxone in the treatment of acute spinal cord injury: results of the Second National Acute Spinal Cord Injury Study. *N Engl J Med*. 1990;322:1405–1411.
13. Bracken MB, Shepard MJ, Holford TR, et al. Administration of methylprednisolone for 24 or 48 hours or tirilazad mesylate for 48 hours in the treatment of acute spinal cord injury: results of the Third National Acute Spinal Cord Injury Randomized Controlled Trial. *JAMA*. 1997;277:1597–1604.
14. Levi AD, Casella G, Green BA, et al. Clinical outcomes using modest intravascular hypothermia after acute cervical spinal cord injury. *Neurosurgery*. 2010;666:670–677.
15. Dietrich WD 3rd. Therapeutic hypothermia for spinal cord injury. *Crit Care Med*. 2009;37(7 suppl):S238–S242.
16. Hawryluk GW, Rowland J, Kwon BK, et al. Protection and repair of the injured spinal cord: a review of completed, ongoing, and planned clinical trials for acute spinal cord injury. *Neurosurg Focus*. 2008;25(5):E14.
17. Sawin PD, Todd MM, Traynelis VC, et al. Cervical spine motion with direct laryngoscopy and orotracheal intubation. *Anesthesiology*. 1996;85:26–36.
18. Turkstra TP, Craen RA, Pelz DM, et al. Cervical spine motion: a fluoroscopic comparison during intubation with lighted stylet, GlideScope and Macintosh laryngoscope. *Anesth Analg*. 2005;101:910–915.
19. Crosby ET. Airway management in adults after cervical spine trauma. *Anesthesiology*. 2006;104:1293–1318.
20. Ball PA. Critical care in spinal cord injury. *Spine*. 2001;26:S27–S30.
21. Winslow C, Rozovsky J. Effect of spinal cord injury on the respiratory system. *Am J Phys Med Rehabil*. 2003;82:803–814.
22. Consortium for Spinal Cord Medicine. Early acute management in adults with spinal cord injury: a clinical practice guideline for health-care professionals. *J Spinal Cord Med*. 2008;31(4):403–479.
23. Estenne M, De Troyer A. Mechanism of the postural dependence of vital capacity in tetraplegic subjects. *Am Rev Respir Dis*. 1987;135(2):367–371.
24. Berlly M, Shem K. Respiratory management during the first five days after spinal cord injury. *J Spinal Cord Med*. 2007;30:309–318.
25. Macias MY, Maiman DJ. Critical care of acute spinal cord injuries. In: Jallo J, Vaccaro AR, eds. *Neurotrauma and Critical Care of the Spine*. New York, NY: Thieme; 2009:171–181.
26. Craven DE. Epidemiology of ventilator-associated pneumonia. *Chest*. 2000;117:186S–187S.
27. Garcia-Leoni ME, Moreno S, Garcia-Garrote F, et al. Ventilator-associated pneumonia in long-term ventilator-assisted individuals. *Spinal Cord*. 2010;48:876–880.
28. Eidelberg EE. Cardiovascular response to experimental spinal cord compression. *J Neurosurg*. 1973;38:326–331.
29. Vale FL, Burns J, Jackson AB, et al. Combined medical and surgical treatment after acute spinal cord injury: Results of a prospective pilot study to assess the merits of aggressive medical resuscitation and blood pressure measurement. *J Neurosurg*. 1997;87:239–246.
30. Hedley MN, et al. Blood pressure management after acute spinal cord injury. *Neurosurgery*. 2002;50(3 suppl):S58–S62.
31. Tuma RF, Vasthare US, Arfors KE, et al. Hypertonic saline administration attenuates spinal cord injury. *J Trauma*. 1997;42:S54–S60.
32. Hedley MN, et al. Deep venous thrombosis and thromboembolism in patients with cervical spinal cord injuries. *Neurosurgery*. 2002;50(3 suppl):S73–S80.
33. Zierler BK. Ultrasonography and diagnosis of venous thromboembolism. *Circulation*. 2004;109(12 suppl 1):I9–I14.
34. Roussi J, Bentolia S, Boudadoud L, et al. Contribution of D-dimer determination in the exclusion of deep vein thrombosis in spinal cord injury patients. *Spinal Cord*. 1999;37:548–552.
35. Roberts A, Young WF. Prophylactic retrievable interior vena cava filters in spinal cord injured patients. *Surg Neurol Int*. 2010;1:68.
36. van Russum AB, Pattynama PM, Ton ER, et al. Pulmonary embolism: validation of spiral CT angiography in 149 patients. *Radiology*. 1996;201:467–470.
37. Lu WY, Rhoney DH, Boling WB, et al. A review of stress ulcer prophylaxis in the neurosurgical intensive care unit. *Neurosurgery*. 1997;41(2):416–426.
38. Herzig SJ, Howell MD, Ngo LH, et al. Acid-suppressive medication use and the risk of hospital-acquired pneumonia. *JAMA*. 2009;301:2120–2128.
39. Burns AS, Rivas DA, Ditunno JF. The management of neurogenic bladder and sexual dysfunction after spinal cord injury. *Spine*. 2001;26(24 suppl):S129–S136.
40. Garcia Leoni ME, Esclarin De Ruz A. Management of urinary tract infection in patients with spinal cord injuries. *Clin Microbiol Infect*. 2003;9:780–785.
41. Young B, Ott L, Rapp RP, et al. The patient with critical neurological disease. *Crit Care Clin*. 1987;3:217–233.
42. Rowan CJ, Gillanders LK, Paice RL, et al. Is early enteral feeding safe in patients who have suffered spinal cord injury? *Injury*. 2004;35:238–242.
43. Marik PE, Vasu T, Hirani A, et al. Stress ulcer prophylaxis in the new millennium: A systematic review and meta-analysis. *Crit Care Med*. 2010;38:2222–2228.

31

Coma and Brain Death

Avinash B. Kumar

KEY POINTS

1. Coma is a disorder of consciousness that is characterized by a state of profound unresponsiveness and a lack of awareness that persists for more than 1 hour.
2. The differential diagnosis of coma should involve ruling out other global disorders of consciousness including vegetative state, locked-in syndrome, akinetic mutism, and catatonia.
3. The initial management of a comatose patient always starts with the ABC approach — airway, breathing, and circulation approach. Once the patient is stabilized, a more thorough history and physical examination may be done to identify causes that are not already apparent and to identify concurrent pathologies.
4. Prompt attention should be paid to the management of potentially reversible causes such as hypoglycemia, electrolyte abnormalities, thiamine deficiency and cerebral edema.
5. A detailed history and neurologic examination along with a noncontrast CT scan is valuable in the initial diagnostic process.
6. Brain death (BD) is the irreversible absence of clinical brain function with the cardinal features of coma, absent brainstem reflexes, and apnea (after excluding reversible confounders).
7. Hemodynamic changes including hypotension, vasopressor-dependent shock, cardiac rhythm abnormalities such as bradycardia, endocrine dysfunction including diabetes insipidus, and thermoregulatory loss are common after progression to brain death.
8. It is crucial to exclude confounding causes such as profound hypothermia, drug and alcohol intoxications, severe metabolic and electrolyte abnormalities, before making a clinical diagnosis of brain death.
9. In the United States, the brain death statutes vary by state and institution, and one must consult with their parent institution about practice patterns.

I. Consciousness and coma

A. **Introduction.** Consciousness is composed of two hierarchical elements (i.e., wakefulness and awareness of self and environment) [1]. Awareness cannot occur without wakefulness, but wakefulness may be observed in the absence of awareness (i.e., vegetative states [VSs]). In coma, the two components of consciousness are affected—wakefulness (i.e., the level of consciousness) and awareness of environment and self (i.e., the content of consciousness)[1]. Neuroanatomically, the levels of arousal or wakefulness are mediated by the reticular activating system (RAS). The RAS is a group of neurons located in the brainstem with projections through the diencephalon and thalamus to the forebrain (Fig. 31.1). Awareness is thought to be related to activity in the cerebral cortices, more specifically the frontoparietal network; the functional connectivity in the network and with the thalami [2]. Coma is a disorder of

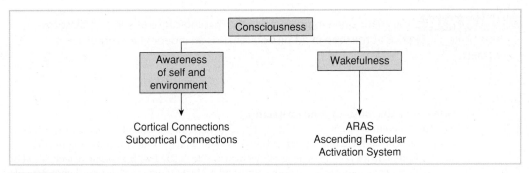

FIGURE 31.1 Components of consciousness.

consciousness that is characterized by a state of profound unresponsiveness and a lack of awareness that persists for more than 1 hour [3]. There is no eye opening and no response to external stimuli. Coma is usually due to insults that impact bilateral cortical structures and/or the RAS. Unilateral lesions may sometimes result in coma if they are large enough to affect the contralateral hemisphere and/or brainstem.

B. Etiology of coma
1. There are several etiologic factors that can result in a comatose state. A simplified approach to the etiology of coma can be classified broadly as intracranial and systemic causes (Table 31.1).
2. Multifocal causes are the most diverse group and account for the largest cohort of cases of coma [4]. Trauma is the leading cause of coma followed by vascular lesions and anoxia. Of the postanoxic causes, the most common are cardiopulmonary arrest, stroke, respiratory arrest, and carbon monoxide poisoning. Other common causes include the postictal state after a seizure, intoxications, and metabolic derangements.

TABLE 31.1   Etiology of coma

Cerebral and intracranial disorders	Systemic causes

• Trauma
  • Traumatic brain injury
  • Cerebral contusions
  • Intracranial hemorrhage—subarachnoid, intraparenchymal, and subdural hemorrhage
• Infections (meningitis and encephalitis)
• Status epilepticus and postictal states
• Increased intracranial pressure and hydrocephalus
• Hypoxic damage (secondary to infarction, cardioembolism, vasculitis, hypercoagulable disorders)
• Malignancy
	• Medication overdose
	  • Opioids
	  • Benzodiazepines
	  • Barbiturates
	  • Tricyclic antidepressants
	  • Aspirin
	  • SSRIs or selective serotonin reuptake inhibitors
	  • Acetaminophen toxicity
	• Drugs of abuse (opioids, alcohol, methanol, ethylene glycol, amphetamines, cocaine)
	• Carbon monoxide toxicity
	• Hypothermia
	• Hypoglycemia; hyperglycemic crises (diabetic ketoacidosis, nonketotic hyperosmolar hyperglycemic state)
	• Advanced hepatic failure
	• Uremia
	• Wernicke's encephalopathy (thiamine deficiency)
	• Endocrine
	  • Panhypopituitarism
	  • Adrenal insufficiency
	  • Myxedema; hyperthyroidism

CLINICAL PEARL Traumatic brain injury remains the leading cause of coma. A Glasgow Coma Scale (GCS) of <8 at the time of admission remains an independent predictor of mortality.

C. Differential diagnosis of comatose states

1. The differential diagnosis of coma should involve ruling out other global disorders of consciousness including VS, locked-in syndrome, akinetic mutism, and catatonia [5].

2. VS is notable for preserved arousal mechanisms associated with a complete lack of self or environmental awareness. Hypothalamic and brainstem function persists; hence patients can survive in these states for prolonged intervals of time. Movements in response to external stimuli can occur but are reflexive and unreproducible. Patients can have spontaneous eye opening but do not track.

3. Akinetic mutism is defined as a state of profound apathy with preserved awareness, revealed by attentive visual pursuit, but a paucity and slowness of voluntary movements not due to paralysis. A distinguishing feature is that these patients do not have spasticity or abnormal reflexes.

4. Locked-in syndrome patients have a largely intact consciousness but a severely limited ability to communicate their awareness due to paralysis of voluntary muscle. It is associated with acute injury to the ventral pons, just below the level of the third nerve nuclei, thus classically sparing vertical eye movements and blinking [6].

5. Catatonia is a complication of psychiatric illnesses such as severe depression, bipolar disorder, or schizophrenia, in which patients have open eyes but do not speak or move spontaneously and do not follow commands, with an otherwise normal neurologic examination and an electroencephalogram showing low voltage but no slowing.

D. Approach and management of a comatose patient

1. **Initial management**

   a. The clinical approach to a comatose patient is outlined in Figure 31.2. Once a patient is established as being unarousable and nonresponsive, the ABCs (airway, breathing, and circulation) are the most important first steps in care. Airway protection by intubation (indicated with a GCS ≤ 8) and circulatory/hemodynamic management are critical to limiting secondary insults.

      (1) Mean arterial pressure (MAP) of less than 70 mm Hg should be treated with volume expansion and/or vasopressors.

      (2) MAPs of greater than 130 mm Hg should be treated with antihypertensives.

      (3) Initial laboratory tests should include a complete blood count, electrolyte panel with chemistries (i.e., magnesium, phosphorus, calcium, BUN, creatinine, lactate, and osmolarity), arterial blood gas, liver functions, PT and PTT, drug screen, and ECG.

      (4) Emperically administer thiamine 100 mg IV in patients who appear malnourished, have strong alcohol abuse history, or have unexplained coma.

      (5) Once vital signs are stabilized, a noncontrast head computed tomography (CT) should be done to assess for intracranial structural changes; for example, intracranial hemorrhage and subarachnoid hemorrhage, acute hydrocephalus, masses, and cerebral edema.

      (6) If there are signs of a herniation syndrome, give 20% mannitol 1 g/kg IV bolus or hypertonic saline.

CLINICAL PEARL Hyperventilation as a routine in the management of cerebral edema is no longer recommended. Normocarbia is the norm.

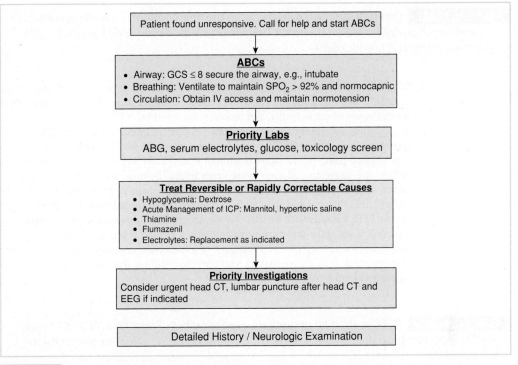

FIGURE 31.2 Clinical approach to a comatose patient.

2. **Secondary evaluation and management**
   a. Once the patient is stabilized, a more thorough history and physical examination may be done to identify causes that are not already apparent and to identify concurrent pathologies. The history of present illness can be obtained from caregivers or family members, witnesses, the emergency medical technicians, clinical records, and medication history. Important elements include the time course, prior focal signs, prior neurologic events, and recent illnesses. Although a complete physical examination is warranted, this chapter will focus on a brief and directed neurologic examination.
   b. By definition, the comatose patient is unarousable and unaware. This is confirmed by the presence or absence of eye opening (awareness) and the response to verbal and somatosensory stimulation (arousability). A noxious stimulus is used to assess arousability. Techniques include squeezing the trapezius, supraorbital pressure, sternal rub, nail bed, or temporomandibular pressure. Reflex responses (i.e., posturing) may be present and arise from subcortical structures.
   c. In the comatose patient the most important cranial nerve reflexes are the pupillary, corneal, and vestibuloocular reflex. Pupil size, position, and reaction to light are individually assessed. Normal pupil size is 3 to 7 mm. A discrepancy of 1 mm in pupil size may be normal. Certain toxidromes are associated with either miosis or mydriasis. For example, the following toxidromes are associated with mydriasis: Sympathomimetic agents, anticholinergic agents, serotonin syndrome, and tricyclic antidepressants. Miosis is associated with opioid agents, sedative-hypnotic agents, and cholinergic agents.
   d. An impaired pupillary response to light, either bilateral or unilateral, usually indicates a primary brainstem lesion or herniation.
3. **Diagnostic testing of coma**
   a. CT scan is sensitive for detecting structural pathology that needs immediate intervention such as cerebral edema, tumor, hemorrhage, and herniation. It is less useful in acute ischemia and toxic metabolic syndromes.

> **CLINICAL PEARL** Cerebral edema is a key factor in the final common pathway in coma due to a number of causes including traumatic brain injury, carbon monoxide toxicity, hepatic encephalopathy, and uremic coma.

    b. Magnetic resonance imaging (MRI) is usually warranted in comatose patients if the initial CT was normal or equivocal. MRI is more sensitive than CT for detecting diffuse axonal injury, acute ischemia, and venous sinus thrombosis [7].

    c. Electroencephalography (EEG) is indicated in cases of unexplained coma. Nonconvulsive status epilepticus (NCSE) has been reported as high as 9% to 18% in patients with unexplained coma [8]. In patients without epilepsy, periodic epileptiform discharges (PEDs) are suggestive of underlying brain injury. In toxic and metabolic causes of coma, as patients progress from lethargy to coma, there is diffuse slowing of background EEG rhythms and changes from alpha to theta and, subsequently, delta activity on the EEG. Patients with hepatic disease, azotemia, and profound hypoglycemia can manifest blunt spike-and-slow wave complexes termed triphasic waves. Though not pathognomonic, they can be suggestive of a metabolic encephalopathy [9]. But the greatest value is in differentiating ictal encephalopathies from psychiatric disease as etiology of coma.

> **CLINICAL PEARL** NCSE is often an underdiagnosed condition. Patients on IV sedation in the ICU including propofol can still have NCSE. Continuous EEG is valuable in establishing the diagnosis.

    d. Lumbar puncture (LP): LP should be considered in suspected infectious and inflammatory causes of coma. However, one must exercise caution that there are no clinical signs of "impending" herniation, and that the CT is negative for potential herniation syndromes before proceeding with the LP [10,11].

4. Assessment of coma: The coma scales

    a. The GCS was initially devised for patients with traumatic brain injury [12], but has gained widespread acceptance and stood the test of time over the past 3 decades as a bedside tool for evaluating the level of consciousness in virtually all acutely ill patients [13]. The Glasgow scale was originally developed using simple parameters for the specific purpose of allowing less experienced doctors and other health professionals to produce an accurate report of a patient's state of consciousness. The Glasgow scale is a composite sum obtained by assessing the following three parameters: Eye opening, best verbal response, and best motor response. The score varies between 3 and 15 points [14] (see chapter 29).

    b. Major limitations of GCS are its inability to accurately assess intubated patients, difficulty in assessing aphasic patients, and limited utility in children, particularly those less than 3 years of age and prior to acquisition of language [15].

    c. Attempts have been made to modify the GCS; however, most of these scales were more complicated and were seldom used outside their countries of origin. Similarly, other scales (e.g., Innsbruck coma scale, reaction level scale (RLS85), FOUR score) have been developed since, yet none have gained similar widespread acceptance like the GCS. The FOUR score was described in 2005 and is composed of four elements (eye response, motor response, brainstem response, and respiration); each with a maximum score of four [16]. It was designed to overcome the shortcomings of the GCS by being able to evaluate intubated patients and evaluate brainstem function. However, it is yet to be validated across multiple centers [15]. A comparison of the GCS and FOUR score are presented in Table 31.2.

TABLE 31.2 Comparing glasgow coma scale and FOUR score coma scale

GCS	FOUR score

• Three major components
  • Eye—4 points
  • Motor—6 points
  • Verbal—5 points
• Limited utility in intubated patients and children with limited language development
• Key component of other ICU severity of illness scales such as acute physiology and chronic health evaluation II score (APACHE-2)
• Widely used and validated for more than 30 years
	• Four components (E_4, M_4, B_4, R_4) with maximum score of 4 points each
	  • Eye response
	  • Motor response
	  • Brainstem reflexes
	  • Respiratory pattern
	• Includes testing for intubated patients and brainstem reflexes
	• Useful in detecting patients with locked-in syndrome and VSs
	• Multicenter trials and validation are pending

   E. **Outcome of coma**

      1. Informed prediction of neurologic outcomes following coma is a key component of management and in many circumstances may help crystallize end-of-life decisions by caregivers of comatose patients. In general, the etiology of coma is a major determinant of prognosis. Toxic and metabolic causes carry a better prognosis compared to anoxic mechanism of coma [17]. Absent pupillary reflex, absent corneal reflex, and a score of 1 on the motor component of GCS on coma day 1 is all associated with a poor prognosis [18]. Interestingly the motor score of the GCS (compared to the eye and verbal scores) has the strongest correlation with outcome from coma [19].

      2. The most widely implemented assessment tool for outcomes following disorders of consciousness is the Glasgow Outcome Scale (GOS). The original GOS was a five-point scale developed in 1975. The original GOS, although it has been utilized extensively, was criticized for being insufficiently sensitive to deficits in cognition, mood, and behavior. Adding a structured interview to accurately categorize patient's disability subsequently led to a modification of the original scale to the GOS-extended (GOSE) [20].

      3. Other scales that assess functional and cognitive disability include Disability rating scale (DRS), Functional Independence Measure (FIM), Community Integration Questionnaire (CIQ), and the Functional Status Examination (FSE).

      4. There has been a growing body of literature about the use of functional neuroimaging (e.g., functional MRI [FMRI] and electrophysiology studies such as evoked potentials (EPs) and event-related potentials [ERPs]) to evaluate residual cortical processing in the absence of the behavioral signs of consciousness. Currently these methods are not widely utilized in everyday neurocritical practice, but are likely to be used in the future [21].

 II. **Brain death**

   A. **Definition of brain death.** BD can be defined as the irreversible absence of clinical brain function with the cardinal features of coma, absent brainstem reflexes, and apnea (after excluding reversible confounders) [22].

   B. **Physiologic changes following brainstem death.** The rostrocaudal spread of irreversible ischemia to different areas of the brain during progression to BD triggers systemic physiologic changes. These changes have been illustrated in Figure 31.3. In the diencephalon, functional components of the hypothalamic pituitary axis are affected leading to loss of regulatory control of hormonal systems. Pontine ischemia manifests as a mixed vagal and sympathetic surge and the Cushing reflex (hypertension, bradycardia, and irregular breathing). With progressive ischemia of the vagal nuclei in the medulla, unopposed sympathetic activity can be seen. With further caudal progression of ischemia, spinal sympathetic pathways are affected ending with total sympathetic denervation. The clinical manifestations are reflective of these changes with hypotension being the most frequently reported hemodynamic abnormality. Increased urine output following BD is most frequently due to diabetes insipidus [23].

      1. **Cardiovascular manifestations following brainstem death**

         a. Progression to BD is accompanied by significant hemodynamic changes. Progressive brainstem ischemia triggers an intense catecholamine storm with plasma catecholamines

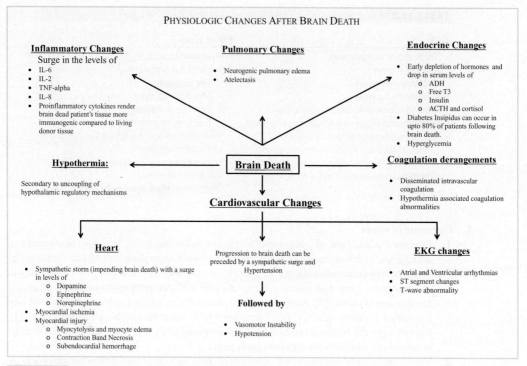

FIGURE 31.3 Physiologic changes after brain death.

increasing by as much as 500% above baseline [24]. This period of autonomic chaos is followed by a combination of increased parasympathetic activity, loss of sympathetic tone, and significant decrease in the peripheral vascular resistance leading to hypotension. Hypotension remains the most consistent hemodynamic change seen in more than 80% of patients following BD [25].

b. Structural myocardial injury can occur even in the absence of coronary artery disease following BD. The spectrum of changes includes myocytolysis, contraction band necrosis (catecholamine-induced hypercontracted state associated with myocyte death, mononuclear infiltration, and early calcification), subendocardial hemorrhages, edema and mononuclear cell infiltration, and early calcification. Cardiac myofibrillar necrosis is histologically identical to the cardiac lesions of catecholamine infusion, hypothalamic stimulation, or reperfusion injury, but the lesions; however, differs from the necrosis seen in classic coronary artery disease due to the rapidity of onset [26].

c. EKG changes are common and thought to be multifactorial in origin following BD. These can include prolongation of QT interval, ST segment changes, T wave abnormalities, ventricular arrhythmias, and conduction abnormalities [26].

2. **Pulmonary changes following brain death.** Pulmonary dysfunction is often seen in severe brain injury patients who progress to BD. These lesions include atelectasis, aspiration, primary pneumonia, ventilator-associated lung injury, and neurogenic pulmonary edema (acute pulmonary edema occurring shortly after a central neurologic insult). Anatomically the posterior hypothalamus and dorsal medulla oblongata are considered the pulmonary edema trigger zones.

3. **Endocrine changes**

a. The onset of anterior and posterior pituitary failure results in a significant proportion of changes in hormonal function following BD.

b. Diabetes insipidus is the most consistently reported (up to 80%) endocrine abnormality following BD [27]. This follows the rapid depletion of antidiuretic hormone (ADH), leading to excessive diuresis, central volume depletion, hypernatremia, and hyper-osmolality. One must be cautious about the use of large volume resuscitation using sodium-containing solutions in the setting of hypernatremia.

c. Free triiodothyronine (T_3) levels drop significantly following BD. The loss of thyroid-stimulating hormone (TSH) from the pituitary and impaired peripheral conversion of T_4 to T_3 accounts for the dramatic drop in the levels [31]. The resultant cardiovascular effect is the loss of inotropy due to the depletion of intracellular high energy phosphates and shift to anaerobic metabolism and lactic acidosis.

d. Insulin levels drop after brainstem death and the resultant drop in intracellular glucose utilization results in a shift toward anaerobic metabolism, lactic acidosis, and systemic hyperglycemia.

e. ACTH and cortisol levels fall within 45 minutes following BD. The significance of a random serum cortisol as a reflection of the hypothalamus–pituitary–adrenal axis in the brain-dead patient remains unclear [28,29].

4. **Pathophysiologic changes in other systems**

a. **Hypothermia.** The uncoupling of hypothalamic thermoregulation combined with loss of compensatory mechanism, such as shivering or vasoconstriction, results in a hypothermic patient following BD. This can be compounded by the use of cold intravenous fluids and blood products during the resuscitation phase. Core body temperature below 35°C can delay the determination of BD examination.

b. **Inflammatory response.** BD is associated with a massive inflammatory response, activation of endothelial cells, platelets, and neutrophils. The immunologic impact is the induction of cytokines, adhesion molecules (E-selectin and ICAM-1), and major histocompatibility complex class II (MHC class II) proteins [30,31]. IL-6, IL-2R, IL-8, and TNF-α levels are elevated following BD and in the future, along with a host of others, these may also serve as a biomarker of potentially successful donor candidates following BD [32]. This inflammatory cytokine surge may, in part, explain the enhanced immunogenicity of transplanted organs from brain-dead donors compared to living donors [32].

C. **Diagnosis of brain death.** Although Mollaret and Goulon first described the clinical concept of BD in 1959, the first push to recognize this irreversible state as a new definition of death was proposed in 1968 by the Ad Hoc Committee of Harvard Medical School [33]. The legal and medical definition of BD was redefined in the landmark President's Commission for the study of Ethical Problems in Medicine and Behavioral Research in 1981, and has continued to be the basis of future reports and consensus guidelines [34]. The American Academy of Neurology, since 1995, has issued practice parameters and evidence-based guideline updates in determining BD [35]. Some of the conditions that can clinically mimic BD are outlined in Table 31.3.

The assessment of BD can be considered in four broad steps as suggested by the AAN guidelines [36].

1. **Step 1.** Establish the cause of the comatose state by history, examination, or neuroimaging. The reversible confounders that can mask a neurologic examination such as hypothermia, drug and alcohol intoxications, and metabolic disturbances should be excluded. The core temperature should be near normal (>36°C) and $PaCO_2$ on the arterial blood gas should be close to normal at baseline. The systolic BP should be maintained avoiding significant

TABLE 31.3 Clinical conditions that can mimic brain death

Clinical conditions that can mimic brain death
High spinal cord injury
Fulminant Guillain–Barre syndrome
Baclofen toxicity
Organophosphate toxicity
Delayed neuromuscular blocker clearance
Profound hypothermia

9

lability during the examination. The detailed clinical examination is a key starting point to determine BD. In the United States, the BD statutes vary by state and institution, and one must consult with their parent institution about practice patterns.

2. **Step 2.** The neurologic examination should demonstrate coma and absence of brainstem reflexes. These include absent corneal and conjunctival reflexes, absence of doll's eye movement, absent eye movements during oculovestibular or cold caloric tests, and absent gag and cough reflex. A key element of the examination is the apnea test. This tests for the absence of a respiratory drive or effort in spite of the built-up of CO_2 exceeding the apneic threshold. In the absence of any respiratory effort over 8 to 10 minutes, the ABG should reflect a $PCO_2 \geq 60$ mm Hg or a 20 mm Hg rise in arterial PCO_2 above baseline.

> **CLINICAL PEARL** The apnea test for BD can be associated with significant hemodynamic changes. It is prudent to abort the apnea test if the patient becomes hemodynamically unstable.

> **CLINICAL PEARL** Clinical features such as fixed, nonreactive pupils, absent gag, and cough reflexes on admission can be misleading and must always be interpreted with caution and reconfirmed after a second detailed neurologic examination in time.

3. **Step 3.** Ancillary or confirmatory testing. Each of these ancillary tests including EEG, cerebral angiography, nuclear medicine perfusion test or cerebral scintigraphy, transcranial Doppler's, and MRI/MRA have been used to substantiate the clinical diagnosis. However, each test can have false positives and should always be interpreted in the correct clinical context by experienced practitioners. Methods for ancillary testing have been outlined in Appendix 1 of the AAN guidelines [36].

> **CLINICAL PEARL** Nuclear medicine confirmatory tests for BD can have false positives such as the "hot nose sign" and EEGs can have blips or interference due to other ICU equipment. Hence they should always be interpreted in the correct clinical context by experienced practitioners.

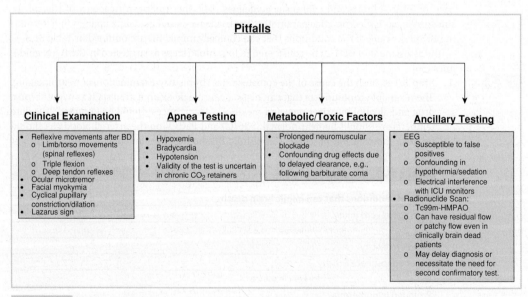

FIGURE 31.4 Pitfalls in the diagnosis of brain death.

4.   **Step 4.** Documentation. The time of death is the time the PCO_2 reaches the target value or when the confirmatory test results have been interpreted.

D.   Pitfalls in the BD examination are outlined in Figure 31.4.

III.   Conclusion. ICUs today can maintain cardiopulmonary function in nonsurvivable brain injury patients for extended periods of time. Death (for the layperson) cannot always be equated to the loss of spontaneous heartbeat. It is the responsibility of the intensivist to discuss prognosis and outcomes in the clearest possible terms to the family members in patient with nonsurvivable injuries to help reach an ethical, humanitarian conclusion to the care of the patient.

REFERENCES

1.   Stevens RD, Bhardwaj A. Approach to the comatose patient. *Crit Care Med.* 2006;34:31–41.
2.   Parvizi J, Damasio AR. Neuroanatomical correlates of brainstem coma. *Brain.* 2003;126:1524–1536.
3.   Medical aspects of the persistent vegetative state. The Multi-Society Task Force on PVS. *N Engl J Med.* 1994;330:1499–1508.
4.   Ropper AH, Brown RJ. *Adams and Victor's Principles of Neurology.* 8th ed. New York, NY: McGraw-Hill; 2005.
5.   Michelson DJ, Ashwal S. Evaluation of coma and brain death. *Semin Pediatr Neurol.* 2004;11(2):105–118.
6.   Smith E, Delargy M. Locked-in syndrome. *BMJ.* 2005;330:406–409.
7.   Yokota H, Kurokawa A, Otsuka T, et al. Significance of magnetic resonance imaging in acute head injury. *J Trauma.* 1991;31:351–357.
8.   Varelas PN, Spanaki MV, Hacein-Bey L, et al. Emergent EEG: Indications and diagnostic yield. *Neurology.* 2003;61:702–704.
9.   Brenner RP. The interpretation of the EEG in stupor and coma. *Neurologist.* 2005;11:271–284.
10.   Hasbun R, Abrahams J, Jekel J, et al. Computed tomography of the head before lumbar puncture in adults with suspected meningitis. *N Engl J Med.* 2001;345:1727–1733.
11.   Joffe AR. Lumbar puncture and brain herniation in acute bacterial meningitis: a review. *J Intensive Care Med.* 2007;22: 194–207.
12.   Teasdale G, Jennett B. Assessment of coma and impaired consciousness. A practical scale. *Lancet.* 1974;2:81–84.
13.   The Brain Trauma Foundation: The American Association of Neurological Surgeons. The Joint Section on Neurotrauma and Critical Care. Glasgow Coma Scale Score . *J Neurotrauma.* 2000;17:563–571.
14.   Bordini AL, Luiz TF, Fernandes M, et al. Coma scales. A historical review. *Arq Neuropsiquiatr.* 2010;68(6):930–937.
15.   Kornbluth J, Bhardwaj A. Evaluation of coma: a critical appraisal of popular scoring systems. *Neurocrit Care.* 2011;14(1): 134–143.
16.   Wijdicks EFM, Bamlet WR, Maramattom BV, et al. Validation of a new coma scale: The FOUR score. *Ann Neurol.* 2005;58: 585–593.
17.   Young GB, Wang JT, Connolly JF. Prognostic determination in anoxic-ischemic and traumatic encephalopathies. *J Clin Neurophysiol.* 2004;21:379–390.
18.   Zandbergen EG, de Haan RJ, Stoutenbeek CP, et al. Systematic review of early prediction of poor outcome in anoxic-ischemic coma. *Lancet.* 1998;352:1808–1812.
19.   Healey C, Osler TM, Rogers FB, et al. Improving the Glasgow Coma Scale score: motor score alone is a better predictor. *J Trauma.* 2003;54:671–678.
20.   Wilson JT, Pettigrew LE, Teasdale GM. Structured interviews for the Glasgow outcome scale and the extended Glasgow outcome scale: guidelines for their use. *J Neurotrauma.* 1998;15:573–585.
21.   Gawryluk JR, D'Arcy RC, Connolly JF, et al. Improving the clinical assessment of consciousness with advances in electrophysiological and neuroimaging techniques. *BMC Neurol.* 2010;10:11.
22.   Busl KM, Greer D. Pitfalls in the diagnosis of brain death. *Neurocritical Care.* 2009;11:276–287.
23.   Smith M. Physiologic changes during brain stem death–lessons for management of the organ donor. *J Heart Lung Transplant.* 2004;23:S217–S222.
24.   Lopau K, Mark J, Schramm L, et al. Hormonal changes in brain death and immune activation in the donor. *Transpl Int.* 2000;13 suppl 1:S282–S285.
25.   Wood KE, Becker BN, McCartney JG, et al. Care of the potential organ donor. *N Engl J Med.* 2004;351:2730–2739.
26.   Kopelnik A, Zaroff JG. Neurocardiogenic injury in neurovascular disorders. *Crit Care Clin.* 2006;22(4):733–752.
27.   Baumann A, Audibert G, McDonnell J, et al. Neurogenic pulmonary edema. *Acta Anaesthesiol Scand.* 2007;51(4):447–455.
28.   Ranasinghe AM, Bonser RS. Endocrine changes in brain death and transplantation. *Best Pract Res Clin Endocrinol Metab.* 2011;25:799–812.
29.   Arafah BM. Hypothalamic pituitary adrenal function during critical illness: limitations of current assessment methods. *J Clin Endocrinol Metab.* 2006;91(10):3725–3745.
30.   Kotsch K, Ulrich F, Reutzel-Selke A, et al. Methylprednisolone therapy in deceased donors reduces inflammation in the donor liver and improves outcome after liver transplantation. *Ann Surg.* 2008;248:1042–1050.
31.   Murugan R, Venkataraman R, HIDonOR Study Investigators, et al. Preload responsiveness is associated with increased interleukin-6 and lower organ yield from brain-dead donors. *Crit Care Med.* 2009;37(8):2387–2393.
32.   de Vries DK, Lindeman JH, Ringers J, et al. Donor brain death predisposes human kidney grafts to a proinflammatory reaction after transplantation. *Am J Transplant.* 2011;11(5):1064–1070.
33.   A definition of irreversible coma. Report of the Ad Hoc Committee of the Harvard Medical School to examine the definition of brain death. *JAMA.* 1968;205:337–340.

34. Guidelines for the determination of death. Report of the medical consultants on the diagnosis of death to the President's Commission for the Study of Ethical Problems in Medicine and Biomedical and Behavioral Research. *JAMA*. 1981;246: 2184–2186.

35. Practice parameters for determining brain death in adults (summary statement). The Quality Standards Subcommittee of the American Academy of Neurology. *Neurology*. 1995;45:1012–1014.

36. Wijdicks EF, Varelas PN, Gronseth GS, et al. American Academy of Neurology. Evidence-based guideline update: determining brain death in adults: report of the Quality Standards Subcommittee of the American Academy of Neurology. *Neurology*. 2010;74(23):1911–1918.

Index

Note: Page number followed by "f" and "t" indicates figure and table respectively.

415